D1560752

Tumour Angiogenesis

Tumour Angiogenesis

Edited by

ROY BICKNELL

Imperial Cancer Research Fund, Institute of Molecular Medicine
University of Oxford, John Radcliffe Hospital
Oxford

CLAIRE E. LEWIS

Department of Pathology
University of Sheffield Medical School
Sheffield

and

NAPOLEONE FERRARA

Department of Cardiovascular Research
Genentech Inc.
South San Francisco
California, USA

Oxford   New York   Tokyo
OXFORD UNIVERSITY PRESS
1997

Oxford University Press, Great Clarendon Street, Oxford OX2 6DP
Oxford   New York
Athens   Auckland   Bangkok   Bogota   Bombay   Buenos Aires
Calcutta   Cape Town   Dar es Salaam   Delhi   Florence   Hong Kong
Istanbul   Karachi   Kuala Lumpur   Madras   Madrid   Melbourne
Mexico City   Nairobi   Paris   Singapore   Taipei   Tokyo   Toronto
and associated companies in
Berlin   Ibadan

Oxford is a trade mark of Oxford University Press

Published in the United States
by Oxford University Press Inc., New York

A catalogue record for this book is available from the British Library

Library of Congress Cataloging in Publication Data
Tumor angiogenesis / edited by Roy Bicknell, Claire E. Lewis, and
Napoleone Ferrara.
1. Tumors–Blood-vessels–Growth.   I. Bicknell, R. J. (R. John)
II. Lewis, Claire E.   III. Ferrara, Napoleone.
RC269.T84   1997   616.99′213—dc21   95–52106

ISBN 0 19 854937 7

Typeset by EXPO Holdings, Malaysia

Printed in Great Britain by
Bookcraft (Bath) Ltd,
Midsomer Norton, Avon.

Acknowledgements

The editors wish to thank the following organizations for their support: the Imperial Cancer Research Fund (RB), Genentech Research (NF), and the Medical Research Council/Breast Cancer Campaign (CEL).

Contents

The plate section is located between pages 376 and 377.

Contributors

A. Agrotis, Cell Biology Laboratory, Baker Medical Research Institute, Alfred Hospital, Prahan, Victoria 3181, Australia.

Anthony C. Allison, Dawa Corporation, Belmont, California 942002, USA.

Frances R. Balkwill, Biological Therapies Laboratory, ICRF Labs, Lincolns Inn Fields, London WC2, UK.

Rachel Bar-Shavit, Department of Oncology, Hadassah-Hebrew University Hospital, Jerusalem 91120, Israel.

Miriam Benezra, Department of Oncology, Hadassah-Hebrew University Hospital, Jerusalem 91120, Israel.

Roy Bicknell, Molecular Angiogenesis Group, Imperial Cancer Research Fund, Institute of Molecular Medicine, University of Oxford, John Radcliffe Hospital, Oxford OX3 9DU, UK.

Andreas Bikfalvi, Growth Factor and Cell Differentiation Laboratory, Université Bordeaux I, 33405, Talence, France.

A. Bobik, Cell Biology Laboratory, Baker Medical Research Institute, Alfred Hospital, Prahan, Victoria 3181, Australia.

Noël Bouck, Department of Microbiology-Immunology, Lurie Cancer Centre, Northwestern University Medical School, Chicago, Illinois, USA.

David J. Chaplin, Tumour Microcirculation Group, Gray Laboratory Cancer Research Trust, Mount Vernon Hospital, Northwood, Middlesex HA6 2JR, UK.

Gerhard Christofori, Research Institute of Molecular Pathology, Dr Bohr-Gasse 7, 1030 Vienna, Austria.

Rangana Choudhuri, Molecular Angiogenesis Group, Imperial Cancer Research Fund, Institute of Molecular Medicine, University of Oxford, John Radcliffe Hospital, Oxford OX3 9DU, UK.

Elaine J. Derbyshire, Department of Pharmacology, Simmons Cancer Centre, The University of Texas Southwestern Medical Centre, 5323 Harry Hines Boulevard, Dallas, Texas 75235-8593, USA.

Graeme J. Dougherty, Gene Therapy Group, Terry Fox Laboratories, BC Cancer Research Centre, 601 West 10th Avenue, Vancouver V5Z 1L3, British Columbia, Canada.

Luis F. Fajardo L.-G., Department of Pathology, Stanford University School of Medicine and Veterans Affairs Medical Centre, Palo Alto, California 94304, USA.

Tai-Ping D. Fan, Department of Pharmacology, University of Cambridge, Tennis Court Road, Cambridge CB2 1QJ, UK.

Napoleone Ferrara, Department of Cardiovascular Research, Genentech Inc., 460 Point San Bruno Boulevard, South San Francisco, California 94080, USA.

F. W. Flitney, Cancer Biology Research Group, School of Biological and Medical Sciences, University of St Andrews, Fife KY16 9TS, Scotland.

Giampietro Gasparini, Department of Oncology, St Bortolo Medical Centre, Vicenza, Italy.

Adrian L. Harris, Molecular Oncology Laboratory, Imperial Cancer Research Fund, Institute of Molecular Medicine, University of Oxford, John Radcliffe Hospital, Oxford, UK.

D. G. Hirst, Radiation Science Research Group, School of Biomedical Sciences, University of Ulster at Jordanstown, Newtonnabey, County Antrim BT37 0QB, Northern Ireland.

Lars Holmgren, Department of Tumour Biology, Karolinska Institute, Stockholm, Sweden.

Rhys T. Jaggar, Molecular Angiogenesis Group, Imperial Cancer Research Fund, Institute of Molecular Medicine, University of Oxford, John Radcliffe Hospital, Oxford OX3 9DU, UK.

Rakesh K. Jain, Edwin L. Steel Lab, Massachusetts General Hospital, Harvard Medical School, Boston 02114, USA.

Eli Keshet, Department of Molecular Biology, Hebrew University – Hadassah Medical School, Jerusalem 91200, Israel.

Sharon Klein, Department of Cell Biology and Kaplan Cancer Centre and Raymond and Beverley Foundation Laboratory, New York University Medical Centre, 550 First Avenue, New York, NY 10016, USA.

Pat Kumar, Metropolitan University of Manchester, Manchester, UK.

Shant Kumar, CRC Paterson Institute, Christie Hospital, Manchester M20 9BX, UK.

Laurence A. Lasky, Department of Molecular Biology, Genentech Inc., 460 Pt San Bruno Boulevard, Southern San Francisco, California 94080, USA.

Russell D. Leek, Molecular Oncology Laboratory, Imperial Cancer Research Fund, Institute of Molecular Medicine, University of Oxford, John Radcliffe Hospital, Oxford, UK.

Claire E. Lewis, Department of Pathology, University of Sheffield Medical School, Beech Hill Road, Sheffield S10 2RX.

Ofer Lider, Department of Immunology, The Weizmann Institute of Science, Rehovot 76100, Israel.

P. J. Little, Cell Biology Laboratory, Baker Medical Research Institute, Alfred Hospital, Prahan, Victoria 3181, Australia.

Joseph A. Madri, Department of Pathology, Yale University School of Medicine, 310 Cedar Street, New Haven, Connecticut 06510, USA.

Hua-Quan Miao, Department of Oncology, Hadassah-Hebrew University Hospital, Jerusalem 91120, Israel.

Amir Moghaddam, Molecular Angiogenesis Group, Imperial Cancer Research Fund, Institute of Molecular Medicine, University of Oxford, John Radcliffe Hospital, Oxford OX3 9DU, UK.

Roberto Montesano, Department of Morphology, University Medical Centre, Geneva, Switzerland.

Michal Neeman, Department of Hormone Research, The Weizmann Institute of Science, Rehovot 76100, Israel.

Michael S. Pepper, Department of Morphology, University Medical Centre, Geneva, Switzerland.

Tamar Peretz, Department of Oncology, Hadassah-Hebrew University Hospital, Jerusalem 91120, Israel.

Guiseppe Pintucci, Department of Dermatology, NYU Medical Center, 550 First Av., New York, NY, USA.

Peter J. Polverini, Department of Oral Medicine, Pathology and Surgery, University of Michigan School of Dentistry, 1011 North University, Room 5217, Ann Arbor, Michigan 48109-1078, USA.

Julie Ponting, CRC Paterson Institute, Christie Hospital, Manchester M20 9BX, UK.

Farzan Rastinejad, Pfizer Inc., Central Research Division, Eastern Point Road, Groton, Connecticut 06340, USA.

Daniel B. Rifkin, Department of Cell Biology and Kaplan Cancer Centre and Raymond and Beverley Foundation Laboratory, New York University Medical Centre, 550 First Avenue, New York, NY 10016, USA.

Paul Rooney, Department of Orthopaedics, Leicester University, Leicester, UK.

T. Kanaga Sabapathy, Institute of Molecular Pathology, Vienna, Austria.

Sabita Sankar, Department of Pathology, Yale University School of Medicine, 310 Cedar Street, New Haven, Connecticut 06510, USA.

Annette Schmidt, Institute for Arteriosclerosis Research, University of Munster, Munster, Germany.

Anke M. Schulte, Lombardi Cancer Centre, Georgetown University, 3970 Reservoir Road NW, Washington DC 20007, USA.

Enzo Spisni, Department of Experimental Biology, University of Bologna, Via Selmi 3, 40126 Bologna, Italy.

Ilan Stein, Department of Molecular Biology, Hebrew University-Hadassah Medical School, Jerusalem 91200, Israel.

Fabienne Tacchini-Cottier, Department of Pathology, University Medical Centre, Geneva, Switzerland.

Philip E. Thorpe, Department of Pharmacology, Simmons Cancer Centre, The University of Texas Southwestern Medical Centre, 5323 Harry Hines Boulevard, Dallas, Texas 75235-8593, USA.

Vittorio Tomasi, Department of Experimental Biology, University of Bologna, Via Selini 3, L0126 Bologna, Italy.

Martin J. Trotter, Pathology Department, Vancouver General Hospital, 855 West 12th Avenue, Vancouver, VSZ IM9 British Colombia, Canada.

Israel Vlodavsky, Department of Oncology, Hadassah-Hebrew University Hospital, Jerusalem 91120, Israel.

Paul E. Young, Department of Molecular Biology, Genentech Inc., 460 Pt San Bruno Boulevard, Southern San Francisco, California 94080, USA.

Erwin F. Wagner, Institute of Molecular Pathology, Vienna, Austria.

Anton Wellstein, Lombardi Cancer Centre, Georgetown University, 3970 Reservoir Road NW, Washington DC 20007, USA.

1. Introduction

Roy Bicknell, Claire E. Lewis, and Napoleone Ferrara

There are two recognized mechanisms by which blood vessels arise that are termed vasculogenesis and angiogenesis. Angiogenesis describes the development of new vessels from existing vessels. The process has been long known; indeed it was certainly recognized as early as 1787 when John Hunter noted that it occurred during the development of reindeer antlers (1). The purpose of this introduction is not to provide a detailed history of the field but to set the scene for the chapters that follow. This book is intended to give a comprehensive review of the state of our current understanding of the field primarily, but not exclusively, in relation to tumour angiogenesis. Each chapter has been written by an acknowledged expert in a specific area. The reason that the volume concentrates on tumour angiogenesis is because studies in this area have dominated the field of angiogenesis over the past 20 years. This is due in part to the work of Petro Gullino at the National Cancer Institute in Frederick and later Judah Folkman at Harvard Medical School. Both have been instrumental in bringing the concept of tumour angiogenesis and its inhibition as a potential anti-cancer therapeutic strategy to the attention of a wide cross-section of the research community. Nevertheless, the contents of the book are of relevance to all researchers interested in blood vessel development, particularly the chapters covering the role of individual cytokines.

Vasculogenesis describes the development of the vasculature from structures that occur in the early embryo known as blood islands (2) (see Chapter 25). Blood islands are composed of cells that develop into the endothelial and haematopoietic systems. The common origin of cells forming the endothelial and haematopoietic systems no doubt accounts for the presence of many common surface antigens in the two different cell types, for example, the CD antigens. During embryogenesis, the endothelial precursors stream into the developing organs and then differentiate into the vascular tree. This process is now known to be controlled exclusively by vascular endothelial growth factor (VEGF). VEGF is the only growth factor gene for which a knockout is known to be lethal, i.e. no other gene product can substitute (3,4). Neither VEGF nor VEGF receptor gene knockout mice develop a vasculature (3–6). There are two VEGF receptors known in mice as flk-1 (KDR in humans) and flt-1. flk-1 gene knockouts fail to develop even blood islands (5), while flt-1 gene knockouts undergo endothelial differentiation but fail to develop an organized vasculature (6). It is of interest that not only do the homozygous VEGF gene knockouts not develop a vasculature but neither do the heterozygous knockouts (3,4). This has been interpreted as a dosing problem, in other words, VEGF transcripts are required from both alleles to give sufficient protein to enable the vascular tree to develop. While this is an interesting possibility, it has not been unequivocally shown that transcription of VEGF from both alleles occurs in the somatic cell. As the endothelial precursors that are found in the blood islands occur only in the embryo, vasculogenesis never occurs in the adult.

Angiogenesis describes the development of new blood vessels from existing vessels. Angiogenesis occurs in both the embryo and the adult. In the developing embryo some organs are vascularized exclusively by vasculogenesis, some by a mixture of vasculogenesis and angiogenesis and others (those that completely lack blood islands) by angiogenesis. Interesting examples of the latter are the brain and kidney. Proliferation of the neuroepithelium leads to thickening of the neural tube, which requires vascularization for continued development. Vascularization occurs as a result of three successive waves of invading capillaries that originate in the perineural vascular plexus. Chick-quail transplantation experiments have shown that without exception the brain capillaries are all derived by invasion (7). The $\alpha_v\beta_3$ integrin has been identified as a marker of angiogenesis (8). It is of interest that α_v gene knockout mice undergo normal vasculogenesis but fail to undergo angiogenesis and the brain and kidney of the developing embryos are not vascularized (9). Important physiological angiogenesis in the adult is found in, for example, wound healing, and in several stages of the female reproductive cycle including development of the ovarian follicle and corpus luteum and in the extensive angiogenesis that occurs in the endometrium during each menstrual cycle. However, in the adult angiogenesis is also a component of many pathologies leading Folkman to collect these together and label them angiogenic diseases. The range of pathologies in which angiogenesis occurs is very diverse but includes the two major killers of Western populations, cancer (tumour angiogenesis), atherosclerosis (hyper-proliferation of the *vasa vasorum* within the athero-sclerotic plaque) as well as diabetic retinopathy, psoriasis, menorrhagia, endometriosis, and many others.

Returning to tumour angiogenesis. It is of interest to consider briefly a number of key observations that have been made over the past few years but without duplicating what is described in later chapters of this volume. Several of the most notable papers in the early 1970s were from Folkman's group. Thus, it was shown that tumours implanted into isolated perfused organs failed to develop (10), but if those same tumours were implanted into the ocular chamber within 6 mm of the iris blood vessels, they induced angiogenesis, grew rapidly and metastasized (11,12). The significance of this observation is that it led Folkman to propose that solid tumours are absolutely dependent on angiogenesis for growth beyond 2 mm and that for every increase in tumour diameter there must be a corresponding increase in vascularization of the growing tumour (13). Another seminal paper was published by Folkman in the *Journal of the National Cancer Institute* in 1990 and was titled 'What is the evidence that tumours are angiogenesis dependent?' (14). In this paper Folkman collected 14 key pieces of evidence that angiogenesis is indeed essential for tumour development. Since the publication of this article, the numbers of new publications in the field has been increasing exponentially each year. Foremost among the most notable observations was the independent discovery of VEGF by at least four groups (15–18), the finding that VEGF is rapidly induced by hypoxia (19) or hypoglycaemia (20), identifying VEGF as a (if not the) stress-induced angiogenic factor (reviewed in Chapter 7 by Keshet *et al.*). The observation that systemic administration of blocking anti-VEGF antibodies inhibit tumour formation by xenografted glioblastoma multiforme (and indeed other tumour types) in nude mice (21). It is now clear that VEGF is a pre-eminent player in tumour angiogenesis. The fibroblast growth factors (FGFs), the first angiogenic peptides discovered, are now known to be heavily sequestered in the extracellular matrix of virtually all tissues. The role of the FGFs in tumour angiogenesis is probably most significant when the tumour becomes large and both invades and degrades the extracellular matrix releasing the sequestered FGF. This would explain why bFGF is detectable in the urine of patients with primary tumours but only when the tumours become large (22). This is yet another indication of the importance of context when considering the regulation and role of individual cytokines in tumour angiogenesis. Each of the polypeptide factors discussed in this volume operates within a dynamic network of interconnected factors, including other cyto-kines, their soluble receptors and antagonists, and a number of proteolytic enzymes regulating their release from the extracellular matrix (see Chapter 10). As this varies from one region of a tumour to another it can make interpretation of the actions of a given factor problematic.

Arguably the most significant clinical observation relating to tumour angiogenesis has been the report that the vascular density of primary human breast carcinomas is an independent prognostic indicator of survival in early-stage breast carcinoma (23). Indeed, the vascular density of primary tumours has now been correlated with survival in many tumour types and the evidence is reviewed by Gasparini in Chapter 4. Later it was shown by ultrasound Doppler imaging that the extent of blood flow within ovarian tumours correlates with malignancy (24).

Finally, turning to the important topic of anti-angiogenesis and other possible strategies for therapeutic intervention. At the time of writing over 200 anti-angiogenic compounds have been described but the reality is that true advances in the use of anti-angiogenics in the clinic remains at a very early stage. A key question here is whether anti-angiogenics at best retard tumour growth or whether they can actually bring about tumour regression. Most of the compounds identified as anti-angiogenics have simply been shown to inhibit angiogenesis and not been shown to have an anti-tumour effect. For very few anti-angiogenics has tumour regression been claimed. Notable among these are antibodies to the $\alpha_v\beta_3$ integrin that as noted above is regarded as a marker of new vessel formation (8,25). Realistically, the primary use of anti-angiogenics for the foreseeable future is most likely to be in the adjuvant situation.

One of the more interesting anti-angiogenic strategies was taken by the groups of Risau and Ullrich (26). In these experiments a dominant negative VEGF receptor (that is one that blocks the growth effects of VEGF on endothelial cells, in this case it was the mouse VEGF receptor flk-1 that lacked a tyrosine kinase signalling domain) was packaged into a retroviral construct such that expression was under control of the retroviral long terminal repeats (LTRs). A viral producer line was then co-xenografted with a glioblastoma into nude mice, and the cells producing virus containing the dominant negative flk-1 shown to inhibit tumour growth. It is thought that virus escaping from the producer line infects the mouse endothelium and blocks the angiogenic activity of VEGF secreted by the glioblastoma. This experiment constitutes the first form of anti-angiogenic gene therapy.

An alternative but related approach to anti-angiogenesis is vascular targeting. The idea here is to damage the tumour vasculature exposing the underlying thrombogenic extracellular matrix in order to bring about blood clot formation in the outer tumour vessels and to subsequently eliminate the tumour by ischaemic necrosis. This approach has been shown to be highly effective in the elegant model system of Thorpe (27) (Chapter 26). In the absence of antibodies that were specific for tumour vasculature, Burrows and Thorpe employed antibodies that recognized mouse major histocompatibility complex (MHC) class II. MHC class II is only expressed on mouse endothelium when it is inflamed. Thus, interferon-γ was transfected into a neuroblastoma line and the interferon-γ expressing transfectants implanted into mice. MHC class II was then only present on the endothelium within the xenografted tumour and delivery of an anti-MHC class II antibody-toxin (ricin) conjugate brought about complete eradication of large solid tumours. The difficulty in obtaining antibodies that are specific for tumour endothelium has led several groups to attempt similar strategies (reviewed in Chapter 27) but involving direct delivery of a toxic gene to the tumour endothelium.

References

1. Hunter, J. (1787). Lectures on the principles of surgery. In *The works of John Hunter* Volume I (ed. J. Palmer), p. 368. London.

2. Noden, D. M. (1989). Embryonic origins and assembly of blood vessels. *Am. Rev. Respir. Dis.*, **140**, 1097–103.

3. Carmeliet, P., Ferreira, V., Breier, G., Pollefeyt, S., Kieckens, I., Gertsenstein, M., *et al.* (1996). Abnormal blood vessel development and lethality in embryos lacking a single VEGF allele. *Nature*, **380**, 435–9.

4. Ferrara, N., Carver-Moore, K., Chen, H., Dowd, M., Lucy Lu, K., O'Shea, S., *et al.* (1996). Heterozygous embryonic lethality induced by targeted inactivation of the VEGF gene. *Nature*, **380**, 439–42.

5. Shalaby, F., Rossant, J., Yamaguchi, T. P., Gertsenstein, M., Wu, X-F., Brietman, M. L., and Schuh, A. C. (1995). Failure of blood-island formation and vasculogenesis in Flk-1-deficient mice. *Nature*, **376**, 62–6.

6. Fong, G. H., Rossant, J., Gertsenstein, M., and Breitman, M. L. (1995) Role of the Flt-1 receptor tyrosine kinase in regulating the assembly of vascular endothelium. *Nature*, **376**, 66–70.

7. Stewart, P. A. and Wiley, M. J. (1981) Developing nervous tissue induces formation of blood–brain characteristics in invading endothelial cells: a study using quail-chick transplantation chimeras. *Dev. Biol.*, **84**, 183–92.

8. Cheresh, D. A. (1987) Human endothelial cells synthesize and express an Arg-Gly-Asp-directed adhesion receptor involved in attachment to fibrinogen and von Willebrand factor. *Proc. Natl Acad. Sci. USA*, **84**, 6471–5.

9. Bader, B. L., Rayburn, H., and Hynes, R. O. (1996) Targeted disruption of the mouse αv integrin gene. In *Integrins and signalling events in cell biology and disease*, Keystone Symposium, Abstract 401.

10. Folkman, J., Long, D. M., and Becker, F. F. (1963) Growth and metastasis of tumours in organ culture. *Cancer*, **16**, 453–67.

11. Gimbrone, M. A., Jr., Leapman, S., Cotran, R. S., and Folkman, J. (1973) Tumour angiogenesis: iris neovascularisation at a distance from intraocular tumours. *J. Natl Cancer Inst.*, **50**, 219–28.

12. Gimbrone, M. A., Leapman, S. B., Cotran, R. S., and Folkman, J. (1972) Tumour dormancy *in vivo* by prevention of neovascularisation. *J. Exp. Med.*, **73**, 461–73.

13. Folkman, J. (1972) Anti-angiogenesis: new concept for therapy of solid tumours. *Ann. Surg.*, **175**, 409–16.

14. Folkman, J. (1990) What is the evidence that tumours are angiogenesis dependent? *J. Natl Cancer Inst.*, **82**, 4–6.

15. Leung, D. W., Cachianes, G., Kuang, W-J., Goeddel, D. V., and Ferrara, N. (1989) Vascular endothelial growth factor is a secreted angiogenic mitogen. *Science*, **246**, 1306–9.

16. Keck, P. J., Hauser, S. D., Krivi, G., Sanzo, K., Warren, T., Feder, J., and Connolly, D. T. (1989) Vascular permeability factor, an endothelial cell mitogen related to PDGF. *Science*, **246**, 1309–12.

17. Gospodarowicz, D., Abraham, J. A., and Schilling, J. (1989) Isolation and characterization of a vascular endothelial cell mitogen produced by pituitary-derived folliculo stellate cells. *Proc. Natl Acad. Sci. USA*, **86**, 7311–15.

18. Conn, G., Soderman, D. D., Schaeffer, M-T., Wile, M., Hatcher, V. B., and Thomas, K. A. (1990) Purification of a glycoprotein vascular endothelial cell mitogen from a rat glioma-derived cell line. *Proc. Natl Acad. Sci. USA*, **87**, 1323–7.

19. Shweiki, D., Itin, A., Soffer, D., and Keshet, E. (1992) Vascular endothelial growth factor induced by hypoxia may mediate hypoxia-initiated angiogenesis. *Nature*, **359**, 843–5.

20. Shweiki, D., Neeman, M., Itin, A., and Keshet, E. (1995) Induction of vascular endothelial growth factor expression by hypoxia and by glucose deficiency in multicell spheroids: implications for tumour angiogenesis. *Proc. Natl Acad. Sci. USA*, **92**, 768–72.

21. Kim, K. J., Li, B., Winer, J., Armanini, M., Gillett, N., Phillips, H. S., and Ferrara, N. (1993) Inhibition of vascular endothelial growth factor-induced angiogenesis suppresses tumour growth *in vivo*. *Nature*, **362**, 841–4.

22. Nguyen, M., Watanabe, H., Budson, A. E., Richie, J. P., Hayes, D. F., and Folkman, J. (1994) Elevated levels of an angiogenic peptide, basic fibroblast growth factor, in the urine of patients with a wide spectrum of cancers. *J. Natl Cancer Inst.*, **86**, 356–61.

23. Weidner, N., Folkman, J., Pozza, F., Bevilacqua, P., Allred, E. N., Moore, D. H., *et al.* (1992) Tumour angiogenesis: a new significant and independent prognostic indicator in early stage breast carcinoma. *J. Natl Cancer Inst.*, **84**, 1875–87.

24. Reynolds, K., Farzaneh, F., Collins, W. P., Campbell, S., Bourne, T. H., Lawton, F., *et al.* (1994) Association of ovarian malignancy with expression of platelet-derived endothelial cell growth factor. *J. Natl Cancer Inst.*, **86**, 1234–8.

25. Brooks, P. C., Montgomery, A. M., Rosenfeld, M., Reisfeld, R. A., Hu, T., Klier, G., and Cheresh, D. A. (1994) Integrin alpha v beta 3 antagonists promote tumour regression by inducing apoptosis of angiogenic blood vessels. *Cell*, **79**, 1157–64.

26. Millauer, B., Shawver, I., Plate, K. H., Risau, W., and Ullrich, A. (1994) Glioblastoma growth inhibited *in vivo* by a dominant-negative FLK-1 mutant. *Nature*, **367**, 576–9.

27. Burrows, F. J. and Thorpe, P. E. (1993) Eradication of large solid tumours in mice with an immunotoxin directed against tumour vasculature. *Proc. Natl Acad. Sci. USA*, **90**, 8996–9000.

2. *In vivo* models of angiogenesis
Tai-Ping D. Fan and Peter J. Polverini

Introduction

To discover and test the efficacy of new anti-angiogenics, it is imperative to have appropriate *in vivo* models. The classical assays for angiogenesis include the hamster cheek pouch (1–4), rabbit ear chamber (5), dorsal skin and air sac (6–8), the chick chorioallantoic membrane (CAM) (8–10), and iris and avascular cornea of rodent eye (11–13). The past 10 years have seen improvements of some of these assays and the introduction of several new models, *e.g.* subcutaneous implantation of plastic chambers (14) or porous polytetrafluoroethylene tubes (15). In particular, techniques involving the subcutaneous implantation of sterile sponges into experimental animals have become popular (16–18). Furthermore, a variety of naturally occurring and chemically modified versions of matrices such as Matrigel (19,20) or fibrin gels (14) that were only used until recently to analyse angiogenesis *in vitro*, have been successfully adapted for the study of angiogenesis *in vivo*. All of these methods allow for direct inspection of an area that is either devoid of blood vessels initially, or has a vascular pattern clearly distinguishable from newly formed capillaries.

As pointed out by Auerbach and his co-workers, 'perhaps the most consistent limitation (to progress in angiogenesis research) has been the availability of simple, reliable, reproducible, quantitative assays of the angiogenic response' (21). This chapter aims to present some of the commonly used *in vivo* assays. Their relative merits and disadvantages are discussed.

Semi-transparent vascularized membranous tissues

Much of our early understanding of the angiogenic response has resulted from the pioneering studies of neovascularization of regenerating tissues. Early studies of angiogenesis were performed by direct observations on live specimens. Using a transparent chamber introduced into a tissue defect, Clark and Clark (22,23) described in detail, the growth of a solid cord of endothelium, from the convex side of a curved vessel, that continued to grow and anastomosed with other endothelial cords or with pre-existing vessels. These observations have been successfully repeated in several other semi-transparent tissues such as the hamster cheek pouch (1,24) and rat mesentery (25,26).

The rat mesenteric-window angiogenesis assay (MWAA) is based on the induction of angiogenesis by activating resident mast cells with intraperitoneal injections of compound 48/80. The window-like membranous parts of the true mesentery is essentially avascular. They measure only 5–10 μm thick and are distinctly outlined by fatty arcades. Neovascularization is quantitated by two technically independent methods (25,26): (i) the number of vessel profiles per unit tissue length (no. UL) of plastic-embedded window cut perpendicular to the surface of 3 μm thick toluidine-blue-stained sections was counted at × 400, and (ii) the vascularized area (VA; as a percentage of the whole window area) in spread preparations of intact mesenteric windows are measured morphometrically by a computerized image analyser. Four to five windows are analysed per animal. The inter- and intrapersonal reproducibility for blind readings was reported to be very high, $r \geqslant 0.99$ using linear regression analysis. The principal advantage of the MWAA is that the test tissue is sparsely vascularized and any neovasculature can be easily recognized. However, relatively large quantities of test material are required.

Dorsal skin and subcutaneous air sac in rodents

The introduction of normal or neoplastic cells or tissue fragments into the dermis of mouse skin and an earlier modified version of this model system, the rat dorsal air sac, were shown to have limited utility as bioassays of angiogenesis. The former model was originally used to demonstrate a role for lymphocytes in dermal angiogenic responses (27,28). The advantage of this system is that it allowed for the use of histocompatible cells and tissues in animals with a genetically defined background. The procedure which simply involved the intradermal injection of cells was proved to be of limited utility due to the inherent inaccuracy of evaluating dermal angiogenic responses. Owing to extreme variability in the macroscopic quantification of vessel counts and the inability to distinguish reliably new vessels from those that became more evident due to vasodilatation, this model has limited application as a routine bioassay. The same holds true for earlier versions of the dorsal air sac (29). In this model, cells or tissue fragments are introduced into an air pocket created on the dorsum of a rat, temporarily creating a thin, isolated vascularized membrane for cells or tissues to establish a new blood supply. This system was severely limited due to the inability of the examiner to monitor the evolution of an angiogenic response. Nevertheless this model system provided the ground work for the eventual development of the corneal bioassay of neovascularization.

The air sac model has recently been improved by Colville-Nash et al. (30) for quantitative studies of pharmacological modulation of angiogenesis in inflammation. Air pouches were induced by the subcutaneous injection of 3 ml of air into anaesthetized mice. Twenty-four hours later, 0.5 ml Freund's complete adjuvant with 0.1% croton oil was injected into the air pouches to elicit granulomatous inflammation. The angiogenic response after 6 days or up to 28 days was quantitated using a modification of the vascular casting method of Kimura et al. (31). To overcome alterations in peripheral vasomotor tone and tissue perfusion related to anaesthesia and ambient temperature that may invalidate the results, mice were placed in a heated jacket at 40°C for 10 min to induce peripheral vasodilatation. Vascular cast was formed by the intravenous injection of 1 ml 5% carmine red in 10% gelatin at 40°C into the warmed mice. This procedure produced an excellent retention of the dye within the vasculature. After chilling the carcasses, the granulomatous air pouch linings were dissected, oven-dried at 56°C for 48 h, weighed, and then digested in papain. The dye was then disssolved in NaOH, and the digests were centrigued and filtered. Finally, the dye content of 200 µl samples was assayed spectrophotometrically and the results were expressed as the VI (vascularity index, µg dye per mg dry weight of tissue). Using this model, the angiostatic steroids tetrahydrocorticol and cortisone were shown to reduce the VI in the absence of heparin. These data suggest that angiostatic steroids may be useful in the treatment of chronic inflammatory disease (30).

Chick chorioallantosis and yolk sac membrane

The CAM was originally used by embryologists to study the developmental potential of embryonic tissue grafts. It was adapted by Folkman's group to study tumour-induced angiogenesis (32). After 72-h incubation, enough albumen was withdrawn to minimize adhesion of the shell membrane. Tissue grafts were then placed on to the CAM through a window made in the eggshell. Three to four days later, a typical radial ('spoke-wheel') arrangement of vessels towards, or a clear increase of vessels around, the graft was taken as evidence of angiogenesis. Blood vessels entering the graft or tumour fragment within the focal plane of the CAM were counted under a stereomicroscope (33).

To assess the angiogenic or anti-angiogenic activity of soluble test substances, they were either prepared in slow-release polymer pellets or air-dried on plastic coverslips and then implanted on to the CAM. A graded scale of 0–4 was used to score the extent of vascularization. Serial dilution assays were then developed to score the number of positives at any particular dilution, using four eggs per assay point. High concentrations of a test substance would show three of four or four of four positive tests. Upon dilution of the test material, the number of positives would decrease until an end-point (none of four) was reached.

Sterile glass-fibre filter paper discs have been used to elicit neovascularization in the CAM. To assess the ability of test compounds to inhibit angiogenesis, they were prepared in 0.5% methylcellulose and air-dried on top of the discs (34). The angiogenic response was assigned scores of 1, 2, 4, 8, 16, or 32 points, with reference to a scoring system. Some investigators induce angiogenesis by filter discs saturated with basic fibroblast growth factor (bFGF) (33). Alternatively, a Silastic ring (diameter 10 mm, weight 17 mg) is placed on the CAM to facilitate local drug administration within the ring. Drugs are applied once daily from day 7 through day 14 within the ring (35). At day 14, the CAM is fixed with buffered formaldehyde, excised, and mounted on a glass slide. Using a 16 × objective, the angiogenic response is quantified by counting the number of blood vessel intersections with an eye-piece rectangular line grid. By standard stereological techniques, the average of four non-overlapping areas can be taken as the microvascular density index for each CAM. Interestingly, angiotensin II stimulates the formation of distinct arteriolar–arteriolar connections ('arcades'), which are different from the typical spoke-wheel arrangement of neovessels induced by growth factors such as bFGF (le Noble, personal communication).

Auerbach et al. have described an alternative CAM assay (9). In this assay, shell-less chick embryos are cultured in Petri dishes. Unlike the original CAM assay where only a small portion of the membrane is exposed in the shell window, the CAM develops on top as a flat membrane, reaching to the edges of the Petri dish and formed a two-dimensional monolayer. Thus, multiple grafts or test substances can be implanted on individual CAMs and the angiogenic responses photographed periodically. The yolk sac assay is a variant of the CAM assay which utilizes early chick embryos removed from their shells and incubated in Petri dishes. The angiogenic agonist or antagonist is placed on the vitelline veins of the yolk sac. Although vessel growth can be analysed and scored by the grading system described above, image analysis is often used to obtain greater accuracy in quantitation (36–38). Here, computer-assisted tracking of images is used to generate both directional vector values and absolute values for the number of individual blood vessels. This approach enables the subtraction of the 'background noise' of resident vessels in the CAM to produce a meaningful assessment of neovascularization.

The principal advantages of the CAM are that it is simple and relatively inexpensive and lends itself to large-scale screening of samples. Also because the CAM can be manipulated outside the egg shell it is possible to monitor and photograph evolving responses on a daily basis. Thus, the CAM assay has been used by numerous investigators in their studies of angiostatic steroids (34,39,40), collagen synthesis inhibitors (41), angiostatic polysaccharides (42), angiostatic antibodies (43), a cartilage-derived inhibitor of angiogenesis (44), retinoids (45), and nitric oxide (NO) releasing vasodilators (46). It is noteworthy that xenografts from mammalian species can become established and grow on the CAM because the early chick embryo lacks a mature immune system. For example, the assay has also been used to demonstrate the effectiveness of anti-integrin $\alpha_v\beta_3$ on angiogenesis induced by fragments of human M21-L melanoma growing on the CAM (33).

The major disadvantage of this assay is that as the CAM already contains a well developed vascular network there may be some difficulty, particularly with inexperienced examiners, in distinguishing vasolidatation that invariably occurs following manipulation of the membrane, from neovascularization. Another common problem is the difficulty in discriminating new capillaries from the background veins, arteries, and non-growing capillaries. In addition, these vessels in the horizontal plane may be falsely affected by contracture of the membrane.

Folkman's group recently developed an ingenious technique to overcome these problems of the CAM (47). The new method is based on the *vertical* growth of new capillary blood vessels into a collagen gel (containing bFGF and sucralfate or tumour cells) through two parallel nylon meshes which align the capillaries for counting (Fig. 2.1). Quantitation of new vessels can be achieved in less than 1 min per embryo, because the top grid positions all of the new vessels in one focal plane. This new assay does not depend on flow, nor does it require injection of dyes, measurement of DNA synthesis, photograph, and image

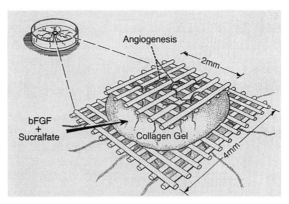

Figure 2.1. Schematic diagram of quantitative angiogenesis bioassay. Basic fibroblast growth factor (bFGF) and sucralfate were mixed in a collagen gel embedded between two pieces of mesh and placed on the chorioallantoic membrane as described in Ngyuyen *et al.* (47). The result was expressed as the percentage of the squares in the top mesh that contained blood vessels.

analysis. Furthermore, it is possible to compare the potency of different angiogenesis inhibitors on a molar basis. This improved CAM assay will no doubt facilitate the discovery of new angiogenesis inhibitors with sufficient potency for clinical applications.

Maragoudakis *et al.* (41) proposed that the rate of basement membrane (BM) biosynthesis can be used as a biochemical index of angiogenesis. To measure the rate of BM biosynthesis in CAM during chick embryo development, [U-¹⁴C]proline and test materials were placed on sterile round plastic discs, dried under sterile condition and then inverted and placed on the surface of CAM. At the end of experiment, the area under the disc was cut off, placed in an appropriate buffer and protein biosynthesis was terminated. After washing with trichloroacetic acid to remove non protein bound radioactivity, discs were subjected to collagenase digestion. The resulting radiolabelled tripeptides corresponding to BM collagen synthesized by the CAM from [U-¹⁴C]proline were counted and expressed as c.p.m./mg protein. It was shown that collagenous proteins represent 80% of the total BM proteins formed by the CAM during the chick embryo development. Furthermore, the rate was maximum between days 8 and 11, which coincided with maximum angiogenesis as determined by morphological evaluation of vascular density. At day 10, collagenous protein synthesis was 11-fold higher than that of day 15 when angiogenesis has reached a plateau. Thus, the extent of their biosynthesis correlated well with new vessel formation. Using substances that modify the rate of BM collagen biosynthesis, these authors demonstrated that monitoring BM formation is a convenient, quantitative method of assessing angiogenesis in the CAM.

The rodent eye: the iris and avascular cornea

The iris and cornea of the rodent eye has proven to be one of the most versatile bioassays for the study of angiogenesis (Fig. 2.2). Initially, these model systems were useful in the study of ocular disease (48,49). However, it soon proved to be an invaluable system to investigate the mechanism of tumour neovascularization. The concept that tumours were angiogenesis dependent was firmly established using these systems in a series of studies from the Folkman laboratory in the early 1970s (6,8,11). These investigators showed that tumour spheroids that were free-floating in the anterior chamber remained biologically dormant. When tumour spheroids contacted the surface of the iris and became vascularized, they rapidly grew as a three-dimensional tumour mass (50). The hypothesis that tumours induced angiogenesis via production of diffusable angiogenic factors was later confirmed using the avascular cornea of the rabbit eye (51).

A wide variety of tissues, cells, and cell extracts or media conditioned by cells grown in culture have been examined for angiogenic stimulatory or inhibitory activity in the cornea. When possible, cell extracts or conditioned media are the preferred form of material to be assayed. One can more accurately determine dosage/potency of a particular test sample and precisely control the quantity and positioning of materials within the corneal stroma, after incorporation into one of several slow-release non-inflammatory polymers. The two most often used materials are poly-2-hydroxylethyl-methacrylate (Hydron® lot No. 110, Interferon Sciences Inc., New Brunswick, NJ) and ethylene-vinyl acetate copolymer (ELVAX, Aldrich Chemical, Milwaukee, WI). Both materials work with equal effectiveness.

The corneal bioassay is best regarded as a qualitative assay, although a number of quantitative measures have been devised for use with this model system. Responses are usually scored on the day animals are killed, 5–7 days after implantation. Positive responses are recorded when sustained ingrowth of capillary loops or sprouts is detected. Negative scores are assigned to responses where either no growth is detected or when an occasional sprout or hairpin loop is detected without evidence of sustained growth. Occasionally (<10% of the time), responses are neither equivocally positive nor negative with samples which are normally positive or inhibitory. In these instances responses are graded as +/−. Several factors account for this, i.e. slight differences in the position of implants within the cornea, variations in the quality and quantity of material being tested. No matter how experienced one is with this technique a certain degree of variability can be expected. Obviously this must be kept at a minimum. Permanent records of vascular response are made following perfusion with India ink. Any commercially available source of waterproof India ink is acceptable. Perfusion via the abdominal aorta is accomplished with a simple pressure vessel capable of maintaining a pressure of 120 mmHg. If so desired, one can quantitate the corneal response. A simple method described by Sholley *et al.* is as follows (52). Vessel length is measured directly using 4 × 5 transilluminated photographic negatives at a magnification of 10 ×. Three radially oriented measurements are taken using a vernier calliper; two of these measurements include vessels present at the periphery of the radius and the third includes the largest vessels along the centre of the radius. The three measurements are averaged to provide a single length of measure for each response.

High-resolution video technology combined with new imaging techniques have been used to quantitate corneal neovascularization, detecting blood vessels down to the size of 8 μm (53). The video recorder enhances the speed of data collection by continuous recording of about 5 min/animal per time point. This non-invasive method enables the investigators to establish the temporal pattern of corneal neovascularization in individual living animals over a period of time. Because multiple data points can be generated from each animal, this method requires fewer animals than studies using a post-mortem quantitation technique.

Now considered the 'gold standard' for the *in vivo* analysis of angiogenesis, the corneal assay has stood the test of time as a reliable and relatively easily interpretable angiogenesis bioassay. Because it is avascular, the cornea avoids the problem of interpretation inherent in the other bioassays. Any vessels penetrating into the corneal stroma can be readily identified as newly formed. With the aid of a stereomicroscope parameters of capillary growth such as sprout and hairpin-loop formation, and the development of corneal oedema and inflammation can be documented in considerable detail (11–13). In comparison with the CAM, this system is technically demanding and relatively expensive. As only one or at most two samples can be evaluated per cornea it is not a practical screening assay.

The rabbit has often been substituted by the mouse (13,72) and the rate (20,54–56) for corneal assay. The availability of an extensive range of inbred strains of mice, the low cost of their maintenance, and reduced amount of space required are obvious advantages. However, the

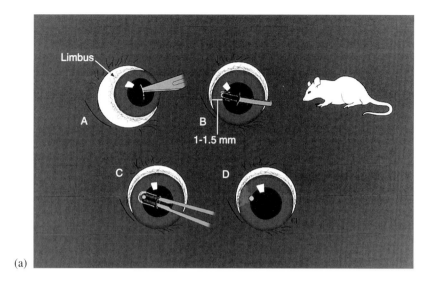

(a)

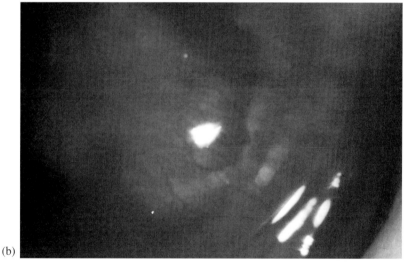

(b)

Figure 2.2. (a) Diagram demonstrating the corneal bioassay of neovascularization. This is one of several bioassays currently used to test cells or compounds for proangiogenic or angiostatic activity. In this diagram, a pellet of Hydron, a slow-release noninflammatory polymer of hydroxyethylmethacrylate, used to incorporate substance for release in the cornea, is being placed within a pocket created in the corneal stroma. This technique was first described by Gimbrone *et al.* (1973) to assay for angiogenic factors produced by tumours and is now one of the most widely used angiogenesis bioassays. (b) This is a photograph of a colloidal carbon perfused cornea seven days after implanting a Hydron pellet containing tumour cell conditioned culture media. Note the brush-like ingrowth of capillary sprouts converging on the implanted pellet (the latter is not visible).

small size of the murine eye makes this model even more technically demanding. Dexterity in microsurgical techniques and implantation of sustained release pellets is critical to obtain reproducible and reliable results.

Recently, the corneal assay has been further modified and adapted in severe combined immunodeficiency (SCID) mice (see later). In one report, such an assay was used to discover circulating angiogenesis inhibitors generated by several human tumours (57). Human tumour cells were injected subcutaneously in SCID mice and allowed to grow until the primary tumours reached ≥ 500 mm^3. Subsequently, corneal pockets were made in the eyes of mice bearing primary subcutaneous tumours and control mice without tumours. A 0.34×0.34 mm sucrose aluminium sulphate pellet coated with Hydron polymer containing bFGF was then implanted into each pocket. The corneas of all mice were routinely examined by slit-lamp biomicroscopy and photographed. From each colour photographic print, the area of new vessel growth was delineated and digitized. Finally, vessel length and clock-hours of neovascularization were measured by computer-assisted image processing. Inhibition of vessel density in corneas of tumour-bearing animals was calculated as a percentage of control values obtained from non-tumour-bearing animals.

Sponge implant models

Subcutaneous implantation of artificial sponges in laboratory animals has become a popular means of studying angiogenesis. Substances to be studied are either injected directly into the sponges (17,58) or incorporated into ELVAX pellets and placed in the centre of the sponge discs (18). Neovascularization of the sponges is commonly assessed histologically (tissue infiltration), morpho-

metrically (vascular density); or biochemically (e.g. DNA, protein, and haemoglobin contents). Different types of sponge materials have been used: polyvinyl alcohol (Ivalon), polyester, polyether polyurethane, and gelatin (Gelfoam). The differences in sponge materials, shape, and size make direct data comparison difficult.

Davidson et al. (16) and Buckley et al. (59) implanted Ivalon sponges subcutaneously in rats to study the angiogenic properties of cartilage-derived growth factor and epidermal growth factor by measuring the DNA, protein, and collagen content of the implants. This group of workers also showed that sponge implants containing slow-release pellets releasing a neutralizing antiserum directed against bFGF significantly reduced content of DNA, protein, and collagen. These data suggest that endogenous bFGF is involved in wound repair (60).

Gelatin sponges (Gelfoam; Upjohn) have been used in mice. These sponges are cut into strips under sterile conditions and then allowed to soak up 1% (w/v) agarose containing growth factors. Two weeks after subcutaneous implantation, the sponge is removed and prepared for histology and haemoglobin measurement. For example, suramin has been shown to prevent neovascularization and tumour growth in such a model (61). Oral administration of an inhibitor of thymidine phosphorylase (6-amino-5-chlorouracil) has also been shown to inhibit angiogenic response elicited by thymidine phosphorylase (62).

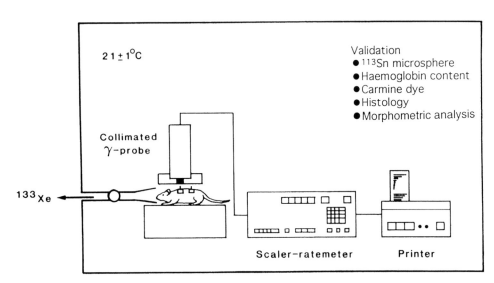

Figure 2.3. The rat sponge model of angiogenesis. Sterile cannulated sponge discs are implanted subcutaneously in rats. Blood flow changes in the sponges are monitored between days 4 and 14 using a ^{133}Xe clearance technique. At fixed time points, the sponges are excised and processed for histological studies and morphometric analysis. The model has been validated by several other techniques as described in Hu et al. (1995). *Lab. Invest.*, **72**, 601–10.

The cannulated sponge model

In 1987, a method of quantitating angiogenesis in sponge implants in rats was described by Andrade and co-workers (17). The method not only allows histological and bio-chemical studies to be made but also has the major advantage of using a simple and rapid ^{133}Xe clearance technique for repeated measurement of relative blood flow changes through the sponges over a period of weeks. As the sponges originally contained no blood vessels, the increase in the rate of ^{133}Xe loss from the sponges was considered to represent neovascularization. To validate this technique, Hu *et al.* (58) carried out comparative studies of 6-min ^{133}Xe clearance measurements with four additional approaches (Fig. 2.3). First, absolute blood flow in the sponges was measured using a standard ^{113}Sn tracer microsphere technique. Second, the amount of neo-vasculature in the sponges was determined by the carmine dye method. Third, the level of haemoglobin and total protein in the implants was tested and finally, histological and morphometric analysis of sponge implants was carried out. Using this model, we have shown that the neovascular responses produced by the inflammatory polypeptides, substance P, and bradykinin, to be inhibited by antagonists for particular receptor subtypes (63,64). Furthermore, it has been shown that the angiogenic responses elicited by cytokines and growth factors can either be neutralized by appropriate antibodies, blocked by receptor antagonists, or reduced by selective signalling pathway inhibitors (65,66). Figure 2.4 shows that the tyrosine kinase inhibitor, laven-dustin A, not only reduced ^{133}Xe clearance from VEGF-treated sponges but also reduced the total fibrovascular growth areas. These investigations consolidate the validity and future applications of this model in angiogenesis research.

In a recent development, Walsh *et al.* (67) used immunohistochemistry and quantitative *in vitro* receptor autoradiography to localize and characterize substance P receptors on developing neovasculature of sponge implants. Furthermore, endothelial proliferation was measured by endothelial proliferating cell nuclear antigen (PCNA) index. It was shown that specific [^{125}I]-substance P binding sites, with characteristics of neurokinin receptors of the NK$_1$ subclass, were localized to micro-vessels in the sponge stroma, progressively increasing in density from day 4 to 14. These data support the hypo-thesis that substance P enhances angiogenesis in this model by a direct action on microvascular NK$_1$ receptors (63).

The cannulated sponge model has been adapted for mice (68). Furthermore, the sponge implants in inbred mice were used to host proliferating tumour cells (69,70). These authors suggest that neoplasms can modulate the synthesis of NO in their vasculature. The increased NO synthesis in cancers could be important in maintaining tumour blood flow.

In comparison with other assays for angiogenesis, several advantages of the cannulated sponge model are apparent.

1. Because the injected ^{133}Xe is cleared by expiration within 2 h, it is possible to make sequential blood flow measurements in the same animal over a period of 2–3 weeks.
2. Owing to the porous nature of the sponge it is possible to retrieve and analyse inflammatory mediators (63), cytokines, and growth factors (93). Such information will help elucidate the role of these factors in angio-genesis.
3. The functional differences of granulation neo-vasculature and tumour neovasculature can be studied in detail.
4. The system allows testing of compounds which can either be administered locally into the sponges or systemically.

The limitations of this system are: (i) unlike the corneal implant assay and CAM assay, gross inspection of sponge neovascularization is not possible; (ii) it is necessary to carry out supporting histological studies on the sponge sections; and (iii) animals have to be kept singly to prevent damage to the cannulae. Therefore, the model uses up experimental animal accommodation.

The disc angiogenesis system

This model system originally described by Fajardo *et al.* (18,71,72) has grown in popularity over the last several years. This implant system consists of a thin wafer of polyvinyl alcohol foam, covered on both sides with Millipore filters leaving only the edges available for cell penetration. Angiogenic factors or antagonists are incorporated into a slow release polymer and placed in the centre of the sponge. The disc is implanted subcutaneously in the host animal through a distal skin incision. The optimal time for retrieval and examination of the sponge varies, depending on the size of the sponge and species of animal. For example in mice, optimal retrieval is 7–21 days after implantation of a 13 mm diameter sponge. To assess cell proliferation, [methyl-^{3}H]-thymidine (^{3}H-TdR) is injected intraperitoneally at 24, 18, and 12 h before euthanasia. Discs are then extracted and prepared for histology and evaluation of angiogenesis. Typically, fifteen 6 mm planar sections are obtained from each disc: three for histological study (haematoxylin and eosin

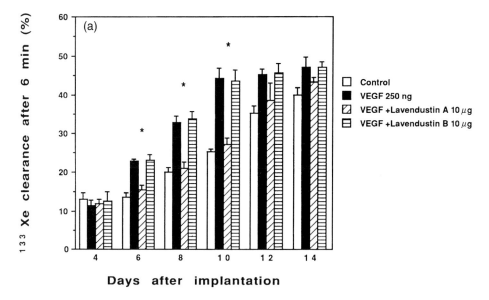

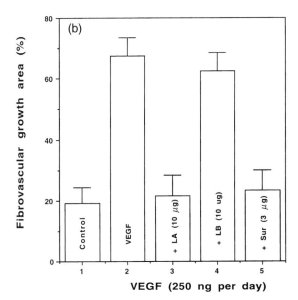

Figure 2.4. Suppression of vascular endothelial growth factor (VEGF)-induced angiogenesis in sponge implants by the receptor tyrosine kinase inhibitor, lavendustin A. (a) Shows lavendustin A (10 μg/day), but not lavendustin B, significantly reduced the ^{133}Xe clearance in the vascularized sponges. (b) Confirms that lavendustin A (LA) and suramin (Sur) completely abolished the fibrovascular growth induced by VEGF.

(H&E)) and measurement of axial growth and one for measurement of total growth area by an automated, computer-assisted image analysis microscopic technique. Ten sections are for scintillation counting and the remaining section for cellular localization of ^{3}H-TdR by autoradiography.

Polakowski *et al.* (73) modified the disc angiogenesis assay and demonstrated the anti-angiogenic properties of

recombinant ribonuclease inhibitor (RNasin). Endothelial cell influx was diminished by RNasin, as shown by lectin-staining of sponge sections and by culturing cells isolated from sponges by collagenase treatment. The anti-angiogenic activity of RNasin was confirmed by implanting Hydron-coated sponges containing bFGF or bFGF plus RNasin into adult mouse corneas. The strong neovascular response elicited by bFGF was almost completely suppressed by RNasin. Most interestingly, a significant reduction in tumour growth was achieved when RNasin-containing ELVAX-coated sponges were implanted subcutaneously underneath an intradermal inoculum of C755 mammary tumour cells.

Similar to the cannulated sponge model discussed earlier, the disc angiogenesis system has been modified to enable the introduction of live cells, i.e. tumour cells or inflammatory cells into the centre of the sponge at various times after implantation (74). It is also possible to retrieve and analyse populations of inflammatory cells and other cell populations that comprise the 'granulation tissue' response that have invaded the sponge. This bioassay offers several advantages over other systems discussed to this point. It is relatively inexpensive and angiogenesis is easily quantitated using standard histological, auto-radiographic, and morphometric methods of analysis. Its chief disadvantage is that one is unable to study the process of angiogenesis, rather one is restricted to an evaluation of the response at fixed time points.

Rat freeze-injured skin graft assay

A novel skin graft model has been developed for the quantitative study of promoters and potential promoters of angiogenesis in wound healing (75). To delay revascularization, full thickness rat skin autografts (2 cm diameter) were subjected to a reproducible and uniform freeze injury. Briefly, the grafts were placed in cryovials and immersed in a cryoprotectant solution [25% dimethyl sulphoxide (DMSO) in Medium 199 (vol./vol.)] and cooled to $-196°C$ in liquid nitrogen. After rapid thawing at 37°C, DMSO was immediately leached out of the skin grafts by immersion in Medium 199. Each graft was then sutured to a 2 cm diameter recipient defect made on the dorsal skin. Candidate angiogenic factors incorporated in ELVAX pellets were implanted at the time of surgery around the perimeter of the graft. Revascularization was assessed quantitatively in terms of blood flow in the grafts using laser Doppler flowmetry and a ^{133}Xe clearance technique. Histological sections were stained for basement membrane laminin for morphometric evaluation of vessel growth. bFGF, thymidine phosphorylase, and angiogenic oligosaccharides of hyaluronan were all found to accelerate healing of freeze-injured grafts (75–77). In contrast, these substances had no effect on either graft blood flow or on vessel growth in uninjured skin grafts. These data support the hypothesis that the potential of a tissue to respond to angiogenic stimuli is related to the integrity of that tissue. Thus, stimulation of wound healing angiogenesis by exogenous growth factors is only possible in the presence of tissue injury, where conditions for healing are suboptimal.

The obvious advantage of this model is that it can provide consistent and reproducible data on the blood flow and vascular changes seen in wound healing. Gross inspection of the graft is possible, which is not true of the various sponge implant and subcutaneous chamber models. Although the model was designed for the study of angiogenic substance, it is predicted that the use of angiogenic inhibitors would lead to graft loss.

Matrigel plugs and alginate-tumour pellets

Matrigel is a laminin-rich reconstituted matrix. It is a mixture of basement membrane components extracted from the Englebreth–Holm–Swarm tumour and found to induce and/or maintain the differentiation of a wide variety of cells (78). It was initially used to investigate capillary tube formation *in vitro* (79). Passaniti *et al.* (19) developed an elegant method of injecting Matrigel-containing bFGF subcutaneously into mice. This model has proved suitable for assessing angiogenesis and anti-angiogenic agents. Grant *et al.* (20) also used this technique to show that scatter factor/hepatocyte growth factor is a potent angiogenic peptide. Briefly, Matrigel in liquid form at 4°C was mixed with scatter factor and injected into the abdominal subcutaneous tissues of mice. At body temperature, Matrigel rapidly formed a solid gel, trapping the growth factor to allow slow release and prolonged exposure to surrounding tissues. The animals were killed on day 10 and the Matrigel plugs excised for histological examination. Angiogenesis was quantitated as total vessel area (mm^2) in the plug sections by image analysis. The main advantage of this method is that, unlike artificial sponge implants, Matrigel provides a more 'natural' micro-environment to initiate an angiogenic response. However, this material is expensive.

A novel means to quantitate tumour-induced angiogenesis was developed by Plunkett and Hailey (80). Tumour cells were mixed in a sterile sodium alginate polymer solution, subjected to a special cell entrapment process and then injected subcutaneously into host animals. The angiogenic response was quantified by measuring the level of haemoglobin or the amount of radiolabelled red blood cells pooled at the injection site of the alginate beads, confirmed by macroscopic photography and microscopic histological examination. More recent studies by Plunkett and co-workers showed that inhibitors of angiogenesis such as protamine sulphate and the angiostatic steroid tetrahydro S inhibited tumour-induced angiogenesis as determined by these two methods and confirmed by gross morphology and histological analysis of the alginate pellet site (81). The distinct merit of this model is that alginate polymer protects the tumour cells from direct contact with the host's immune system, enabling them to induce neovascularization in a syngeneic, allogeneic, or xenogeneic system.

Conventional tumour models and transfectants

Numerous animal tumour models have been developed to test the anti-angiogenic and anti-cancer effects of drugs. Most investigators inject tumour cells (*e.g.* C6 rat glioblastoma, human large cell adenocarcinoma) subcutaneously into the flank of BALB/c nude mice. Drugs are often administered intravenously. After regular intervals, tumour measurements are made in three dimensions with a vernier calliper. Assuming the tumour to be an ellipsoid, the volume is calculated using the equation: volume (mm^3) = $\pi/6 \times d_1 \times d_2 \times d_3$, where d_1, d_2, and d_3 are the measured tumour dimensions in millimetres. For example, subcutaneous injection of TNP-470 (AGM-1470) has been shown to inhibit tumour growth in a dose-dependent manner, and the tumour sizes of B16BL6 melanoma, M5076 reticulum cell sarcoma, Lewis lung carcinoma, and Walker 256 carcinoma were maximally reduced to 16, 10, 17, and 4% of that in the respective control. Furthermore, TNP-470 reduced the number of pulmonary metastatic foci of intravenously inoculated B16BL6 melanoma in a dose-dependent manner, and the number of metastatic foci was reduced to 10% of that in the control by treatment with TNP-470 at 60 mg/kg, three times/week (82). To mimic human glioblastoma multiforme, other investigators have established VX2 carcinoma in rabbit brains or C6 glioblastoma in rat brains, respectively (83,84). To quantitate S-phase fraction of tumour and endothelial cells and the vascular density, tumour sections are stained simultaneously for bromodeoxyuridine and laminin or fibronectin.

To test whether VEGF may be a tumour angiogenesis factor *in vivo*, Kim *et al.* (85) injected human rhabdomyosarcoma, glioblastoma multiforme, or leiomyosarcoma cell lines into nude mice. They showed that treatment with a monoclonal antibody specific for VEGF inhibited the neovascularization and growth of the tumours, but had no effect on the growth rate of the tumour cells *in vitro*. These findings demonstrate that inhibition of the action of an angiogenic factor spontaneously produced by tumour cells may suppress tumour growth *in vivo*.

Transfection experiments have become popular to test the effects of overexpressing candidate genes on angiogenesis and tumour growth in nude mice. For example, the thymidine phosphorylase (TP) gene under control of the cytomegalovirus promoter in plasmid pcDNA-1-neo (Invitogen) was transfected into MCF-7 breast carcinoma cells (76). Overexpression of TP in MCF-7 cells had no effect on growth *in vitro*. In contrast, xenografts of the MCF-7 transfectants in ovariectomized BALB/c *nu/nu* mice markedly enhanced tumour growth *in vivo*. This model could be used to examine the anti-angiogenic/anti-cancer activities of selective inhibitors of TP.

Human severe combined immunodeficiency (SCID) mouse chimera

The use of SCID mice as an immunological sanctuary for human skin xenografts provides an excellent environment for the analysis of human skin biology and pathology (86–91). The SCID mouse mutation is a result of alterations in the DNA recombinase system that is necessary for rearranging the variable diversity joint of immunoglobulins and T-cell receptors leading to a failure of both T and B cells to differentiate (86); however, these mice have a functional complement of circulating platelets, neutrophils, monocytes, and natural killer cells. Furthermore, this model allows for standardization and reproducibility of results for the study of human tumours and chronic inflammatory diseases such as psoriasis in the context of both active disease and during periods of remission without the ethical or logistical concerns associated with repeated serial biopsies. This model system has only recently been used for the study of angiogenesis, but will no doubt prove to be invaluable for the study of many human angiogenesis dependent diseases.

In an exciting development, Brooks *et al.* (92) used a SCID mouse/human chimeric model to study the functional role of vascular integrin $\alpha_v\beta_3$ in human breast tumour-induced angiogenesis in the microenvironment of the human skin. First of all, they transplanted full-thickness human foreskin graft on to SCID mice. When the skin graft had healed, $\alpha_v\beta_3$-negative MCF-7PB human breast carcinoma cells were injected intradermally within the human skin. Over a period of 3 weeks, these cells formed well-defined solid tumours containing numerous blood vessels infiltrating the central mass of these tumours.

To determine the origin of the tumour-associated blood vessels, frozen tumour sections were stained with antibodies that react specifically with human but not murine blood vessels. Using anti-human CD31 monoclonal antibody and a polyconal antibody directed to human or mouse factor VIII, these authors provided unequivocal evidence that integrin $\alpha_v\beta_3$ was highly expressed on human angiogenic blood vessels associated with malignant human breast carcinoma. Most importantly, systemic administration of monoclonal antibody LM609 directed to integrin $\alpha_v\beta_3$ not only disrupted human angiogenesis but reduced the growth and invasive properties of human breast carcinoma in the SCID mouse/human chimeric model. These data show that $\alpha_v\beta_3$ antagonists have therapeutic potential in the treatment of human breast cancer.

Conclusions

A better understanding of the angiogenic process and its subversion in disease states should reveal specific targets for pharmacological interventions. The variety of *in vivo* bioassays of angiogenesis have enabled investigators to make rapid progress in elucidating the mechanism of action of a variety of angiogenic factors and inhibitors. Cost, simplicity, reproducibility, and reliability are important determinants dictating the choice of methods. Some of the assays are quantitative while others are qualitative. Some assays (*e.g.* the CAM) are suitable for large-scale screening of anti-angiogenic compounds, others (*e.g.* sponge models) are capable of handling small to medium-scale assessment of drugs. The corneal assay is a reliable and relatively easily interpretable angiogenesis bioassay. However, because the corneal assay is technically demanding, its usefulness as a screening assay by the pharmaceutical industry may be limited. In choosing a particular assay, the investigator should consider the suitability of different model systems to answer specific questions. Ideally, two different assays should be performed in parallel to confirm the angiogenic or anti-angiogenic activities of test substances. To evaluate their potential anti-cancer activities, anti-angiogenic compounds are invariably tested in animal tumour models. The advent of human SCID mouse chimera is expected to facilitate development of clinically relevant models of human angiogenic diseases. Such models would predict the efficacy and specificity of novel anti-angiogenic agents before clinical trials.

References

1. Klintworth, G. K. (1973). The hamster cheek pouch; an experimental model of corneal neovascularization. *Am. J. Pathol.*, **73**, 691–710.
2. Greenblatt, M. and Shubik, P. (1968). Tumor angiogenesis: transfilter diffusion studies in the hamster by the transparent chamber technique. *J. Natl Cancer Inst.*, **41**, 111–24.
3. Sanders, A. G. and Shubik, P. (1964). A transparent window for use in the Syrian hamster. *Isr. J. Exp. Med.*, **11**, 118.
4. Greenblatt, M., Choudair, K. V. R. T., Sanders, A. G., and Shubik, P. (1969). Mammalian microcirculation in the living animal: methodologic considerations. *Microvasc. Res.*, **1**, 420–32.
5. Sandison, J. C. (1924). A new method for the microscopic study of living growing tissue by the introduction of a transparent chamber in the rabbit's ear. *Anat. Rec.*, **28**, 281–7.
6. Folkman, J. and Cotran, R. S. (1976). Relation of vascular proliferation of tumor growth. *Int. Rev. Exp. Pathol.*, **16**, 207–48.
7. Folkman, J., Merler, E., Abernathy, C., and Williams, G. (1971). Isolation of tumor factor responsible for angiogenesis. *J. Exp. Med.*, **133**, 275–88.
8. Folkman, J. (1974). Tumor angiogenesis factor. *Cancer Res.*, **34**, 2109–13.
9. Auerbach, R., Kubai, L., Knighton, D., and Folkman, J. (1974). A simple procedure for the long term cultivation of chicken embryos. *Dev. Biol.*, **41**, 391–4.
10. Knighton, D., Ausprunk, D., Tapper, D., and Folkman, J. (1977). Avascular and vascular phases of tumor growth. *Br. J. Cancer*, **35**, 347–56.
11. Gimbrone, M. A., Jr., Cotran, R. S., Leapman, S. B., and Folkman, J. (1974). Tumor growth and neovascularization: an experimental model using the rabbit cornea. *J. Natl Cancer Inst.*, **52**, 413–27.
12. Polverini, P. J., Cotran, R. S., Gimbrone, M. A., Jr., and Unanue, E. R. (1977). Activated macrophages induce vascular proliferation. *Nature*, **269**, 804–6.
13. Muthukkaruppan, V. and Auerbach, R. (1979). Angiogenesis in the mouse cornea. *Science*, **205**, 1416–18.
14. Dvorak, H. F., Harvey, V. S., Estrella, P., Brown, L. F., McDonagh, J. and Dvorak, A. M. (1987). Fibrin containing gels induce angiogenesis: implications for tumor stroma generation and wound healing. *Lab. Invest.*, **57**, 673–86.
15. Sprugel, K. H., McPherson, J. M., Clowes, A. W., and Ross, R. (1987). Effects of growth factors *in vivo*. I. Cell ingrowth into porous subcutaneous chambers. *Am. J. Pathol*, **129**, 601–13.
16. Davidson, J. M., Klagsbrun, M., Hill, K. E., Buckley, A., Sullivan, R., Brewer, P. S., and Woodward, S. C. (1985). Accelerated wound repair, cell proliferation and collagen accumulation are produced by a cartilage-derived growth factor. *J. Cell Biol.*, **199**, 1219–27.
17. Andrade, S. P., Fan, T-P. D., and Lewis, G. P. (1987). Quantitative *in vivo* studies on angiogenesis in a rat sponge model. *Br. J. Exp. Pathol.* **68**, 755–66.
18. Fajardo, L. F., Kowalski, J., Kwan, H. H., Prionas, S. D., and Allison, A. C. (1988). The disc angiogenesis system. *Lab. Invest.*, **58**, 718–34.
19. Passaniti, A., Taylor, R. M., Pili, R., Guo, Y., Long, P. V., Haney, J. A., Pauly, R. R., Grant, D. S., and Martin, G. R. (1992). A simple, quantitative method for assessing angiogenesis and antiangiogenic agents using reconstituted basement membrane, heparin, and fibroblast growth factor. *Lab. Invest.*, **67**, 519–28.
20. Grant, D. S., Keinman, H. K., Goldberg, I. D., Bhargava, M., Nickoloff, B. J., Polverini, P., and Rosen, E. M. (1993). Scatter factor induces blood vessel formation *in vivo*. *Proc. Natl Acad. Sci. USA*, **90**, 1937–41.
21. Auerbach, R., Auerbach, W., and Polakowski, I. (1991). Assays for angiogenesis: a review. *Pharmacol. Ther.*, **51**, 1–11.

22. Clark, E. R. (1939). Microscopic observations on the growth of blood capillaries in the living animal. *Am. J. Anat.*, **64**, 251–9.

23. Clark, R. A., Stone, R. D., Leung, D. Y. K., Silver, I., Hohn, D. D., and Hunt, T. K. (1976). Role of macrophages in wound healing. *Surg. Forum*, **27**, 16–18.

24. Schreiber, A. B., Winkler, M. E., and Derynck, R. (1986). Transforming growth factor-α: a more potent angiogenic mediator than epidermal growth factor. *Science*, **232**, 1250–3.

25. Norrby, K., Jakobsson, A., and Sorbo, J. (1990). Quantitative angiogenesis in spreads of intact rat mesenteric windows. *Microvasc. Res.*, **39**, 341–8.

26. Norrby, K. (1994). Basic fibroblast growth factor and *de novo* mammalian angiogenesis. *Microvasc. Res.*, **48**, 96–113.

27. Sidky, Y. A. and Auerbach, R. (1975). Lymphocyte-induced angiogenesis: a quantitative and sensitive assay of the graft-vs-host reaction. *J. Exp. Med.*, **141**, 1084–100.

28. Sidky, Y. A. and Auerbach, R. (1976). Lymphocyte-induced angiogenesis in tumor-bearing mice. *Science*, **192**, 1237–8.

29. Selye, H. (1953). On the mechanism through which hydrocortisone affects the resistance of tissues to injury. *J. Am. Med. Assoc.*, **152**, 1207–13.

30. Colville-Nash, P. R., Alam, C., Appleton, I., Brown, J. R., Seed, M. P., and Willoughby, D. A. (1995). The pharmacological modulation of angiogenesis in chronic granulomatous inflammation. *J. Pharmacol. Exp. Ther.*, **274**, 1463–72.

31. Kimura, M., Amemiya, K., Yamada, T., and Suzuki, J. (1986). Quantitative method for measuring adjuvant-induced angiogenesis in insulin-treated diabetic mice. *J. Pharmacobiodyn.*, **9**, 442–6.

32. Folkman, J. (1975). Tumor angiogenesis. *Adv. Cancer Res.*, **43**, 175–203.

33. Brooks, P. C., Clark, R. F., and Cheresh, D. A., (1994). Requirement of vascular integrin $\alpha_v\beta_3$ for angiogenesis. *Science*, **264**, 569–71.

34. Wilks, J. W., Scott, P. S., Vrba, L. K., and Cocuzza, J. M. (1991). Inhibition of angiogenesis with combination treatments of angiostatic steroids and suramin. *Int. J. Radiat. Biol.*, **60**, 73–7.

35. le Noble, F. A. C., Schreurs, N. H. J. S., Van Straaten, H. W. M., Slaaf, D. W., Smits, J. F. M., Rogg, H., and Struijker-Boudier, H. A. J. (1993). Evidence for a novel angiotensin II receptor involved in angiogenesis in chick embryo chorioallantoic membrane. *Am. J. Physiol.*, **264**, R460–5.

36. Voss, K., Jakob, W., and Roth, K. (1984). A new image analysis method for the quantification of neovascularization. *Exp. Pathol.*, **26**, 155–61.

37. Vu, M., Smith, C., Burger, P., and Klintworth, G. (1985). Methods in laboratory investigation: an evaluation of methods to quantitate the chick chorioallantoic membrane assay in angiogenesis. *Lab. Invest.*, **53**, 499–508.

38. Strick, D. M., Waycaster, R. L., Montani, J., Gay, W. J., and Adair T. H. (1991). Morphometric measurements of chorioallantoic membrane vascularity: effects of hypoxia and hyperoxia. *Am. J. Physiol.*, **29**, H1385–9.

39. Crum, R., Szabo, S., and Folkman, J. (1985). A new class of steroids inhibits angiogenesis in the presence of heparin or a heparin fragment. *Science*, **230**, 1375–8.

40. Ingber, D. E., Madri, J. A., and Folkman, J. (1986). A possible mechanism for inhibition of angiogenesis by angiostatic steroids: induction of capillary basement membrane dissolution. *Endocrinology*, **119**, 1768–75.

41. Maragoudakis, M. E., Panoutsacopoulou, M., and Sarmonika, M. (1988). Rate of basement membrane biosynthesis as an index to angiogenesis. *Tissue Cell*, **20**, 531–9.

42. Tanaka, N. G., Sakamoto, A., Inoue, K., Korenaga, H., Kadoya, S., Ogawa, H., and Osada, Y. (1989). Antitumor effects of an antiangiogenic polysaccharide from an *Arthrobacter* species with or without a steroid. *Cancer Res.*, **49**, 6727–30.

43. Oikawa, T., Hirotani, K., Shimamura, M., Ashino-Fuse, H., and Iwaguchi, T. (1989). Powerful antiangiogenic activity of herbimycin A (named angiostatic antibiotic). *J. Antibiotics*, **42**, 1202–4.

44. Moses, M. A., Sudhalter, J., and Langer, R. (1990). Identification of an inhibitor of neovascularization from cartilage. *Science*, **248**, 1408–10.

45. Oikawa, T., Hirotani, K., Nakamura, O., Shudo, K., Hiragun, A., and Iwaguchi, T. (1989). A highly potent antiangiogenic activity of retinoids. *Cancer Lett.*, **48**, 157–62.

46. Pipili-Synetos, E., Papageorgiou, A., Sakkoula, E., Sotiropoulou, G., Fotsis, T., Karakiulakis, G., and Maragoudakis, M. E. (1995). Inhibition of angiogenesis, tumour growth and metastasis by the NO-releasing vasolidators, isosorbide mononitrate and dinitrate. *Br. J. Pharmacol.* **116**, 1829–34.

47. Nguyen, M., Shing, Y., and Folkman, J. (1994). Quantitation of angiogenesis and antiangiogenesis in the chick embryo chorioallantoic membrane. *Microvasc. Res.*, **47**, 31–40.

48. Cogan, D. G., (1962). Corneal vascularization. *Invest. Ophthalmol.*, **1**, 253–9.

49. Levine, R., Shapiro, A., and Baum, J. (1963). Experimental corneal neovascularization. *Arch. Ophthalmol.*, 242–9.

50. Gimbrone, M. A., Jr., Leapman, S., Cotran, R. S., and Folkman, J. (1973). Tumor angiogenesis: iris neovascularization at distance from experimental intraocular tumors. *J. Natl Cancer Inst.*, **50**, 219–18.

51. Gimbrone, M. A., Jr., Cotran, R. S., Leapman, S. B., and Folkman, J. (1974). Tumor growth and neovascularization: an experimental model using the rabbit cornea. *J. Natl Cancer Inst.*, **52**, 413–27.

52. Sholley, M. M., Ferguson, G. P., Seibel, H. R., Montour, J. L. and Wilson, J. D. (1984). Mechanisms of neovascularization: vascular sprouting can occur without proliferation of endothelial cells. *Lab. Invest.*, **51**, 624–34.

53. Conrad, T. J., Chandler, D. B., Corless, J. M., and Klintworth, G. K. (1994). *In vivo* measurement of corneal angiogenesis with video data acquisition and computerized image analysis. *Lab. Invest.*, **70**, 426–34.

54. Polverini, P. J. and Leibovich, S. J. (1984). Induction of neovascularization *in vivo* and endothelial cell proliferation *in vitro* by tumor-associated macrophages. *Lab. Invest.*, **51**, 635–42.

55. Leibovich, S. J., Polverini, P. J., Shepard, H. M., Wiseman, D. M., Shively, V., and Nuseir, N. (1987). Macrophage-induced angiogenesis is mediated by tumor necrosis factor-alpha. *Nature*, **329**, 630–2.

56. Van Meir, E. G., Polverini, P. J., Chazin, V. R., Su Huang, H-J., de Tribolet, N., and Cavanee, W. K. (1994). Release of an inhibitor of angiogenesis upon induction of wild type p53 expression in glioblastoma cells. *Nature Genet.*, **8**, 171–6.

57. Chen, C., Parangi, S., Tolentino, M. J., and Folkman, J. (1995). A strategy to discover circulating angiogenesis inhibitors generated by human tumors. *Cancer Res.*, **55**, 4230–3.

58. Hu, D. E., Hiley, C. R., Smither, R. L., Gresham, G. A., and Fan, T.-P. D. (1995). Correlation of ^{133}Xe clearance, blood flow and histology in the rat sponge model for angiogenesis. Further studies with angiogenic modifiers. *Lab. Invest.*, **72**, 601–10.

59. Buckley, A., Davidson, J. M., Kamerath, C. D., Wolt, T. B., and Woodward, S. C. (1985). Sustained release of epidermal growth factor accelerates wound repair. *Proc. Natl. Acad. Sci. USA*, **82**, 7340–4.

60. Broadley, K. N., Aquino, A. M., Woodward, S. C., Buckley-Stuttock, A., Sato, Y., Rifkin, D., and Davidson, J. M. (1989). Monospecific antibodies implicate basic fibroblast growth factor in normal would repair. *Lab. Invest.*, **61**, 571–5.

61. Pesenti, E., Sola, F., Mongelli, N., Grandi, M., and Spreafico, F. (1992). Suramin prevents neovascularization and tumor growth through blocking of basic fibroblast growth factor activity. *Br. J. Cancer*, **66**, 367–72.

62. Miyadera, K., Sumizawa, T., Haraguchi, M., Yoshida, H., Konstanty, W., Yamada, Y., and Akiyama, S. (1995). Role of thymidine phosphorylase activity in the angiogenic effect of platelet derived endothelial cell growth factor/thymidine phosphorylase. *Cancer Res.*, **55**, 1687–90.

63. Fan, T.-P. D., Hu, D. E., Guard, S., Gresham G. A., and Watling, K. J. (1993). Stimulation of angiogenesis by substance P and interleukin-1 in the rat and its inhibition by NK$_1$ or interleukin-1 receptor antagonists. *Br. J. Pharmacol.*, **110**, 43–9.

64. Hu, D. E. and Fan, T.-P. D. (1993). [Leu^8]des-Arg^9-bradykinin inhibits the synergistic interaction between bradykinin and interleukin-1 in angiogenesis. *Br. J. Pharmacol.*, **109**, 14–17.

65. Hu, D. E., Hori, Y., Presta, M., Gresham, G. A., and Fan, T-P. D. (1994). Inhibition of angiogenesis by IL-1 receptor antagonist and selected cytokine antibodies in rats. *Inflammation*, **18**, 45–58.

66. Hu, D. E. and Fan, T.-P. D. (1995). Suppression of VEGF-induced angiogenesis by the protein tyrosine kinase inhibitor, lavendustin A. *Br. J. Pharmacol.* **114**, 262–8.

67. Walsh, D. A., Hu, D.-E., Mapp, P. I., Polak, J. M., Blake, D. R., and Fan, T.-P. D. (1996). Innervation and neurokinin receptors during angiogenesis in the rat sponge granuloma. *Histochem. J.*, **28**, 759–69.

68. Mahadevan, V., Hart, I. R., and Lewis, G. P. (1989). Factors influencing blood supply in wound granuloma quantiated by a new *in vivo* technique. *Cancer Res.*, **49**, 415–19.

69. Andrade, S. P., Hart, I., and Piper, P. J. (1992). Inhibitors of nitric oxide synthase selectively reduce flow in tumour-associated neovasculature. *Br. J. Pharmacol.*, **107**, 1092–5.

70. Buttery, L. D. K., Springall, D. R., Andrade, S. P., Riveros-Moreno, V., Hart, I., Piper, P. J., and Polak, J. M. (1993). Induction of nitric oxide synthase in the neo-vasculature of experimental tumours in mice. *J. Pathol.*, **171**, 311–19.

71. Fajardo, L. F., Kwan, H. H., Kowalski, J., Prionas, S. D., and Allison, A. C. (1992). Dual role of tumor necrosis factor-α in angiogenesis. *Am. J. Pathol.*, **140**, 539–44.

72. Kowalski, J., Kwan, H. H., Prionas, S. D., Allison, A. C., and Fajardo, L. F. (1992). Characterization and application of the disk angiogenesis system. *Exp. Mol. Pathol.*, **56**, 1–19.

73. Polakowski, I. J., Lewis, M. K., Muthukkaruppan, V. R., Erdman, B., Kubai, L., and Auerbach, R. (1993).A ribonuclease inhibitor expresses anti-angiogenic properties and

74. Nelson, M. J., Conley, P. K., and Fajardo, L. F. (1993). Application of the disc angiogenesis system to tumor-induced neovascularization. *Exp. Mol. Pathol.*, **58**, 105–13.

75. Lees, V. C. and Fan, T.-P. D. (1994). A freeze-injured skin graft model for the quantitative study of basic fibroblast growth factor and other promoters of angiogenesis in wound healing. *Br. J. Plast. Surg.*, **47**, 349–59.

76. Moghaddam, A., Zhang, H-T., Fan, T.-P. D., Hu, D.-E., Lees, V. C., Turley, H., *et al.* (1995). Thymidine phosphorylase is angiogenic and promotes tumour growth. *Proc. Natl Acad. Sci. USA*, **92**, 998–1002.

77. Lees, V. C., Fan, T.-P. D., and West, D. C. (1995). Angiogenesis in a delayed revascularization model is accelerated by angiogenic oligosaccharides of hyaluronan. *Lab. Invest.*, **73**, 259–66.

78. Kleinman, H. K., Graf, J., Iwamoto, Y., Kitten, G. T., Ogle, R. C., Sasaki, M., *et al.* (1987). Role of basement membranes in cell differentiation. *Ann. N. Y. Acad. Sci.*, **513**, 134–45.

79. Kubota, Y., Kleinman, H. K., Martin, G. R., and Lawley, T. J. (1988). The role of laminin and basement membrane in the morphological differentiation of human endothelial cells into capillary-like structures. *J. Cell Biol.*, **107**, 1589–98.

80. Plunkett, M. L. and Hailey, J. A. (1990). An *in vivo* quantitative angiogenesis model using tumor cells entrapped alginate. *Lab. Invest.*, **62**, 510–7.

81. Robertson, N. E., Discafani, C. M., Downs, E. C., Hailey, J. A., Sarre, O., Runkle, R. L. *et al.* (1991). A quantitative *in vivo* mouse model used to assay inhibitors of tumor-induced angiogenesis. *Cancer Res.*, **51**, 1339–44.

82. Yamaoka, M., Yamamoto, T., Masaki, T., Ikeyama, S., Sudo, K., and Fujita, T. (1993). Inhibition of tumor growth and metastasis of rodent tumors by the angiogenesis inhibitor O-(chloroacetyl-carbamoyl)fumagillol (TNP-470; AGM-1470). *Cancer Res.*, **53**, 4262–7.

83. Zagzag, D., Brem, S., and Robert, F. (1988). Neovascularization and tumour growth in the rabbit brain. A model for experimental studies of angiogenesis and the blood–brain barrier. *Am. J. Pathol.*, **131**, 361–72.

84. Brem, S. S., Zagzag, D., Tsanaclis, A. M. C., Gateley, S., Elkouby, M.-P., and Brien, S. E. (1990). Inhibition of angiogenesis and tumour growth in the brain. Suppression of endothelial cell turnover by penicillamine and the depletion of copper, and angiogenic cofactor. *Am. J. Pathol.*, **137**, 1121–42.

85. Kim, K. J., Li, B., Winer, J., Armaninim M., Gillett, N., Phillips, H. S., and Ferrara, N. (1993). Inhibition of vascular endothelial growth factor-induced angiogenesis suppresses tumour growth *in vivo*. *Nature*, **362**, 841–4.

86. Bosma, G. C. I., Custer, R. P., and Bosma, M. J. (1983). A severe combined immunodeficiency mutation in the mouse. *Nature*, **301**, 527–30.

87. Bosma, M. J. and Carrol, A. M. (1991). The SCID mouse mutant: definition, characterization and potential uses. *Annu. Rev. Immunol.*, **9**, 323–50.

88. Hendrickson, E. A. (1993). The SCID mouse: relevance as an animal model system for studying human disease. *Am. J. Pathol.*, **143**, 1511–22.

89. Vaporciyan, A. A., Delisser, H. M., Yan, H. C., Mendiguren, I. I., Thom, S. R., Jones, M. I., *et al.* (1993). Involvement of platelet-endothelial cell adhesion molecule-1 in neutrophil recruitment *in vivo*. *Science*, **262**, 1580–2.

leads to reduced tumor growth in mice. *Am. J. Pathol.*, **143**, 507–17.

90. Yan, H.-C., Juhasz, I., Pilewski, J., Murphy, G. F., Herlyn, M., and Albelda, S. M. (1993). Human/severe combined immunodeficient mouse chimeras. An experimental *in vivo* model to study the regulation of human endothelial cell–leukocyte adhesion molecules. *J. Clin. Invest.*, **91**, 986–96.

91. Nickoloff, B. I., Kunkel, S. L., Burdick, M., and Strieter, R. M. (1995). Severe combined immunodeficiency mouse and human psoriatic skin chimeras. *Am. J. Pathol.*, **46**, 580–8.

92. Brooks, P. C., Stromblad, S., Klemke, R., Visscher, D., Sarkar, F. H. and Cheresh, D. A. (1995). Antiintegrin blocks human breast cancer growth and angiogenesis in human skin. *J. Clin. Invest.*, **96**, 1815–22.

93. Hori, Y., Hu, D.-E., Yasui, K., Smither, R. L., Gresham, G. A., and Fan, T.-P. D. (1996). Differential effects of angiostatic steroids and dexamethasone on angiogenesis and cytokine levels in rat sponge implants. *Br. J. Pharmacol.*, **118**, 1584–91.

3. Mechanistic insights into tumour angiogenesis

Roy Bicknell

Angiogenesis

As outlined in Chapter 1 there are two recognized processes by which new blood vessels are formed. These are called vasculogenesis and angiogenesis. Vasculogenesis describes the formation of new vessels from the endothelial presursors that are present in the blood islands of the developing embryo. Angiogenesis is the development of new blood vessels from pre-existing blood vessels. In the adult, all new blood vessels arise by angiogenesis.

Angiogenesis is, nevertheless, a complex process that involves many sequential steps. In response to an angiogenic stimulus released from, for example a tumour, a sequence of events occurs that culminates in the formation of new vessels. Prominent among these steps in sequential order are: (i) retraction of pericytes from the ablumenal surface of the capillary; (ii) release of proteases, *e.g.* urokinase plasminogen activator, from 'activated' endothelial cells; (iii) degradation of the extracellular matrix surrounding the existing capillary; (iv) endothelial cell migration and possibly proliferation; (v) alignment of the migrating endothelial cells into tube-like structures; (vi) anastomoses (or fusion) of the newly formed vessels; and (vii) initiation of blood flow in the newly formed capillaries (Fig. 3.1.). While much is now known about the early steps in the process, comparatively little is known about what controls the later stages such as anastomoses and initiation of blood flow. This is because as yet, good models with which to study them have not been developed. A possible exception is that involving implantation of sections of rat aorta into an extracellular matrix (1). Following embedding into fibrin small vessels comprised of endothelial cells grow out into the matrix from the microvasculature that normally provides nutrients for the aortic smooth muscle over a period of several days (Fig. 3.2.). Close inspection reveals that these vessels will occasionally fuse and use of polymerase chain reaction could permit characterization of gene expression in the anastomosing cells.

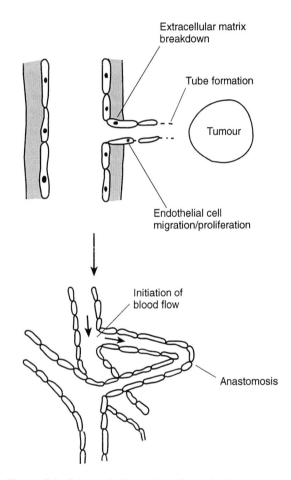

Figure 3.1. Schematic illustration of steps in the angiogenic process.

Growth of solid tumours is angiogenesis dependent

There now exists much evidence that growth of solid tumours is angiogenesis dependent. Early evidence was collected by Folkman in an article published in the *Journal of the National Cancer Institute* in 1990 (2). The following is taken verbatim from this important paper.

The hypothesis that tumour growth is angiogenesis dependent rests in part on the following evidence:

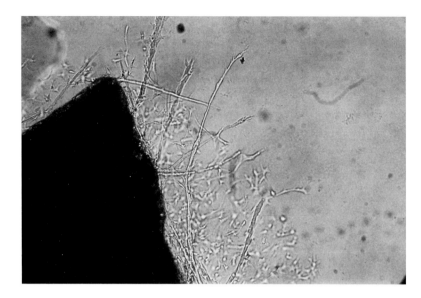

Figure 3.2. Microvessels growing out of a rat aorta embedded within a fibrin matrix (see reference 1).

(a) The growth rate of tumors implanted in subcutaneous transplant chambers in mice is slow and linear before vascularization and rapid and nearly exponential after vascularization.

(b) Tumors grown in isolated perfused organs where blood vessels do not proliferate are limited to 1–2 mm³ but expand rapidly to 1–2 cm³ after vascularization on transplantation to mice.

(c) Tumor growth in the avascular cornea proceeds slowly and at a linear rate but switches to exponential growth after vascularization.

(d) Tumors suspended in the aqueous fluid of the anterior chamber of the eye remain viable, avascular, and limited in size (<1 mm³). Once they are implanted on the iris vessels, however, they induce neovascularization and grow rapidly, reaching 16,000 times their original volume within 2 weeks.

(e) Human retinoblastomas metastic to the vitreous or the anterior chamber are similarly avascular, viable and growth restricted.

(f) Within a solid tumor, the [³H]thymidine labeling index of tumor cells decreases with increasing distance from the nearest open capillary. The mean labelling index for a given tumor is a function of the labeling index of the vascular endothelial cells in that tumor.

(g) Tumors implanted on the choriollantoic membrane of the chick embryo are often restricted in growth during the avascular phase (≥72 hr), but rapid growth begins within 24 hours after vascularization. In one study, tumors did not exceed a mean diameter of 0.93 ± 0.29 (SD) mm during the avascular phase, but after vascularization, tumors reached a mean diameter of 8.0 ± 2.5 mm by day 7.

(h) The chorioallantoic membrane appears on day 5 in the chick embryo, and the [³H]thymidine labeling index of its vascular endothelial cells decreases with age, with an abrupt reduction on day 11. Tumors implanted on the chorioallantoic membrane in successively older embryos grow at slower rates in parallel with the reduced rates of endothelial cell growth.

(i) Vascular casts of metastases to the rabbit liver show that these tumors are avascular up to 1 mm in diameter. Beyond that size, the tumors are vascularized.

(j) Carcinoma of the ovary metastasizes to the peritoneal membrane as tiny avascular seeds, which rarely grow beyond a limited size until after vascularization.

(k) Angiogenesis inhibitors that are not cytostatic to tumor cells in vitro inhibit tumor growth in vivo.

(l) The appearance of neovascularization at the base of a human melanoma is associated with increased growth and metastasis. Metastasis is rare prior to neovascularization.

(m) In one study of transgenic mice that develop carcinomas of the pancreatic islets (beta cells), large tumors arose from a subset of preneoplastic hyperplastic islets that had become vascularized.

(n) After subcutaneous injection of tumor cells into mice, tumors have become vascularized at about 0.4 mm³. With increasing tumor size, the blood vessels occupied approximately 1.5% of the tumor volume, a 400% increase over normal subcutaneous tissue. The tumor infiltrated surrounding connective tissue and expanded into the newly formed vessels in that tissue.

More recent developments in our understanding of tumour angiogenesis will now be discussed.

Expression of polypeptide angiogenic factors in tumours

Glioblastoma multiforme is unusual among solid tumour types in that the major angiogenic activity present in the glioblastoma is vascular endothelial growth factor (VEGF) (3). This contrasts with, for example, primary human breast carcinomas, which are known to produce a wide range of polypeptide angiogenic factors. For example, an examination of 84 primary human breast tumours for expression of messenger RNAs of seven angiogenic polypeptides — VEGF, platelet-derived endothelial cell growth factor (PDECGF) thymidine phosphorylase (TP), acidic and basic fibroblast growth factor (aFGF and bFGF), pleiotrophin (PTN), midkine (MK), placental growth factor, and transforming growth factor β_1 (TGF-β_1) revealed that most tumours produced multiple factors and in no case was a tumour found that expressed a single angiogenic factor (Bicknell *et al.*, unpublished observations). It is possible to conceive of tumour angiogenic factor profiles that are very likely to differ between solid tumour types. Such profiles may be simple, as for glioblastoma, where expression of one angiogenic factor predominates or complex as in breast carcinomas where expression of multiple factors is found. Much work is yet required to obtain detailed angiogenic profiles of most tumour types.

Whether tumours express predominantly a single or in contrast multiple angiogenic activities has implications for possible strategies for intervention in the angiogenic process. In 1993 it was shown that intraperitoneal administration of monoclonal antibodies that blocked the endothelial growth stimulating activity of VEGF markedly retarded the growth of a human glioblastoma cell line that had been subcutaneously xenografted into mice (4). The same treatment was shown to inhibit the *in vivo* growth of several other xenografted cell lines and clearly the blocking of a polypeptide angiogenic factor is able to retard the growth of some tumour lines *in vivo*. However, in no case did administration of anti-VEGF antibodies completely block tumour growth. Similar observations were made when glioblastoma and other cell line initiated VEGF-induced angiogenesis was abrogated by retroviral delivery of a dominant negative VEGF receptor (5,6). It follows that where the angiogenic activity of a tumour is initiated by primarily one factor, specific blocking of that factor holds promise of anti-angiogenic therapy. If, however, multiple factors mediated the angiogenic activity of a particular tumour alternative strategies of intervention will be required (for further discussion of this problem see Chapter 23).

A case in which an anti-angiogenic strategy has been shown to bring about tumour regression is in the use of antibodies to the $\alpha_v\beta_3$ integrin dimer that block binding to its ligands. These studies will now be discussed.

The involvement of cell adhesion molecules in angiogenesis

The role of $\alpha_v\beta_3$ and $\alpha_v\beta_5$ integrins in angiogenesis

In the last couple of years, several papers from the laboratory of David Cheresh at the Scripps Research Institute in La Jolla have implicated a critical role for the α_v integrin in angiogenesis. The original observation that prompted these studies was that the $\alpha_v\beta_3$ dimer is markedly more strongly expressed on the vessels in healing wounds than it is on vessels in healthy tissues. This prompted Cheresh to propose that the $\alpha_v\beta_3$ dimer is a marker of active 'angiogenesis', i.e. that it is strongly expressed on blood vessels that are undergoing angiogenesis. The expression of the α_v integrin is known to be far more restricted than is that of many other members of the integrin family. α_v integrin expression appears to occur primarily on vascular smooth muscle and endothelial cells, melanomas, glioblastomas, monocytes, and on macrophages where it constitutes part of the receptor that recognizes apoptotic cells prior to their engulfment by the macrophage.

Subsequent to showing that the $\alpha_v\beta_3$ integrin is an angiogenic marker, the Scripps group employed a monoclonal antibody (LM609) (7) that is known to block the interaction of the $\alpha_v\beta_3$ molecule with its cognate ligands (ligands include vitronectin, fibrinogen, von Willibrand factor, and CD31/PECAM-1) (7,8) to show that the antibody was able to block tumour-induced angiogenesis on the chick chorioallantoic membrane (CAM) (9). It was then shown that the LM609 antibody efficiently blocks not only tumour-induced angiogenesis that also tumour growth (10). It appears that the 'activated' endothelial cell that is undergoing angiogenesis utilizes the $\alpha_v\beta_3$ integrin to adhere to the extracellular matrix during the angiogenic process. The LM609 antibody blocks this adherence and the 'angiogenic' endothelial cells apoptose with the resulting collapse of the newly forming tumour vasculature and tumour regression. It has recently been shown that VEGF and bFGF induce angiogenesis by different mechanistic pathways involving either the $\alpha_v\beta_3$ or the $\alpha_v\beta_5$ integrins. Thus, antibody to $\alpha_v\beta_3$ integrin (LM609) was able to block VEGF but not bFGF-induced angiogenesis in both the CAM and the rabbit corneal assay, whereas monoclonal antibody (P1F6) to the $\alpha_v\beta_5$ integrin blocked bFGF but not

VEGF-induced angiogenesis in the same two assays (11). Tumour necrosis factor-α-induced angiogenesis was, like VEGF-induced angiogenesis shown to utilize the $\alpha_v\beta_3$ integrin, while in contrast that induced by TGF-α or phorbol ester was mediated by the $\alpha_v\beta_5$ integrin. Use of the protein kinase C inhibitor calphostin C showed that this enzyme was involved in the $\alpha_v\beta_5$ pathway but not the $\alpha_v\beta_3$ pathway (11). It will be of interest to see whether all angiogenic factors follow one or other of these two pathways or whether other as yet unidentified pathways exist. The number of distinct mechanistic angiogenic pathways that may exist has clear implications for the development of anti-angiogenic strategies (see Chapter 23).

E-selectin and vascular endothelial growth factor (VCAM) in angiogenesis

It was recently shown (12) that in addition to a role for integrins in angiogenesis, that angiogenesis is induced in the rabbit cornea by soluble E-selectin and soluble VCAM, molecules that are intimately involved in inflammatory diapedesis. In addition to clear induction of angiogenesis *in vivo*, the soluble adhesion molecules were chemotactic for human umbilical endothelial (HUVEC) cells in a Boyden chamber assay. Antibodies to the known ligands of E-selectin and VCAM, anti-sialyl Lewis X and anti-VLA-4 blocked HUVEC cell migration in response to soluble E-selection or soluble VCAM, respectively. The antibodies were also shown to block corneal angiogenesis induced by synovial fluid from patients with rheumatoid arthritis, anti-sialyl Lewis X more efficiently than did anti-VCAM. The role (if any) of soluble E-selectin or soluble-VCAM in tumour angiogenesis is as yet unclear as is the mechanism by which they induce angiogenesis.

Angiogenic factor transfection followed by xenograft experiments

Background

Numerous studies have reported the effect of transfection of an angiogenic factor into a given cell line followed by subsequent study of the effect of the transfection on tumorigenesis by xenografting into nude mice. Angiogenic factors that have been studied in this way include aFGF/bFGF, VEGF, the neurokines MK and PTN, PDECGF/TP and TGF-β_1. As several different model systems have been used by researchers it is at present somewhat difficult to compare the biological effects of transfection of different factors. The most significant dif-

ference between the model systems used is in that of the cell line that was transfected. However, an overriding conclusion from these studies is that expression of a 'pure' angiogenic factor (that is one that stimulates growth of endothelial cells but not other cell types, for example VEGF) confers a growth advantage *in vivo* but not *in vitro*. This supports the idea that the rate of growth of (at least some) solid tumours is limited by angiogenesis. In an attempt to develop a standardized model that will permit a direct comparison of the effect of transfection of a given angiogenic factor on tumour growth we have over several years used a transfection and xenograft model that utilizes the human MCF-7 breast carcinoma cell line. Studies with the MCF-7 line will be discussed below.

Acidic and basic fibroblast growth factors

Several studies have examined the effect of transfection of members of the FGF family on tumour growth. A favoured cell type for these studies has been the immortal mouse 3T3 fibroblast. aFGF and bFGF lack a classic secretion peptide and an interesting approach has been the fusion of a secretion peptide to the native FGF gene. Thus, chimeras have been made with the secretion peptides from IgG (13) and growth hormone (14) to bFGF and γ-interferon (15) and FGF3 (*hst*) (16) to aFGF. The transfectants having the γ-interferon secretion signal fused to aFGF have not been studied *in vivo* and will not be discussed further.

While transfection of aFGF or bFGF in the absence of an artificially fused secretion signal had little or no phenotypic effect on the transfectants, when a secretion signal was fused to the gene then dramatic effects on the behaviour of the cells was seen. The result has been referred to as 'transformation' in that the FGF-transfected cells exhibited unusual morphological features *in vitro*. Thus, when the IgG promoter was fused to the bFGF gene and the chimera expressed in 3T3 cells, the cells formed large stellate clumps in culture rather than growing as a monolayer (13). The transfectants did not, however, grow in soft agar (13). This contrasts with the report of Blam *et al.* (14) who fused the growth hormone secretion signal to bFGF and also expressed the construct on 3T3 cells. These workers observed not only the 'transformed morphology' of the cells but that they also readily formed colonies in soft agar (14). Arguably the most significant observation in these two papers is that when a secretion signal was fused to bFGF and the gene transfected into the non-tumorigenic 3T3 cell, the resulting transfectants were highly tumorigenic. Transfectants lacking a secretion signal did not form tumours.

Another paper concerned fusion of the FGF4 (*hst*) secretion signal to aFGF followed by transfection into 3T3 cells (16). The transfectants, unlike control cells, were not only strongly tumorigenic but also showed what were described as 'vascular nests' and exaggerated haemangiectasia. The vascular nests comprised ectactic spaces into which tumour cells projected. The clumps of tumour cells were covered by a layer of endothelium. That expression of an angiogenic factor should have profound effects on the vasculature is not surprising but is interesting to contrast with the effect of expression of VEGF on tumour vasculature described below. Expression of VEGF had a much less profound effect on the vasculature, giving rise to vascular hot spots but not haemangiectasia. It is accepted, however, that the differences could be the result of a dosage effect.

Fibroblast growth factor-4 (FGF-4/hst)

Transfection of FGF-4 (that has a secretion signal) into MCF-7 cells followed by xenografting has been performed by Kerns group in Washington (17,18). The resulting cell line was called MKS-1 cells. It was found that expression of FGF-4 promoted metastasis and unexpectedly the tumours were oestrogen independent but required tamoxifen. The mechanism by which expression of FGF-4 has such an effect on the hormone responsiveness of the cells remains unknown.

Vascular endothelial growth factor

Studies on the biological effects of VEGF transfection are easier to interpret in their relevance to tumour angiogenesis than those of transfection of aFGF or bFGF in view of the fact that VEGF is restricted as a growth factor to endothelial cells. The first reported transfection of VEGF followed by xenograft studies was that of Ferrara et al. in 1993 (19). The line chosen for transfection was the Chinese hamster ovary (CHO) cell line. CHO cells do not form tumours when xenografted into nude mice. By contrast, transfected CHO cells expressing either the 121 or 165 splice variants of VEGF readily formed tumours when xenografted. The tumours were described as 'benign' and did not show an aggressive phenotype. However, these studies revealed the important observation that elevated expression of an angiogenic factor in at least some immortalized but non-tumorigenic cell lines can alone confer tumorigenicity. In view of the fact that the wild-type cells are not tumorigenic it was not possible to compare tumours from wild-type cells and transfectants histochemically as has been done for VEGF transfection in the MCF-7 model (20; also see below). A second study described transfection of $VEGF_{165}$ into HeLa cells followed by xenograft into nude mice (21). In this study it was

claimed that the VEGF-transfected cells gave rise to more rapidly growing and more vascular tumours than did wild-type cells but no data were given to support this (21).

The neurokines midkine and pleiotrophin

PTN has previously been transfected into non-tumorigenic 3T3 fibroblasts (22). Unlike the wild-type 3T3 cells, the transfected fibroblasts were not only tumorigenic in nude mice, but when injected subcutaneously into the mice showed extensive metastasis to the liver, brain, and lung (22). No other information was given.

In a separate study, Wellsteins group transfected PTN into the adrenocortical line SW13 (23). Similar to the VEGF/CHO studies of Ferrara described above, transfection of PTN into SW13 cells conferred tumorigenicity on to an otherwise immortal but non-tumorigenic cell line. Further studies showed that the PTN induced tumorigenicity in the line could be reversed by administration of the anti-angiogenic drug pentosan polysulphate (24). No studies have yet reported transfection of MK. Both MK and PTN have been transfected into the MCF-7 cell line and the results are discussed below.

Platelet-derived endothelial cell growth factor/thymidine phosphorylase

In the original report of the isolation of PDECGF/TP as platelet-derived endothelial cell growth factor (25) the gene was transfected into a1-1 cells (Harvey-ras transformed 3T3 fibroblasts) and the PDECGF/TP expressing transfectants shown to give rise to more highly vascular tumours when implanted into nude mice (25). It is noteworthy that the transfected gene was, like the wild-type gene without a classic secretion peptide. Similar observations have been made by our group in the MCF-7 model (26) and are discussed below.

Transforming growth factor β1

TGF-β1 is a strong inhibitor of endothelial cell growth in vitro but paradoxically is angiogenic in vivo. Chang et al. transfected TGF-β1 into meth A sarcoma cells and examined the effect of expression on tumorigenesis (27). It is interesting that expression of TGF-β1 converted the meth A cells that normally grow as a floating suspension to an adhesive population that exhibited dendritic processes. Their growth rate in vitro was also three- to five-fold lower than the wild-type cells. Despite this, it was found that expression of TGF-β1 increased tumorigenicity of the meth A sarcoma as assessed by both tumour incidence and tumour growth. Thus, it was concluded that expression of the TGF-β1 confers a growth advantage which overrules any direct anti-proliferative effects. The nature of this growth advantage has not been elucidated, it remains possible that it may be due to the increased angiogenic activity of the transfected cells.

Nitric oxide (NO) synthase

NO is a potent vasodilator (the so-called endothelial-derived relaxing factor) that mediates endothelial cell growth and migration *in vitro* in response to (for example) the angiogenic peptide, Substance P (28). To examine a potential role for NO in tumour growth, the group of Moncada transfected a subclone of the tumorigenic human colon carcinoma cell line DLD-1 with the inducible NO synthase (iNOS) gene (29). A transfectant clone called iNOS-19 was shown to produce about 20-fold more NO over an 8-day period compared with that produced by the wild-type sub-clone of DLD-1. Despite the fact that iNOS-19 cells grew significantly slower *in vitro* than did the wild-type cells, they were shown to form much more rapidly growing tumours when xenografted into nude mice. An estimation of the vascular density of the tumours by counting erythrocyte positive areas suggested that the overall vascular density of the iNOS-19 tumours was significantly greater than that in controls. The presence or absence of vascular hot spots was not reported.

The MCF-7 breast carcinoma cell model

Vascular endothelial growth factor

The MCF-7 cell line was chosen (see reference 20) to study the effect of transfection of angiogenic factors on tumour behaviour for the following reasons: when xenografted subcutaneously into nude mice early passage MCF-7 cells form: (i) slow growing; (ii) poorly vascularized; (iii) hormone (oestrogen) dependent; (iv) tamoxifen sensitive tumours that (v) do not metastasize. Thus, the effect of transfection of any single gene on each of these parameters may be examined. Zhang *et al.* (20) first used $VEGF_{121}$ as a control. $VEGF_{121}$ was chosen for several reasons. First, there was rapidly increasing evidence that VEGF played an important part in tumour angiogenesis including the observation that its expression was induced in carcinoma lines by hypoxia (30) and indeed that VEGF is probably a 'physiological' stress-response angiogenic factor (see chapter by Keshet). Secondly, in the screen of angiogenic factor mRNA expression in primary human breast carcinomas described above, the $VEGF_{121}$ splice variant was found to be the most highly expressed of the VEGF isoforms. Thus, expression of the $VEGF_{121}$ splice variant was placed under control of the cytomegalovirus

(CMV) promoter in the plasmid pCDNAneo-1 to ensure constitutive high-level expression.

Transfection and xenograft studies (20) showed that $VEGF_{121}$ expressing cells gave rise to: (i) more rapidly growing and (ii) more highly vacularized tumours (see Fig. 3.3, in the plate section) than did the wild-type cells. There were no effects on hormone dependence or tamoxifen sensitivity and no evidence of metastasis was seen. [It is noted in passing that the most straightforward and reliable way to visualize mouse microvasculature is to use the rat monoclonal antibody to mouse CD3 (31). CD31 has been known for several years to be an excellent pan-endothelial marker (31–33)].

Although the vasculature in the wild-type tumours was remarkably homogeneous throughout the tumour that in the VEGF expressing tumours was not showing the existence of vascular 'hot-spots'. The vascular 'hot-spots' are very similar to those that have been shown to correlate with lymph node metastasis in primary human breast carcinomas (see Chapter 4); however, despite this no evidence of lymph node metastasis was observed. It is also notable that the vascular 'hot spots' were often found to be closely associated with larger vessels. Larger vessels were rarely, if ever, seen in sections of the wild-type tumours. The increased vascular density and presence of larger vessels so increased the haemoglobin content of the VEGF expressing tumours that they appeared pink (Fig. 3.3.; H-T. Zhang and R. Bicknell, unpublished observations). Note the large vessels apparent just under the surface of the skin in the VEGF expressing tumours (Fig. 3.3.), such vessels were never seen in the control tumours.

Of all the transfections and xenografts that we have so far performed, only $VEGF_{121}$ transfectants have given rise to vascular 'hot-spots'. This, is believed to be due to the fact that $VEGF_{121}$ is the only factor transfected that is freely diffusible from the cells that make it (the others either tightly binding to heparin on the cell surface such as $VEGF_{165}$, $VEGF_{189}$, MK and PTN or being intracellular PDECGF/TP). This is in accord with predictions from reaction–diffusion pre-patterning models such as those discussed by Chaplin (34). A second unexpected result was that despite the appearance of vascular 'hotspots' in the $VEGF_{121}$ expressing tumours no evidence of metastasis was found. I suspect that this is because in the primary human breast tumours exhibiting metastases it occurs into the lymphatics and not into the vasculature. Thus, it may be that tumours having a high vascular density have a higher interstitial pressure and that this forces the carcinoma cells at the periphery of the tumour into the existing lymphatics, leading to lymphatic spread. In the xenografted tumours lymphatics are sparse and this cannot occur. It would be interesting to measure the interstitial pressure of poorly and highly vascularized primary human breast carcinomas.

Preliminary experiments with MCF-7 cells expressing comparable amounts of $VEGF_{165}$ or $VEGF_{189}$ have shown that the effects on tumour growth are much less than those of $VEGF_{121}$. Thus, expression of $VEGF_{189}$ had virtually no effect on tumour growth and that of $VEGF_{165}$ was much delayed compared with that of $VEGF_{121}$ (P. A. E. Scott et al., unpublished observations).

Platelet-derived endothelial cell growth factor/thymidine phosphorylase

MCF-7 transfectants overexpressing PDECGF/TP have been prepared such that studies with them are directly comparable with the $VEGF_{121}$ transfectants described above. Two sets of transfectants were prepared, namely, those with the native PDECGF/TP gene (26) as used by Ishikawa et al. (25) in their transfection of a1-1 cells but also transfectants in which the IgG secretion signal had been fused to the PDECGF/TP gene such that the PDECGF/TP protein would be efficiently secreted from the MCF-7 cell (26; H-T. Zhang and R. Bicknell, unpublished observations). Overexpression of PDECGF/TP had no effect on in vitro growth under any of the conditions examined. Transfectants with the gene lacking a secretion signal were found to form much more rapidly growing tumours in athymic mice (26). However, despite the 10-fold more rapid growth of the tumours the vascular density was identical to that of the wild-type tumours. There were no effects on hormone dependence, tamoxifen sensitivity, or metastasis. Transfectants in which the PDECGF/TP was actively secreted showed no difference in either in vitro or in vivo growth to that of wild-type cells (35). These studies are in agreement with those of Ishikawa et al. and show that it is imperative that PDECGF/TP be retained within the cell that is overexpressing for it to have an effect on tumour growth. These observations will be discussed further below.

Midkine and pleiotrophin

MCF-7 transfectants overexpressing mouse MK and human PTN have been prepared such that they are again directly comparable with those overexpressing VEGF and PDECGF/TP (R. Choudhuri, H-T. Zhang and R. Bicknell, unpublished observations). Overexpression of MK and PTN again gave more rapidly growing tumours in vivo but without effects on growth in vitro. Growth in vivo of the two sets of transfectants was virtually indistinguishable from each other and also from that of the $VEGF_{121}$ trans-fectants. Again there were no effects on either hormone

dependence, tamoxifen sensitivity or metastasis. In contrast to the $VEGF_{121}$ expressing tumours, vascular 'hot-spots' were absent but the overall vascular density of the tumours was significantly greater than that of wild-type or control transfectants. MK and PTN transfectant tumours were also 'pink' and showed the presence of larger vessels as described for the $VEGF_{121}$ expressing tumours above.

Some general comments on results from the MCF-7 cell model

Figure 3.4 summarizes diagramatically the growth and vascular density data from the MCF-7 studies described above. Unlike the transfection studies in MCF-7 cells of members of the FGF family that have been described by researchers from Georgetown University reviewed above, no effects on hormone dependence, tamoxifen sensitivity, or metastasis have been observed. It appears from the data presented that growth of the subcutaneously xenografted early passage MCF-7 cell is rate limited by angiogenesis. $VEGF_{121}$, MK, or PTN overexpression overcomes this rate limitation to growth, the tumour growth is now rate limited by some other factor. In contrast, PDECGF/TP overcomes this other rate limitation as well and these transfectants form much more rapidly growing tumours. I propose that these exceptionally fast growing tumours are also rate limited by angiogenesis and that is why the vascular density of these very fast growing tumours is identical to that of the slowest growing wild-type or mock-transfected

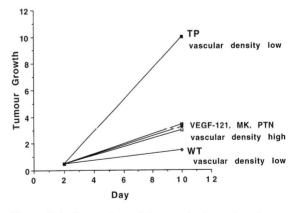

Figure 3.4. Comparison of the growth of transfected MCF-7 cells when xenografted into nude mice. In no case did transfection have any effect of the rate of cell growth as a two-dimensional monolayer in vitro. Vascular densities: low ~ 8 vessels per 0.159 mm^2 field, high ~ 12 vessels per 0.159 mm^2 field. TP, thymidine kinase; MK, midkine; PTN, pleiotrophin; VEGF, vascular endothelial growth factor; WT, wild type.

tumours. Thus, this particular vascular density (7.6 ± 0.9 vessels per 0.159 mm² field) represents rate limiting angiogenesis. It is proposed that the $VEGF_{121}$, MK and PTN overexpressing tumours have an excess of angiogenic activity and that their growth *in vivo* is not rate limited by angiogenesis. It is the excess of angiogenic activity that leads to the extensive vascularization that is characterized by the presence of either the vascular 'hot-spots' and larger vessels. (in the case of $VEGF_{121}$ expressing tumours) or an increased vascular density above that of wild-type or mock-transfected tumours (in the case of MK and PTN expressing tumours).

Insights into the role of angiogenesis of tumorigenesis

Background

Several strains of transgenic mice have provided useful insights into the role of angiogenesis in tumour development. Among these are the studies in Hanahan's laboratory at UCSF with a strain of mice in which expression of the SV40 large T oncoprotein is under control of the rat insulin gene regulatory region [the so-called RIP1-Tag2 mice) (36) and in two transgenic strains that develop fibrosarcomas of the skin [one carries the transforming genes of bovine papilloma virus (37) and a second expressing the oncogene v-*jun* under the control of the H2K promoter (38).] Another transgenic line of interest is that in which the Fps/Fes protein-tyrosine kinase has been constitutively activated by mutation and then introduced into the germ line (39). Relevant studies with these mice will now be discussed.

SV40 large T oncoprotein under control of the rat insulin promoter transgenic mice (RIP1-Tag2 mice)

It was found that all RIP1-Tag2 mice develop carcinoma of the pancreas by 12 weeks of age. Further examination showed that hyperplasia of the β-cells became apparent at 4–6 weeks of age and by 9.5 weeks 50% of the islets showed hyperproliferation of the β-cells. Despite this only a minor population of the hyperplastic islets had progressed to carcinomas by 12 weeks. To examine the hypothesis that expression of an angiogenic factor may be an essential event in the progression, islets were isolated from the pancreas by collagenase digestion and purified on a 'Ficoll' gradient. The isolated islets were then placed into tissue culture wells containing capillary endothelial cells embedded within a collagen matrix. With islets iso-

lated from normal mice no locomotion or proliferation of the endothelial cells was observed. In contrast, every β-cell carcinoma induced a rapid radial alignment of the endothelial cells within the gel in a pattern that converged towards the implanted tumour. Following radial alignment, cells migrated towards the islet and formed endothelial cell sprouts and occasional capillary tubes consistent with *in vitro* angiogenesis.

Isolated islets from RIP1-Tag2 mice of various ages were then examined in this assay. Islets from 5-week-old mice had no effect on the endothelial cells embedded in the matrix. In contrast, a small subset of islets from older transgenic mice induced radial endothelial alignment followed by the other events induced by the carcinomas. These results were interpreted as showing that the onset of angiogenic activity occurs in hyperplastic islets before tumour formation. Analysis of 1900 transgenic islets showed that the percentage that elicited angiogenesis *in vitro* was 0% at 4–5 weeks, 0.57 ± 0.35% at 6–7 weeks, 2.8 ± 0.6% at 8–10 weeks, and 3.6 ± 0.39% at 11–12 weeks. There was found to be a strong correlation between the increasing incidence of angiogenic transgenic islets and the rising frequency of tumour formation with age. It was concluded that the induction of angiogenesis is an important step in tumorigenesis.

The angiogenic activity secreted from the islets has been analysed. Cell lines have been derived from both the hyperplastic islets (40) and from the carcinomas. Both secrete angiogenic factors such as bFGF and VEGF but it has not yet proven possible to pin-down precisely which single factor, if any, is responsible for the angiogenic transformation. It may be due to several factors that differ between individual islets.

BPV-1 mice: transgenics that develop fibrosarcomas of the skin

Hanahan's group have also studied transgenic mice harbouring the bovine papilloma virus 1 genome. These mice ultimately develop skin tumours but there is a long latency period. About 8–9 months mild or aggressive hyperplasia of the dermal layer is seen. The aggressive form of fibromatosis is characterized by an increased overall skin thickness, an increased density of fibroblasts and with angiogenesis. Subsequently, fibrosarcomas that are locally invasive but benign arise from these hyperplastic regions. Fibroblast lines isolated from the aggressive fibromatosis or from fibrosarcomas were spindle shaped, showed anchorage independent growth and were tumorigenic.

As the transition from mild fibromatosis to aggressive fibromatosis was accompanied by a dramatic increase in vascular density, further studies of the cell lines isolated from BPV-1 mice have focused on the angiogenic activity of these lines (41). Cell lines derived from aggressive fibromatosis or fibrosarcomas, unlike those from normal tissue or tissue showing mild fibromatosis were found to secrete endothelial growth factors into the conditioned media. One of these factors was bFGF. In view of the fact that bFGF does not have a classic secretion signal it is not clear how it passes into the conditioned media. There was no evidence of cell death or lysis. It appears instead that a switch in the subcellular localization of bFGF in the cell lines corresponds to a 'switch' to the angiogenic phenotype.

Activated Fps/Fes protein-tyrosine kinase transgenic mice (MF1 mice). Angiogenesis in transgenic mice.

The Fps/Fes proto-oncogene is known to encode a cytoplasmic protein tyrosine kinase that is highly expressed in haematopoietic cells. Following mutation to give a constitutively activated kinase the gene was inserted into the germline of mice (39). The genomic fragment used had previously been shown to contain all of the transcriptional elements required by physiological Fps/Fes expression (42). The transgenic mice were found to display widespread hypervascularity that often progressed to multifocal haemangiomas. An abnormally high degree of vascularity was found in the subcutaneous brown adipose tissue that gave the young transgenic mice a darker colour. All MF1 mice eventually became anaemic and succumbed to the systemic effects of vascular hyperplasia such as internal haemorrhaging. In many aspects these mice are similar to those carrying the polyoma middle T oncogene that also develop spontaneous haemangiomas (43,44). The latter mice are discussed in detail in Chapter 24 by Pepper et al.

Transgenic angiogenic factor mice: VEGF transgenic mice

Somewhat surprisingly there have to date been few studies involving engineering of transgenic mice with angiogenic factors. One of these is the preparation of an angiogenic mouse expressing VEGF under the control of the human keratin 4 promoter to target overexpression of mouse VEGF to basal epidermal keratinocytes and to the follicle of the outer root sheath (45). The transgenic mice showed visibly enhanced skin vascularization, particularly in the ears (that were bright pink). Interestingly, enhanced expression of both of the mouse VEGF receptors flk-1 and flt-1 was detected on skin microvessels in the upper dermis and surrounding hair follicles of the VEGF transgenic mice. As

yet there have been no reports of the expression of an angiogenic factor in a transgenic affecting tumorigenesis.

References

1. Nicosia, R. F. and Ottinetti, A. (1990). Growth of microvessels in serum-free matrix culture of rat aorta. *Lab. Invest.*, **63**, 115–122.
2. Folkman, J. (1990). What is the evidence that tumors are angiogenesis dependent? *J. Natl Cancer Inst.*, **82**, 4–6.
3. Plate, K. H., Breier, G., Weich, H. A., and Risau, W. (1992). Vascular endothelial growth factor is a potential tumour angiogenesis factor in human gliomas *in vivo*. *Nature*, **359**, 845–8.
4. Kim, K. J., Li, B., Winer, J., Armanini, M., Gillet, N., Phillips, H. S., and Ferrara, N. (1993). Inhibition of vascular endothelial growth factor-induced angiogenesis suppresses tumour growth *in vivo*. *Nature*, **362**, 841–4.
5. Millauer, B., Shawver, L. K., Plate, K. H., Risau, W., and Ulrich, A. (1994). Glioblastoma growth inhibited *in vivo* by a dominant-negative Flk-1 mutant. *Nature*, **367**, 576–9.
6. Millauer, B., Longhi, M. P., Plate, K. H., Shawver, L. K., Risau, W., Ullrich, A., and Strawn, L. M. (1996). Dominant-negative inhibition of flk-1 suppresses the growth of many tumour types *in vivo*. *Cancer Res.*, **56**, 1615–20.
7. Cheresh, D. A. (1987). Human endothelial cells synthesize and express an Arg-Gly-Asp-directed adhesion receptor involved in attachment to fibrinogen and von Willebrand factor. *Proc. Natl Acad. Sci. USA*, **84**, 6471–5.
8. Buckley, C. D., Doyonnas, R., Newton, J. P., Blystone, S. D., Brown, E. J., Watt, S. M., and Simmons, D. L. (1996). Identification of $\alpha_v\beta_3$ as a heterotypic ligand for CD31/PECAM-1. *J. Cell Sci.*, **109**, 437–45.
9. Brooks, P. C., Clark, R. A. F., and Cheresh, D. A. (1994). Requirement of vascular integrin $\alpha_v\beta_3$ for angiogenesis. *Science*, **264**, 569–71.
10. Brooks, P. C., Montgomery, A. M. P., Rosenfeld, M., Reisfeld, R. A., Hu, T., Klier, G. and Cheresh, D. A. (1994). Integrin $\alpha_v\beta_3$ antagonists promote tumor regression by inducing apoptosis of angiogenic blood vessels. *Cell*, **79**, 1157–64.
11. Friedlander, M., Brooks, P. C., Shaffer, R. W., Kincaid, C. M., Varner, J. A., and Cheresh, D. A. (1995). Definition of two angiogenic pathways by distinct α_v integrins. *Science*, **270**, 1500–2.
12. Koch, A. E., Halloran, M. M., Haskell, C. J., Shah, M. R., and Polverini, P. J. (1995). Angiogenesis mediated by soluble forms of E-selectin and vascular cell adhesion molecule-1. *Nature*, **376**, 517–19.
13. Rogelj, S., Weinberg, R. A., Fanning, P., and Klagsbrun, M. (1988). Basic fibroblast growth factor fused to a signal peptide transforms cells. *Nature*, **331**, 173–5.
14. Blam, S. B., Mitchell, R., Tischer, E., Rubin, J. S., Silva, M., Silver, S., et al. (1988). *Oncogene*, **3**, 129–36.
15. Jouanneau, J., Gavrilovic, J., Caruelle, D., Jaye, M., Moens, G., Caruelle, J-P., and Thiery, J-P. (1991). Secreted or nonsecreted forms of acidic fibroblast growth factor produced by transfected epithelial cells influence cell morphology, motility and invasive potential. *Proc. Natl Acad. Sci. USA*, **88**, 2893–7.
16. Forough, R., Zhan, X., MacPhee, M., Friedman, S., Engleka, K. A., Sayers, T., et al. (1993). Differential transforming

abilities of non-secreted forms of human fibroblast growth factor-1. *J. Biol. Chem.*, **268**, 2960–8.

17. McLeskey, S. W., Kurebayashi, J., Honig, S. F., Zwiebel, J., Lippman, M. E., Dickson, R. B., and Kern, F. G. (1993). Fibroblast growth factor 4 transfection of MCF-7 cells produces cell lines that are tumorigenic and metastatic in ovariectomised or tamoxifen-treated athymic nude mice. *Cancer Res.*, **53**, 2168–77.

18. Kurebayashi, I., McClesky, S. W., Johnson, M. D., Lippman, M. E., Dickson, R. B., and Kern, F. G. (1993). Quantitative demonstration of spontaneous metastasis by MCF-7 human breast cancer cells cotransfected with fibroblast growth factor 4 and *Lacz. Cancer, Res.*, **53**, 2178–87.

19. Ferrara, N., Winer, J., Burton, T., Rowland, A., Siegel, M., Phillips, H. S., *et al.* (1993). Expression of vascular endothelial growth factor does not promote transformation but confers a growth advantage *in vivo* to Chinese hamster ovary cells. *J. Clin. Invest.*, **91**, 160–70.

20. Zhang, H-T., Craft, P., Scott, P. A. E., Ziche, M., Weich, H. A., Harris, A. L., and Bicknell, R. (1995). Enhancement of tumour growth and vascular density by transfection of vascular endothelial cell growth factor into MCF-7 human breast carcinoma cells. *J. Natl Cancer Inst.*, **87**, 213–19.

21. Kondo, S., Asano, M., and Suzuki, H. (1993). Significance of vascular endothelial growth factor/vascular permeability factor for solid tumor growth and its inhibition by the antibody. *Biochem. Biophys. Res. Commun.*, **194**, 1234–41.

22. Chauhan, A. K., Li, Y-S., and Deuel, T. F. (1993). Pleiotrophin transforms NIH 3T3 cells and induces tumours in nude mice. *Proc. Natl Acad. Sci. USA*, **90**, 679–682.

23. Fang, W. J., Hartmann, N., Chow, D., Riegel, A. T., and Wellstein, A. (1992). Pleiotrophin stimulates fibroblasts, endothelial and epithelial cells and is expressed in human cancer. *J. Biol. Chem.*, **267**, 25889–97.

24. Zugmaier, A., Lippman, M. E., and Wellstein, A. (1992). Inhibition by pentosan polysulfate (PPS) of heparin-binding growth factors released from tumour cells and blockage by PPS of tumour growth in animals. *J. Natl Cancer Inst.*, **84**, 1716–24.

25. Ishikawa, F., Miyazono, K., Hellman, U., Drexler, C., Wernstedt, C., Hagiwara, K., *et al.* (1989). Identification and angiogenic activity and the cloning and expression of platelet-derived endothelial cell growth factor. *Nature*, **338**, 557–62.

26. Moghaddam, A., Zhang, H-T., Fan, T-P. D., Hu, D-E., Lees, V. C., Turley, H., *et al.* (1995). Thymidine phosphorylase is angiogenic and promotes tumour growth. *Proc. Natl Acad. Sci. USA*, **92**, 998–1002.

27. Chang, H.-L., Gillet, N., Figari, I., Lopez, A. R., Palladino, M. A., and Derynck, R. (1993). Increased transforming growth factor β expression inhibits cell proliferation *in vitro*, yet increases tumorigenicity and tumour growth of meth A sarcoma cells. *Cancer Res.*, **53**, 4391–8.

28. Ziche, M., Morbidelli, L., Masini, E., Amerini, S., Granger, H. J., Maggi, C. A., *et al.* (1994). Nitric oxide mediates angiogenesis *in vivo* and endothelial cell growth and migration *in vitro* promoted by substance P. *J. Clin. Invest.*, **94**, 2036–44.

29. Jenkins, D. C., Charles, I. G., Thomsen, L. L., Moss, D. W., Holmes, L. S., Baylis, S. A., *et al.* (1995). Roles of nitric oxide in tumor growth. *Proc. Natl Acad. Sci. USA*, **492**, 4392–6.

30. Shweiki, D., Itin, A., Soffer, D., and Keshet, E. (1992). Vascular endothelial growth factor induced by hypoxia may mediate hypoxia-initiated angiogenesis. *Nature*, **359**, 843–5.

31. Vecchi, A., Garlanda, C., Lampugnani, M. G., Resnati, M., Stoppacciaro, A., Ruco, L., *et al.* (1994). Monoclonal antibodies specific for endothelial cells of mouse blood vessels. *Eur. J. Cell Biol.*, **63**, 247–54.

32. Parums, D. V., Cordell, J. L., Micklem, K., Heryet, A. R., Gatter, K. C., and Mason, D. Y. (1990) JC70: a new monoclonal antibody that detects vascular endothelium associated antigen on routinely processed tissue sections. *J. Clin. Pathol.*, **43**, 752–7.

33. Kuzu, I., Bicknell, R., Harris, A. L., Jones, M., Gatter, K. C., and Mason, D. Y. (1992). Heterogeneity of vascular endothelial cells with relevance to diagnosis of vascular tumours. *J. Clin. Pathol.*, **45**, 143–8.

34. Chaplain, M. A. J. (1995). Reaction–diffusion prepatterning and its potential role in tumour invasion. *J. Biol. Syst.*, **3**, 929–36.

35. Zhang, H-T. (1995). Transfection of angiogenic factors into human MCF-7 breast carcinoma cells: effects on growth *in vivo*. DPhil. thesis, University of Oxford.

36. Folkman, J., Watson, K., Ingber, D., and Hanahan, D. (1989). Induction of angiogenesis during the transition from hyperplasia to neoplasia. *Nature*, **339**, 58–61.

37. Lacey, M., Alpert, S., and Hanahan, D. (1986). Bovine papillomavirus elicits skin tumours in transgenic mice. *Nature*, **322**, 609–12.

38. Schuh, A. C., Keating, S. J., Monteclaro, F. S., Vogt, P. K., and Breitman, M. L. (1990). Obligatory wounding requirement for tumourigenesis in v-jun transgenic mice. *Nature*, **346**, 756–60.

39. Greer, P., Haigh, J., Mbamalu, G., Khoo, W., Bernstein, A., and Pawson, T. (1994). The Fps/Fes protein-tyrosine kinase promotes angiogenesis in transgenic mice. *Mol. Cell. Biol.*, **14**, 6755–63.

40. Radvanyi, F., Christgau, S., Baekkeskov, S., Jolicoeur, C., and Hanahan, D. (1993). Pancreatic β cells cultured from individual preneoplastic foci in a multistage tumorigenesis pathway: a potentially general technique for isolating physiologically representative cell lines. *Mol. Cell. Biol.*, **13**, 4223–32.

41. Kandel, J., Bossy-Wetzel, E., Radvanyi, F., Klagsbrun, M., Folkman, J., and Hanahan, D. (1991). Neovascularisation is associated with a switch to the export of bFGF in the multistep development of fibrosarcoma. *Cell*, **66**, 1095–104.

42. Greer, P., Maltby, J., Rossant, J., Bernstein, A., and Pawson, T. (1990). Myeloid expression of the human c-fps/fes proto-oncogene in transgenic mice. *Mol. Cell. Biol.*, **10**, 2521–7.

43. Williams, R. L., Courtneidge, S. A., and Wagner, E. R. (1988). Embryonic lethalities and endothelial tumours in chimeric mice expressing polyoma virus middle T oncogene. *Cell*, **52**, 121–31.

44. Williams, R. L., Risau, W., Zerwes, H.-G., Drexler, H., Aguzzi, A., and Wagner, E. (1989). Endothelioma cells expressing the polyoma middle T oncogene induce haemangiomas by host cell recruitment. *Cell*, **57**, 1053–63.

45. Detmar, M., Brown, L. F., Dvorak, H. F., and Claffey, K. P. (1995). Overexpression of VPF/VEGF in the skin of transgenic mice leads to increased skin vascularization. *J. Invest. Dermatol.*, **105**, 448 (Abstr.).

4. Prognostic and predictive value of intra-tumoral microvessel density in human solid tumours

Giampietro Gasparini

Introduction

The majority of human solid tumours are heterogeneous diseases, made up of multiple cell clones with diverse biological aggressiveness (1,2). The tumour cell heterogeneity is the result of the genomic instability (3) due to genetic alterations that may include: mutations, deletions, chromosomal rearrangements, activation of oncogenes, downregulation of tumour suppressor genes, and gene amplification (4–7). Tumour cell heterogeneity may confer different properties of growth, immunogenicity, ability to metastatize, and sensitivity to treatments to the diverse cell clones. Tumour cell genomic instability and heterogeneity are the biological basis of the clinical observation that both the outcome of the patients and their responsiveness to anti-cancer therapy may be different among tumours classified as having the same pathological or clinical stage. Thus, for several solid tumours it is difficult, by using conventional clinicopathological criteria, to assess the prognosis or the likelihood of response to a specific form of anti-cancer treatment of any single patient.

This important clinical problem stimulated the search for several novel markers to obtain more precise and selective prognostic information, as well as the development of markers related to responsiveness or resistance to specific forms of anti-cancer treatments to predict the likelihood of their efficacy (8).

Among the new biological prognostic and predictive markers that have been developed and tested for their clinical usefulness, angiogenesis is emerging as one of the more potentially useful. This is not surprising taking into account the biological role played by neovascularization in tumour transformation, progression, and metastasis (9). There are now a large amount of experimental (10) and clinical data (11,12) demonstrating that growth of solid tumours is angiogenesis-dependent (13).

In this chapter I will review the methods to assess the vascular density of human solid tumours, the relationship between vascularization of primary tumours, metastasis, and the clinicopathological studies correlating the degree of intra-tumoral microvessel density (IMD) with prognosis and responsiveness to anti-cancer therapy that have been published to date.

Methods to assess the vascular density of human solid tumours

Angiogenesis is a very complex phenomenon that is generally inhibited in normal tissues of the adult (14–16), but is activated in some pathological diseases, for example cancer (17–20). In each tumour the angiogenic activity, at a certain time, is the result of the net balance between angiogenic stimuli and natural angiogenesis inhibitors (21). This balance is critical, may change in time, and may be regulated at different steps: cellular (*e.g.* by pericytes, macrophages, fibroblasts, mast cells, etc.) (22–28), genetic (*e.g.* the control of wild-type p53 on thrombospondin-1) (29,30), biochemical (31–35), or mechanical (36–40).

Therefore it is not easy to develop a single method able to detect such a complex biological phenomenon. At present the most widely used method to assess angiogenesis in human neoplasia is the quantification of IMD of primary tumours by using specific markers for endothelial cells, these include factor VIII-related antigen (fVIII-RA), CD31 (platelet/endothelial cell adhesion molecule/PECAM) and CD34, and using a standard immunoperoxidase technique to stain microvessels (41–43).

To date anti-CD31 is the most sensitive pan-endothelial marker available which recognizes a greater number of microvessels than the other endothelial markers tested such as fVIII-RA or CD34 (41,44). These two latter antibodies may therefore underestimate the extent of intra-tumoral vascularization (45), and fVIII-RA also recognizes lymphatics (46). On the other hand, the specificity of the antibody to CD31 is not absolute because it reacts with cells other than endothelial, for example plasma cells (47). Nevertheless, two studies comparing the prognostic value of IMD assessed using either CD31 or fVIII-RA found that both the markers provided significant prognostic information (44,48). It is noteworthy to emphasize that all the above markers are not able to discriminate between quiescent versus activated/proliferating endothelium. Three recently developed antibodies, namely, E-9 (49,50), TEC-11 to endoglin (51), and LM-609 to integrin αvβ3 (52) seem to be specific for activated/proliferating endothelial cells. Comparative studies are needed to establish whether the use of these markers will have a better prognostic value than CD31 or fVIII-RA.

With immunocytochemistry, intra-tumoral capillaries and small venules can be identified and counted by light microscopic analysis in those representative areas of tissue block of the invasive tumour component chosen by a careful examination of haematoxylin and eosin stained sections. As the common finding is that the distribution of IMD is heterogeneous, it has been suggested that the area of highest microvessel count (what has become known as the vascular 'hot spot') should be identified and used to assess the IMD of each tumour (43). This being based on the hypothesis that the most angiogenic tumour cell clones are those that are most aggressive and that influence the biological behaviour of the tumour (53) (see Fig. 4.1, in the plate section).

A fundamental question concerning this method is: Is the assessment of IMD a real static quantitative measure of the angiogenic activity of a tumour? At least three studies provide information on this. Li et al. (54) found a strong association between IMD, assessed in primary cerebral tumours of infancy, and the levels of basic fibroblast growth factor (bFGF) in the liquor. Furthermore, both these methods correlated with the prognosis of the patients. Toi et al. (55) in a large study involving more than 300 breast cancer patients, showed that IMD and the expression of vascular endothelial growth factor (VEGF) detected in the primary tumours by immunocytochemical methods, are closely associated, and that both have prognostic value in univariate analysis. A third study by Fox et al. (56) reported that IMD is associated with urokinase-type plasminogen activator (uPA) and plasminogen activator inhibitor 1 (PAI-1), enzymes involved in the early steps of the process of angiogenesis. Overall, the results of these three studies demonstrate that IMD is a marker of the angiogenic activity, being strictly related to angiogenic peptides and to enzymes involved in the degradation of extracellular matrix and of the basal lamina of vessels.

Some methodological recommendations to assess properly IMD have been reviewed by several authors (11,53).

Table 4.1. Potential methodological pitfalls for the determination of intra-tumoral microvessel density by using immunocytochemical methods

Use of insufficiently specific or sensitive markers for vascular endothelial cells (e.g. vimentin, Ulex europaeus-I agglutinin, collagen IV).

Unsatisfactory intensity of staining. This may be related to the use of insufficient primary antibody concentration or to unsuitable methods of fixation or immunostaining.

Microvessel counts not performed in the invasive component of the tumour. This may be due to the lack of careful histological control of the section to be used (by using haematoxylin and eosin staining).

Incorrect identification of the 'hot spot' area within each tumour.

Incorrect evaluation of each element that should be considered a single, countable microvessel.

Insufficient extended field in which to perform the evaluation.

Using the method suggested by Weidner et al. (43) several independent studies have shown that a high degree of IMD is significantly associated with metastasis, prognosis, and responsiveness to anti-cancer therapy in different human tumour types (reviewed in references 11,12,53,57). However, not all investigators have been able to confirm a significant association of vascularization with clinical outcome (58–60) and metastatic spread (59). The results of these negative studies are likely to be due in part to bias in the clinical study design, or to methodological problems (Table 4.1). Some studies were also not supported by suitable statistical analysis correlating the pathological results with the clinical end-points (see below). However, the immunopathological methods up to now used to assess IMD, even if of clinical value, are suboptimal because the counting of microvessels is laborious and the identification of the 'hot spot' may present interobserver variability (61,62). Furthermore, some steps of the method need more standardization, validation procedures, and quality control protocols (53, 63).

In order to improve the reproducibility of the pathological evaluation of IMD, at least two new methods are under evaluation. The first consists of using a multiparametric computerized image analysis system (CIAS) that can be employed to measure concurrently more parameters related to the vascularization such as: intensity of the staining, microvessel number, and total endothelial area and perimeter. Two studies found this methodology is feasible and able to improve the objectivity of microvessel evaluation (61,62).

The second technique is under application at the University of Oxford and is based on the Chalkley point method coupled with a visual 'eyeballing' vascular grading system. Fox *et al.* (62) found a significant correlation between Chalkley counting and the manual method (Weidner's) and prognosis. Other potentially useful pathological methods to detect angiogenic activity in human tumour pathology are the intra-tumoral determination, by immunocytochemical or *in situ* hybridization or immunoenzymatic techniques, of angiogenic peptides (e.g. bFGF or VEGF) and/or natural angiogenesis inhibitors (thrombospondin 1) or enzymes related to the proteolytic degradation of extracellular matrix and of the basal lamina of vessels (such as uPA or PAI-1) (see reference 64 for a review). However, these methods are still in the preliminary phase of their development and are not suitable for routine clinical use.

Recently, it has been demonstrated that it is possible to measure serum and urine levels of bFGF, and it has been shown that the concentrations of this angiogenic peptide correlate with the status of disease and prognosis (65). Similarly, it is possible to determine the concentrations of thrombospondin 1 in body fluids, but the clinical meaning of this assessment is not yet clear (66).

The association of vascular density of primary tumours with metastasis

Biological rationale

There is growing experimental evidence that angiogenesis is involved both at the beginning and at the end of the development of metastasis (67–69). To be able to metastasize via blood vessels tumour cells need to adhere to endothelial cells, penetrate into the vessel lumen, survive in the circulation, undergo extravasation, and arrest in the target distant tissue to establish a viable secondary (70).

The Folkman group have recently demonstrated a biological mechanism explaining why the removal of a primary tumour can be followed by a stimulation of growth of distant metastases. The transplantable murine Lewis lung carcinoma (3LL) produces a potent natural angiogenesis inhibitor, angiostatin, that has a long half-life in the circulation and acts like a hormone to inhibit systemically the proliferation of endothelial cells. The resection of the primary tumour depletes angiostatin and thus induces rapid growth of distant metastases (71). In

another study the same group have found that micrometastases remain dormant when the local tumour cell proliferation is balanced by an equivalent rate of apoptosis in the presence of angio-inhibition. Conversely, micrometastases exhibited rapid growth when the inhibition of angiogenesis was removed and this was accompanied by a threefold decreased rate of apoptosis with an unaffected tumour cell proliferation rate (72).

Studies correlating the degree of intra-tumoral microvessel density in primary tumours with metastasis

Tumour metastasis is the major cause of mortality in cancer patients, so the identification of a marker strictly associated with the metastatic potential of each single tumour is of clinical relevance for the management and therapy of cancer patients (63). Sixteen studies have been up to now specifically designed in order to verify whether IMD, determined in the primary tumour, correlates with local (lymph nodal) or distant metastasis in different types of human solid tumours (Table 4.2). Irrespective of the tumour type studied, 77% of the studies (10 of 13) found that highly vascularized tumours have a significantly higher likelihood to present locoregional lymph nodal metastasis than those poorly vascularized. Similarly, 77% of the studies (10 of 13) found a significant correlation between IMD in the primary tumour and the development of distant metastasis. Overall, the studies here considered have been performed using different methods and include a total of 1153 patients, and nine different types of tumours with a different clinical or pathological stage. However, also taking into account the heterogeneity of the series analysed, the clinical findings seem to confirm the results of experimental studies showing a close relationship between angiogenic activity and metastatic spread (67–72). Each single study includes quite a small number of cases; however, a large study performed by Gasparini *et al.* (73) in a series of node-negative breast cancer patients confirms this observation. By using the anti-CD31 antibody and an immunocytochemical method to assess IMD, the authors (73) found that IMD was significantly predictive for all the sites recurrence, stratified in three dominant sites: viscera, bone, and soft tissue metastasis.

Angiogenesis and prognosis

Biological rationale

McGuire proposed that the most important requirement for a new prognostic indicator is that it be a marker with a

Table 4.2. Clinicopathological studies assessing the relationship of intra-tumoral microvessel density with metastasis

Author (year)	Reference	Endothelial marker	Tumour type	No. of patients	Association with metastasis	
					Nodal P	Distant P
Srivastava (1988)	74	Ulex-europaeus-I* agglutinin	malignant melanoma	20	both sites =	0.025
Carnochan (1991)	60	Ulex-europaeus-I* agglutinin	malignant melanoma	107	NS	NS
Weidner (1991)	43	fVIII-RA	breast cancer	49	both sites =	0.003
Wakui (1992)	75	vimentin	prostatic carcinoma	101	ND	<0.0001†
Macchiarini (1992)	76	fVIII-RA	non-small cell lung cancer	87	both sites =	<0.0001
Sneige (1992)	77	fVIII-RA	breast cancer	138	<0.05	ND
Sahin (1992)	78	fVIII-RA	breast cancer	81	ND	0.07
Hall (1992)	79	fVIII-RA	breast cancer	87	both sites =	NS
Weidner (1993)	80	fVIII-RA	prostatic carcinoma	74	ND	<0.0001†
Gasparini (1993)	81	CD-31	head and neck squamous cell carcinoma	70	both sites =	0.004
Olivarez (1994)	82	fVIII-RA	testicular germ cell tumour (stage A)	65	0.011	ND
Saclarides (1994)	83	fVIII-RA	rectal carcinoma	48	both sides =	0.06
Graham (1994)	84	fVIII-RA / CD-34	malignant melanoma	20‡	both sides =	0.035 (fVIII-RA) 0.049 (CD-31)
Yamazaki (1994)	85	fVIII-RA	lung adenocarcinoma	42	NS	0.027
Jaeger (1994)	86	fVIII-RA	bladder cancer	40	<0.0001	ND
Maeda (1995)	87	fVIII-RA	gastric carcinoma	124	<0.01	NS

ND, not done; NS, not significant.   * By using the percentage vascular area at the tumour base
† Only metastasts in bone marrow are considered   ‡ By comparing matched groups by sex, age, stage, and treatment.

clear biological background, strictly related to the aggressiveness of each single tumour (88). A marker of angiogenesis, as IMD is, fully agrees with such a requirement for the following reasons:

1. Angiogenesis is necessary for the progression from the pre-invasive (e.g. in situ carcinoma) to the invasive phase of a primary tumour (89,90).

2. In invasive tumours, even in the same histotype, the angiogenic activity is heterogeneous and in invasive breast carcinoma it has been demonstrated that IMD is a continuous variable (73). This allows the possibility to stratify the angiogenic activity of tumours in different subgroups.

3. Several clinicopathological studies have found that IMD is not associated with the expression of several other biological markers including: p53, c-erbB-2, epidermal growth factor receptor, and hormone receptors (44,91). This is the biological basis which allows one

to ascertain that IMD is an independent marker of prognosis.

4. A high angiogenic activity of a primary tumour facilitates the development of locoregional and distant metastasis (Table 4.2).

Clinicopathological studies on breast carcinoma

Breast carcinoma is the tumour type on which more independent studies have been performed to verify the prognostic value of IMD. The clinical importance of the determination of tumour angiogenesis in such a neoplasm has been recently reviewed (11), hence the results of the studies up to now published or presented at scientific meetings have been updated (Table 4.3). Eighteen studies (44,55,58,62,73,91–103) are considered including 2770 breast cancer patients and 1502 with node-negative tumours, the latter being the subgroup of major clinical interest (8). In fact, about 70% of patients with node-negative breast carcinoma have a favourable long-term outcome, but the remaining proportion is at high risk of recurrence and death (8). Following the evaluation guidelines suggested by Gasparini *et al.* (8) 1738 patients (888 with node-negative tumours) have been enrolled in pilot or yet to be completed studies (those presented at meetings, but not finalized in publications) and 1032 (724 with node-negative tumours) in four confirmatory studies (55,73,96,103). Considering the results obtained in univariate analysis as a first step, 10 of 14 (71.5%) evaluable studies found that IMD is significantly associated with relapse-free survival (RFS), and nine of 13 (69.2%) evaluable studies showed a significant association with overall survival (OS).

In 13 of the 18 considered studies a multivariate analysis was performed in order to see whether IMD is an independent prognostic factor when other variables are concurrently evaluated (Table 4.3). Ten studies had a multivariate analysis on RFS and six (60%) demonstrated that IMD is a significant and independent prognostic indicator for recurrence. Ten studies had a multivariate analysis on OS and six (60%) demonstrated that IMD is a significant and independent marker for survival.

Overall, about three-quarters of the studies found that IMD is of prognostic value; however, six studies are negative and do not find a significant association between the determination of angiogenesis and the clinical outcome of the patients. Four of these studies included small series of patients: 93 (58), 92 (97), 84 (98), and 40 (102), respectively, and four of these six trials included both node-positive and node-negative patients. From a methodological point of view, only three of these six negative studies included a multivariate analysis (58,94,103). In five studies the endothelial marker used was fVIII-RA (58,94,97,102,103) and in the last one it was CD31 (98).

Van Hoef *et al.* (58) using fVIII-RA counted a median number of intra-tumoral vessels higher than that found in all the other studies employing the same marker suggesting methodological problems in the criteria of microvessel counts. The studies by Conner *et al.* (97) and Sightler *et al.* (98) were presented at a meeting and have not yet been published, so there is no detailed information on how they have been performed. Finally, the studies by Vermeulen *et al.* (102) and Axelsson *et al.* (103) were performed on selected cohorts of patients. This procedure to assess prognosis in a non-consecutive series, may be impaired by serious bias related to the selection procedure (*e.g.* the use of pathological blocks fixed in different manners, different surgical techniques to remove the primary tumour, different schedules of postsurgical treatment and follow-up, etc.). Thus in at least three of the negative studies a methodological bias is present, that may explain the lack of correlation between the prognostic variable under evaluation and clinical outcome.

Taking into account the heterogeneity of the series studied, that different endothelial markers have been used and that non-homogeneous criteria have been employed to stratify the tumours between high versus low vascularized, the assessment of IMD is equally emerging as one of the most powerful prognostic indicators for operable breast cancer. At present, this should not mean that this marker is to be regularly used to select high-risk patients with operable breast cancer. In fact, prior to a wide use of IMD and its possible routine clinical application, prospective randomized clinical trials are needed to verify the results observed in the retrospective studies here reported. Furthermore, the method of assessment of IMD is still suboptimal and needs to be standardized and made more objective.

Clinicopathological studies on other solid tumours

Angiogenic activity, measured by counting IMD, has been studied to assess the prognosis of a number of solid tumours other than breast cancer. Carnochan *et al.* (60), using the endothelial marker lectin, *Ulex europaeus*-I, assessed the vascularization of 107 primary cutaneous malignant melanomas of intermediate thickness. After 5 years no significant association was found with both RFS and OS. Vesalainen *et al.* (104) used an antibody to collagen IV to determine the vascularization in 88 early-stage prostatic adenocarcinomas. After a long period of observation the degree of angiogenesis significantly predicted OS. Saclarides *et al.* (83), using a fVIII-RA staining, found a significant association between IMD and OS in a small series of patients with various stages of rectal cancer.

The study of Li *et al.* (54) was performed in a series of 26 patients with brain tumours of the infancy. A strict correlation was observed between IMD (factor VIII-RA or CD34) and both RFS and OS. Furthermore, the degree of vascularization of the primary tumour was significantly associated with the liquor levels of bFGF. Yamazaki *et al.* (85) did not observe a significant correlation between IMD and prognosis in 42 patients with various stages of lung adenocarcinoma. The prognostic value of IMD was also studied in gastric carcinoma by Maeda *et al.* (87) and in transitional cell bladder cancer by Bochner *et al.* (105). Both the studies found a significant association of IMD with both RFS and OS.

Two investigators studied the prognostic value of IMD in head and neck cancer patients. Using the anti-CD31

Table 4.3. Intra-tumoral microvessel density and prognosis in operable breast carcinoma

Author (year)	Ref.	Endothelial marker	No. of pts	Tumour stage	No. of node-negative patients	Association with metastasis Nodal P	Distant P	Association with RFS	Association with OS	Multivariate analysis RFSp	OSp	Median follow-up (years)
Pilot Studies												
Horak (1992)	44	CD31	103	I–II	64	<0.01	ND	ND	0.006	ND	ND	2.5
Weidner (1992)	91	fVIII-RA	165	I–II	83	0.017	<0.001	<0.001	0.001	<0.001	<0.001	4.0
Bosari (1992)	92	fVIII-RA	180	I–II	151	<0.01	<0.01	<0.004	<0.008	<0.03	<0.03	9.0
Visscher (1993)	93	Type IV collagenase	58	I to IV	28	0.02	0.001	0.001	ND	NS	ND	5.1
van Hoef (1993)	58	fVIII-RA	93	I	93	ND	NS	NS	NS	NS	NS	13.0
Khanuia (1993)	94	fVIII-RA	164	I–II	125	NS	NS	NS	ND	ND	NS	8.0
Obermair (1994)	95	fVIII-RA	64	I–II	32	0.03	<0.01	<0.01	ND	<0.01	ND	4.1
Conner (1994)	97	fVIII-RA	92	ND	ND	ND	ND	ND	NS	ND	NS	16
Sighter (1994)	98	CD-31	84	ND	ND	ND	ND	ND	NS	ND	ND	ND
Simpson (1994)	99	CD-34	178	I–II	ND	ND	0.004	0.004	0.004	NS	NS	6.0
Bundred (1994)	100	fVIII-RA	151	I–II	ND	ND	<0.0001	<0.001	<0.001	ND	ND	ND
Ogawa (1995)	101	fVIII-RA	155	I–II–III	91	NS	<0.001	<0.001	0.025	<0.002	<0.001	7.0
Vermuelen (1995)	102	fVIII-RA	40	I	40	ND	NS	NS	ND	ND	ND	Cohort1 = 3.0 Cohort2 = 11.3
Fox (1995)	62	CD31	211	I–II	112	0.05	ND	ND	0.02	ND	0.05	3.5

Table 4.3. *cont.*

Author (year)	Ref.	Endothelial marker	No. of pts	Tumour stage	No. of node-negative patients	Association with metastasis		Association with RFS	Association with OS	Multi-variate analysis		Median follow-up (years)
						Nodal P	Distant P			RFSp	OSp	
Confirmatory Studies												
Gasparini (1994)	73	CD31	254	I	254	ND	0.0001	0.0001	0.012	0.004	0.047	5.1
Toi (1995)	55	fVIII-RA	328	I–II	130	<0.01	<0.001	<0.001	ND	<0.0001	ND	4.6
Obermair (1995)	96	fVIII-RA	230	I	230	ND	ND	<0.0001	<0.0001	ND	<0.001	ND 4.6
Axelsson (1995)	103	fVIII-RA	220	I–II	110	NS	NS	NS	NS	NS	NS	NS 11.5

ND, not done; NS, not significant. Modified from reference 11.

antibody our group determined vascularization in a series of 73 stage II–IV head and neck squamous cell carcinoma enrolled in a randomized clinical trial which compared two different schedules of concurrent chemoradiation therapy (cisplatin versus carboplatin and conventional dosage of radiation therapy). After 2 years, IMD did not correlate with RFS and OS; however, this marker significantly predicted the likelihood to obtain clinical complete remission. Low vascularized tumours had a significantly higher probability of responding to such treatment, irrespective of the schedule used (106).

The second study by Williams *et al.* (107) was performed in a series of 66 patients with T1-3No carcinomas of the oral cavity. A significant association was found between the percentage of vascularity, using fVIII-RA, and RFS and OS. The different results obtained in these two studies can be explained by the following features.

1. Williams *et al.* (107) selected a more homogeneous group of patients with regard to the site of the primary tumour and all the tumours were node-negative at diagnosis.

2. The treatments were different: only surgery in Williams' series (107) and chemoradiation therapy in Gasparini's series (106).

3. The median follow-up time of observation was significantly longer in the American study (4.5 years versus 1.5 years).

4. The study by Gasparini *et al.* (106) was mainly designed to assess the responsiveness to therapy.

Finally, Hollingsworth *et al.* (108) and van Diest (109) studied the correlation between angiogenesis (CD34 staining and lectin *Ulex europaeus*-1, respectively) and prognosis in advanced stages of ovarian cancer. Hollingsworth *et al.* (108) found a significant association between IMD and prognosis, while in the study by van Diest *et al.* (109) a tendency for worse prognosis with higher microvessel count was found, but a statistical significance level was not reached. In the study the patients were treated with debulking surgery and platinum-based chemotherapy.

Overall, 792 patients and nine different tumour types have been studied to verify the prognostic value of intra-

Table 4.4. Intra-tumoral microvessel density and prognosis in solid tumours other than breast cancer

Author (year)	Reference	Endothelial marker	Tumour type	Stage	No. of patients	Median follow-up	Association with prognosis RFSp	OSp	Multivariate analysis
Carnochan (1991)	60	lectin *Ulex europaeus*-I	malignant melanoma	0.85–1.25 mm	107	5	NS	NS	ND
Vesalainen (1994)	104	collagen IV	prostatic adenocarcinoma	T1–2Mo	88	12	ND	0.026	ND
Saclarides (1994)	83	fVIII-RA	rectal cancer	A–D	48	4.1	ND	0.013	ND
Li (1994)	54	fVIII-RA / CD-34	brain tumours in children	various	26	1.2	0.005	0.02	ND
Yamazaki (1994)	85	fVIII-RA	lung adeno carcinoma	I–IV	42	6	0.027	NS	ND
Williams (1994)	107	fVIII-RA	oral cavity carcinoma	T1–3 NoMo	66	5	<0.0001	0.07	ND
Maeda (1995)	87	fVIII-RA	gastric carcinoma	I–IV	124	5	ND	<0.05	0.048
Hollingsworth (1995)	108	CD34	ovarian cancer	III–IV	43	2.5	0.064	0.0036	0.030
van Diest (1995)	109	lectin *Ulex europaeus*-I	ovarian cancer	III–IV	49	3.8	ND	0.25	NS
Bochner (1995)	105	fVIII-RA	bladder cancer	invasive	126	6.5	0.004	0.0001	<0.05
Gasparini (1995)	106	CD31	head and neck cancer	II–IV	73	2.0	NS	NS	NS

NS, not significant; ND, not done.

tumoral vascularization. Five of the seven evaluable studies (71%) found a significant association between IMD and RFS and seven of the 10 evaluable studies (70%) with OS (Table 4.4). However, only in five studies was a multivariate analysis carried out (87,105,106,108,109), and only three studies had more than 100 patients included in the analysis (60,87,105). Thus, although the overall trend is that the assessment of IMD retains a prognostic value in the majority of the solid tumours considered, no definitive conclusion can be drawn at present on the real clinical usefulness of this marker. Prior to performing prospective studies and to using IMD to assess prognosis in solid tumours in clinical practice, a more homogeneous and larger series of patients for each tumour type need to be studied in retrospective studies.

Angiogenesis and prediction of response to anti-cancer therapy

Biological and pharmacological rationale

Tumour-cell–stromal interaction constitutes the microenvironment of tumour growth and contributes to tumour progression and metastasis (110–112). The relationship between the parenchymal and stromal components of a solid tumour is dynamic and complex. The stromal structures and cells play an active part in providing vascular supply, regulating permeability to gas and nutrients, immunological response, and cell to cell adhesion mechanisms. Moreover, they mediate intercellular communications by diffusible factors that act by autocrine and paracrine mechanisms (113).

Folkman was the first to hypothesize in 1971 (114) that a structure of the stroma of solid tumours, namely the vascular endothelium, may represent a target for novel anti-cancer therapeutical approaches.

There is recent evidence that the stromal components of solid tumours may play a part in determining the efficacy of conventional anti-cancer treatments. Contrary to expectation, the onset of vascularization gradually makes a tumour more inaccessible to drugs. In fact, while earlier stages of the cancers are well perfused, further tumour growth causes an enhanced interstitial pressure related both to the pressure exerted by proliferating parenchymal cells and to the lack of a functional intra-tumoral network of lymphatics. These phenomena cause vascular compression, necrosis and reduce the blood supply (115–118). Furthermore, normal endothelial cells within some normal and neoplastic tissues express the P170-glycoprotein, that relates to multidrug resistance (119). Thus, the vascular component of the tumours, even if actively proliferating,

may be resistant to the action of some chemotherapeutic agents. Two recent experimental studies found that, via a paracrine effect, bFGF mediates resistance to some cytotoxic agents *in vitro* (120) and to tamoxifen *in vivo* (121). Teicher *et al.* (122) showed that the concurrent use of cytotoxic therapy and anti-angiogenesis produces a potentiation of the anti-tumoral effect *in vivo*. Similar results have been observed by combining radiation therapy and angiogenesis inhibitors (123). Yamaoka *et al.* (124) found that the anti-tumoral effect of an angiogenesis inhibitor, TNP-470 (AGM-1470, a synthetic analogue of fumagillin) is mediated through the inhibition of endothelial cell proliferation. Furthermore, there is experimental evidence that tumour cells and vascular endothelial cells within a solid tumour may stimulate each other by paracrine factors (113) and that a better control of tumour growth may be obtained by using specific treatments targeting both cell populations. While chemotherapy, hormone therapy, and radiation therapy affect tumour cell proliferation, angiogenesis inhibitors are experimentally capable of inhibiting endothelial cell proliferation or migration to form new capillaries (125,126).

These pre-clinical findings support the importance of the quantification of angiogenic activity as a surrogate marker to predict the responsiveness to conventional anti-cancer treatments and in the future, perhaps, to assess the responsiveness to the pharmacological modulation of angiogenesis.

Early clinical studies on angiogenesis as a predictive marker for responsiveness to conventional anti-cancer therapy

The first study we performed to assess the prognostic value of IMD in operable breast carcinoma, done in collaboration with Weidner and Folkman, showed that this marker is a new significant and independent prognostic indicator in operable breast carcinoma (91).

By analysing separately the group of node-negative tumours (*n* = 82) from node-positive (*n* = 83), we found that the significance of IMD was retained in both the groups in univariate and multivariate analysis. The patients with node-positive disease received heterogeneous forms of adjuvant therapy, mainly tamoxifen for 3 years for those postmenopausal patients with oestrogen-positive tumours, and chemotherapy (CMF schedule) for the premenopausal women or for those that were postmenopausal oestrogen receptor negative. Thus it was not possible to establish a direct correlation between IMD and efficacy of a specific form of adjuvant treatment in this study. In order to answer this important question we undertook a second study restricted to a series of nearly 200 node-positive breast cancer patients treated with either adjuvant chemotherapy (CMF schedule) or hormone therapy (tamoxifen). The findings of this more recent study show that, irrespective of the adjuvant treatment administered, only those patients with poorly vascularized cancers gained some benefit from adjuvant therapy. In fact, we found a strong inverse relationship between probability of RFS and OS with the degree of vascularization of the primary tumour (127). Also Toi et al. (55) who analysed separately a group of 198 node-positive breast cancers treated with diverse adjuvant treatments found an inverse significant association between microvessel counts and RFS.

In two studies on breast cancer patients treated with adjuvant tamoxifen, Macaulay et al. (128) and Gasparini et al. (129) found that the patients with highly vascularized tumours had a statistically significant poorer outcome than those with tumours poorly vascularized.

Overall, the results of these five studies evaluating the predictive value of angiogenesis in node-positive operable breast cancer, suggest that IMD seems to be potentially useful to select those patients who are more likely to gain a benefit from adjuvant therapy. This important observation needs to be tested in randomized prospective clinical trials prior to a potential use in clinical practice. Gasparini et al. (130) also studied the degree of vascularization in a series of breast cancer patients with advanced disease (stages III–IV). By using fVIII-RA it was observed that the median number of microvessels at 'hot spots' in this series was higher than that observed in early stages using the same endothelial cell marker (91). However, in this small series, IMD did not correlate with clinical outcome or response to chemotherapy.

Vacca et al. (131) assessed vascularization of bone marrow in 46 patients with multiple myeloma. By comparing IMD between the group of patients with active or progressive disease versus non-active disease, a statistically significant difference was found. As all the patients received chemotherapy, this study also demonstrated an inverse relationship between the degree of vascularization and the efficacy of chemotherapy. In particular those eight patients who had progressive disease during therapy were those with the highest absolute microvessel counts in bone marrow.

Another study by Gasparini et al. (106) evaluated angiogenesis in patients with advanced stages of head and neck squamous cell carcinoma treated with concurrent chemoradiation therapy. The degree of IMD was significantly predictive of poor response to platinum-based chemotherapy and radiation therapy, in terms of complete remission (Table 4.5). A similar finding has been observed by Hollingsworth et al. (108) and Gasparini et al. (132) in

series of epithelial ovarian cancers in patients treated with platinum-based combined chemotherapy.

The general finding is that the more a solid tumour is vascularized, the lower the likelihood is that it may be responsive to adjuvant or palliative conventional anti-cancer treatments. This opens new relevant potential clinical applications of the determination of angiogenesis in solid tumours. Larger new studies should be specifically designed in the future in order to verify whether IMD predicts responsiveness to specific forms of anti-cancer treatments or, on the contrary, if this finding can be generalized.

Summary and conclusions

An optimal method to assess the complex processes related to angiogenesis has not yet been developed. However, there is sufficient evidence to consider that the determination of IMD is a feasible measure of the angiogenic activity in human solid tumours (54–56). This method may be improved by using:

1. More specific and selective markers for activated/proliferating microvessels (49–52).

2. By improving the techniques of staining.

3. By using more objective and reproducible methods for microvessel count (61,62,133).

4. By a standardization of the criteria of evaluation of IMD and of the identification of the neovascular 'hot spot' within each single tumour. (53)

Furthermore, as alternative methods are available to assess angiogenesis (reviewed in references 11, 64) at this time, perhaps, the concurrent use of more of these may enhance the accuracy of the measurement of the angiogenic activity (63). In any case, the determination of angiogenesis by IMD in human neoplasia has permitted an increase in our understanding of the role of angiogenesis in human tumour growth, progression, and metastasis. The most important findings are:

1. Approximately three-quarters of the clinicopathological studies confirmed that a strict association exists between the degree of angiogenic activity of a primary tumour and its potential to develop locoregional or distant metastasis. These clinical data agree with those observed in experimental models.

2. The results of 18 retrospective studies that determined IMD in more than 2700 breast cancers, show that angiogenesis is one of the most powerful prognostic indicators available. In fact, more than 70% of the

Table 4.5. Intra-tumoral microvessel density and prediction of efficacy of anti-cancer therapy

Author (year)	Reference	Endothelial marker	Tumour type	Stage	No. of patients	Treatment	Prediction of efficacy (P)
Weidner (1992)	91	fVIII-RA	Breast cancer	II	82	Heterogenefous adjuvant treatments	yes (<0.001 for both RFS and OS)
Gasparini (1993)	130	fVIII-RA	Breast cancer	III–IV	42	Neoadjuvant chemotherapy (stage III) or palliative chemotherapy (stage IV)	no
Toi (1995)	55	fVIII-RA	Breast cancer	II	198	Heterogeneous adjuvant treatments	yes (<0.05 for RFS)
Gasparini (1995)	127	CD31	Breast cancer	II	191	Adjuvant chemotherapy or hormone therapy	yes (<0.01 for RFS and OS in both the treatment groups)
Macaulay (1995)	128	CD31	Breast cancer	I–II	88	Adjuvant tamoxifen	yes for RFS in ER-positive cases (0.022)
Gasparini (1996)	129	CD31	Breast cancer	II	178	Adjuvant tamoxifan	yes (<0.01 for RFS and OS)
Vacca (1994)	131	fVIII-RA	Multiple myeloma	various	46	Various schedules of chemotherapy	yes (active vs non active disease 0.001)
Gasparini (1995)	106	CD31	Head and neck squamous cell carcinoma	II–IV	73	Concurrent chemo-radiation therapy	yes (CR vs non response = 0.045)
Hollingsworth (1995)	108	CD34	Ovarian cancer	III–IV	43	Platinum-based chemotherapy	yes (0.064 for OS and 0.0036 for RFS)
Van Diest (1995)	109	lectin-Ulex europaeus-I	Ovarian cancer	III–IV	49	Platinum-based chemotherapy	no (only a trend for worse OS = 0.25)
Gasparini (1996)	132	CD31	Ovarian cancer	III–IV	60	Platinum-based chemotherapy	yes (<0.01 for poor response)

studies found a significant association between vascularization and clinical outcome of the patients. Sixty % of the studies in which a multivariate analysis was performed demonstrated that IMD is an independent prognostic marker. On the basis of these results the determination of angiogenesis should be evaluated in prospective controlled clinical trials in order to verify the real prognostic value of this marker prior to potential use in clinical practice.

3. The results of 11 retrospective studies suggest that IMD may be a prognostic marker of general value also in other solid tumours. In fact, irrespectively of the tumour type studied, a significant association between IMD and prognosis has been found in the majority of the studies.

4 Preliminary studies suggest that the determination of angiogenesis may be a marker able to predict responsiveness to some forms of conventional anti-cancer therapy. An inverse relationship between the degree of vascularization and responsiveness to anti-cancer treatments has been shown both in the adjuvant setting (55,91,127,128,129) and in palliative therapy in advanced tumours (106,108,131,132).

It will be important to verify in clinical prospective and controlled clinical trials whether angiogenesis is really capable of identifying the patients with high-risk breast cancer who have the highest likelihood to benefit from adjuvant therapy. A proof of this may open the possibility to enhance the selection of patients for current conventional adjuvant treatments and, in the future, to enhance efficacy of the adjuvant therapy for breast cancer by the administration of anti-angiogenic agents (126).

Pre-clinical studies of Teicher *et al.* (122) shows that the 'two-compartment' therapy of cancer, by targeting simultaneously both parenchymal and stromal cells using conventional anti-cancer drugs and with angio-inhibitors, respectively, leads to a potentiation of the anti-tumoral activity.

In conclusion, translational research on tumour angiogenesis holds promise for a better management and for novel therapeutic approaches in patients with solid tumours (134–138).

Acknowledgements

Studies supported in part by a grant from the Associazione Italiana per la Ricerca sul Cancro (A. I. R. C.) — Milan.

References

1. Heppner, G. H. (1989). Tumor cell societies. *J. Natl Cancer Inst.*, **81**, 648–9.
2. Heppner, G. H. (1984). Tumor heterogeneity. *Cancer Res.*, **44**, 2259–65.
3. Callahan, R. and Campbell, G. (1989). Mutations in human breast cancer: an overview. *J. Natl Cancer Inst.*, **81**, 1780–1786.
4. Editorial (1987). Gene amplification in malignancy. *Lancet*, **i**, 839–40.
5. Prehen, R. T. (1994). Cancers beget mutations *versus* mutations beget cancers. *Cancer Res.*, **54**, 5296–300.
6. Nicolson, G. L. (1987). Tumor cell instability, diversification, and progression to the metastatic phenotype: from oncogene to oncofetal expression. *Cancer Res.*, **47**, 1473–87.
7. Liu, V., Farrington, S. M., Petersen, G. M., Hamilton, S. R., Persons, R., Papadopoulus, N., *et al.* (1995). Genetic instability occurs in the majority of young patients with colorectal cancer. *Nature Med.*, **1**, 348–52.
8. Gasparini, G., Pozza, F., and Harris, A. L. (1993). Evaluating the potential usefulness of new prognostic and predictive indicators in node-negative breast cancer patients. *J. Natl Cancer Inst.*, **85**, 1206–19.
9. Folkman, J. (1992). The role of angiogenesis in tumor growth. *Semin. Cancer Biol.*, **3**, 65–72.
10. Folkman, J. (1993). Tumor angiogenesis. In *Cancer medicine*, IV edn (ed. J. Holland, E. Frei, R. C. Bast, *et al.*), pp. 153–71. Lea and Febiger, Melbourne, PA.
11. Gasparini, G. and Harris, A. L. (1995). Clinical importance of the determination of tumor angiogenesis in breast carcinoma: much more than a new prognostic tool. *J. Clin. Oncol.*, **13**, 765–82.
12. Gasparini, G. (1994). Quantification of intratumoral vascularization predicts metastasis in human invasive solid tumours. *Oncol. Rep.*, **1**, 7–12.
13. Folkman, J. (1989). What is the evidence that tumors are angiogenesis dependent? *J. Natl Cancer Inst.*, **82**, 4–6.
14. RayChaudhury, A., Frazer, W. A., and D'Amore, P. A. (1994). Comparison of normal and tumorigenic endothelial cells: differences in thrombospondin production and responses to transforming growth factor-beta. *J. Cell Sci.*, **107**, 39–46.
15. Mumby, S. M., Abbott-Brown, D., Raugi, G. J., Bornstein, P. (1984). Regulation of thrombospondin secretion by cells in culture. *J. Cell Physiol.*, **120**, 280–8.
16. Wong, S. Y., Purdie, A. T., and Han, P. (1992). Thrombospondin and other possible related matrix proteins in malignant and benign breast disease. *Am. J. Pathol.*, **140**, 1473–82.
17. Brem, S. S., Gullino, P. M., and Medina, D. (1977). Angiogenesis: a marker for neoplastic transformation of mammary papillary hyperplasia. *Science*, **195**, 880–1.
18. McLeskey, S. W., Kurebayashi, J., Honig, S. F., Zwiebel, J., Lippman, M. E., Dickson, R. B., and Kern, F. G. (1993). Fibroblast growth factor 4 transfection of MCF-7 cells produces cell lines that are tumorigenic and metastatic in ovariectomized or tamoxifen-treated athymic nude mice. *Cancer Res.*, **53**, 2168–77.
19. Kandel, J., Bossy-Wetzel, E., Radvanyi, F., Klagsbrun, M., Folkman, J., and Hanahan, D. (1991). Neovascularization is associated with a switch to the export of bFGF in the multi-step development of fibrosarcoma. *Cell*, **66**, 1095–104.
20. Zhang, H-T., Craft, P., Scott, P. A. E., Ziche, M., Weilch, H. A., Harris, A. L., and Bicknell, R. (1995). Enhancement of tumor growth and vascular density by transfection of vascular endothelial cell growth factor into MCF-7 human breast carcinoma cells. *J. Natl Cancer Inst.*, **87**, 213–19.
21. Folkman, J. and Shing, Y. (1992). Angiogenesis. *J. Biol. Chem.*, **267**, 10931–4.
22. D'Amore, P. A. (1992). Capillary growth: a two-cell system. *Cancer Biol.*, **3**, 49–56.
23. Schlingemann, R. O., Rietveld, F. J. R., de Wall, R. M. W., Ferrone, S., and Ruiter, D. J. (1990). Expression of the high molecular weight melanoma-associated antigen by pericytes during angiogenesis in tumors and in healing wounds. *Am. J. Pathol.*, **136**, 1393–405.
24. Marks, R. M., Roche, W. R., Czerniecki, M., Penny, R., and Nelson, D. S. (1986). Mast cell granules cause proliferation of human microvascular endothelial cells. *Lab. Invest.*, **55**, 289–94.
25. Leibovich, S. J., Polverini, P. J., Shepard, H. M., Wiseman, D. M., Shively, V., and Nuseir, N. (1987). Macrophage-induced angiogenesis is mediated by tumour necrosis factor-α. *Nature*, **329**, 630–2.
26. Vignaud, J. M., Marie, B., Klein, N., Plenat, F., Pech, M., Borrelly, J., *et al.* (1994). The role of platelet-derived growth factor production by tumor-associated macrophages in tumor stroma formation in lung cancer. *Cancer Res.*, **54**, 5455–63.
27. Hlatky, L., Tsionou, C., Hahnfeldt, P. H., and Coleman, C. N. (1994). Mammary fibroblasts may influence breast tumor angiogenesis via hypoxia-induced vascular endothelial growth factor up-regulation and protein expression. *Cancer Res.*, **54**, 6083–6.
28. Pertovaara, L., Kaipainen, A., Mustonen, T., Orpana, A., Ferrara, N., Saksela, O., and Alitalo, K. (1994). Vascular

endothelial growth factor is induced in response to transforming growth factor-β in fibroblastic and epithelial cells. *J. Biol. Chem.*, **269**, 6271–4.

29. Dameron, K. M., Volpert, O. V., Tainsky, M. A., and Bouck, N. (1994). Control of angiogenesis in fibroblasts by p53 regulation of thrombospondin-1. *Science*, **265**, 1582–5.

30. Kieser, A., Wiech, H. A., Brandner, G., Marmé D., and Kolch, W. (1994). Mutant p53 potentiates protein kinase C induction of vascular endothelial growth factor expression. *Oncogene*, **9**, 963–9.

31. Okamura, K., Sato, Y., Matsuda, T., Hamanaka, R., Ono, M., Kohno, K., and Kuwano, M. (1991). Endogeneous basic fibroblast growth factor-dependent induction of collagenase and interleukin-6 in tumor necrosis factor-treated human microvascular endothelial cells. *J. Biol. Chem.*, **266**, 19162–5.

32. Mason, I. J. (1994). The ins and outs of fibroblast growth factors. *Cell*, **78**, 547–52.

33. Tuszynski, G. P., Rothman, V., Murphy, A., Siegler, K., Smith, L., Smith, S., *et al.* (1987). Thrombospondin promotes cell-substratum adhesion. *Science*, **236**, 1570–3.

34. Mumby, S. M., Abbott-Brown, D., Raugi, G. J., and Bornstein, P. (1984). Regulation of thrombospondin secretion by cells in culture. *J. Cell. Physiol.*, **120**, 280–8.

35. D'Amore, P. A. and Smith, S. R. (1993). Growth factor effects on cells of the vascular wall: a survey. *Growth Factors*, **8**, 61–75.

36. Ingber, D. E. (1991). Control of capillary growth and differentiation by extracellular matrix. Use of a tensegrity (tensional integrity) mechanism for signal processing. *Chest*, **99**, 34–40.

37. Stetler-Stevenson, W. G., Aznavoorian, S., and Liotta, L. A. (1993). Tumor cell interactions with the extracellular matrix during invasion and metastasis. *Annu. Rev. Cell Biol.*, **9**, 541–73.

38. Terranova, V. P., Hujanen, E. S., and Martin, G. R. (1986). Basement membrane and the invasive activity of metastatic tumor cells. *J. Natl Cancer Inst.*, **77**, 311–16.

39. Dvorak, H. F., Magy, J. A., Dvorak, A. M. (1991). Structure of solid tumors and their vasculature: implications for therapy with monoclonal antibodies. *Cancer Cells*, **3**, 77–84.

40. Hynes, R. O. and Lander, A. D. (1992). Contact and adhesive specificities in the associations, migrations, and targeting of cells and axons. *Cell*, **68**, 303–22.

41 Parıms, D. V., Cordell, J. L., Micklem, K., Heryet, A. R., Gatte, K. C., and Mason, D. Y. (1990). JC70: a new monoclonal antibody that detects vascular endothelium associated antigen on routinely processed tissue sections. *J. Clin. Pathol.*, **43**, 752–7.

42. Jahroudi, N. and Lynch, D. C. (1994). Endothelial-cell-specific regulation of von Willebrand factor gene expression. *Mol. Cell Biol.*, **14**, 999–1008.

43. Weidner, N., Semple, J. P., Welch, W. R., and Folkman, J. (1991). Tumor angiogenesis and metastasis — correlation in invasive breast carcinoma. *N. Engl. J. Med.*, **324**, 1–8.

44. Horak, E. R., Leek, R., Klenk, N., LeJeune, S., Smith, K., Stuart, N., *et al.* (1992). Angiogenesis, assessed by platelet/endothelial cell adhesion molecule antibodies, as indicator of node metastases and survival in breast cancer. *Lancet*, **340**, 1120–24.

45. Miettinen, M., Lindenmayer, A. E., and Chaubal, A. (1994). Endothelial cell markers CD31, CD34, and BNH9 antibody to H- and Y-antigens — evaluation of their specificity and sensitivity in the diagnosis of vascular tumors and comparison with von Willebrand factor. *Modern Pathol.*, **7**, 82–90.

46. Dumont, A. E. (1993). Factor VIII-related antigen. *J. Natl Cancer Inst.*, **85**, 674 (letter).

47. Weidner, N. (1993). Factor VIII-related antigen. *J. Natl Cancer Inst.*, **85**, 674–5 (letter).

48. Toi, M., Kashitani, J., and Tominaga, T. (1993). Tumor angiogenesis is an independent prognostic indicator in primary breast carcinoma. *Int. J. Cancer*, **55**, 371–4.

49. Wang, J. M., Kumar, S., Pye, D., Van Agthoven, A. J., Krupinski, J., and Hunter, R. D. (1993). A monoclonal antibody detects heterogeneity in vascular endothelium of tumours and normal tissues. *Int. J. Cancer*, **54**, 363–70.

50. Wang, J. M., Kumar, S., Pye, D., Haboubi, N., and Al-Nakib, L. (1994). Breast carcinoma: comparative study of tumor vasculature using two endothelial cell markers. *J. Natl Cancer Inst.*, **86**, 386–8.

51. Burrows, F. J., Derbyshire, E. J., Tazzari, P. L., Amlot, P., Gazdar, A. F., King, S. W. *et al.* (1995). Up-regulation of endoglin on vascular endothelial cells in human solid tumors: Implications for diagnosis and therapy. *Clin. Cancer Res.*, **1**, 1623–34.

52. Thorpe, P. E., Derbyshire, E. J., King, S. W., and Burrows, F. J. (1994). Targeting the vasculature of carcinoma and other solid tumors. *Proc. Am. Assoc. Cancer Res.*, **35**, 379 (Abstr. 2260).

53. Vermeulen, P. B., Gasparini, G., Fox, S. B., Toi, M., Martin, L., McCulloch, P., *et al.* (1996). Quantification of angiogenesis in solid human tumours: An international consensus on the methodology and criteria of evaluation. *Eur. J. Cancer*, **32A**, 2474–84.

54. Li, V. W., Folkerth, R. D., Watanabe, H., Yu, C., Rupnick, M., Barnes, P., *et al.* (1994). Microvessel count and cerebrospinal fluid basic fibroblast growth factor in children with brain tumours. *Lancet*, **344**, 82–6.

55. Toi, M., Inada, K., Suzuki, H., and Tominaga, T. (1995). Tumor angiogenesis in breast cancer: its importance as a prognostic indicator and the association with vascular endothelial growth factor expression. *Breast Cancer Res. Treatment*, **36**, 193–204.

56. Fox, S. B., Stuart, N., Smith, K., Brunner, N., and Harris, A. L. (1993). High levels of uPA and PAI-1 are associated with highly angiogenic breast carcinoma. *J. Pathol.*, **170** (Suppl.), 388 (Abstr.).

57. Gasparini, G. (1996). Clinical significance of the determination of angiogenesis in human breast cancer. Update of the biological background and overview of the Vicenza studies. *Eur. J. Cancer*, **32A**, 2485–93.

58. Van Hoef, M. E. H. N., Knox, W. F., Dhesi, S. S., Howell, A., and Schor, A. M. (1993). Assessment of tumour vascularity as a prognostic factor in lymph node negative invasive breast cancer. *Eur. J. Cancer*, **29A**, 1141–5.

59. Weidner, N. (1995). Intratumoral microvessel density as a prognostic factor in cancer. *Am. J. Pathol.*, **147**, 1–11.

60. Carnochan, P., Briggs, J. C., Westbury, G., and Davies, A. J. S. (1991). The vascularity of cutaneous melanoma: a quantitative histological study of lesions 0.85–1.25 mm in thickness. *Br. J. Cancer*, **67**, 102–7.

61. Barbareschi, M., Gasparini, G., Weidner, N., Morelli, L., Forti, S., Eccher, C., *et al.* (1995). Microvessel density quantification in breast carcinomas: assessment by light

microscopy vs a computer-aided image analysis system. *Appl. Immunohistochem.*, **3**, 75–84.

62. Fox, S. B., Leek, R. D., Weekes, M. P., Whitehouse, R. M., Gatter, K. C., and Harris, A. L. (1995). Quantitation and prognostic value of breast cancer angiogenesis: Comparison of microvessel density, Chalkley count and computer image analysis. *J. Pathol.*, **177**, 275–83.

63. Gasparini, G. (1995). Biological and clinical role of angiogenesis in breast cancer. *Breast Cancer Res. Treatment*, **36**, 103–7.

64. Barbareschi, M., Gasparini, G., Morelli, L., Forti, S., and Dalla Palma, P. (1995). Novel methods for the determination of the angiogenic activity of human tumors. *Breast Cancer Res. Treatment*, **36**, 181–92.

65. Nguyen, M., Watanabe, H., Budson, A. E., Richie, J. P., Hayes, D. F., and Folkman, J. (1994). Elevated levels of an angiogenic peptide, basic fibroblast growth factor, in the urine of patients with a wide spectrum of cancers. *J. Natl Cancer Inst.*, **86**, 356–61.

66. Nathan, F. E., Hernandez, E., Dunton, C. J., Treat, J., Switalska, H. I., Joseph, R. R., and Tsuzynski, G. P. (1994). Plasma thrombospondin levels in patients with gynecologic malignancies. *Cancer*, **73**, 2853–8.

67. Mahadevan, V. and Hart, I. R. (1991). Tumour angiogenesis and metastasis. *Eur. J. Cancer*, **27**, 679–80.

68. Zetter, B. R. (1988). Angiogenesis. State of the art. *Chest*, **93**, 15S–66S.

69. Weinstat-Saslow, D., and Steeg, P. S. (1994). Angiogenesis and colonization in the tumor metastatic process: basic and applied advances. *FASEB J.*, **8**, 401–7.

70. Fidler, I. J. and Ellis, L. M. (1994). The implications of angiogenesis for the biology and therapy of cancer metastasis. *Cell*, **79**, 185–8.

71. O'Reilly, M. S., Holmgren, L., Shing, Y., Chen, C., Rosenthal, R. A., Moses, M., *et al.* (1994). Angiostatin: a novel angiogenesis inhibitor that mediates the suppression of metastases by Lewis lung carcinoma. *Cell*, **79**, 315–28.

72. Holmgren, L., O'Reilly, M. S., and Folkman, J. (1995). Dormancy of micrometastases: Balanced proliferation and apoptosis in the presence of angiogenesis suppression. *Nature Med.*, **1**, 149–53.

73. Gasparini, G., Weidner, N., Bevilacqua, P., Maluta, S., Dalla Palma, P., Caffo, O., *et al.* (1994). Tumor microvessel density, p53 expression, tumor size and peritumoral lymphatic vessel invasion are relevant prognostic markers in node-negative breast carcinoma. *J. Clin. Oncol.*, **12**, 454–66.

74. Srivastava, S., Laidler, P., Davies, R. P., Horgan, K., and Hughes, L. E. (1988). The prognostic significance of tumor vascularity in intermediate-thickness (0.76–4.0 mm thick) skin melanoma. *Am. J. Pathol.*, **133**, 419–23.

75. Wakui, S., Furusato, M., Itoh, T., Sasaki, H., Akiyama, A., Kinoshita, I., *et al.* (1992). Tumour angiogenesis in prostatic carcinoma with and without bone marrow metastasis: a morphometric study. *J. Pathol.*, **168**, 257–62.

76. Macchiarini, P., Fontanini, G., Hardin, M. J., Squartini, F., and Angeletti, C. A. (1992). Relation of neovascularisation to metastasis of non-small-cell lung cancer. *Lancet*, **340**, 145–6.

77. Sneige, N., Singletary, E., Sahin, A., and El-Nagger, A. (1992). Multiparameter analysis of potential prognostic factors in node negative breast cancer patients. 1992 Annual Meeting of the US and Canadian Academy of Pathology. *Modern Pathol.*, **1**, 18A (Abstr. 96).

78. Sahin, A., Sneige, N., Singletary, E., and Ayala, A. (1992). Tumor angiogenesis detected by factor-VIII immunostaining in node-negative breast carcinoma (NNBC): a possible predictor of distant metastasis. Annual Meeting of the US and Canadian Academy of Pathology. *Modern Pathol.*, **1**, 17A (Abstr. 93).

79. Hall, N. R., Fish, D. E., Hunt, N., Goldin, R. D., Gullino, P. J., and Monson, J. R. T. (1992). Is the relationship between angiogenesis and metastasis real? *Surg. Oncol.*, **1**, 223–9.

80. Weidner, N., Carroll, P. R., Flax, J., Blumenfeld, W., and Folkman, J. (1993). Tumor angiogenesis correlates with metastasis in invasive prostate carcinoma. *Am. J. Pathol.*, **143**, 401–9.

81. Gasparini, G., Weidner, N., Maluta, S., Pozza, F., Boracchi, P., Mezzetti, M., *et al.* (1993). Intratumoral microvessel density and p53 protein: Correlation with metastasis in head-and-neck squamous-cell carcinoma. *Int. J. Cancer*, **55**, 739–44.

82. Olivarez, D., Ulbright, T., DeRiese, W., Foster, R., Reister, T., Einhorn, L., and Sledge, G. (1994). Neovascularization in clinical stage A testicular germ cell tumor: prediction of metastatic disease. *Cancer Res.*, **54**, 2800–2.

83. Saclarides, T. J., Speziale, N. J., Drab, E., Szeluga, D. J., and Rubin, D. B. (1994). Tumor angiogenesis and rectal carcinoma. *Dis. Colon Rectum*, **37**, 921–6.

84. Graham, C. H., Rivers, J., Kerbel, R. S., Stankiewicz, K. S., and White, W. L. (1994). Extent of vascularization as a prognostic indicator in thin (<0.76 mm) malignant melanomas. *Am. J. Pathol.*, **145**, 510–14.

85. Yamazaki, K., Abe, S., Takekawa, H., Sukoh, N., Watanabe, N., Ogura, S., *et al.* (1994). Tumor angiogenesis in human lung adenocarcinoma. *Cancer*, **74**, 2245–50.

86. Jaeger, T. M., Weidner, N., Chew, K., Moore, D. H., Kerschmann, R. L., Waldman, F. M., and Carroll, P. R. (1994). Tumor angiogenesis and lymph node metastases in invasive bladder carcinoma. *J. Urol.*, **151**, 348a (Abstr. 482).

87. Maeda, K., Chung, Y-S., Takasuka, S., Ogawa, Y., Sawada, T., Yamashita, Y., *et al.* (1995). Tumor angiogenesis as a predictor of recurrence in gastric carcinoma. *J. Clin. Oncol.*, **13**, 477–81.

88. McGuire, W. L. (1991). Breast cancer prognostic factors: Evaluation guidelines. *J. Natl Cancer Inst.*, **83**, 154–5.

89. Guidi, A. J., Fisher, L., Harris, J. R., and Schnitt, S. J. (1994). Microvessel density and distribution in ductal carcinoma *in situ* of the breast. *J. Natl Cancer Inst.*, **86**, 614–19.

90. Folkman, J., Watson, K., Ingber, D., and Hanahan, D. (1989). Induction of angiogenesis during the transition from hyperplasia to neoplasia. *Nature*, **339**, 58–61.

91. Weidner, N., Folkman, J., Pozza, F., Bevilacqua, P., Allred, E. N., Moore, D. H., Meli, S., and Gasparini, G. (1992). Tumor angiogenesis: a new significant and independent prognostic indicator in early-stage breast carcinoma. *J. Natl Cancer Inst.*, **84**, 1875–87.

92. Bosari, A., Lee, K. C., DeLellis, R. A., Wiley, B. D., Heatley, G. J., and Silverman, M. L. (1992). Microvessel quantification and prognosis in invasive breast carcinoma. *Hum. Pathol.*, **23**, 755–61.

93. Visscher, D. W., Smilanetz, S., Drozdowicz, S., and Wykes, S. M. (1993). Prognostic significance of image

morphometric microvessel enumeration in breast carcinoma. *Anal. Quant. Cytol. Histol.*, **15**, 88–92.

94. Khanuja, P. S., Gimotty, P., Fregene, T., George, J., and Pienta, K. J. (1993). Angiogenesis quantitation as a prognostic factor for primary breast carcinoma 2 cms or less. In *Adjuvant therapy of cancer*, VII (ed. S. E. Salmon), pp. 226–32. J. B. Lippincott, Philadelphia.

95. Obermair, A., Czerwenka, K., Kurz, C., Buxhaum, P., Schemper, M., and Sevelda, P. (1994). Influence of tumoral microvessel density on the recurrence-free survival in human breast cancer: preliminary results. *Onkologie*, **17**, 44–49.

96. Obermair, A., Kurz, C., Czerwenka, K., Thoma, M., Kaider, A., Wagner, T., *et al.* (1995). Microvessel density and vessel invasion in lymph-node negative breast cancer: Effect on recurrence-free survival. *Int. J. Cancer*, **62**, 126–31.

97. Conner, M. G., Crowe, D. R., Sellers, M. T., Beenken, S. W., Soong, S. J., Urist, M., *et al.* (1994). Pathologic and molecular prognostic factors in breast carcinoma: a 16 year follow-up. Proceedings of the 1994 Annual Meeting of the US and Canadian Academy of Pathology. *Modern Pathol.*, **7**, 14 (Abstr. 61).

98. Sightler, H. E., Borowsky, A. D., Dupont, W. D., Page, D. L., and Jensen, R. A. (1994). Evaluation of tumor angiogenesis as a prognostic marker in breast cancer. Proceedings of the 1994 Annual Meeting of the US and Canadian Academy of Pathology. *Modern Pathol.*, **7**, 22 (Abstr. 107).

99. Simpson, J. F., Ahn, C., Battifora, H., and Esteban, J. M. (1994). Vascular surface area as a prognostic indicator in invasive breast carcinoma. Proceedings of the 1994 Annual Meeting of the US and Canadian Academy of Pathology. *Modern Pathol.*, 7, 22 (Abstr. 108).

100. Bundred, N. J., Bowcott, M., Walls, J., Faragher, E. B., and Knox, F. (1994). Angiogenesis in breast cancer predicts node metastases and survival. *Br. J. Surg.*, **81**, 768 (Abstr.).

101. Ogawa, Y., Chung, Y-S., Nakata, B., Takatsuka, S., Maeda, K., Saeada, T., *et al.* (1995). Microvessel quantitation in invasive breast cancer by staining for factor VIII-related antigen. *Br. J. Cancer*, **71**, 1297–301.

102. Vermeulen, P. B., Hellemans, P., Verhoeven, D., VanDam, P., Goovaerts, G., Van Marck, E., *et al.* (1995). Determination of tumor microvessel density in lymph-node negative breast carcinoma. Does it have prognostic value? *Proc. Am. Assoc. Cancer Res.*, **36**, 87 (Abstr. 522).

103. Axelsson, K., Ljung, B-M. E., Moore II, D. H., Thor, A. D., Chew, K. L., Edgerton, S. M., *et al.* (1995). Tumor angiogenesis as a prognostic assay for invasive ductal breast carcinoma. *J. Natl Cancer Inst.*, **87**, 997–1008.

104. Vesalainen, S., Lipponen, P., Talja, M., Alhava, E., and Syrjanen, K. (1994). Tumor vascularity and basement membrane structure as prognostic factors in T1-2MO prostatic adenocarcinoma. *Anticancer Res.*, **14**, 709–14.

105. Bochner, B. H., Cote, R. J., Weidner, N., Groshen, S., Chen, S-C., Skinner, D. G., *et al.* (1995). Angiogenesis in bladder cancer: relationship between microvessel density and tumor prognosis. *J. Natl Cancer Inst.*, **87**, 1603–12.

106. Gasparini, G., Bevilacqua, P., Bonoldi, E., Testolin, A., Galassi, A., Verderio, P., *et al.* (1995). Predictive and prognostic markers in a series of patients with head and neck squamous-cell invasive carcinoma treated with concurrent chemoradiation-therapy. *Clin. Cancer Res.*, **1** 1375–83.

107. Williams, J. K., Carlson, G. W., Cohen, C., Derose, P. B., Hunter, S., and Jurkiewicz, M. J. (1994). Tumor angiogenesis as prognostic factor in oral cavity tumors. *Am. J. Surg.*, **168**, 373–80.

108. Hollingsworth, H. C., Kohn, E. C., Steinberg, S. M., Rothenberg, M. L., and Merino, M. J. (1995). Tumor angiogenesis in advanced stage ovarian carcinoma. *Am. J. Pathol.*, **147**, 33–41.

109. Van Diest, P. J., Zevering, J. P., Zevering, L. C., and Baak, J. P. A. (1995). Prognostic value of microvessel quantitation in cisplatin treated Figs 3 and 4 ovarian cancer patients. *Pathol. Res. Pract.*, **191**, 25–30.

110. Horwitz, A. F. and Thiery, J. P. (1994). Cell-to-cell contact and extracellular matrix. *Cell Biol.*, **6**, 645–7.

111. Van den Hoof, A. (1991). The role of stromal cells in tumor metastasis: a new link. *Cancer Cells*, **3**, 186–7.

112. Liotta, L. A. (1986). Tumor invasion and metastases — role of the extracellular matrix: Rhoads Memorial Award Lecture. *Cancer Res.*, **46**, 1–7.

113. Rak, J. W., and Kerbel, R. S. (1996). Reciprocal paracrine interactions between tumour cells and endothelial cells: The 'angiogenesis progression' hypothesis. *Eur. J. Cancer*, **32A**, 2438–50.

114. Folkman, J. (1971). Tumor angiogenesis: therapeutic implications. *N. Engl. J. Med.*, **285**, 1182–6.

115. Gullino, P. M., Clark, S. H., and Grantham, F. H. (1964). The interstitial fluid of solid tumors. *Cancer Res.*, **5**, 780–98.

116. Jain, R. K. (1987). Transport of molecules in the tumor interstitium: a review. *Cancer Res.*, **47**, 3039–51.

117. Butler, T. P. and Guillino, P. M. (1975). Quantitation of cell shedding into efferent blood of mammary adenocarcinoma. *Cancer Res.*, **35**, 512–16.

118. Dvorak, H. F., Magy, J. A., and Dvorak, A. M. (1991). Structure of solid tumors and their vasculature: implications for therapy with monoclonal antibodies. *Cancer Cells*, **3**, 77–84.

119. Cordon-Cardo, C., O'Brien, J. P., Boccia, J., Casals, D., Bertino, J. R., and Melaned, M. R. (1990). Expression of the multidrug resistance gene product (P-glycoprotein) in human normal and tumor tissues. *J. Histochem. Cytochem.*, **38**, 1277–87.

120. Huang, A. and Wright, J. A. (1994). Fibroblast growth factor mediated alterations in drug resistance, and evidence of gene amplification. *Oncogene*, **9**, 491–9.

121. Mc Leskey, S. W., Kurebeyashi, J., and Honig, S. F. (1993). Fibroblast growth factor-4 transfection of MCF-7 cells produces cell lines that are tumorigenic and metastatic in ovariectomized and on tamoxiten-treated athymic nude mice. *Cancer Res.*, **53**, 2168–77.

122. Teicher, B. A., Sotomayor, E. A., and Huang, Z. D. (1992). Antiangiogenic agents potentiate cytotoxic cancer therapies against primary and metastatic disease. *Cancer Res*, **52**, 6702–4.

123. Teicher, B. A., Holden, S. A., Dupuis, N. P., Kakeji, Y., Ikebe, M., Emi, Y., and Goff, D. (1995). Potentiation of cytotoxic therapies by TNP-470 and minocycline in mice bearing EMT-6 mammary carcinoma. *Breast Cancer Res. Treatment*, **36**, 227–36.

124. Yamaoka, M., Yamamoto, T., Masaki, T., Ikeyama, S., Sudo, M., Fujita, T. (1993). Inhibition of tumor growth and metastasis of rodent tumors by the angiogenesis inhibitor O-(chlorocetyl-carbomoyl)fumagillol (TNP-470; AGM-1470). *Cancer Res.*, **53**, 4262–7.

125. Gasparini, G. and Harris, A. L. (1994). Does improved control of tumour growth require an anti-cancer therapy targeting both neoplastic and intratumoral endothelial cells? *Eur. J. Cancer*, **30A**, 201–6.

126. Folkman, J. (1995). Tumor angiogenesis in women with node-positive breast cancer. *Cancer J. Sci. Am.*, **1**, 106–8.

127. Gasparini, G., Barbareschi, M., Boracchi, P., Verderio, P., Caffo, O., Meli, S., *et al.* (1995). Tumor angiogenesis predicts clinical outcome of node-positive breast cancer patients treated either with adjuvant hormone therapy or chemotherapy. *Cancer J. Sci. Am.*, **1**, 131–41.

128. Macaulay, V. M., Fox, S. B., Zhang, H., Whitehouse, R. M., Leek, R. D., Gatter, K. C., *et al.* (1995). Breast cancer angiogenesis and tamoxifen resistance. *Endocrine-related Cancer*, **2**, 97–103.

129. Gasparini, G., Fox, S. B., Verderio, P., Bonoldi, E., Bevilacqua, P., Boracchi, P., *et al.* (1996). Angiogenesis adds information to estrogen receptor status in predicting the efficacy of adjuvant tamoxifen in node-positive breast cancer patients. *Clin. Cancer Res.*, **2**, 1191–8.

130. Gasparini, G., Bevilacqua, P., Pozza, F., Meli, S., and Weidner, N. (1993). P-glycoprotein expression predicts response to chemotherapy in previously untreated advanced breast cancer. *Breast*, **2**, 27–32.

131. Vacca, A., Ribatti, D., Roncati, L., Ranier, G., Serio, G., Silvestrini, F., and Dammacco, F. (1994). Bone marrow angiogenesis and progression in multiple myeloma. *Br. J. Haematol.*, **87**, 503–8.

132. Gasparini, G., Bonoldi, E., Viale, G., Verderio, P., Boracchi, P., Panizzoni, G. A., *et al.* (1996). Prognostic and predictive value of tumour angiogenesis in ovarian carcinomas. *Int. J. Cancer (Pred. Oncol.)*, **69**, 205–11.

133. Simpson, J. F. and Battifora, H. (1995). Angiogenesis as a prognostic factor in breast cancer: Can we count on it? *Appl. Immunoistochem.*, **3**, 73–4.

134. Gasparini, G. (1995). Angiogenesis in preneoplastic and neoplastic lesions. *Cancer J.*, **8**, 91–3.

135. Ellis, L. M. and Fidler, I. J. (1995). Angiogenesis and breast cancer metastasis. *Lancet*, **346**, 388–90.

136. Fan, T-P. D., Jaggar, R., and Bicknell, R. (1995). Controlling the vasculature: Angiogenesis, anti-angiogenesis and vascular targeting of gene therapy. *TIPS*, **16**, 57–66.

137. Gasparini, G. (1996). Angiogenesis research up to 1996. A commentary on the state of the art and suggestions for future studies. *Eur. J. Cancer*, **32A**, 2379–85.

138. Folkman, J. (1995). Clinical applications of research on angiogenesis. *N. Engl. J. Med.*, **333**, 1757–63.

5. Vascular and interstitial physiology of tumours: role in cancer detection and treatment

Rakesh K. Jain

Introduction

Cancer is the second leading cause of death in the United States and in many industrialized countries (1). After the primary tumour has been surgically removed and/or sterilized by radiation, the residual disease is usually managed with a variety of systemic therapies (Table 5.1). For these therapies to be successful, they must satisfy two requirements: (i) the relevant agent must be effective in the *in vivo* microenvironment of tumours, and (ii) this agent must reach the target cells *in vivo* in optimal quantities. The goal of this article is to examine the latter issue. More specifically, I will discuss the pathophysiology of the tumour vasculature and interstitium, and the important part it plays in the delivery of diagnostic and therapeutic agents to solid tumours.

All conventional and novel therapeutic agents can be divided into three categories: molecules, particles and cells (Table 5.1). A blood-borne molecule or particle that enters the tumour vasculature reaches cancer cells via dis-

tribution through the vascular compartment, transport across the microvascular wall, and transport through the interstitial compartment. For a molecule of given size, charge, and configuration, each of these transport processes may involve diffusion and convection. In addition, during the journey the molecule may bind non-specifically to proteins or other tissue components, bind specifically to the target(s), or be metabolized (2). Although lymphokine-activated killer (LAK) cells [lymphocytes activated by the lymphokine interleukin (IL) 2] or tumour-infiltrating lymphocytes (TIL) are capable of deformation, adhesion, and migration, they encounter the same barriers that restrict their movement in tumours. Some of these physiological parameters are also important for heat transfer in normal and tumour tissues during hyperthermic treatment of cancer (3).

The overall aim of this chapter is to discuss how the tumour pathophysiology affects each of the above-mentioned steps involved in the delivery of various agents. More specifically, I will describe recent findings on: (i) how angiogenic vessels function and what determines blood flow heterogeneities in tumours; (ii) how blood flow influences the metabolic microenvironment in tumours, and how microenvironment affects the physiological properties of tumours (*e.g.* vascular permeability); (iii) how material moves across the microvascular wall; and (iv) how it moves through the interstitial compartment and the lymphatics. In addition, I will point out the role of cell deformation and adhesion in the delivery of cells. Following analysis of these processes for molecules, particles and cells, I will integrate this information in a unified framework for scale-up from mice to humans (Fig. 5.1). In this article, I will briefly describe various experimental and theoretical approaches, recent findings in these six areas, and finally, how we can take some of these concepts from bench to bedside for potential improvement in cancer detection and treatment.

Table 5.1 Systemic therapy of cancer. Agents used in various conventional and novel therapies can be divided into three categories: molecules, particles, and cells.

Therapy	Agent		
	Molecules	Particles	Cells
Radiotherapy	✓	✓	
Chemotherapy	✓	✓	
Immunotherapy	✓	✓	✓
Gene therapy	✓	✓	✓
Hyperthermia	✓		
Photodynamictherapy	✓	✓	

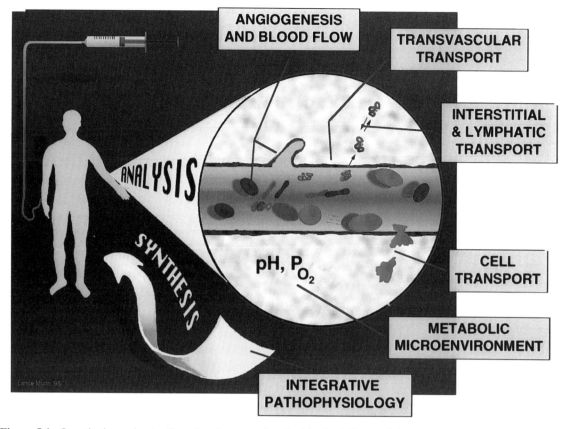

Figure 5.1. Quantitative understanding of various steps involved in the delivery of therapeutic agents can be achieved by analysing the underlying processes and then integrating the resulting information in a unified framework.

Experimental and theoretical approaches

The following four approaches have been used by various investigators to gain insight into the pathophysiology of solid tumours:

1. A tissue-isolated tumour which is connected to the host's circulation by a single artery and a single vein (4,5). This technique was originally developed by P. M. Gullino at the National Cancer Institute in 1961 for rat (6); we have recently adapted it to mice (7,8) and humans (9).

2. A modified Sandison rabbit ear chamber (10,11), a modified Algire mouse dorsal chamber (12,13), and a cranial window in mice and rats (14). The ear chamber has the advantage of superior optical quality and the mice of working with immunodeficient and genetically engineered animals. Recently, we have developed a quantitative angiogenesis assay using these windows to study the physiology of vessels modified by individual growth factors (15) (Fig. 5.2). One can also perfuse single vessels of tumours in these windows (16).

3. *In vitro* methods to assess the deformability and adhesion of normal and neoplastic cells (17–20), as well as measurements of adhesion molecules' expression in intact monolayers (21) (Fig. 5.3).

4. Mathematical models to describe and integrate the data obtained from the above three approaches, to scale up biodistribution data from mice to humans, and to design future experiments (22–35).

While each of these approaches has its limitations, it is their combination that has permitted us to develop the framework for tumour pathophysiology described in this article.

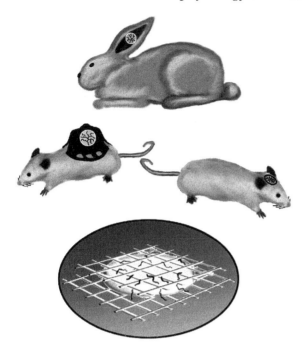

Figure 5.2. Various microcirculatory preparations used to study delivery of therapeutic agents in solid tumours: (a) Sandison window in the rabbit ear (11); (b) Algire window in the dorsal skin of rodents (12); (c) cranial window in rodents (14); and (d) collagen I gel, containing angiogenic factors, sandwiched between nylon mesh (3 × 3 mm) to permit the growth of blood vessels (15). These preparations allow non-invasive, continuous measurement of angiogenesis and blood flow; metabolites, such as pH, P_{O_2}; transport of molecules and particles; and cell-cell interactions *in vivo*.

Distribution through vascular space

The tumour vasculature consists of both vessels recruited from the pre-existing network of the host vasculature, and vessels resulting from the angiogenic response of host vessels to cancer cells (36,37). Movement of molecules through the vasculature is governed by the vascular morphology (*i.e.* the number, length, diameter, and geometric arrangement of various blood vessels) and the blood flow rate (27,38–40).

Although the tumour vasculature originates from the host vasculature and the mechanisms of angiogenesis are similar (37,41), its organization may be completely different depending on the tumour type, its growth rate, and its location (40). The fractal dimensions and minimum path lengths of tumour vasculature are different from those of the normal host vessels (38). The architecture and blood flow are different not only among various tumour types but also between a spontaneous tumour and its transplants (36,42). For example, unlike normal tissue, where red blood cell (RBC) velocity is dependent on vessel diameter, there is no such dependence in tumours (12,14). Furthermore, the RBC velocity may be an order of magnitude lower in tumours compared with the host vessels (Fig. 5.4). The temporal and spatial heterogeneity in tumour blood flow may, in part, be a result of elevated geometric and viscous resistance in tumour vessels (5,43,44), as well as coupling between high vascular permeability and elevated interstitial fluid pressure (35).

Based on perfusion rates, four regions can be recognized in a tumour: an avascular, necrotic region, a seminecrotic region, a stabilized microcirculation region, and an advancing front (45) (Fig. 5.5a). Intratumour blood flow distributions in spontaneous animal and human tumours are now being investigated using nuclear magnetic resonance, positron emission tomography, and functional computerized tomography (32,42,46–48). While limited, these results are in concert with the transplanted tumour studies: blood flow rates in necrotic and seminecrotic regions of tumours are low, while those in non-necrotic regions are variable and can be substantially higher than in surrounding (contralateral) host normal tissues (48). Considering these spatial and temporal heterogeneities in blood supply coupled with variations in the vascular morphology at both microscopic and macroscopic levels, it is not surprising that the spatial distribution of therapeutic agents in tumours is heterogeneous and that the average uptake decreases, in general, with an increase in tumour weight. This perfusion heterogeneity also makes it difficult to heat the high perfusion regions of a tumour during hyperthermia (3).

Metabolic microenvironment

The temporal and spatial heterogeneities in blood flow are expected to lead to a compromised metabolic microenvironment in tumours. To quantify the spatial gradients of key metabolites, we have recently adapted two optical techniques: fluorescence ratio-imaging microscopy (FRIM) and phosphorescence quenching (49–52). As shown in Fig. 5.6, both pH and P_{O_2} decrease as one moves away from tumour vessels leading to acidic and hypoxic regions in tumours. While low P_{O_2} and pH are detrimental to some therapies (*e.g.* radiation, hyperthermia), they might enhance the effect of certain drugs, if the drug could be delivered in adequate quantities in those regions (53,54).

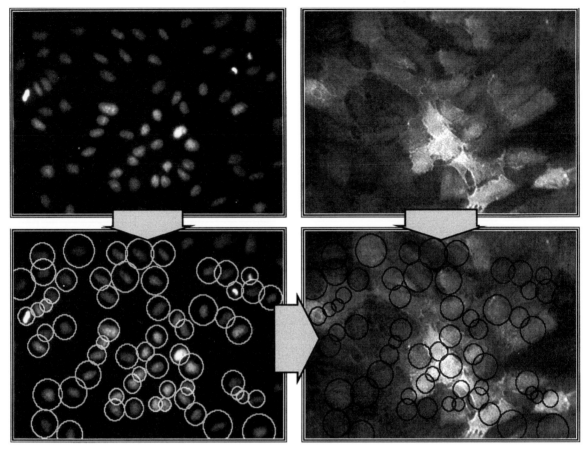

Figure 5.3. Targeted sampling fluorometry (TSF) allows the quantification of adhesion molecule expression over an intact cell monolayer on a cell-by-cell basis. At top are the two images acquired for analysis: the nuclei are stained with propidium iodide and the adhesion molecule is labelled with fluorescein using double immunostaining. The nuclei are first located in the propidium iodide channel, and regions of interest (ROIs) formed around each nucleus (bottom left); these ROIs are then applied to the immunostain image to find the fluorescence intensity in each region, corresponding to one cell. The procedure yields a histogram of intensities for the monolayer. (Adapted from reference 21.)

To gain further insight into tumour metabolism, we have combined two powerful approaches: magnetic resonance spectroscopy and tissue isolated tumours. The former allows us to measure the energy level in tumours while the latter allows us to control the supply of individual substrates (*e.g.* glucose, oxygen) to the tumour. Using this approach, we have recently shown that solid tumours depend more on glucose than oxygen to maintain their ATP level (55).

Transport across the microvascular wall

Once a blood-borne molecule has reached an exchange vessel, its extravasation, J_s (g/s), occurs by diffusion and convection and, to some extent, presumably by transcytosis (56). Diffusive flux is proportional to the exchange vessel's surface area, S (cm^2), and the difference between the plasma and interstitial concentrations, $C_p - C_i$ (g/m). Convection is proportional to the rate of fluid leakage, J_f (m/s), from the vessel. J_f, in turn, is proportional to S and the difference between the vascular and interstitial hydrostatic pressures, $P_v - P_i$ (mmHg), minus the osmotic reflection coefficient (σ) times the difference between the vascular and interstitial osmotic pressures $\pi_v - \pi_i$ (mmHg). The proportionality constant that relates transluminal diffusion flux to concentration gradients, $(C_p - C_i)$, is referred to as the vascular permeability coefficient, P (cm/s), and the constant that relates fluid leakage to pressure gradients is referred to as the hydraulic con-

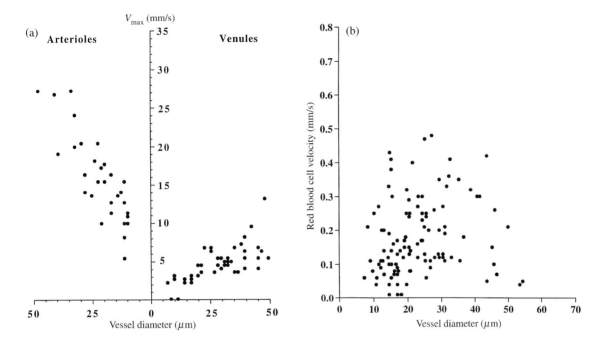

Figure 5.4. Blood velocity as a function of vessel diameter in (a) normal pial vessels, and (b) a human glioma (U87) xenograft on the pial surface. Note that in normal microcirculation, blood velocity is dependent on vessel diameter, whereas in tumours there is no such dependence. Furthermore, the blood velocity in tumour vessels is about an order of magnitude lower than in host vessels. (Adapted from reference 14.)

ductivity, L_p (cm/mmHg • s). The effectiveness of the transluminal osmotic pressure difference in producing fluid movement across a vessel wall is characterized by σ, which is close to 1 for a macromolecule and close to zero for a small molecule. Thus, the transport of a molecule across normal or tumour vessels is governed by three transport parameters (P, L_p, and σ), the surface area for exchange, and the transvascular concentration and pressure gradients.

Vascular permeability and hydraulic conductivity of tumours in general is significantly higher than that of various normal tissues (14,56–61), and hence, these vessels may lack permselectivity (62) (see Fig. 5.7a,b, in the plate section). Despite increased overall permeability, not all blood vessels of a tumour are leaky (Fig. 5.7b). Even the leaky vessels have a finite pore size, which we have been able to measure in a human colon carcinoma (LS174T) xenografted in the dorsal window (see Fig. 5.7c,d, in the plate section). Not only does the vascular permeability vary from one tumour to the next, but within the same tumour it varies both spatially and temporally (56). The local microenvironment plays an important part in controlling vascular permeability. For example, a human glioma (HGL21) is fairly leaky when grown subcutaneously in

immunodeficient mice, but it exhibits blood–brain barrier properties in the cranial window (see Fig. 5.7e,f, in the plate section). We have not seen such site-dependent differences for other tumours. Our working hypothesis is that the host–tumour interactions control the production and secretion of cytokines associated with permeability changes (e.g. vascular permeability factor (VPF) or vascular endothelial growth factor (VEGF)). A better understanding of the molecular mechanisms of permeability regulation in tumours will possibly yield strategies for improved drug delivery.

If tumour vessels are indeed 'leaky' to fluid and macromolecules, then what leads to the poor extravasation of these agents in various regions of tumours? As shown by us and others (63–75), experimental and human tumours exhibit high interstitial fluid pressure (IFP) (Table 5.2). Furthermore, the uniformly high pressure drops precipitously to normal values in the tumour's periphery or in the peritumour region (25,26,64). This may lower fluid extravasation in the high pressure regions, especially because the oncotic and hydrostatic pressures are also equal between the intravascular and extravascular space (66,76). Because the transvascular transport of macromolecules in normal tissues occurs primarily by convection (56,77),

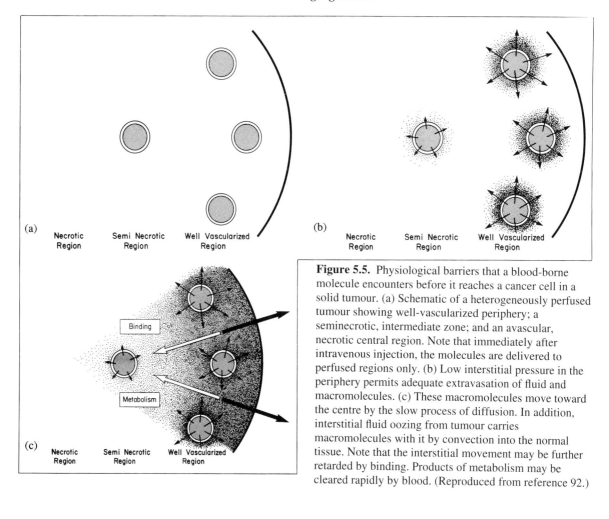

Figure 5.5. Physiological barriers that a blood-borne molecule encounters before it reaches a cancer cell in a solid tumour. (a) Schematic of a heterogeneously perfused tumour showing well-vascularized periphery; a seminecrotic, intermediate zone; and an avascular, necrotic central region. Note that immediately after intravenous injection, the molecules are delivered to perfused regions only. (b) Low interstitial pressure in the periphery permits adequate extravasation of fluid and macromolecules. (c) These macromolecules move toward the centre by the slow process of diffusion. In addition, interstitial fluid oozing from tumour carries macromolecules with it by convection into the normal tissue. Note that the interstitial movement may be further retarded by binding. Products of metabolism may be cleared rapidly by blood. (Reproduced from reference 92.)

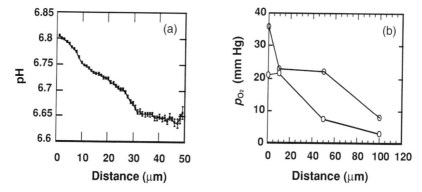

Figure 5.6. Spatial gradients of metabolites in tumours. (a) pH gradients measured using fluorescence ratio-imaging microscopy. (Adapted from reference 51.) (b) P_{O_2} gradients measured using phosphorescence quenching (Adapted from reference 52.) Distance from the vessel wall, in microns, is shown on the x-axis, with zero being the vessel wall.

Table 5.2. Interstitial fluid pressure (mmHg) in normal and neoplastic tissues in patients.

Tissue type	N	Mean	Range
Normal skin	5	0.4	−1.0–3.0
Normal breast	8	0.0	−0.5–3.0
Head/neck carcinomas	27	19.0	1.5–79.0
Cervical carcinomas	26	23.0	6.0–94.0
Lung carcinomas	26	10.0	1.0–27.0
Metastatic melanomas	14	21.0	0.0–60.0
Metastatic melanomas	12	14.5	2.0–41.0
Breast carcinomas	13	29.0	5.0–53.0
Breast carcinomas	8	15.0	4.0–33.0
Brain tumors*	17	7.0	2.0–15.0
Brain tumors*	11	1.0	−0.5–8.0
Colorectal liver mets	8	21.0	6.0–45.0
Lymphomas	7	4.5	1.0–12.5
Renal cell carcinoma	1	38.0	—

* Patients were treated with anti-edema therapy.

convective transport of macromolecules in the centre of tumours may be less than in the tumour periphery (25,26). Additionally, the average vascular surface area per unit tissue weight decreases with tumour growth, hence reduced transvascular exchange would be expected in large tumours compared with small tumours (26,27).

Transport through interstitial space and lymphatics

Once a molecule has extravasated, its movement through the interstitial space occurs by diffusion and convection (63). Diffusion is proportional to the concentration gradient in the interstitium, and convection is proportional to the interstitial fluid velocity, u_i (cm/s). The latter, in turn, is proportional to the pressure gradient in the interstitium. Just as the interstitial diffusion coefficient, D (cm^2/s), relates the diffusive flux to the concentration gradient, the interstitial hydraulic conductivity, K (cm^2/mmHg • s), relates the interstitial velocity to the pressure gradient (63). Values of these transport coefficients are determined by the structure and composition of the interstitial compartment as well as the physicochemical properties of the solute molecule (78–83).

Using fluorescence recovery after photobleaching (FRAP) D of various molecules was found to be about one-third that in water (84) and similar to that in the host tissue (83). Similarly, the value of K for a human colon carcinoma xenograft (LS174T) measured using two differ-

ent methods (85,86) was found to be higher than that of a hepatoma (78), which in turn was higher than that of the liver. Given these relatively high values of D and K, why do exogenously injected macromolecules not distribute uniformly in tumours? As discussed next, there are two reasons for this apparent paradox.

The time constant for a molecule with diffusion coefficient D to diffuse across distance L is approximately $L^2/4D$. For diffusion of immunoglobulin IgG in tumours, this time constant is on the order of 1 h for a 100-μm distance, days for a 1-mm distance, and months for a 1-cm distance. So for a 1-mm tumour, diffusional transport would take days and for a 1-cm tumour, it would take months. If the central vessels have collapsed completely due to cellular proliferation and interstitial matrix re-arrangement there would be no delivery of macromolecules by blood flow to this necrotic centre. Binding may further retard the transport in tumours (28,29,84,87–91). The role of binding is illustrated in Fig. 5.8, (see the plate section), which compares the rate of fluorescence recovery of a photobleached spot in tumour tissue injected with a non-specific vessus specific IgG. In addition to the heterogeneity in D in tumours, the most unexpected result of these photobleaching studies was the large extent (30–40%) of non-specific binding (84).

As mentioned earlier, interstitial fluid pressure is high in the centre of tumours and low in the periphery and surrounding tissue (25,26,64). Therefore, one would expect interstitial fluid motion from the tumour's periphery into the surrounding normal tissue (Fig. 5.5b,c). In various animal and human (xenograft) tumours studied to date, 6–14% of plasma entering the tumour has been found to leave from the tumour's periphery (56,92). This fluid leakage leads to a radially outward interstitial fluid velocity of 0.1–0.2 μm/s at the periphery of 1 cm 'tissue-isolated' tumour (56). (The radially outward velocity is likely to be an order of magnitude lower in a tumour grown in the subcutaneous tissue or muscle (26).) A macromolecule at the tumour periphery has to overcome this outward convection to diffuse into the tumour. The relative contribution of this mechanism of heterogeneous distribution of antibodies in tumours may be smaller than the contribution of heterogeneous extravasation due to elevated pressure and necrosis (26).

In most normal tissues, extravasated macromolecules are taken up by the lymphatics and brought back to the central circulation. Because of the lack of functional lymphatics within the tumour, the fluid and macromolecules oozing from the tumour surface must be picked by the peritumour host lymphatics (27). To characterize the transport into and within the lymphatic capillaries, a mouse tail model was recently developed (93). The uptake and transport in this model using a macroscopic approach (RTD analysis) and a microscopic approach (FRAP) have also been measured (94,95). There is a definite need to understand changes in lymphatic transport in the presence of a tumour.

Transport of cells

So far we have discussed the vascular and interstitial parameters that govern the transport of molecules and particles (*e.g.* liposomes) in tumours. When a leucocyte enters a blood vessel, it may continue to move with flowing blood, collide with the vessel wall, adhere transiently or stably, and finally extravasate. These interactions are governed by both local hydrodynamic forces and adhesive forces. The former are determined by the vessel diameter, fluid velocity, and haematocrit, and the latter by the expression, strength and kinetics of bond formation between adhesion molecules and by surface area of contact (96). Deformability of cells affects both types of forces. Despite their importance in immunotherapy and gene therapy, the determinants of cell transport in tumours have not been examined.

Using intravital microscopy, rolling of endogenous leucocytes was shown to be generally low in tumour vessels, whereas stable adhesion (≥30 s) was found to be comparable between normal and tumour vessels (Fig. 5.9a,b) (97). On the other hand, both rolling and stable adhesion are nearly zero in angiogenic vessels induced in collagen gels by bFGF or VEGF/VPF, two of the most potent angiogenic factors (15). Whether the latter is due to a low flux of leucocytes into angiogenic vessels and/or down-regulation of adhesion molecules in these immature vessels is currently not known. The age of the animal also plays an important part in leucocyte–endothelial interactions (98).

To gain further insight into the type of cells that adhere to tumour vessels, the localization of IL-2 activated natural killer (A-NK) cells in normal and tumour tissues in mice was examined using positron emission tomography (19,99). Following systemic injection, these cells localized primarily in the lungs immediately after injection and a non-detectable number of cells arrived in the tumour (19). These findings were consistent with the previous work on the deformability of these cells using micropipette aspiration technique, which showed that IL-2 activation makes these cells rigid and should lead to their mechanical entrapment in the lung microcirculation (18,100).

One approach to reduce lung entrapent is to reduce the rigidity of these cells (101). Another approach to circumvent the lung is to inject ANK cells into the blood supply of tumours. In the latter case, A-NK cells, both

Rolling leukocytes at different sites

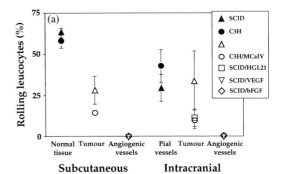

Leukocyte adherence at different sites

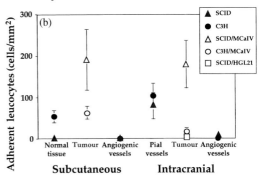

Figure 5.9. Leucocyte–endothelial interactions in normal and tumour (97) and angiogenic (15) vessels in the dorsal skin window and the cranial window: (a) rolling and (b) adhesion. Note that rolling is significantly reduced in tumour vessels compared with host vessels, while stable adhesion is similar in both vessel types. Both rolling and adhesion are negligible in angiogenic vessels.

xenogeneic and syngeneic, adhered to blood vessels in three different tumour models (19,102,103). These results also supported the hypothesis that the endogenous cells that adhere to tumour vessels after systemic IL-2 injection are mostly activated lymphocytes (104).

To find out the adhesion molecules involved in the A-NK cell adhesion to tumour vessels, two *in vitro* approaches were used. In the first approach, the tumour vasculature was simulated *in vitro*, by incubating the human umbilical vein endothelial cells (HUVECs) in the tumour interstitial fluid collected using a micropore chamber (6,24,53,105). Using targeted sampling fluorometry (Fig. 5.3), the expression of relevant adhesion molecules on the HUVEC monolayers was quantified (21). A flow chamber was utilized to determine the relative contributions of these molecules in adhesion under physiological flow conditions (20). Molecules up-regulated on the HUVECs include ICAM-1 and VCAM-1, which bind to CD18 and VLA-4 on the A-NK cells. Sporadic upregulation of E-selection was also observed. The role of these molecules *in vivo* was confirmed by treating A-NK cells with antibodies against CD18 and VLA-4 prior to injecting them into the arterial supply of tumours. As in the *in vitro* studies, blocking these adhesion molecules nearly eliminated the adhesion of A-NK cells to tumour vessels (105).

What leads to the up-regulation of these molecules in the tumour vasculature? These molecules can be up-regulated by tumour necrosis factor (TNF) α and a protein of 90 kDa molecular weight (p90) secreted by some neoplastic cells (96,106), and down-regulated by transforming growth factor (TGB) β (107–109). Are there other molecules present in the tumour milieu that are also inducing this up-regulation? As tumour growth and metastasis are angiogenesis dependent, two most potent angiogenic molecules — basic fibroblast growth factor (bFGF) and VEGF/VPF — were investigated (37,110). VEGF was found to mimic tumour interstitial fluid, and up-regulate these molecules. bFGF, on the other hand, exhibited no effect when used alone, but abrogated the up-regulation induced by VEGF or TNF-α (105). These findings are in concert with earlier reports that bFGF retards the transmigration of lymphocytes across the endothelial monolayer (111) and reduces adhesion of endothelial cells to collagen (112). They also offer a possible explanation for lower leucocyte–endothelial interactions in tumours; bFGF might have down-regulated adhesion molecules in these tumours. More efforts are now needed for defining interactions between angiogenic and adhesion molecules using various *in vitro* and *in vivo* approaches, including genetically engineered mice (113).

Pharmacokinetic modelling

So far we have analysed each of the steps in the delivery of molecules and cells to and within solid tumours. Can we take this information and integrate it in a unified framework? We and others have been successful to some extent in this endeavour, using physiologically based pharmacokinetic modelling. This approach, pioneered by K. Bischoff and R. L. Dedrick in the 1960s, has been applied successfully to describe and scale up the biodistribution of low molecular weight agents [for a review, see references (3,114,115)]. Recently, this approach has been extended to macromolecules and cells (31,33,116).

In this approach, a mammalian body is represented by a number of physiological compartments interconnected anatomically (Fig. 5.10). The volume and blood flow rate

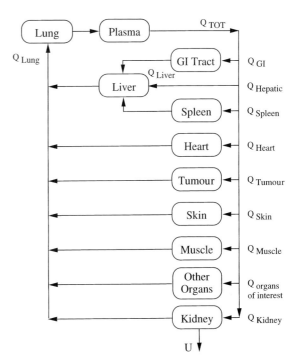

Figure 5.10. Schematic of physiologically based kinetic model to describe the biodistribution of molecules and cells in a mammalian system. Such an approach permits interspecies scale-up of biodistribution. (Adapted from reference 33.)

to each of these compartments/organs are known or can be measured. The parameters that characterize transport across the subcompartments (i.e. vascular, interstitial and cellular) and the metabolism of various agents are not generally known and cannot be easily measured. The usual approach is to use as many measured parameters as possible and estimate the remaining parameters by fitting the model to the murine biodistribution data. By scaling-up the parameters using well-defined scale-up laws (114), one can then predict the biodistribution in human patients and compare with clinical data. Discrepancies between predictions and actual data can help in identifying interspecies differences and to question the model assumptions. This is an evolutionary process — as the understanding of underlying physiology and biochemistry improves, the relevant parameters are modified and the model is refined further. The model is useful not only for designing murine experiments and/or clinical trials, but also in identifying the sensitive parameters that need careful measurement and analysis. If one needs detailed spatial information about a tissue/organ, then a distributed parameter model for that organ, *e.g.* tumour (22,26–29,31,33,117,118) is developed.

While simple in principle, this cyclic approach of analysis and synthesis has served as a useful paradigm for developing a deeper understanding of drug and cell distribution in normal and malignant tissues. The level of sophistication of these models is likely to improve with the understanding of underlying principles (39).

Bench to bedside

The vascular and interstitial factors that contribute to the poor delivery of therapeutic agents to tumours include heterogeneous blood supply, interstitial hypertension, relatively long transport distances in the interstitium, and cellular heterogeneities (Fig. 5.5). How can these physiological barriers be exploited or overcome? Can we take our findings about these barriers from the bench to the bedside? Two recently developed strategies that have the potential to improve the detection and treatment of solid tumours in patients are described here.

As stated earlier, all solid tumours in patients exhibit interstitial hypertension (Table 5.2), provided the patient has not received any anti-oedema treatment (72). We have also shown theoretically and confirmed experimentally that IFP rises quite steeply in the tumour boundary (25,64). We have used this knowledge in improving the design of the needle used by radiologists to localize the tumour for sur-

gical excision (119). We can facilitate the needle placement in a tumour by placing a pressure-sensor in the needle. As tumours begin to exhibit interstitial hypertension almost from the onset of angiogenesis, this needle may be able to help in localizing early disease. The same concept may be useful in optimizing location and infusion pressure of needles employed in intratumour infusion of therapeutic agents (86), and for monitoring the response to therapy (73).

Several physical (*e.g.* radiation, heat) and chemical (*e.g.* vasoactive drugs) agents may lead to an increase in tumour blood flow or vascular permeability (42,56,120,121), or lower pH (53,54). Another approach may be based on increasing the interstitial transport rate of molecules by increasing K or D enzymatically (78,86,92) or using multistep approaches (30,31,122). Several physical and chemical agents have been used to lower IFP in tumours (12,85,123–128). As microvascular and interstitial pressure in tumours are approximately equal, any change in one is followed rapidly by a similar change in the other, and thus the convective enhancement disappears rapidly (34,66,129,130). By adapting a poroelastic model to solid tumours, we have calculated theoretically and confirmed experimentally that the time constant of pressure transmission across the tumour vasculature is on the order of 10 s (34). During such a short time the convective enhancement is calculated to be very small (~ 1%). However, if the vas-

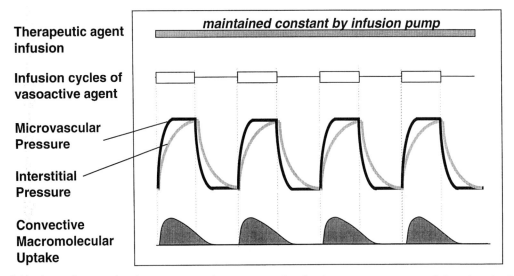

Figure 5.11. A novel approach to increase convective transport of molecules across tumour vessels based on the finding that there is a ~ 10 second delay in the transmission of intravascular pressure to the interstitial compartment. For this approach to work, the transvascular transport has to be unidirectional *or* the extravasated molecule must bind avidly so that it does not intravasate when the intravascular pressure is lower than interstitial pressure. (Adapted from reference 34.)

cular pressure is increased repeatedly and if the trans-vascular transport is unidirectional or if the molecule binds avidly in the extravascular region, then one can, in principle, increase drug delivery to solid tumours significantly (Fig. 5.11).

In contrast, the physiological barriers discussed here may be less of a problem for: (i) radioimmunodetection; (ii) treating leukaemias, lymphomas, and small tumours (*e.g.* micrometastases), in which the physiological barriers are not yet fully established; (iii) treatment of adequately perfused, low-pressure regions of large tumours; and (iv) treatment with antibodies or other agents directed against the host cells (*e.g.* tumour endothelial cells, fibroblasts) or the subendothelial matrix. These physiological barriers also may pose less problems for treatment with a molecule or cell that has nearly 100% specificity for cancer cells. While such selective molecules or cells are being developed, methods are urgently needed to overcome or exploit these physiological barriers in tumours. It is hoped that an improved understanding of the pathophysiology of tumours will help in developing these strategies.

Summary and conclusions

To reach cancer cells in a tumour, a blood-borne diagnostic or therapeutic agent must make its way into the blood vessels of the tumour and across the vessel wall into the interstitium, and finally migrate through the interstitium. Unfortunately, solid tumours often develop in ways that hinder each of these steps. Our research goals are to analyse each of these steps experimentally and theoretically, and then integrate the resulting information in a unified theoretical framework. This paradigm of analysis and synthesis has allowed us to obtain a better understanding of physiological barriers in solid tumours, and to develop novel strategies to exploit and/or overcome these barriers for improved cancer detection and treatment.

Acknowledgements

A slightly modified version of this article was published as the Whitaker Distinguished Lecture in the *Annals of Biomedical Engineering*, **24**, 457–73, 1996. I thank Blackwell Science Ltd and the Biomedical Engineering Society for allowing me to reproduce this article. I also thank Carol Lyons and Gerry Mullouny for typing this manuscript, Larry Baxter and Yuval Gazit for their help with the references, Lance Munn for his help with Figs 5.1–5.3, Fan Yuan with Figs 5.4 and 5.7, Gabriel Helmlinger with Fig. 5.6, David Berk with Fig. 5.8, Marc Dellian with Fig. 5.9, Larry Baxter with Fig. 5.10, Paolo Netti with Fig. 5.11, and Yves Boucher with Table 5.2. Research described here was primarily supported by grants from the National Cancer Institute, the National Science Foundation, and the American Cancer Society.

References

1. Beardsley, T. (1994). Trends in cancer epidemiology: a war not won. *Scientific Am.*, **270**, 118–26.
2. Jain, R. K. (1994). Barriers to drug delivery in solid tumors. *Scientific Am.*, **271**, 58–65.
3. Jain, R. K. (1994). Transport phenomena in tumors. *Adv. Chem. Eng.*, **20**, 129–200.
4. Sevick, E. M. and Jain, R. K. (1988). Blood flow and venous pH of tissue-isolated Walker 256 carcinoma during hyperglycemia. *Cancer Res.*, **48**, 1201–7.
5. Sevick, E. M. and Jain, R. K. (1989). Geometric resistance to blood flow in solid tumors perfused *ex vivo*: effects of tumor size and perfusion pressure. *Cancer Res.*, **49**, 3506–12.
6. Gullino, P. M. (1970). Techniques in tumor pathophysiology. In *Methods in cancer research* (ed. H. Busch), pp. 45–92. Academic Press, New York.
7. Kristjansen, P. E., Roberge, S., Lee, I., and Jain, R. K. (1994). Tissue-isolated human tumor xenografts in athymic nude mice. *Microvasc. Res.*, **48**, 389–402.
8. Kristjansen, P. E. G., Brown, T. J., Shipley, L. A., and Jain, R. K. (1996). Intratumor pharmacokinetics, flow resistance, and metabolism during gemcitabine infusion in *ex vivo* perfused human small cell lung cancer. *Clin. Cancer Res.*, **2**, 359–67.
9. Less, J. R., Posner, M. C., Wolmark, N., and Jain, R. K. (1996). Geometric resistance to blood flow and vascular network architecture in human colorectal carcinoma. *Microcirculation* (in press).
10. Dudar, T. E. and Jain, R. K. (1983). Microcirculatory flow changes during tissue growth. *Microvasc. Res.*, **25**, 1–21.
11. Zawicki, D. F., Jain, R. K., Schmid-Schoenbein, G. W., and Chien, S. (1981). Dynamics of neovascularization in normal tissue. *Microvasc. Res.*, **21**, 27–47.
12. Leunig, M., Yuan, F., Menger, M. D., Boucher, Y., Goetz, A. E., Messmer, K., and Jain, R. K. (1992). Angiogenesis, microvascular architecture, microhemodynamics, and interstitial fluid pressure during early growth of human adenocarcinoma LS174T in SCID mice. *Cancer Res.*, **52**, 6553–60.
13. Leunig, M., Yuan, F., Berk, D. A., Gerweck, L. E., and Jain, R. K. (1994). Angiogenesis and growth of isografted bone: quantitative *in vivo* assay in nude mice. *Lab. Invest.*, **71**, 300–7.
14. Yuan, F., Salehi, H. A., Boucher, Y., Vasthare, U. S., Tuma, R. F., and Jain, R. K. (1994). Vascular permeability and microcirculation of gliomas and mammary carcinomas transplanted in rat and mouse cranial windows. *Cancer Res.*, **54**, 4564–8.
15. Dellian, M., Witwer, B. P., Salehi, H., Yuan, F., and Jain, R. K. (1996). Quantitation and physiological characterization of bFGF and VEGF/VPF induced vessels in mice:

effect of microenvironment on angiogenesis. *Am. J. Pathology*, **149**, 59–72.

16. Lichtenbeld, H., Yuan, F., Michel, C. C., and Jain, R. K. (1996). Perfusion of single tumor microvessels. *Microcirculation* (in press).

17. Traykov, T. T. and Jain, R. K. (1987). Effect of glucose and galactose on red blood cell membrane deformability. *Int. J. Microcirc.: Clin. Exp.*, **6**, 35–44.

18. Sasaki, A., Jain, R. K., Maghazachi, A. A., Goldfarb, R. H., and Herberman, R. B. (1989). Low deformability of lymphokine-activated killer cells as a possible determinant of *in vivo* distribution. *Cancer Res.*, **49**, 3742–6.

19. Melder, R. J., Brownell, A. L., Shoup, T. M., Brownell, G. L., and Jain, R. K. (1993). Imaging of activated natural killer cells in mice by positron emission tomography: preferential uptake in tumors. *Cancer Res.*, **53**, 5867–71.

20. Munn, L. L., Melder, R. J., and Jain, R. K. (1994). Analysis of cell flux in the parallel plate flow chamber: implications for cell capture studies. *Biophys. J.*, **67**, 889–95.

21. Munn, L., Koenig, G. C., Jain, R. K., and Melder, R. J. (1995). Kinetics of adhesion molecule expression and spatial organization using targeted sampling fluorometry. *BioTechniques*, **19**, 622–31.

22. Jain, R. K. and Wei, J. (1977). Dynamics of drug transport in solid tumors: Distributed parameter model. *J. Bioeng.*, **1**, 313–29.

23. Pierson, R. N., Price, D. C., Wang, J., and Jain, R. K. (1978). Extracellular water measurements: organ tracer kinetics of bromide and sucrose in rats and man. *Am. J. Physiol.*, **235**, 254–64.

24. Jain, R. K., Wei, J., and Gullino, P. M. (1979). Pharmacokinetics of methotrexate in solid tumors. *J. Pharmacokinet. Biopharm.*, **7**, 181–94.

25. Jain, R. K. and Baxter, L. T. (1988). Mechanisms of heterogeneous distribution of monoclonal antibodies and other macromolecules in tumors: significance of elevated interstitial pressure. *Cancer Res.*, **48**, 7022–32.

26. Baxter, L. T. and Jain, R. K. (1989). Transport of fluid and macromolecules in tumors. I. Role of interstitial pressure and convection. *Microvasc. Res.*, **37**, 77–104.

27. Baxter, L. T. and Jain, R. K. (1990). Transport of fluid and macromolecules in tumors. II. Role of heterogeneous perfusion and lymphatics. *Microvasc. Res.*, **40**, 246–63.

28. Baxter, L. T. and Jain, R. K. (1991). Transport of fluid and macromolecules in tumors. III. Role of binding and metabolism. *Microvasc. Res.*, **41**, 5–23.

29. Baxter, L. T. and Jain, R. K. (1991). Transport of fluid and macromolecules in tumors. IV. A microscopic model of the perivascular distribution. *Microvasc. Res.*, **41**, 252–72.

30. Yuan, F., Baxter, L. T., and Jain, R. K. (1991). Pharmacokinetic analysis of two-step approaches using bifunctional and enzyme-conjugated antibodies. *Cancer Res.*, **51**, 3119–30.

31. Baxter, L. T., Zhu, H., Mackensen, D. G., and Jain, R. K. (1994). Physiologically based pharmacokinetic model for specific and nonspecific monoclonal antibodies and fragments in normal tissues and human tumor xenografts in nude mice. *Cancer Res.*, **54**, 1517–28.

32. Eskey, C. J., Wolmark, N., McDowell, C. L., Domach, M. M., and Jain, R. K. (1994). Residence time distributions of various tracers in tumors: implications for drug delivery and blood flow measurement. *J. Natl Cancer Inst.*, **86**, 293–9.

33. Baxter, L. T., Zhu, H., Mackensen, D. G., Butler, W. F., and Jain, R. K. (1995). Biodistribution of monoclonal antibodies: scale-up from mouse to man using a physiologically based pharmacokinetic model. *Cancer Res.*, **55**, 4611–22.

34. Netti, P. A., Baxter, L. T., Boucher, Y., Skalak, R., and Jain, R. K. (1995). Time dependent behavior of interstitial fluid pressure in solid tumors: Implications for drug delivery. *Cancer Res.* **55**, 5451–8.

35. Netti, P. A., Baxter, L. T., Boucher, Y., and Jain, R. K. (1996). Effect of transvascular fluid exchange on arteriovenous pressure relationship: implication for temporal and spatial heterogeneities in tumor blood flow *Microvasc. Res.*, **52**, 27–46.

36. Jain, R. K. (1988). Determinants of tumor blood flow: a review. *Cancer Res.*, **48**, 2641–58.

37. Folkman, J. (1995). Tumor angiogenesis. In *The molecular basis of cancer* (ed. Mendelsohn, P. M., Howley, M. A. P. and Liotta, L. A.), pp. 206–32. W. B. Saunders, Philadephia.

38. Gazit, Y., Berk, D. A., Leunig, M., Baxter, L. T., and Jain, R. K. (1995). Scale-invariant behavior and vascular network formation in normal and tumor tissue. *Phys. Rev. Lett.*, **75**, 2428–31.

39. Baish, J. W., Gazit, Y., Berk, D. A., Nozue, M., Baxter, L. T., and Jain, R. K. (1996). A novel approach to examine the role of vascular heterogeneity in nutrient and drug delivery for tumors: an invasion percolation model. *Microvasc. Res.*, **51**, 327–46.

40. Less, J. R., Skalak, T. C., Sevick, E. M., and Jain, R. K. (1991). Microvascular architecture in a mammary carcinoma: branching patterns and vessel dimensions. *Cancer Res.*, **51**, 265–73.

41. Patan, S., Munn, L. L., and Jain, R. K. (1996). Intussusceptive microvascular growth in solid tumors: a novel mechanism of tumor angiogenesis. *Microvasc. Res.*, **51**, 260–72.

42. Jain, R. K. and Ward-Hartley, K. A. (1984). Tumor blood flow: Characterization, modifications and role in hyperthermia. *IEEE Trans. Sonics Ultrasonics*, **31**, 504–26.

43. Sevick, E. M. and Jain, R. K. (1989). Viscous resistance to blood flow in solid tumors: effect of hematocrit on intratumor blood viscosity. *Cancer Res.*, **49**, 3513–19.

44. Sevick, E. M. and Jain, R. K. (1991). Effect of red blood cell rigidity on tumor blood flow: increase in viscous resistance during hyperglycemia. *Cancer Res.*, **51**, 2727–30.

45. Endrich, B., Reinhold, H. S., Gross, J. F., and Intaglietta, M. (1979). Tissue perfusion inhomogeneity during early tumor growth in rats. *J. Natl Cancer Inst.*, **62**, 387–95.

46. Eskey, C. J., Koretsky, A. P., Domach, M. M., and Jain, R. K. (1992). 2H-nuclear magnetic resonance imaging of tumor blood flow: spatial and temporal heterogeneity in a tissue-isolated mammary adenocarcinoma. *Cancer Res.*, **52**, 6010–19.

47. Hamberg, L. M., Kristjansen, P. E., Hunter, G. J., Wolf, G. L., and Jain, R. K. (1994). Spatial heterogeneity in tumor perfusion measured with functional computed tomography at 0.05 microliter resolution. *Cancer Res.*, **54**, 6032–6.

48. Vaupel, P. and Jain, R. K. (ed.) (1991). *Tumor blood supply and metabolic environment*. Gustav Fischer Verlag, Stuttgart.

49. Dellian, M., Helmlinger, G., Yuan, F., and Jain, R. K. (1996). Interstitial pH in solid tumors measured by fluorescence ratio imaging and optical sectioning: effect of glucose

on spatial and temporal gradients. *Br. J. Cancer*, **74**, 1206–15.

50. Martin, G. R. and Jain, R. K. (1993). Fluorescence ratio imaging measurement of pH gradients: calibration and application in normal and tumor tissues. *Microvasc. Res.*, **46**, 216–30.

51. Martin, G. R. and Jain, R. K. (1994). Noninvasive measurement of interstitial pH profiles in normal and neoplastic tissue using fluorescence ratio imaging microscopy. *Cancer Res.*, **54**, 5670–4.

52. Torres-Filho, I. P., Leunig, M., Yuan, F., Intaglietta, M., and Jain, R. K. (1994). Noninvasive measurement of microvascular and interstitial oxygen profiles in a human tumor in SCID mice. *Proc. Natl Acad. Sci. USA*, **91**, 2081–5.

53. Jain, R. K., Shah, S. A., and Finney, P. L. (1984). Continuous noninvasive monitoring of pH and temperature in rat Walker 256 carcinoma during normoglycemia and hyperglycemia. *J. Natl Cancer Inst.*, **73**, 429–36.

54. Ward, K. A. and Jain, R. K. (1988). Response of tumours to hyperglycaemia: characterization, significance and role in hyperthermia. *Int. J. Hyperthermia*, **4**, 223–50.

55. Eskey, C. J., Koretsky, A. P., Domach, M. M., and Jain, R. K. (1993). Role of oxygen vs. glucose in energy metabolism in a mammary carcinoma perfused *ex vivo*: direct measurement by 31P NMR. *Proc. Natl Acad. Sci. USA*, **90**, 2646–50.

56. Jain, R. K. (1987). Transport of molecules across tumor vasculature. *Cancer Metastasis Rev.*, **6**, 559–93.

57. Gerlowski, L. E., and Jain, R. K. (1986). Microvascular permeability of normal and neoplastic tissues. *Microvasc. Res.*, **31**, 288–305.

58. Yuan, F., Leunig, M., Berk, D. A., and Jain, R. K. (1993). Microvascular permeability of albumin, vascular surface area, and vascular volume measured in human adenocarcinoma LS174T using dorsal chamber in SCID mice. *Microvasc. Res.*, **45**, 269–89.

59. Yuan, F., Leunig, M., Huang, S. K., Berk, D. A., Papahadjopoulos, D., and Jain, R. K. (1994). Microvascular permeability and interstitial penetration of sterically stabilized (stealth) liposomes in a human tumor xenograft. *Cancer Res.*, **54**, 3352–6.

60. Sevick, E. M. and Jain, R. K. (1991). Measurement of capillary filtration coefficient in a solid tumor. *Cancer Res.*, **51**, 1352–5.

61. Dvorak, H. F., Brown, L. F., Detmar, M., and Dvorak, A. M. (1995). Vascular permeability factor/vascular endothelial growth factor, microvascular hyperpermeability, and angiogenesis. *Am. J. Physiol.*, **146**, 1029–39.

62. Yuan, F., Dellian, M., Fukumura, D., Leunig, M., Berk, D. A., Torchillin, V. P., and Jain, R. K. (1995). Vascular permeability in a human tumor xenograft: Molecular size-dependence and cut-off size. *Cancer Res.*, **55**, 3752–6.

63. Jain, R. K. (1987). Transport of molecules in the tumor interstitium: a review. *Cancer Res.*, **47**, 3039–51.

64. Boucher, Y., Baxter, L. T., and Jain, R. K. (1990). Interstitial pressure gradients in tissue-isolated and subcutaneous tumors: implications for therapy. *Cancer Res.*, **50**, 4478–84.

65. Boucher, Y., Kirkwood, J. M., Opacic, D., Desantis, M., and Jain, R. K. (1991). Interstitial hypertension in superficial metastatic melanomas in humans. *Cancer Res.*, **51**, 6691–4.

66. Boucher, Y. and Jain, R. K. (1992). Microvascular pressure is the principal driving force for interstitial hypertension in solid tumors: implications for vascular collapse. *Cancer Res.*, **52**, 5110–14.

67. Roh, H. D., Boucher, Y., Kalnicki, S., Buchsbaum, R., Bloomer, W. D., and Jain, R. K. (1991). Interstitial hypertension in carcinoma of uterine cervix in patients: possible correlation with tumor oxygenation and radiation response. *Cancer Res.*, **51**, 6695–8.

68. Gutmann, R., Leunig, M., Feyh, J., Goetz, A. E., Messmer, K., Kastenbauer, E., and Jain, R. K. (1992). Interstitial hypertension in head and neck tumors in patients: correlation with tumor size. *Cancer Res.*, **52**, 1993–5.

69. Less, J. R., Posner, M. C., Boucher, Y., Borochovitz, D., Wolmark, N., and Jain, R. K. (1992). Interstitial hypertension in human breast and colorectal tumors. *Cancer Res.*, **52**, 6371–4.

70. Curti, B. D., Urba, W. J., Alvord, W. G., Janik, J. E., Smith, J. W., Madara, K., and Longo, D. L. (1993). Interstitial pressure of subcutaneous nodules in melanoma and lymphoma patients: changes during treatment. *Cancer Res.*, **53**, 2204–7s.

71. Nathanson, S. D. and Nelson, L. (1994). Interstitial fluid pressure in breast cancer, benighn breast conditions, and breast parenchyma. *Ann. Surg. Oncol.*, **1**, 333–8.

72. Boucher, Y., Salehi, H., Witwer, B. P., Harsh, G. R., and Jain, R. K. (1996). Interstitial fluid pressure in intracranial tumors in patients and in rodents. *Br. J. Cancer* (in press).

73. Znati, C. A., Karasek, K., Faul, C., Roh, H.-D., Boucher, Y., Rosenstein, M. *et al.* (1997). Interstitial fluid pressure changes in cervical carcinoma patients undergoing radiation therapy: a potential prognostic factor (submitted).

74. Znati, C. A., Rosenstein, M., Boucher, Y., Epperly, M. W., Bloomer, W. D. and Jain, R. K. (1996). Effect of radiation on interstitial fluid pressure and oxygenation in a human colon carcinoma xenograft. *Cancer Res.*, **56**, 964–8.

75. Arbit, E., Lee, J., and DiResta, G. (1994). *Interstitial hypertension in human brain tumors: possible role in peritumoral edema formulation*. Springer-Verlag; Tokyo.

76. Stohrer, M., Boucher, Y., Stangassinger, M., and Jain, R. K. (1995). Oncotic pressure in human tumor xenografts. *Proc. AACR*, (Abstr.).

77. Rippe, B. and Haraldsson. (1987). Fluid and protein fluxes across small and large pores in the microvasculature. Application of two-pore equations. *Acta Physiol. Scand.*, **131**, 411.

78. Swabb, E. A., Wei, J., and Gullino, P. M. (1974). Diffusion and convection in normal and neoplastic tissues. *Cancer Res.*, **34**, 2814.

79. Berk, D. A., Yuan, F., Leunig, M., and Jain, R. K. (1993). Fluorescence photobleaching with spatial Fourier analysis: measurement of diffusion in light-scattering media. *Biophys. J.*, **65**, 2428–36.

80. Johnson, E. M., Berk, D. A., Jain, R. K., and Deen, W. M. (1995). Diffusion and partitioning of proteins in charged agarose gels. *Biophys. J.*, **68**, 1561–8.

81. Johnson, E. M., Berk, D. A., Jain, R. K. and Deen, W. M. (1996). Hindered diffusion in agarose gels: test of effective medium model. *Biophys. J.*, **70**, 1017–26.

82. Nugent, L. J. and Jain, R. K. (1984). Extravascular diffusion in normal and neoplastic tissues. *Cancer Res.*, **44**, 238–44.

83. Chary, S. R. and Jain, R. K. (1989). Direct measurement of interstitial convection and diffusion of albumin in normal and neoplastic tissues by fluorescence photobleaching. *Proc. Natl Acad. Sci. USA*, **86**, 5385–9.

84. Berk, D. A., Yuan, F., Leunig, M., and Jain, R. K. (1997). Interstitial protein transport in a human tumor xenograft: direct *in vivo* measurement of specific and nonspecific binding. *Proc. Natl Acad. Sci. USA* (in press).

85. Znati, C. A., Boucher, Y., Rosenstein, M., Turner, D., Watkins, S., and Jain, R. K. (1997). Effect of radiation on the interstitial matrix and hydraulic conductivity of tumors (submitted).

86. Boucher, Y., Brekken, C., Netti, P. A., Baxter, L. T., and Jain, R. K. (1995). Hydraulic conductivity of solid tumors: A novel *in vivo* measurement technique and implications for drug delivery (submitted).

87. Kaufman, E. N. and Jain, R. K. (1990). Quantification of transport and binding parameters using fluorescence recovery after photobleaching. Potential for *in vivo* applications. *Biophys. J.*, **58**, 873–85.

88. Kaufman, E. N. and Jain, R. K. (1991). Measurement of mass transport and reaction parameters in bulk solution using photobleaching. Reaction limited binding regime. *Biophys. J.*, **60**, 596–610.

89. Kaufman, E. N. and Jain, R. K. (1992). *In vitro* measurement and screening of monoclonal antibody affinity using fluorescence photobleaching. *J. Immunol. Methods*, **155**, 1–17.

90. Kaufman, E. N. and Jain, R. K. (1992). Effect of bivalent interaction upon apparent antibody affinity: experimental confirmation of theory using fluorescence photobleaching and implications for antibody binding assays. *Cancer Res.*, **52**, 4157–67.

91. Juweid, M., Neumann, R., Paik, C., Perez-Bacete, M. J., Sato, J., Van Osdol, W., and Weinstein, J. N. (1992). Micropharmacology of monoclonal antibodies in solid tumor: direct experimental evidence for a binding site barrier. *Cancer Res.*, **52**, 5144.

92. Jain, R. K. (1989). Delivery of novel therapeutic agents in tumors: physiological barriers and strategies. *J. Natl Cancer Inst.*, **81**, 570–6.

93. Leu, A. J., Berk, D. A., Yuan, F., and Jain, R. K. (1994). Flow velocity in the superficial lymphatic network of the mouse tail. *Am. J. Physiol.*, **267**, H1507–13.

94. Berk, D. A., Swartz, M. A., Leu, A. J., and Jain, R. K. (1996). Transport in lymphatic capillaries: II. Microscopic velocity measurement with fluorescence recovery after photobleaching. *Am. J. Physiol.*, **270**, H330–7.

95. Swartz, M. A., Berk, D. A., and Jain, R. K. (1996). Transport in lymphatic capillaries: I. Macroscopic measurements using residence time distribution theory. *Am. J. Physiol.*, **270**, H324–9.

96. Melder, R. J., Munn, L. L., Yamada, S., Ohkubo, C., and Jain, R. K. (1995). Selectin and integrin mediated T lymphocyte rolling and arrest on TNFα-activated endothelium is augmented by erythrocytes. *Biophys. J.*, **69**, 2131–8.

97. Fukumura, D., Salehi, H. A., Witwer, B., Tuma, R. F., Melder, R. J. and Jain, R. K. (1995). TNFα-induced leukocyte-adhesion in normal and tumor vessels: effect of tumor type, transplantation site and host. *Cancer Res.*, **55**, 4824–9.

98. Yamada, S., Melder, R. J., Leunig, M., Ohkubo, C., and Jain, R. K. (1995). Leukocyte-rolling increases with age. *Blood*, **86**, 4707–8.

99. Melder, R. J., Elmaleh, D., Brownell, A. L., Brownell, G. L., and Jain, R. K. (1994). A method for labeling cells for positron emission tomography (PET) studies. *J. Immunol. Methods*, **175**, 79–87.

100. Melder, R. J. and Jain, R. K. (1992). Kinetics of inter-leukin-2 induced changes in rigidity of human natural killer cells. *Cell Biophysics*, **20**, 161–76.

101. Melder, R. J. and Jain, R. K. (1994). Reduction of rigidity in human activated natural killer cells by thioglycollate treatment. *J. Immunol. Methods*, **175**, 69–77.

102. Melder, R. J., Salehi, H. A., and Jain, R. K. (1995). Localiztion of activated natural killer cells in MCaIV mammary carcinoma grown in cranial windows in C3H mice. *Microvasc. Res.*, **50**, 35–44.

103. Sasaki, A., Melder, R. J., Whiteside, T. L., Herberman, R. B., and Jain, R. K. (1991). Preferential localization of human adherent lymphokine-activated killer cells in tumor microcirculation. *J. Natl Cancer Inst.*, **83**, 433–37.

104. Ohkubo, C., Bigos, D., and Jain, R. K. (1991). Interleukin 2 induced leukocyte adhesion to the normal and tumor microvascular endothelium *in vivo* and its inhibition by dextran sulfate: implications for vascular leak syndrome. *Cancer Res.*, **51**, 1561–63.

105. Melder, R. J., Koenig, G., Witwer, B., Safabakhsh, N., Munn, L. L., and Jain, R. K. (1996). Activated natural killer cells bind angiogenic vessels through CD 18 and VLA4 dependent adhesion. *Nat. Med.*, **2**, 992–7.

106. Jallal, B., Powell, F., Zachwieja, J., Brakebusch, C., Germain, L., Jacobs, J., Iacobelli, S. and Ullrich, A. (1995). Suppression of tumor growth *in vivo* by local and systemic 90K level increase. *Cancer Res.*, **55**, 3223–7.

107. Gamble, J. R. and Vadas, M. A. (1988). Endothelial adhesiveness for blood neutrophils is inhibited by transforming growth factor-beta. *Science*, **242**, 97–9.

108. Gamble, J. R. and Vadas, M. A. (1991). Endothelial cell adhesiveness for human T lymphocytes is inhibited by transforming growth factor-beta. *J. Immunol.*, **146**, 1149–54.

109. Gamble, J. R. and Khew-Goodall, Y. (1993). Transforming growth factor-beta inhibits E-selectin expression on human endothelial cells. *J. Immunol.*, **150**, 4494–503.

110. Fidler, I. J. and Ellis, L. M. (1994). The implications of angiogenesis for biology and therapy of cancer metastasis. *Cell*, **79**, 185–88.

111. Kitayama, J., Nagawa, J., Yasuhara, H., Tsuno, N., Kimura, W., Shibata, Y., and Muto, T. (1994). Suppressive effect of basic fibroblast growth factor on transendothelial emigration of CD4(+) T-lymphocyte. *Cancer Res.*, **54**, 4729–33.

112. Haying, J. B. and Williams, S. K. (1994). Reduced adhesion of human microvascular endothelial cells to collagen in response to basic FGF is mediated by β1 integrin. *FASEB J.*, **8**, (Abstr. 263).

113. Yamada, S., Mayadas, T. M., Yuan, F., Wagner, D. D., Hynes, R. O., Melder, R. J., and Jain, R. K. (1995). Rolling in P-selectin deficient mice is reduced but not eliminated in the dorsal skin. *Blood*, **86**, 3487–92.

114. Dedrick, R. L. (1973). Animal scale-up. *J. Pharmacokinet. Biopharm.*, **1**, 435–61.

115. Gerlowski, L. E. and Jain, R. K. (1983). Physiologically based pharmacokinetic modeling: principles and applications. *J. Pharmaceut. Sci.*, **72**, 1103–27.

116. Zhu, H., Melder, R., Baxter, L., and Jain, R. K. (1996). Physiologically based kinetic model of effector cell bio-

distribution: implications for adoptive immunotherapy. *Cancer Res.*, **56**, 3771–81.

117. Jain, R. K. (1979). Transient temperature distributions in an infinite perfused medium due to a time-dependent, spherical heat source. *Trans. ASME J. Biomech. Eng.*, **101**, 82–6.

118. Jain, R. K. (1978). Effect of inhomogeneities and finite boundaries on temperature distribution in a perfused medium with application to tumors. *Trans. ASME J. Biomech. Eng.*, **100**, 235–41.

119. Jain, R. K., Boucher, Y., Stacey-Clear, A., Moore, R. and Kopans, D. (1995). Method for locating tumors prior to needle biopsy, U.S. Patent Number 5,396,897, March 14.

120. Gerlowski, L. E. and Jain, R. K. (1985). Effect of hyperthermia on microvascular permeability to macromolecules in normal and tumor tissues. *Int. J. Microcric.: Clin. Exp.*, **4**, 363–72.

121. Dudar, T. E. and Jain, R. K. (1984). Differential response of normal and tumor microcirculation to hyperthermia. *Cancer Res.*, **44**, 605–12.

122. Baxter, L. T., Yuan, F., and Jain, R. K. (1992). Pharmacokinetic analysis of the perivascular distribution of bifunctional antibodies and haptens: comparison with experimental data. *Cancer Res.*, **52**, 5838–44.

123. Kristjansen, P. E., Boucher, Y., and Jain, R. K. (1993). Dexamethasone reduces the interstitial fluid pressure in a human colon adenocarcinoma xenograft. *Cancer Res.*, **53**, 4764–6.

124. Lee, I., Boucher, Y., and Jain, R. K. (1992). Nicotinamide can lower tumor interstitial fluid pressure: mechanistic and therapeutic implications. *Cancer Res.*, **52**, 3237–40.

125. Lee, I., Boucher, Y., Demhartner, T. J., and Jain, R. K. (1994). Changes in tumour blood flow, oxygenation and interstitial fluid pressure induced by pentoxifylline. *Br. J. Cancer*, **69**, 492–6.

126. Lee, I., Demhartner, T. J., Boucher, Y., Jain, R. K., and Intaglietta, M. (1994). Effect of hemodilution and resuscitation on tumor interstitial fluid pressure, blood flow, and oxygenation. *Microvasc. Res.*, **48**, 1–12.

127. Leunig, M., Goetz, A. E., Dellian, M., Zetterer, G., Gamarra, F., Jain, R. K., and Messmer, K. (1992). Interstitial fluid pressure in solid tumors following hyperthermia: possible correlation with therapeutic response. *Cancer Res.*, **52**, 487–90.

128. Leunig, M., Goetz, A. E., Gamarra, F., Zetterer, G., Messmer, K., and Jain, R. K. (1994). Photodynamic therapy-induced alterations in interstitial fluid pressure, volume and water content of an amelanotic melanoma in the hamster. *Br. J. Cancer*, **69**, 101–3.

129. Zlotecki, R. A., Boucher, Y., Lee, I., Baxter, L. T., and Jain, R. K. (1993). Effect of angiotensin II induced hypertension on tumor blood flow and interstitial fluid pressure. *Cancer Res.*, **53**, 2466–8.

130. Zlotecki, R. A., Baxter, L. T., Boucher, Y., and Jain, R. K. (1995). Pharmacologic modification of tumor blood flow and interstitial fluid pressure in a human tumor xenograft: network analysis and mechanistic interpretation. *Microvasc. Res.* **50**, 429–43.

6. Microregional tumour blood flow: heterogeneity and therapeutic significance

David J. Chaplin, Martin J. Trotter, and Graeme J. Dougherty

Introduction

The continued proliferation of tumour cells depends on an adequate supply of oxygen and nutrients and removal of the waste products of cellular metabolism. These 'services' are provided by blood vessels. Thus, expansion of a solid tumour requires the acquisition of a vascular supply. There is evidence that tumours can acquire their vascularity, at least in part, by incorporation of existing host vessels, particularly arteriolar vessels (1–3). However, it is now evident that the majority of tumour vessels are acquired by angiogenesis and that this process is a prerequisite for the continued rapid growth of solid tumours beyond a size of 1 mm³ (4,5).

The strong and continuous angiogenic stimulus in tumour tissue results in new blood vessels which differ in many respects to those in normal tissues. These differences include a lack of smooth muscle, abnormal branching patterns, absence of nervous innervation, channels without a continuous endothelial lining and lack of a collateral supply (6–11). In addition to structural abnormalities the apparent absence of a lymphatic system to assist interstitial fluid drainage, in many solid tumours, results in abnormally high interstitial fluid pressures (12,13).

The abnormalities of tumour blood supply can be summarized as: (i) abnormal vascular network; (ii) spatial and temporal heterogeneity in tumour perfusion; and (iii) loss of intrinsic control mechanisms. All three are interrelated and can influence therapeutically relevant parameters such as tumour oxygen distribution, nutrient supply, metabolic microenvironment (*e.g.* pH distribution and bioenergetic status), and response to vasoactive drugs designed to manipulate tumour blood flow. In this chapter we will focus on the heterogeneity in microregional flow within tumours and its consequence for therapeutic approaches to the treatment of solid tumours.

Vascular network in tumours

In very general terms, the purpose of the microcirculation is to deliver blood to tissue parenchyma in balance with the metabolic needs of the cells. Each normal tissue in the body has its own characteristic vascular system but all circulatory beds share certain common structural features, which are modified by the particular arrangement and function of the parenchymal tissue. Malignant tissue, as a consequence of abnormal morphogenesis, has a structurally abnormal blood supply. Lewis (1927) noted that each tumour type had a characteristic vascular pattern and that 'the blood vessels do not determine the growth of the tumour; but the tumour determines the growth and pattern of blood vessels' (14). The structurally diverse nature of neoplastic growth leads to a wide variation in the organization of tumour vasculature and a common pattern cannot be recognized. In his exhaustive review, Warren (7) concludes, '... each tumour type, and in some cases each tumour, tends to be a law unto itself. It has to be recognized, therefore, that the vascular morphology of tumours, like other characteristics, has to be studied for each tumour type and that generalizations may be difficult to make'. Differences in the vascular patterns of various tumours are governed by a combination of at least three factors (15): (i) the growth pattern and growth rate of the tumour cells; (ii) the effectiveness of the angiogenic stimulus released by the tumour; and (iii) the influence of tumour interstitial pressure on compression of blood vessels.

As a malignant tumour is an expansile, growing mass, its vascular supply is constantly changing, adapting to requirements of the tumour or being compressed and destroyed by the tumour cells (16). Tumour vascular architecture, then, is difficult to depict accurately in static, permanent terms but, rather must be envisioned as a dynamic entity involving development, destruction, and rearrangement of blood vessels.

In a typical vascular tree, blood flows successively through arteries, arterioles, terminal arterioles, capillaries, postcapillary venules, venules, and veins. In malignant tissue, this hierarchy is often lost and the vessel network is most commonly described as 'chaotic' (16). It is also known that tumours can possess a significant number of arteriovenous shunts. These are a category of tumour vessels with very low resistance to flow. These vessels facilitate the direct passage of blood from the arterial supply to the venous drainage without passage through the exchange vessels (capillaries). Flow through these shunts has been estimated at up to 30% of total tumour flow (17,19). Thus, measurements of overall tumour blood flow may well overestimate nutritive flow to the tumour itself.

Intrinsic control of tumour blood flow

In the circulatory system as a whole, several different mechanisms are provided (local, nervous, and humoral) to control blood flow to different parts of the body. At the microcirculatory level, control is almost entirely local, that is, flow is controlled by intrinsic mechanisms in proportion to the tissue's need for perfusion. Local control of microcirculatory flow is mediated via vascular smooth muscle, which dictates vessel 'tone' at the arteriolar or pre-capillary sphincter level. Two important mechanisms are thought to be involved (20): (i) metabolic control, i.e. the capacity to adjust flow as tissue metabolic requirements change, and (ii) myogenic control, i.e. local autoregulatory adjustments that stabilize flow and intravascular pressure, factors crucial in control of transcapillary fluid and solute exchange.

Abnormalities of tumour vascular architecture and vessel wall structure, specifically an apparent lack of smooth muscle in newly formed tumour vessels (10), seriously disturb microcirculatory control mechanisms. Active vasomotor adjustments within the microcirculation occur only in vessels with smooth muscle in their walls, although the possibility that endothelial cells (21) or pericytes (22) with contractile properties might also play a part cannot be discounted. Thus, incorporated host arterioles will be the only tumour vessels involved directly in local control of blood flow and unlike normal tissues such vessels are in the minority among the predominantly capillary/venous tumour circulation.

Lack of a well defined system of local microcirculatory control in tumour tissue leads to several important differences between tumour vasculature and that of normal tissue. Tumour microcirculation can be characterized as a 'passive' system, lacking the ability to autoregulate flow in response to changes in perfusion pressure. Absence of autoregulation in tumours, as evidenced by a linear pressure-flow relationship, has been demonstrated on several occasions (23,24).

Loss of local microcirculatory control mechanisms in tumour tissue is based not only on structural derangements (lack of vascular smooth muscle) but also on functional considerations. As outlined by Intaglietta and Mirhashemi (25) in reference to ischaemic states, an inert microvascular network, with arterioles maximally dilated to serve a high metabolic demand, is characterized by: low arteriolar–venular pressure gradient, low flow velocity, higher blood viscosity, and non-selective capillary perfusion. 'In this situation capillary perfusion becomes heterogeneous and only the microvessels with low hydraulic resistance maintain flow' (26). The similarities to tumour microcirculation are clear and thus, it may be possible to think of regions within tumours as representing a form of 'ischaemic' or 'shock' state.

Spatial and temporal heterogeneities in tumour perfusion

Several quantitative studies showed that for many experimental tumours at least, blood flow is often higher in the tumour periphery than in central regions (27–29). Endrich et al. (27) measured perfusion in five tumour 'zones' defined as necrotic, semi-necrotic, stabilized tumour circulation, advancing tumour front, and normal tissue. Blood flow in peripheral tumour regions (advancing front) was significantly higher than that of surrounding normal tissue.

Tumour blood flow is also characterized by temporal heterogeneity at a fixed location. Over the long term, as a tumour grows, the vascular pattern constantly changes due to variable rates of angiogenesis, vessel collapse and destruction, and formation of necrosis. A quantitative study of these temporal changes was performed by Endrich et al. (27) using tumours grown in transparent chambers. In addition to flow changes which occur as a tumour grows, local, transient changes in perfusion have been shown to occur in tumours growing as thin two-dimensional sheets in observation chambers. Based on observations made of tumours grown in transparent chambers, Gullino (30) proposed that 'regurgitation and intermittent circulation (i.e. periods of stasis) followed by resumption of blood flow, sometimes in a direction opposite to the previous one, are probably the "normal" features of the vascular transport system of tumours'. Other similar studies supported this hypothesis: Yamaura and Sato (31) noted that blood flow in tumour vessels was unstable and changed even with the animal's movement or respiration; Endrich *et al.* (27) also described 'regurgitation and intermittent flow' and Reinhold (32) observed differences in flow rates of a factor of 5–10, even in adjacent capillaries. Flow intermittency has been assessed quantitatively in two-dimensional tumours by measuring red blood cell (RBC) velocity in single vessels (33–35). Arterioles 20–40 μm in diameter supplying the tumour microvasculature exhibited strong vasomotor activity in approximately 50–60% of the vessels observed and this results in flow fluctuations in downstream tumour vessels. The periodicity of this flow intermittency was 2–3 min (32).

Assessment of microregional heterogeneity in perfusion in three-dimensional solid tumours *in situ* has been made possible in recent years by the identification of fluorescent dyes which can demarcate functional vasculature following intravenous administration (36–40). One technique involves the use of Hoechst 33342 in conjunction with fluorescence-activated cell sorting. The methods and rationale of the sorting procedure have been described in detail elsewhere (36,37). Intravenous injection of Hoechst 33342 results in selective distribution of the stain in the perivascular tumour cells. Such cells are well oxygenated and are sensitive to radiation delivered simultaneously with Hoechst 33342 administration. As Hoechst 33342 has a very short plasma half-life, when injection of this vascular marker is divorced by several minutes from the start of irradiation, the vessels which become non-perfused in this time, will result in cells which are brightly stained with Hoechst exhibiting a radiobiologically hypoxic response. This scenario has been observed in several experimental tumours. A second technique involves the sequential intravenous injection of two fluorescent vascular markers. The stains employed are Hoechst 33342 and the carbocyanine dye DiOC$_7$ (3), both of which have short (<3 min) circulation half-lives and preferentially stain cells adjacent to perfused blood vessels. When injections of the vascular markers are separated by some interval, each stain defines only those tumour vessels which were perfused during the few minutes immediately post-injection; thus, two 'pictures' of tumour perfusion are obtained and tumour vessels subject to periods of non-perfusion can be easily visualized in frozen sections as they are outlined by one stain but not the other (39). Intermittent flow elucidated by this double staining method has been shown to be a common feature of many experimental rodent tumours and human tumour xenografts (25).

It should be emphasized that the use of plasma-borne perfusion probes could underestimate the temporal heterogeneity in oxygen delivery. For example, if a vessel within the tumour became partially occluded reducing or even preventing the passage of RBCs but, still facilitating plasma perfusion, the vessel in question would receive the vascular stain but no oxygen delivery. Indeed, the availability of a multi-channel laser Doppler flowmeter which facilitates the monitoring of erythrocyte flux simultaneously within several microregions of tissue, has demonstrated that fluctuations of erythrocyte flux by a factor of two or more occur in ~50% of the microregions monitored in an experimental tumour over a period of 1 h (40). More recent studies with the laser Doppler system have demonstrated that microregional fluctuations in erythrocyte flux also occur in primary human malignancies (Fig. 6.1). Evidence from histological studies using fluorescent perfusion probes indicates that such changes do not occur just in single isolated vessels, but many vessels can be involved resulting in large microregions being subjected to hypoxia and/or reperfusion (41).

Tumour oxygenation and its therapeutic implications

There are several therapeutic implications of heterogeneous tumour blood flow. Uptake and distribution of blood-borne anti-cancer agents including chemicals, antibodies, and gene delivery systems such as liposomes or virus particles will be compromised. In addition, many regions within the tumour will be subjected to an altered microenvironment. Indeed, regions of hypoxia, acidosis, and nutrient depletion are common features of both experimental and primary human malignancies (42–46). Although each of these parameters can influence cellular function and response to therapy, the emphasis of the remainder of this chapter will focus on tumour oxygenation.

Oxygen tension in tumours

The Eppendorf PO_2 histograph represents the current state-of-the-art machine for measuring oxygen partial pressures in tissues. The 300 μm hypodermic needle electrode is moved in a succession of rapid forward and backward steps through the tumour tissue. A large number of readings, acquired at many different locations, allows reproducible frequency distributions to be obtained, which have proved to be a sensitive indicator of tissue oxygen supply and the function of the microcirculation. This technique therefore provides a reliable method of directly measuring tumour oxygenation, which is applicable to both experimental and clinical use; its advent has resulted in a dramatic increase in the availability of detailed information concerning both rodent and human tumour oxygenation. These data confirm that hypoxia is a feature of experimen-

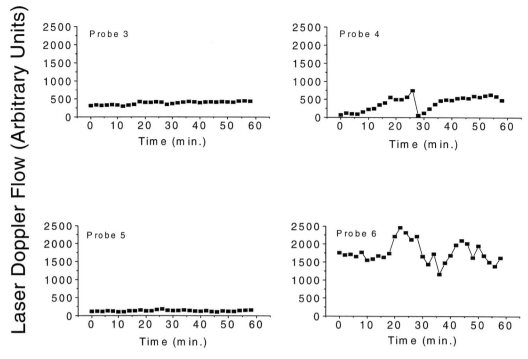

Figure 6.1. Examples of microregional flow fluctuations detected in four microregions ($<10^{-2}$ mm^3) of a primary human breast tumour using laser Doppler microprobes. It can be seen that even over the 1 h monitoring period fluctuations in erythrocyte flow can be detected in two of the regions sampled. As the signal reflects the flow in several capillaries in front of the probe, a change in flux by a factor of two could represent an equal reduction in all capillaries or complete stoppage of flow in half of them.

tal tumours. Regional Po_2 values of 15 mmHg (~2% O$_2$) appear to be common in human malignancies but infrequent or absent in normal tissues. Values of <2.5 mmHg have also been detected in primary human tumours, a level of hypoxia consistent with radiation resistance (46,47). An example of oxygen tension distributions in subcutaneous HT-29 colonic adenocarcinoma and in normal subcutis in severe combined immunodeficient mice is shown in Fig. 6.2. It can be seen that the tumour tissue is subjected to much lower oxygen tension than the subcutis.

The nature of hypoxia within tumours

If we consider a microregion within a tumour such as that shown in Fig. 6.3, how do regions of low oxygen tension occur? Thomlinson and Gray originally proposed a model of 'diffusion limited' hypoxic cells existing distant from blood vessels (48). In a system with constant blood flow and oxygen delivery capacity, the utilization of oxygen by cells close to the blood vessel results in a gradual decline in the oxygenation and nutritional status of cells distant

from the vessel. Such cells would be subjected to hypoxia or even anoxia for many hours, be nutrient deprived and presumably, non-proliferating. Although this model was considered to describe the major cause of hypoxia for many years, other contributory mechanisms are now thought to play a significant part. Temporal changes in erythrocyte flux will alter oxygen delivery to cells at a fixed distance from blood vessels. In Fig. 6.4a–d we have depicted four of the many possible scenarios that could exist in a vessel at a given instant in time. Figure 6.4a (see the plate section) depicts the classical model of diffusion limited hypoxia. The light blue shaded area depicts the cells at a nominal oxygen tension (< 2.5 mmHg) for illustrative purposes. However, if the flux of RBCs within the vessel is reduced the rim of hypoxic cells will increase (Fig. 6.4b,d, plate section). If the flow is completely stopped, even the endothelium will become hypoxic. A hypoxic region of perivascular and endothelial cells may also occur at the venous end of a tumour vessel even in the presence of flowing erythrocytes if the erythrocytes are deoxygenated (Fig. 6.4c). Evidence in support of the latter

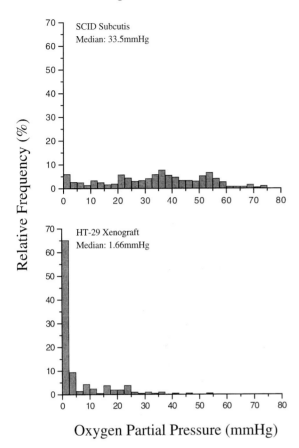

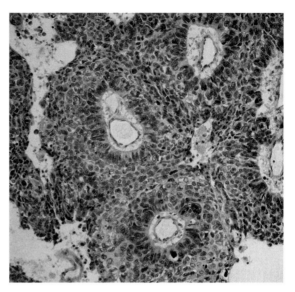

Figure 6.3. Histological section of a primary human squamous cell carcinoma of the lung. The cuff of viable tumour cells surrounding each vessel can be seen in this section.

Oxygen Partial Pressure (mmHg)

Figure 6.2. Histograms of measured Po$_2$ values in the normal subcutis over the sacral region of the back of SCID mice (upper panel) and in subcutaneously growing HT-29 adenocarcinomas (lower panel).

has been gained using cryospectrophotometry. This technique which enables the amount of oxyhaemoglobin present within red cells to be determined, has shown that in contrast to normal tissues, a large percentage of intravascular erythrocytes in experimental rodent and primary human tumours are deoxygenated (45,46). Thus, at any time, different oxygenation scenarios exist in and around different vessels and at different locations along a given vessel. Moreover, the scenario at any location will change over minutes, hours, and days.

Biological consequences of tumour hypoxia

Cell survival

It is well established, using cell lines *in vitro* that cells can survive in anoxic conditions for many hours or even days when provided with glucose and maintained at a pH close

to 7 (49–51). Rotin and colleagues showed that if oxygen tension was maintained at 0.2% (1.5 mmHg) cell survival was not significantly reduced from normal even following a 6 h incubation at pH 6.2. However, if anoxia was combined with incubation at pH 6.0 in the absence of glucose, cell survival was rapidly compromised, although, even under these extreme conditions, 20% of the cells survived a 2 h exposure period.

Cell proliferation

Under essentially anoxic conditions cellular proliferation is compromised or even cessated (49,52,53). However, Koch and colleagues showed that in a fibroblast cell line cellular proliferation was not greatly impaired as long as the oxygen content remained above 500 p.p.m. (i.e. ~0.4 mmHg, 0.05% O$_2$). Again it has to be remembered that these studies were carried out at pH 7.4 and with availability of glucose and other nutrients. Work with EMT6 tumour cells has shown that cell growth may be arrested at higher oxygen concentrations if the pH of the incubating media is reduced (54).

Gene expression

Over the last few years interest has been growing in investigating the molecular response to oxygen deprivation. Hypoxia has now been shown to induce increased expression of several mammalian genes including erythropoietin (Epo) (55), endothelin (56) interleukin (IL) 1 α (57), vascular endothelial cell growth factor (VEGF) (58–60), platelet-derived growth factor B chain (61), IL-8 (62), tumour necrosis factor (63), and metallothionein IIA (64). It has to be emphasized that the level and duration of hypoxia used in individual experiments varied as did the cell types. For example, oxygen tensions of 1–2% were used to show induction of VEGF in glioma cells (60) and for induction of IL-8 and IL-1 in endothelial cells (57,62). However, conditions of 0.01% O_2 followed by 24 h of re-oxygenation were used in the study by Murphy and colleagues investigating the induction of metallothionein in human squamous carcinoma cells (64).

It is clear from these studies that gene expression is altered when cells are incubated under tumour relevant oxygen tensions rather than under aerobic tissue culture conditions (21% O_2). Important questions are raised by these findings: (i) Does the change in gene expression persist under continuous passage of the cells or is it a response to the stress of changing oxygen tension? (ii) Are similar patterns of gene expression induced by an acute reduction in oxygenation as are induced by an increase in oxygenation in previously anoxic areas? With the dynamic heterogeneity in flow that exists within solid tumours, increases and decreases in oxygenation are undoubtedly a routine feature of tumour cell physiology.

The hypoxia-induced up-regulation of angiogenic growth factor (VEGF) could be an important event for continued tumour growth since, as the tumour cells outgrow their blood supply, hypoxia will develop and via increased expression of VEGF will stimulate new vessel growth into the hypoxic region.

In addition to being a key physiological factor that drives angiogenesis, hypoxia has also been shown to increase metastatic potential (65) and has recently been associated with the acquisition of a more malignant phenotype in experimental melanoma (66). Molecular changes associated with these events have not been elucidated. However, it is of interest to note that the expression of the hypoxia-induced cytokine IL-8 has been correlated with metastatic potential of human melanoma cells in nude mice (67). In addition, an anoxia inducible endonuclease and the associated enhanced DNA breakage has been implicated in modulating genomic instability (68).

Therapeutic consequences of tumour hypoxia

Radiation

It is well established that as the oxygen tension of cells *in vitro* is reduced below 10 mmHg (1.5% O_2) cells become increasingly resistant to radiation (69). It is the amount of oxygen present at the time of irradiation or a few milliseconds after which is important (70,71). This reflects the fact that free radicals produced in DNA, either by the direct action of radiation on the DNA or by the free radicals produced in the surrounding aqueous solution can be repaired under hypoxia, but are fixed in the presence of oxygen (69).

Chemotherapy

It is obvious that the heterogeneous blood flow within tumours will profoundly influence drug delivery. However, the hypoxia produced as a result of this chaotic blood flow can also have effects on the cellular response to certain chemotherapeutic drugs. Studies by Roizen-Towle and Hall in 1978 demonstrated that exponentially growing cells in a culture which is rendered chronically hypoxic show more resistance to bleomycin than normally proliferating cells (72). Studies with multicellular spheroids indicated that factors, in addition to drug penetration, drug uptake, and cell cycle effects, were responsible for the resistance to Adriamycin in the centre of the spheroid (73). The effect of chronic hypoxia on the response of cells *in vitro* to Adriamycin demonstrated that large increases in resistance were obtained if cells were maintained in hypoxic conditions for several hours prior to drug treatment (74,75). Martin and McNally showed that cells *in vitro*, treated with the concentration of drug attained in the same cells grown as a solid tumour *in vivo*, were much more sensitive and associated this discrepancy at least in part to hypoxia (76). Subsequent studies with a range of drugs demonstrated that oxygenation was an important factor influencing the cytoxicity of many established chemotherapeutic drugs (77). In general, the effect induced by hypoxic preincubation was drug resistance.

Biological therapies

Although much experimental effort has been afforded to evaluating biological therapies *in vitro* and *in vivo*, relatively little attention has focused on how the complex microenvironmental and physiological features influence treatment efficiency. However, it is now evident that tumour relevant oxygen tensions can dramatically alter the potency of certain cytokines. Studies by Aune and Pogue in 1989 demonstrated that changing the oxygen tension of the cellular environment from 12 to 4% reduced the anti-proliferative effects of interferon (IFN) γ (78). The induction of lymphokine-activated killer (LAK) cell activity by IL-2 in human peripheral blood mononuclear cells is critically dependent on the oxygen tension in culture conditions (79). This study showed that for a given degree of target cell killing the IL-2 activated effector to target cell ratio had to be increased by a factor of 3 if the effector cells were incubated with IL-2 at 5% instead of 21% oxygen and a factor of 20 if the incubation with IL-2 was carried out at 2% oxygen. Several studies have demonstrated the critical importance of oxygen tension in determining the cytotoxic/anti-proliferative effects of tumour necrosis factor (TNF) α (80–83). In our own studies we have shown that exposure to 2% oxygen for 24 h, prior to TNF treatment, induces a four-to 50-fold increase in resistance compared with cells incubated at 21% oxygen (80,81). Moreover, continued passage of cells at tumour relevant oxygen tensions, prior to additions of TNF, further increased cellular resistance (81). These latter studies showed that preincubation oxygen tension is the important determining factor for the response to subsequent exposure to TNF. The underlying mechanism responsible for the induction of resistance has not yet been elucidated, although cell cycle effects are not responsible (81). Several mechanisms can be postulated. First, there is convincing evidence that reactive oxygen species mediate, at least in part, the cytotoxic activities of TNF (82–84,85). Thus, if hypoxia induces the production of proteins that protect the cell against such species, increased resistance would be evident. One such protein could be manganese superoxide dismutase (MnSOD), high levels of which are known to protect cells from TNF-induced cytotoxicity (86,87). Secondly, endogenous TNF production has been reported to protect cells against exposure to exogenous TNF (88,89). Recent reports indicate that incubating macrophages in an atmosphere containing 2% oxygen can dramatically up-regulate the endogenous production of both TNF and its soluble receptors (63). A third explanation is that receptor number, affinity, or rate of internalization of the receptor–ligand complex is altered by prior exposure to low oxygen environments.

Hypoxia as a target for therapy

The compromised oxygenation status existing in many regions of solid tumours can be a major cause of resistance to existing therapies. However, over recent years several chemical agents have been identified and developed which have greater toxicity towards hypoxic compared with aerobic cells. These compounds can therefore selectively target hypoxic tumour cells which are resistant to other therapies. The leading classes of compounds are: (i) the benzotriazone-di-*N*-oxides; (ii) 'dual function' alkylating nitroimidazoles; and (iii) quionones. The development and activity of these compounds has been recently reviewed (90). In brief, these drugs undergo metabolic reduction, facilitated by bioreductive enzymes and lower oxygen con-

ditions present in solid tumours, to generate cytotoxic metabolites. The use of these compounds in conjunction with radiation and drug therapy has elicited promising results in experimental systems and clinical studies are underway.

As is evident from the preceding section, a large number of hypoxia-regulated genes have already been identified. The hypoxia sensitive promoter elements of such genes could be used in a gene construct to drive the expression of a toxic gene or other genes such as nitroreductase, thymidine kinase, or cytosine deaminase. Following successful gene transfer to the tumour-bearing host, the latter genes would allow selective activation of prodrugs in the hypoxic tumour regions.

One problem with systemically administered gene delivery systems, such as retroviruses or adenoviruses, is that their access to cancer cells distant from the blood vessels will be compromised by the high interstitial pressure that exists within tumour tissue (12,13). Moreover, for delivery systems which have a short circulation time, access to some tumour regions may be prevented by temporary occlusion or reduction in blood flow. However, several procedures can be used to prolong circulation time including prolonged infusions or multiple injections. Poor access to tumour cells distant from blood vessels would probably severely limit the use of systemically administered gene delivery systems for hypoxia targeted gene therapy if hypoxia was caused simply by diffusion limitations as depicted in Fig. 6.4a. However, the evidence for acute changes in blood flow and for deoxygenated erythrocytes causing perivascular hypoxia indicates that hypoxia could be a very useful target for gene therapy approaches, including those directed against the endothelium.

Summary and conclusions

The angiogenic stimulus in tumours results in an abnormal and chaotic blood supply which does not adequately and consistently supply all the tumour cells with oxygen and nutrients. Indeed, there is convincing evidence that reduced oxygen tensions (P_{O_2} <15 mmHg) are a common feature of solid tumours. These hypoxic regions arise not only from diffusion limitations but from temporal changes in blood flow, such that even the endothelium may be subject to hypoxic or even anoxic conditions. The instability of microregional flow has the implication that a large proportion of the tumour cell and associated host cell populations could be subjected to hypoxia and nutrient deprivation for varying periods of time. Evidence from *in vitro* studies indicate that these cells will retain their clonogenic and proliferative capacity. Cellular response to radiation, chemotherapy, and cytokines can be severely compromised by exposure to reduced oxygen tension. Moreover, it is becoming evident that the expression of a large number of genes can be upregulated by hypoxia and by the subsequent reoxygenation. These gene products include those which influence angiogenesis, metastasis, and response to oxidative stress. This provides evidence that hypoxia maybe a fundamental driving force for many of the key biological processes occurring within tumour tissue. Because of its preferential occurrence in tumours, hypoxia is receiving attention as a potential target for therapy utilizing drug and gene-therapy based approaches.

Although not emphasized in this chapter, concomitant changes in nutrient delivery (*e.g.* glucose) and the acidic pH associated with inadequate blood flow are also known to influence biological processes, gene expression, and therapeutic response. The dynamics of tumour blood flow will also influence the access of systemically administered therapeutics to the tumour tissue particularly those with short plasma half-lives.

In conclusion, the unique pathophysiology of tumours has a profound influence on the molecular and cellular processes which occur in tumour cells and their associated stroma. Structure/function abnormalities of neoplasia at the tissue level still remain only partly understood as do the biological and molecular consequences of the dependent tissue environment and thus continued research in these areas is essential. Indeed, therapeutic exploitation of aberrant solid tumour structure, physiology, and metabolism may provide important adjuncts to conventional and novel treatment modalities.

References

1. Gullino, P. M. and Grantham, F. H. (1962). Studies on the exchange of fluids between host and tumour III. Regulation of blood flow in hepatomas and other rat tumour. *J. Natl Cancer Inst.*, **28**, 211–229.
2. Peter, W., Teixeira, M., Intaglietta, M., and Gross, J. F. (1980). Microcirculatory studies in rat mammary carcinoma I. Transparent chamber method, development of microvasculature and pressure in tumour vessels. *J. Natl Cancer*, **65**, 631–42.
3. Thompson, W. D., Shiach, K. J., Fraser, R. A., McIntosh, L. C., and Simpson, J. G. (1987). Tumours acquire their vascularity by vessel incorporation, not vessel ingrowth. *J. Pathol.*, **151**, 323–32.
4. Folkman, J. (1986). How is blood vessel growth regulated in normal and neoplastic tissue? — G. H. A. Clowes Memorial Award Lecture. *Cancer Res.*, **46**, 467–73.
5. Folkman, J. (1990). What is the evidence that tumour are angiogenesis dependent? *J. Natl Cancer Inst.*, **82**, 4–6.
6. Mattsson, J., Appelgren, L., Hamberger, B., and Peterson, H. I. (1977). Adrenergic innervation of tumour blood vessels. *Cancer Lett.*, **3**, 347–351.

7. Warren, B. A. (1979). The vascular morphology of tumours. In *Tumour blood circulation: angiogenesis, vascular morphology and blood flow of experimental tumours* (ed. H. I. Peterson), pp. 1–47. CRC Press, Boca Raton.
8. Grunt, T. W., Lametschwandtner, A., and Karrer, K. (1986). The characteristic structural features of the blood vessels of the Lewis lung carcinoma. *Scanning Electron Microsc.*, **11**, 575–89.
9. Tsukamoto, H., Mishima, Y., Hayashibe, K., and Sasase, A. (1992). α-smooth muscle actin expression in tumour and stromal cells of benign and malignant human pigment cell tumours. *J. Invest. Dermatol.*, **98**, 116–20.
10. Kobayashi, H., Tsuruchi, N., Sugihara, K., Kaku, T., Saito, T., Kamura, T., *et al.* (1993). Expression of α-smooth muscle actin in benign or malignant ovarian tumours. *Gynaecol. Oncol.*, **48**, 308–13.
11. Jain, R. K. (1988). Determinants of tumour blood flow: a review. *Cancer Res.*, **48**, 2641–58.
12. Boucher, Y., Baxter, L. T., and Jain, R. K. (1990). Interstitial pressure gradients in tissue isolated and subcutaneous tumours implications for therapy. *Cancer Res.*, **50**, 4478–84.
13. Jain, R. K. (1994). Barriers to drug delivery in solid tumours. *Scientific Am.*, **271**, 58–65.
14. Lewis, W. H. (1927). The vascular pattern of tumours. *Johns Hopkins Hosp. Bull.*, **41**, 156–73.
15. Falk, P. (1978). Patterns of vasculature in two pairs of related fibrosarcomas in the rat and their relation to tumour responses to single large doses of radiation. *Eur. J. Cancer*, **14**, 237–50.
16. Reinhold, H. S., and van den Berg-Blok, A. (1983). Vascularization of experimental tumours. In *Development of the vascular system* (Ciba Foundation Symposium 100), pp. 100–19. Pitman Books, London.
17. Vaupel, P., Kallinowski, F., and Okunieff, P. (1989). Blood flow, oxygen and nutrient supply and metabolic microenvironment of human tumours: a review. *Cancer Res.*, **49**, 6449–65.
18. Tozer, G. M., Shaffi, K. M., Prise, V. E., and Cunningham, J. J. (1994). Characterisation of tumour blood flow using a 'tissue-isolated' preparation. *Br. J. Cancer*, **70**, 1040–1046.
19. Wheeler, R. H., Ziessman, H. A., Medvec, B. R., Juni, J. E., Thrall, J. H., Keyes, J. W., *et al.* (1986). Tumour blood flow and systemic shunting in patients receiving intraarterial chemotherapy for head and neck cancer. *Cancer Res.*, **46**, 4200–4.
20. Granger, H. J., Borders, J. L., Meininger, G. A., Goodman, A. H., and Barnes, G. E. Microcirculatory control systems. In *The physiology and pharmacology of the microcirculation* (ed. N. A. Mortillaro), pp. 209–35, Vol. 1. Academic Press, New York.
21. Ragan, D. M. S., Schmidt, E. E., MacDonald, I. C., and Groom, A. C. (1988). Spontaneous cyclic contractions of the capillary wall *in vivo*, impeding red cell flow: a quantitative analysis. Evidence for endothelial cell contractility. *Microvasc. Res.*, **36**, 13–30.
22. Sims, D. E. (1986). The pericyte — a review. *Tissue Cell*, **18**, 153–74.
23. Vaupel, P. (1975). Interrelationship between mean arterial blood pressure, blood flow and vascular resistance in solid tumour tissue of DS-carcinosarcoma. *Experientia*, **31**, 587–9.
24. Chaplin, D. J. and Trotter, M. J. (1991). Chemical modifiers of tumour blood flow. In *Tumour blood supply and metabolic*

microenvironment (ed. P. Vaupel and R. K. Jain), pp. 65–85. Gustav Fisher Verlag, Stuttgart.

25. Intaglietta, M. and Mirhashemi, S. (1987). Reactivation of the microcirculation in ischemia. In *Microcirculation — an update* (ed. M. Tsuchiya, M. Asano, Y. Mishima and M. Oda), pp. 545–6, Vol. 1. Elsevier, Amsterdam.

26. Intaglietta, M. and Meyer, J. U. (1987). Vasomotion, the treatment of ischemia with vasoactive materials and the reversal of the microcirculatory 'steal' effect. In *Microcirculation — an update* (ed. M. Tsuchiya, M. Asano, Y. Mishima and M. Oda), pp. 223–4, Vol. 2. Elsevier, Amsterdam.

27. Endrich, B., Reinhold, H. S., Gross, J. F., and Intaglietta, M. (1979). Tissue perfusion inhomogeneity during early tumour growth in rats. *J. Natl Cancer Inst.*, **62**, 387–95.

28. Jirtle, R. A. and Hinshaw, W. M. (1981). Estimation of malignant tissue blood flow with radioactively labelled microspheres. *Eur. J. Cancer Clin. Oncol.*, **17**, 1353–5.

29. Tozer, G. M., Lewis, S., Michalowski, A., and Aber, V. (1990). The relationship between regional variations in blood flow and histology in a transplanted rat fibrosarcoma. *Br. J. Cancer*, **61**, 250–7.

30. Gullino, P. M. (1975). Extracellular compartments of solid tumours. In *Methods in cancer research* (ed. F. F. Becker), pp. 327–54. *Cancer*, Vol. 3. Plenum Press, New York.

31. Yamaura, H. and Sato, H. (1974). Quantitative studies on the developing vascular system of rat hepatoma. *J. Natl Cancer Inst.*, **53**, 1229–40.

32. Reinhold, H. S. (1971). Improved microcirculation in irradiated tumours. *Eur. J. Cancer*, **7**, 273–80.

33. Intaglietta, M., Myers, R. R., Gross, J. F., and Reinhold, H. S. (1977). Dynamics of microvascular flow in implanted mouse mammary tumours. *Bibl. Anat.*, **15**, 273–6.

34. Reinhold, H. S., Blachiwiecz, B., and Blok, A. (1977). Oxygenation and reoxygenation in 'sandwich' tumours. *Bibl. Anat.*, **15**, 270–2.

35. Endrich, B., Hammersen, F., Gotz, A., and Messmer, K. (1982). Microcirculatory blood flow, capillary morphology and local oxygen pressure of the hamster amelanotic melanoma A-Mel-3. *J. Natl Cancer Inst.*, **68**, 475–85.

36. Chaplin, D. J., Durand, R. E., and Olive, P. L. (1985). Cell selection from a murine tumour using the fluorescent perfusion probe Hoechst 33342. *Br. J. Cancer*, **51**, 569–72.

37. Chaplin, D. J., Durand, R. E., and Olive, P. L. (1986). Acute hypoxia in tumours: implications for modifiers of radiation effects. *Int. J. Radiat. Oncol. Biol. Phys.*, **12**, 1279–82.

38. Chaplin, D. J., Olive, P. L., and Durand, R. E. (1987). Intermittent blood flow in a murine tumour: radiobiological effects. *Cancer Res.*, **47**, 597–601.

39. Trotter, M. J., Chaplin, D. J., Durand, R. E., and Olive, P. L. (1989). The use of fluorescent probes to identify regions of transient perfusion in murine tumours. *Int. J. Radiat. Oncol. Biol. Phys.*, **16**, 931–4.

40. Chaplin, D. J. and Hill, S. A. (1995). Temporal heterogeneity in microregional erythrocyte flux within experimental tumours. *Br. J. Cancer*, **71**, 1210–13.

41. Trotter, M. J., Chaplin, D. J., and Olive, P. L. (1991). Possible mechanisms for intermittent blood flow in the murine SCCVII carcinoma. *Int. J. Radiat. Biol.*, **60**, 139–46.

42. Vaupel, P., Frinak, S., and Bicher, H. I. (1981). Heterogenous oxygen partial pressure and pH distribution in C3H mouse mammary adenocarcinoma. *Cancer Res.*, **41**, 2008–13.

43. Wike-Hooley, J. L., Haveman, J., and Reinhold, H. S. (1984). The relevance of tumour pH to the treatment of malignant disease. *Radiother. Oncol.*, **2**, 343–66.

44. Kallinowski, F., Schlenger, K. H., Runkel, S., Kloes, M., Stohrer, M., Okunieff, P., and Vaupel, P. (1989). Blood flow, metabolism, cellular microenvironment and growth rate of human tumour xenografts. *Cancer Res.*, **49**, 3759–64.

45. Mueller-Klieser, W., Vaupel, P., Manz, R., and Schmidseder, R. (1981). Intracapillary oxyhemoglobin saturation of malignant tumours in humans. *Int. J. Radiat. Oncol. Biol. Phys.*, **7**, 1397–404.

46. Vaupel, P. (1994). *Blood flow, oxygenation, tissue pH distribution and bioenergetic status of tumours*, pp. 1–77, Vol. 23. Ernest Schering Research Foundation.

47. Hockel, M., Knoop, C., Schlenger, K., Vorndran, B., Bassman, E., Mitze, M. (1993). Intratumoral pO_2 predicts survival in advanced cancer of the uterine cervix. *Radiother. Oncol.*, **26**, 45–50.

48. Thomlinson, R. H. and Gray, L. H. (1955). The histological structure of some human lung cancers and the possible implications for radiotherapy. *Br. J. Cancer*, **9**, 539–49.

49. Shrieve, D. C., Deen, D. F., and Horns, J. W. (1983). Effects of extreme hypoxia on the growth and viability of EMT6/SF mouse tumour cells *in vitro*. *Cancer Res.*, **43**, 3521–7.

50. Rotin, D., Robinson, B., and Tannock, I. F. (1986). Influence of hypoxia and an acidic environment on the metabolism and viability of cultured cells: potential implications for cell death in tumours. *Cancer Res.*, **46**, 2821–6.

51. Yao, K. S., Clayton, M., and O'Dwyer, P. J. (1995). Apoptosis in human adenocarcinoma HT-29 cells induced by exposure to hypoxia. *J. Natl Cancer Inst.*, **87**, 117–22.

52. Koch, C. J., Kruuv, J., and Frey, H. E. (1973). The effect of hypoxia on the generation time of mammalian cells. *Radiat. Res.*, **53**, 43–8.

53. Born, R., Hug, O., and Trott, K. R. (1976). The effect of prolonged hypoxia on growth and viability of Chinese hamster cells. *Int. J. Radiat. Oncol. Biol. Phys.*, **1**, 687–97.

54. Casciari, J. J., Sotirchos, S. V., and Sutherland, R. M. (1992). Variations in tumour cell growth rates and metabolism with oxygen concentrations, glucose concentration and extracellular pH. *J. Cell. Physiol.*, **151**, 386–94.

55. Beru, N., McDonald, J., Lacombe, C., and Goldwasser, E. (1986). Expression of the erythropoietin gene. *Mol. Cell. Biol.*, **6**, 2571–5.

56. Kourembanas, S., Marsden, P. A., McQuillan, L. P., and Faller, D. V. (1991). Hypoxia induces endothelin gene expression in cultured human endothelium. *J. Clin. Invest.*, **88**, 1054–7.

57. Shreeniwas, R., Koga, S., Karakurum, M., Pinsky, D., Kaiser, E., Brett, J., *et al.* (1992). Hypoxia mediated induction of endothelial cell interleukin Iα. *J. Clin. Invest.*, **90**, 2333–9.

58. Plate, K. H. Breier, G., Weich, H. A., and Risau, W. (1992). Vascular endothelial growth factor is a potential tumour angiogenesis factor in human gliomas *in vivo*. *Nature*, **359**, 845–8.

59. Shweiki, D., Itin, A., Soffer, D., and Keshet, E. (1992). Vascular endothelial growth factor induced by hypoxia may mediate hypoxia-initiated angiogenesis. *Nature*, **359**, 843–5.

60. Goldberg, M. A. and Schneider, T. J. (1994). Similarities between the oxygen sensing mechanisms regulating the expression of vascular endothelial growth factor and erythro-

poietin. *J. Biol. Chem.*, **269**, 4355–9.

61. Kourembanas, S., Hannan, R. L., and Faller, D. V. (1990). Oxygen tension regulates the expression of the platelet derived growth factor-β chain in human endothelial cells. *J. Clin. Invest.*, **86**, 670–4.

62. Karakurum, M., Shreeniwas, R., Chen, J., Pinsky, D., Yan, S. D., Anderson, M., *et al.* (1994). Hypoxic induction of interleukin-8 gene expression in human endothelial cells. *J. Clin. Invest.*, **93**, 1564–70.

63. Scannel, G., Waxman, K., Kaeml, G. J., Ioli, G., Gatanga, T., Yamamoto, R., and Granger, G. A. (1993). Hypoxia induces a human macrophage cell line to release tumour necrosis factor α and its soluble receptors *in vitro*. J. Surg. Res., **54**, 281–5.

64. Murphy, B. J., Laderoute, K. R., Chin, R. J., and Sutherland, R. M. (1994). Metallothionen IIA is up-regulated by hypoxia in human A431 squamous carcinoma cells. *Cancer Res.*, **54**, 5808–10.

65. Young, S. D., Marshall, R. S., and Hill, R. P. Hypoxia induces DNA over-replication and enhances metastatic potential of murine tumour cells. *Proc. Natl Acad. Sci. USA*, **85**, 9533–8.

66. Stackpole, C. W., Groszek, L., and Kalbag, S. (1994). Benign to malignant B16 melanoma progression induced in two stages *in vitro* by exposure to hypoxia. *J Natl Cancer Inst.*, **86**, 361–7.

67. Singh, R. K., Gutman, M., Radinsky, R., Bucana, C. D., and Fidler, I. J. (1994). Expression of interleukin 8 correlates with the metastatic potential of human melanoma cells in nude mice. *Cancer Res.*, **54**, 3242–7.

68. Russo, C. A., Weber, T. K., Volpe, C. M., Stoler, D. L., Petrelli, N. J., Rodriguez-Biggs, M., *et al.* (1995). An anoxia inducible endonuclease and enhanced DNA breakage as contributors to genomic instability in cancer. *Cancer Res.*, **55**, 1122–8.

69. Hall, E. J. (1988). *Radiobiology for the radiologist*. Harper and Row, Philadelphia.

70. Howard-Flanders, P. and Moore, D. (1958). The time interval after pulsed irradiation within which injury in bacteria can be modified by dissolved oxygen. I. A search for an effect of oxygen 0.02 seconds after pulsed irradiation. *Radiat. Res.*, **9**, 422–37.

71. Michael, B. D., Adams, G. E., Hewitt, H. B., Jones, W. B. G. and Watts, M. E. (1973). A post-effect of oxygen in irradiated bacteria: a submillisecond fast mixing study. *Radiat. Res.*, **54**, 239–51.

72. Roizen-Towle, L. and Hall, E. J. (1978). Studies with bleomycin and misonidazole on aerated and hypoxic cells. *Br. J. Cancer*, **37**, 254–60.

73. Sutherland, R. M., Eddy, H. A., Bareham, B., Reich, K., and Vanantwerp, D. (1979). Resistance to adriamycin in multicellular spheroids. *Int. J. Radiat. Oncol. Biol. Phys.*, **5**, 1225.

74. Smith, E., Stratford, I. J., and Adams, G. E. (1980). Cytotoxicity of adriamycin on aerobic and hypoxic Chinese hamster V79 cells *in vitro*. *Br. J. Cancer*, **41**, 568–72.

75. Born, R. and Eichholtz-Wirth, H. (1981). Effect of different physiological conditions on the action of adriamycin on Chinese hamster cells *in vitro*. *Br. J. Cancer*, **44**, 241–6.

76. Martin, W. M. C. and McNally, N. J. (1980). Cytotoxicity of adriamycin to tumour cells *in vivo*. *Br. J. Cancer*, **42**, 881–9.

77. Teicher, B. A., Lazo, J. S., and Sartorelli, A. C. (1981). Classification of antineoplastic agents by their selective toxicities towards oxygenated and hypoxic tumour cells. *Cancer Res.*, **41**, 73–81.

78. Aune, T. M. and Pogue, S. (1989). Inhibition of tumour cell growth by Interferon-γ is mediated by two distinct mechanisms, dependent on tumour oxygenation, induction of tryptophan degradation and depletion of intracellular nicotinamide adenine dinucleotide. *J. Clin. Invest.*, **84**, 863–75.

79. Ishizaka, S., Kimoto, M., and Tsujii, T. (1992). Defect in generation of LAK cell activity under oxygen-limited conditions. *Immunol. Lett.*, **32**, 209–14.

80. Sampson, L. E. and Chaplin, D. J. (1994). The influence of microenvironment on the cytotoxicity of TNFα *in vitro*. *Int. J. Radiat. Oncol. Biol. Phys.*, **29**, 467–71.

81. Lynch, E. M., Sampson, L. E., Khalil, A. A., Horsman, M. R., and Chaplin, D. J. (1995). Cytotoxic effect of tumour necrosis factor-alpha on sarcoma F cells at tumour relevant oxygen tension. *Acta Oncol.*, **34**, 423–7.

82. Park, Y. M. K., Anderson, R. L., Spitz, D. R., and Hahn, G. M. (1992). Hypoxia and resistance to hydrogen peroxide confer resistance to tumour necrosis factor in murine L929 cells. *Radiat. Res.*, **131**, 162–8.

83. Naldini, A., Cesari, S., and Bocci, V. (1994). Effects of hypoxia on the cytotoxicity mediated by tumour necrosis factor α. *Lymphokine Cytokine*, **13**, 233–7.

84. Zimmerman, R. J., Chan, A., and Leadon, S. A. (1989). Oxidative damage in murine tumour cells treated *in vitro* by recombinant human tumour necrosis factor. *Cancer Res.*, **49**, 1644–8.

85. Yamauchi, N., Kuriyama, H., Watanabe, N., Neda, H., Maeda, M., and Niitsu, Y. (1989). Intracellular hydroxyl radical production induced by recombinant tumour necrosis factor and its implication in the killing of tumour cells *in vitro*. *Cancer Res.*, **49**, 1671–5.

86. Wong, C. H. W., Elwell, J. H., Oberley, L. W., and Geoddel, D. V. (1989). Manganous superoxide dismutase is essential for cellular resistance to cytotoxicity of tumour necrosis factor. *Cell*, **58**, 923–31.

87. Zyad, A., Benard, J., Tursz, Clarke, R., and Chouaib, S. (1994). Resistance to TNF α and Adriamycin in the human breast cancer MCF-7 cell line: relationship to MDR1, MnSOD and TNF gene expression. *Cancer Res.*, **54**, 825–31.

88. Vanhaesebroeck, B., Decoster, E., Van Ostade X, Van Bladel, S., Lenaerts, A., Van Roy F., and Fiers, W. (1992). Expression of an exogenous tumour necrosis factor (TNF) gene in TNF sensitive cell lines confers resistance to TNF mediated cell lysis. *J. Immunol.*, **148**, 2785–94.

89. Himeno, T., Watanabe, N., Yamauchi, N., Maeda, M., Tsuji, Y., Okamoto, T., *et al.* (1990). Expression of endogenous TNF as a protective protein against the cytotoxicity of exogenous TNF. *Cancer Res.*, **50**, 4941–5.

90. Workman, R. and Stratford, I. J. (1993). The experimental development of bioreductive drugs and their role in cancer therapy. *Cancer Metastasis Rev.*, **12**, 73–82.

7. Mechanisms of stress-induced angiogenesis in tumours

Eli Keshet, Ilan Stein, and Michal Neeman

Introduction

Tumour angiogenesis is generally viewed as the conse-quence of an 'angiogenic switch', i.e. a genetic event that endows the tumour with the ability to recruit blood vessels from the neighbouring tissue. Whether the up-regulation of angiogenesis stimulators (1) or the down-regulation of angiogenesis inhibitors (2), the 'angiogenic switch' is con-ceived as a stochastic event in the succession of genetic hits that underlie tumour progression.

In contrast to the stochastic nature of the tumour angio-genic switch, physiological angiogenesis represents a tissue response to either an hormonal stimulation (*e.g.* an-giogenesis in the reproductive system) or an environmen-tal insult. Of utmost importance is the ability of a tissue to expand its vasculature in response to insufficient perfusion (ischaemia). Recent studies have shown that ischaemia-driven angiogenesis is a fundamental process operating to match the vasculature to the metabolic requirements of the tissue under different physiological settings as well as in some cases of developmentally programmed angiogenesis. These studies have further shown that this adaptive, feed-back response is mediated by induced expression of vascu-lar endothelial growth factor (VEGF) in response to a deficiency in oxygen (hypoxia) or glucose (hypogly-caemia). Findings concerning ischaemia-driven angiogen-esis in non-tumour tissues are reviewed in the next section.

The concept highlighted in this review is that tumour cells, like their normal counterparts, are able to 'sense' is-chaemia and react by eliciting a compensatory angiogene-sis. Therefore, stress-induced angiogenesis is likely to be an important component of tumour neovascularization, in-dependent of angiogenic activities produced by a genetic switch. This hypothesis is based on two suppositions. First, that tumour cells can respond to an ischaemic insult, i.e. that the ability to regulate angiogenic factor expression was not lost concomitantly with cellular transformation. Second, that stress conditions conductive for augmented expression of angiogenic factors develop during growth of natural tumours. Evidence that a number of natural human tumours indeed up-regulate VEGF, specifically in hypoxic microenvironments is provided later.

The complex multicellular organization of primary tumours makes it difficult, however, to distinguish stress-induced expression from expression associated with the emergence of new tumour genotypes. To overcome this difficulty, patterns of angiogenic factor expression were also studied in multicell spheroids. Representing a genetic-ally homogeneous population of tumour cells in which a continuum of different microenvironments develops due to limited availability of oxygen and nutrients, spheroids are particularly useful for determining the effects of environ-mental factors. Results obtained from the spheroid model are outlined in the section on 'Angiogenic switch versus stress-induced angiogenesis', p. 73.

One implication of the fact that tumour neovasculariza-tion is affected by environmental factors is that the overall angiogenic output of a tumour cell may constantly change during tumour growth. Furthermore, stress-induced angio-genesis may become a predominant factor when other sources of angiogenic activity are blocked in attempts to inhibit tumour growth. These considerations are discussed in the section on 'Genetic and environmental factors in tumour angiogenesis', p. 75.

The central role of VEGF as a mediator of ischaemia-induced angiogenesis and relevant aspects of VEGF regu-lation are further discussed later in this chapter. First, it is shown that two different consequences of tissue ischaemia namely, hypoxia and hypoglycaemia act as a trigger for VEGF induction. Second, viewing VEGF as a stress-induced gene, its mode of regulation is compared with that of other oxygen-regulated proteins (ORPs) and glucose-regulated proteins (GRPs). Third, available data con-cerning molecular mechanisms of VEGF regulation by hypoxia and hypoglycaemia are presented.

Physiological and developmental angiogenesis as an adaptive response to oxygen deficiency

To assure efficient exchange of oxygen and nutrients, every cell of the body needs to be sufficiently close to a blood capillary. Accordingly, the process of capillary sprouting continues until sufficient proximity has been at-tained. Thereafter, angiogenesis enters a state of quies-cence (with the exception of angiogenic cycles in the female reproductive system). Yet, every increase in tissue mass is matched by neovascularization, securing that ade-quate vascular density is maintained. In addition, increase in the work-load of an organ often leads to a compensatory angiogenesis. For example, regions of the brain with intense neuronal activity have a higher vascular density than less active regions (3,4). Thus, angiogenesis seems to be induced when the metabolic requirements of the tissue exceed the perfusion capability of existing vessels. A likely mechanism of this adaptive, feedback response is that a relative deficiency of oxygen leads to up-regulation of angiogenesis stimulator(s). Therefore, a search for hypoxia-inducible angiogenic factor expression was carried out, examining a number of candidate genes whose angiogenic potential was previously demonstrated in ex-perimental models.

In the initial experiments, cells of a rat glioma line were cultured under normoxic and hypoxic conditions, and steady-state levels of the respective mRNAs were subse-quently measured by RNA-blot analysis. Of the mRNAs analysed, steady-state levels of VEGF mRNA were significantly increased within a few hours of growth under low oxygen tensions, with a maximal, over 10-fold induc-tion measured after 18 h of severe hypoxia. The increase in VEGF mRNA levels was reversible. Upon re-exposure of cells to normal oxygen tension, VEGF expression re-turned to its low constitutive level (5). These experiments suggested for the first time that levels of VEGF expression are inversely modulated by changes in tissue oxygen. Another hypoxia-inducible factor with angiogenic poten-tial is platelet-derived growth factor BB (PDGF-BB) (6). However, VEGF has so far received most of the attention because of a large body of findings (not yet available for PDGF) showing that VEGF is a key player in natural angiogenesis.

VEGF is a secreted, 46 kDa dimeric protein that is active as an endothelial cell-specific mitogen, as a potent angiogenic factor, and as a vascular permeability factor. VEGF is thought to act as a paracrine angiogenic factor, i.e. it is produced and secreted by the tissue to which the new capillaries grow. This conclusion is supported by studies showing that VEGF is transiently up-regulated in tissues engaged in active angiogenesis, while its cognate receptors are expressed on target endothelial cells in nearby blood vessels (see Chapter 16 for references).

A paracrine mechanism of VEGF function fits the sup-position that VEGF acts to direct growth of new blood vessels to under-perfused tissues. It is envisaged that cells in the ischaemic tissue up-regulate VEGF expression. The

secreted VEGF isoforms generate a gradient that instructs the growth of capillary sprouts (expressing VEGF recep-tors) towards the site from which VEGF emanates. To evaluate in which tissues this regulatory response might take place, the ability to up-regulate VEGF in response to hypoxia was examined in different cell types. The list of cells shown to up-regulate VEGF in vitro during hypoxia includes fibroblasts, muscle cells, myocytes, retinal pig-mented epithelium, astrocytes, and endothelial cells (5,7–10), as well as a number of tumour cells (see below). Thus, it seems that VEGF is induced by hypoxia in most, if not all cells in vitro.

Hypoxic regulation of VEGF in vivo was demonstrated, however, in only few cases. Of particular interest is VEGF regulation in the ischaemic myocardium, as the develop-ment of coronary collateral vessels represents, at least in part, a process of ischaemia-induced neovascularization (11). We have shown that multiple forms of differentially spliced VEGF mRNA are induced in ischaemic territories of a porcine myocardium shortly after experimental occlu-sion of a major coronary artery (7). Therefore, it is likely that VEGF plays a part in the natural process of ischaemia-induced collateral formation. The notion that up-regulation of endogenous VEGF may indeed result in collateral for-mation is supported by studies showing that exogenous VEGF induces collateral formation in animal models of both myocardial ischaemia and hindlimb ischaemia (12,13). The retina is another system where experimental occlusion of blood vessels has led to up-regulation of en-dogenous VEGF (14,15). These studies demonstrate that when homeostasis in a well-vascularized organ is impaired (e.g. due to vessel occlusion) VEGF is induced in order to elicit compensatory angiogenesis.

Angiogenic responses to insufficient perfusion also take place during normal development, particularly during organogenesis. A striking example is development of the vasa vasorum, i.e. blood vessels that nourish blood vessels. The fact that vasa vasorum only penetrate the walls of those vessels that are too thick to be adequately perfused from within, argue for an hypoxia-driven mechanism. Increased demand for oxygen and nutrients, imposed by an increase in tissue mass or the onset of specialized activi-ties that consume much oxygen has to be matched by a parallel increase in perfusion capability. To examine the hypothesis that a low, sub-pathological level of hypoxia might serve as a trigger for developmental angiogensis, normal development of the retina vasculature was studied. It was shown that 'physiological' hypoxia caused by the onset of neuronal activity is detected by strategically located populations of neuroglia, first astrocytes, then Müller cells. In response they secrete VEGF, inducing for-mation of the superficial and deep layers of retinal vessels, respectively. As the vessels become patent, and the hypoxic stimulus is relieved, VEGF is down-regulated. A direct role for hypoxia-induced VEGF in the intact developing retina was demonstrated by showing that vessel formation was inhibited in animals grown under an oxygen-enriched atmosphere that suppresses endogenous VEGF production (9). In this way vessel formation is matched to oxygen demand.

The notion that 'physiological' levels of hypoxia act as a trigger for some developmental angiogenesis requires that restoration of normoxia will take place before oxygen deprivation will cause a significant damage. This is of particular significance in neuronal tissues where even short ischaemic episodes may cause irreversible damage. It is possible, therefore, that certain cells within the brain function as sensitive hypoxia 'sensors' by virtue of having a low threshold of response to low oxygen tensions. In keeping with this suggestion are the findings that a mild retinal ischaemia, caused by laser-driven occlusion of selected veins of a rabbit retina, leads to up-regulation of VEGF specifically in astrocytes, i.e. the same cells that up-regulate VEGF during development of superficial retinal vessels (9,15). In contrast, severe retinal ischaemia, caused by obliteration of retinal vessels in animal models of retinopathy of prematurity (16) or in patients with proliferative diabetic retinopathy (15,17) results in up-regulation of VEGF expression by additional cell types.

Augmented vascular endothelial growth factor expression in hypoxic microenvironments of natural tumours

A microtumour reaching a detectable size (over a millimetre in diameter) contains substantial heterogeneous microenvironments. It has been argued that multiple tumour microenvironments in which there may be major gradients of critical metabolites, nutrients, hormones, and growth factors, are a major factor facilitating further emergence of new and diverse cell phenotypes (18). A major cause of the emergence of diverse microenvironments is imbalanced vascularization. Tumour neovascularization often lacks the precision inherent to developmentally programmed angiogenesis where vascular supply is constantly adjusted to changes in tissue needs. In tumours, in particular in fast-growing tumours, vascular development often lags behind the rapid increase in tumour mass. The result is the emergence of progressively stressed microenvironments that, unless neovascularized in time, undergo necrosis. The gap between tumour growth and vascular growth and, accordingly, the degree of tumour hypoxia and necrosis is highly variable among different types of tumours.

Glioblastoma is an example of a highly angiogenic tumour with imbalanced vascularity. Glioblastoma multiforme (GM) is the most malignant tumour of astrocytic origin in humans. High malignancy grade gliomas mostly develop by progression from astrocytomas of low malignancy grade and the switch to an angiogenic phenotype is thought to occur during progression from low-grade to high-grade glioma (19). A characteristic feature of GM is that, despite extensive microvascular proliferation, extensive areas undergo necrosis, presumably due to insufficient perfusion. Glioblastoma biopsies were analysed by *in situ* hybridization, with the expectation that a stress-induced angiogenic factor will be predominantly expressed in a restricted subpopulation of tumour cells, reflecting the localization of hypoxic microregions. These experiments revealed that VEGF expression is dramatically up-regulated in a small fraction of tumour cells alongside the periphery of necrotic regions, i.e. in cells subjected to a severe hypoxia. Highest mRNA levels were detected in the tumour cells juxtaposed to cells undergoing necrosis, cells known as palisading cells due to their morphology (5,20).

Progression from a low-grade glioma to glioblastoma is also associated with a co-ordinate up-regulation of the two VEGF receptors, *flt-1* and *flk-1* in the tumour vascular endothelial cells (21). Thus, VEGF is likely to act in a paracrine fashion on nearby blood vessels. Co-visualization of VEGF producing cells and blood vessels in GM tumours has shown that capillary bundles are preferentially clustered alongside the regions of VEGF-expressing cells (5,20). This pattern suggests that the pathognomonic vascular glomeruli characteristic of GM are formed by focal angiogenic responses elicited by exceedingly high amounts of stress-induced VEGF. It is possible that uneven distribution of blood vessels in tumours, in general, is the result of the regional nature of environmentally regulated angiogenesis. Induction of large amounts of VEGF — a potent vascular permeability factor (hence also known as VPF) (22,23) — may also account for the apparent leakiness of blood vessels in GM tumours. Up-regulation of VEGF in hypoxic tumour microenvironments is not limited to tumours of astrocytic origin and was also demonstrated in other natural tumours as well as in a number of transplanted tumour xenografts (24–26). Thus, stress-induced angiogenesis is a common occurrence in actively growing tumours.

Angiogenic switch versus stress-induced angiogenesis

Analysis of spontaneous or experimental tumours is limited in the sense that the cause of altered expression is unknown. For example, up-regulated expression of VEGF in palisading cells in GM tumours can be equally attributed to the fact that these cells may represent dedifferentiated anaplastic glioma cells (27), or to hypoxic regulation of VEGF, or to a paracrine effect of necrosis factors. On the other hand, analysis of monolayer cultures is short of reproducing the complexity of ecological niches developing in a three-dimensional mass. To overcome these shortcomings, researchers have resorted to analysis of three-dimensional multicell spheroids. Spheroids grown from established cell lines represent a clonal cell population in which gradients of oxygen, glucose, and other nutrients create a continuum of different microenvironments (18,28,29). The spheroid system thus simulates microregions that develop in under-vascularized tumours at various distances from capillaries. Alternatively, the spheroid can be viewed as a model of the initial, avascular phase of tumour progression. Implantation of multicellular spheroids in experimental animals can be used to study in detail the avascular–vascular transition in tumour progression (30,31).

Multicellular spheroids can be derived from almost any anchorage-dependent tumorigenic cell line, by continuous culture as a stirred suspension. The spheroid develops during its growth a necrotic centre surrounded by a zone of quiescent cells while cell proliferation continues in the outer rim (32). The proliferative capacity of cells at different regions of the spheroid was probed by selective dissociation showing a fraction of quiescent cells in the inner region of the viable rim (33). These inner cell layers also exhibit a significant fraction of hypoxic cells that are resistant to radiation (34,35) and chemotherapy (36–38).

The development of microenvironmental heterogeneity within the spheroids stems from insufficient rate of nutrient diffusion and clearance of waste products (36–38). Diffusion across different zones of spheroids was characterized by nuclear magnetic resonance (NMR) microscopy, showing 10-fold lower diffusion in the viable rim relative to the extracellular water (39,40). Consequently, significant gradients of oxygen, pH, and different metabolites are created. These gradients were measured across multicellular spheroids using microelectrodes (41,42), chemiluminescence (43), electron spin resonance (44), and NMR microscopy (37). In accord with the wide range of metabolic milieu, inner regions of spheroids show elevated expression of ORP and GRP, respectively (18). Thus this system proves an efficient in vitro experimental tool for molecular analysis of stress-regulated genes. In contrast with in vivo models of tumour xenografts, multicellular spheroids can be exposed to acute or chronic alteration of the external medium conditions thus expanding the range of microenvironmental conditions even further and providing mechanistic information on key regulatory pathways. Spheroids have been particularly useful in addressing four issues relevant to this discussion: (i) distinguishing a direct stress-induced expression from a genetic alteration or an indirect paracrine effect of necrotic factors; (ii) comparing different stress challenges, particularly hypoglycaemia versus hypoxia; (iii) comparing expression of VEGF with the expression of other stress proteins; and (iv) monitoring the actual angiogenic capacity and the effect of vascularization on VEGF expression in implanted spheroids in vivo.

1. Expression of VEGF is greatly up-regulated in quiescent cells occupying the inner layers of C6 spheroids. When hypoxia in the inner core is abolished by acute hyperoxygenation, VEGF is down-regulated to the same low level of expression detected in non-stressed, dividing cells occupying the outer layers (26; also see Fig. 7.1). Comparison of spheroids derived from different tumour cell lines have shown that tumours that do not express VEGF intrinsically are as efficient as tumours producing VEGF constitutively in their ability to up-regulate VEGF when subjected to stress.

2. Acute glucose deprivation — another consequence of vascular insufficiency — also activates VEGF expression (26). Experiments carried out in cell monolayers established that VEGF can be independently induced by hypoxia or by hypoglycaemia. Interestingly, no induction of VEGF occurs in cultured glioma cells deprived of both oxygen and glucose. Up-regulation of VEGF expression requires protein synthesis (26,45) which perhaps cannot be carried out during the double stress. Notably, situations of chronic or acute hypoglycaemia may develop in certain microregions due to hypovascularity and due to recurrent, transient closures of tumour vessels (46,47). Multicell spheroids have been used to produce a gradient of suboptimal glucose concentrations superimposed on an oxygen gradient. Under these conditions, VEGF was induced in two distinct, non-contiguous regions, suggesting that different stress combinations are conductive to VEGF induction (26; also see Fig. 7.1). Measurements of actual oxygen and glucose concentrations across the spheroid, in conjunction with in situ hybridization analysis, will enable definition of these combinations. Future studies should uncover additional stress conditions frequently encountered in unperfused regions of tumours, including temperature gradients, pH, lactate, interstitial pressure and deficiency in amino acids and essential trace elements.

3. Many oxygen and glucose response proteins are induced in inner regions of multicellular spheroids (18). The expression of VEGF and other stress-regulated genes

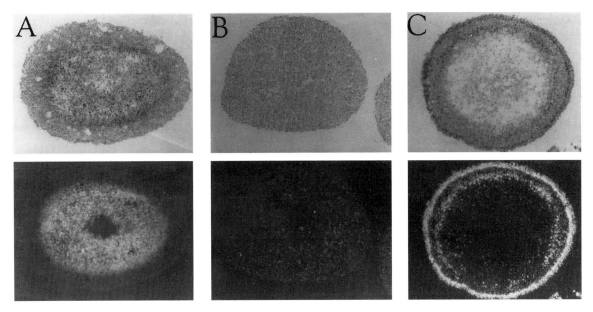

Figure 7.1. Vascular endothelia growth factor (VEGF) expression by hypoxia and hypoglycaemia in multicell spheroids. C6 glioma spheroids were sectioned and hybridized *in situ* with a VEGF-specific probe. (a) A spheroid (approximately 800 mm in diameter) cultured in a standard medium (4.5 g/l glucose) saturated with a mixture of 95% air/5% CO_2. (b) Hyperoxygenated spheroid, exposed for 16 h to a mixture of 95% oxygen/5% CO_2. (c) A spheroid cultured under standard conditions (4.5 g/l glucose) and transferred to a low glucose medium (0.1 g/l glucose) for 6 h prior to fixation. To visualize autoradiographic grains better, slides were photographed under brightfield (top) and darkfield (bottom) illuminations.

can be compared in consecutive slices of spheroids at a wide range of acute and chronic stress conditions. Using this methodology, the regulatory mechanisms of activation of these genes can be evaluated and the ORP/GRPs can be sorted to groups which are co-expressed at all stress conditions (45). This aspect will be discussed in the section on 'VEGF as an ORP'.

4. Upon implantation in nude mice, spheroids are efficiently neovascularized. This provides a convenient *in vivo* model that, in conjunction with magnetic resonance imaging (MRI) enables continuous and simultaneous non-invasive monitoring of a developing tumour and, independently, of its vasculature. The model provides defined initial conditions of tumour geometry, simulating further expansion of a small, avascular nodule. Vessel growth towards C6 spheroids is induced within 4 days after implantation, during which time a lag in tumour growth is consistently observed (31). These findings provide further evidence for the concept that tumour growth is angiogenesis-dependent (48). Actual tumour perfusion was followed by intravenous injection of the MRI contrast reagent Gd-DTPA to tumour-bearing mice 15 days after spheroid implantation. A transient rise in signal intensity was

observed for the large blood vessels remote from the tumour, followed by a quick clearance. Signal enhancement in peripheral regions of the tumour due to new vessels that have already penetrated the tumour was slow and also the rate of clearance was slow implying that blood vessels in close proximity to the tumour were highly permeable (31). This increased permeability correlates well with the activity of VEGF as a vascular permeability factor.

Concomitant with invasion of blood vessels and restoration of normoxia to the spheroid core, VEGF expression is gradually down-regulated to a constitutive low level of expression, representing the output of non-stressed glioma cells (26). This experimental system permits an assessment *in vivo* of the relative contributions of stress-induced angiogenesis and angiogenesis induced by the tumour 'angiogenic switch'.

Genetic and environmental factors in tumour angiogenesis

The angiogenic power of a tumour is determined by the sum of angiogenic stimuli arising from the angiogenic switch and angiogenic stimuli arising from environmental stress. The relative significance of the two sources of angiogenic factors may vary at different stages of tumour growth. Angiogenic factors might be induced by stress even at stages preceding a genetic switch, once the avascular tumour has grown beyond a size of a few millimetres in diameter. This argues that, in principle, stress-induced production of angiogenic factors might be sufficient to induce angiogenesis in avascular tumours. Yet, a large body of evidence suggests that a genetic switch is essential for the transition from the avascular to the vascular phase (see reference 49 for a recent review). Recent studies have also shown that neovascularization of distant micrometastases is promoted by removal of a source of a circulating inhibitor of angiogenesis (50). It is possible that stress-induced VEGF is not sufficient to counteract the effect of negative regulators and that removal of this barrier is the key event in the genetic switch. Indeed, recent studies have emphasized that down-regulation of natural angiogenesis inhibitors is an important component of the angiogenic switch (51,52). At certain stages of tumour progression, presumably after down-regulation of negative regulators, augmented VEGF expression should be sufficient to elicit neovascularization. For example, in MCF-7 human breast carcinoma cells transfected with a VEGF-producing vector, augmented VEGF expression is sufficient to cause enhanced tumour, growth and vascular density (53).

Increased levels of VEGF mRNA and protein were detected in many tumours, including tumours of astrocytic origin (21), haemangioblastoma (54), breast carcinoma (24), ovarian carcinoma (55), colon cancers (56), and renal cancer (57). In the first three cases, up-regulation of VEGF receptors by the tumour endothelial cells was also reported. These increases may be due to genetic changes in tumour cells. The nature of genetic changes leading to increased VEGF production is not known. Transfecting a mutated form of the tumour suppressor gene p53 into cultured fibroblasts induced expression of VEGF mRNA (58). Interestingly, a mutation in a single tumour suppressor gene may activate angiogenesis by both down-regulating angiogenesis inhibitors (51,52) as well as by up-regulating a major angiogenesis stimulator. Indeed, restoration of wildtype p53 DNA to breast tumours grown in nude mice resulted in a marked reduction in both the number of tumour blood vessels and the overall rate of tumour growth (59).

The important role of VEGF in tumour angiogenesis prompted attempts to inhibit tumour growth by inhibiting VEGF action. Two different approaches to inhibit VEGF action were used: the use of neutralizing monoclonal antibody to VEGF (25) and the strategy of dominant-negative inhibition of the VEGF receptor *flk-1* (60). In both cases these treatments resulted in inhibition of vascularization and, thereby growth of glioma cells xenografted into nude mice. Thus, anti-VEGF modality was both necessary and sufficient to inhibit angiogenesis, presumably because VEGF is both the major angiogenic factor produced constitutively by glioma cells and induced by stress. A more complex situation might exist, however, when an angiogenic factor other than VEGF is the predominant factor produced constitutively by the tumour and hence chosen as a therapeutic target. We argue that in this case, impairment of vascular function will cause severe ischaemic stress and, as a result, induction of VEGF and compensatory angiogenesis will follow. Thus, irrespective of the identity of the angiogenic factors activated by a genetic change, any attempt to inhibit tumour neovascularization needs to consider stress-induced angiogenesis mediated by VEGF.

Stress-induced angiogenesis may become a major factor also during other modalities of cancer therapy. This was illustrated in a system of human breast carcinoma cells inoculated in nude mice and subjected to anti-oestrogen therapy. Oestrogen-responsive MCF-7 tumours treated with the anti-oestrogen tamoxifen undergo rapid necrosis. The finding that tamoxifen-induced death of tumour cells is preceded by a marked decrease in vascular density prompted the suggestion that the tumour vasculature is a primary target of tamoxifen (61). Irrespective of cause, extensive ischaemia leads to a dramatic induction of VEGF and a second wave of angiogenesis, culminating in formation of large clusters of leaky vessels around the necrotic areas (Degani and E. Keshet, in preparation). A third wave of angiogenesis is associated with tissue repair and replacement of the necrotic regions with a fibrotic tissues. Non-invasive procedures of monitoring blood flow and vascular permeability (62) have shown that dynamic changes in vascular distribution and permeability take place as a result of tamoxifen treatment. Notably, ischaemia-induced angiogenesis may result in re-distribution and increased leakiness of tumour vessels.

Another consideration concerns the fact that hypoxic tumour cells are more resistant to radiotherapy. Tumours in which vascularization depends on stress-induced VEGF expression will maintain, during their growth, a significant fraction of hypoxic, radio-resistant cells. In contrast, no radio-resistant cells are expected in tumours in which vascular growth is not lagging behind tumour growth. The prevalence of solid tumours phenotypically belonging to the first group, reinforce the notion that stress-induced angiogenesis is a common component of tumour neovascularization.

Vascular endothelial growth factor as an oxygen-regulated protein and glucose-regulated protein

Studies summarized above support the conclusion that VEGF behaves as a classical stress-induced gene and specifically, as an ORP/GRP. The ability to 'sense' hypoxia and, independently, hypoglycaemia is an advantage in the natural situation where a deficiency in only one of these key metabolites might develop. It is not clear, however, whether the two responses proceed through totally independent pathways or alternatively, that both forms of stress converge in the accumulation of a common mediator acting as the proximal VEGF inducer. Examination of different metabolites known to accumulate during hypoxia and hypoglycaemia, with respect to their ability to directly induce VEGF, has not yielded conclusive results. It has been shown that VEGF is induced by adenosine (63,64) as well as by cobalt ions (65). The later finding suggests that a haem protein might be involved.

To date, there is no evidence for translational or post-translational control of VEGF expression. In all cases examined, stress-induced increases in steady-state levels of VEGF mRNA were accompanied by parallel increases in VEGF protein secreted into the culture medium. Therefore, effects of hypoxia and hypoglycaemia were examined at the levels of transcription initiation and mRNA stabilization. Increase in steady-state levels of VEGF mRNA is partly due to transcriptional activation but mostly due to an increase in mRNA stability (45,66). Both oxygen and glucose deficiencies lead to the extension of a VEGF mRNA half-life, in a protein synthesis-dependent manner (45).

Regulatory proteins known as early response genes (ERGs) or immediate early genes, (such as c-*myc*, c-*fos*, and certain cytokines and mediators of inflammation) are induced within minutes after cells are exposed to extra-cellular stimuli, and are encoded by unstable mRNAs with a half-life of 10–30 min. The half-life of VEGF is approximately 40 min (in C6 cells), i.e. longer than ERG mRNAs but significantly shorter than most mammalian mRNAs, which typically survive for hours or days. In this respect VEGF is similar to mRNAs encoding for a number of soluble growth factors that are intrinsically unstable with a half-life of <1 h, and that their increased steady-state level is primarily due to decreased mRNA degradation (see reference 67 for a recent review). A high rate of turnover permits rapid cessation of the production of the respective protein when it is no longer needed, *e.g.* when the ischaemic stress is relieved. The regulated turnover of short-lived mRNAs is known to be determined by the presence of AU-rich elements (AREs) in the 3′ untranslated region (UTR) functioning as destabilizing determinants. Likewise, the 3′ UTR of VEGF mRNAs contains the destabilizing AUUUA motif in the context of an AU-rich region.

Among the ORP/GRPs identified, only in a few the biological significance of stress-induced expression is known and compatible with a role in relieving the stress. These include hypoxia-induced expression of erythropoietin (68,69) which acts to generate more oxygen-carrying erythrocytes, and hypoglycaemia-induced expression of glucose transporter type 1 (GLUT-1) (70) which acts to improve uptake of available glucose, and haem oxygenase (71). Hypoxia-induced expression of erythropoietin is primarily at the level of increased transcription and only in part due to mRNA stabilization (68). A major difference from VEGF regulation is that erythropoietin production is regulated by hypoxia only in the liver and kidney, whereas VEGF is hypoxia-inducible in most, if not all tissues. GLUT-1 shares with VEGF the same short half-life under non-stressed condition that is extended more than eight fold when cells are deprived of either oxygen or glucose. VEGF is differently regulated, however, than the ORP/GRPs grp78 and HSP70 whose mRNAs are not stabilized by these insults.

To show that VEGF and GLUT-1 are co-induced in differentially stressed microenvironments, multicell spheroids were analysed by *in situ* hybridization. Cellular microenvironments conducive to induction of VEGF and GLUT-1 were completely coincidental (45). The concerted regulation of these two genes under many different forms of ischaemic stress suggests that both genes might be downstream targets of the same immediate response protein. Such a mechanism may assure a co-ordinate up-regulation of different genes which may functionally complement each other in relieving the ischaemic stress.

It should be pointed-out that, while mRNA stabilization accounts for the majority of up-regulated VEGF expression under ischaemia, this stress also causes a slight increase in the transcription rate (45,66). Initial attempts to delineate *cis*-acting elements necessary for hypoxic regulation of VEGF have shown that hypoxia-responsive enhancer elements are present in both the 5′ and 3′ flanking regions of the VEGF gene (72). Moreover, recent studies have shown that hypoxia inducibility is confirmed on the VEGF gene by a 5′-promoter sequence which binds hypoxia-inducible factor-1 (HIF-1) (reviewed in ref. 73), a protein which is itself upregulated and stabilized by hypoxia (74). Interestingly, endothelial cells express another hypoxia-inducible transcription factor (with 48% sequence homology to HIF-1) which activates expression of the endothelial tyrosine kinase gene, Tie-2 (75). This raises the possibility that hypoxia may both induce VGF and regulate the response(s) of endothelial cells to such growth factors.

An increased rate of transcription might be the predominant mode of VEGF regulation in response to other stimuli. VEGF expression is also induced by oestrogens (76,77) and by a number of cytokine and and growth factors, including EGF, PDGF-BB, bFGF, and IL-1 beta (73–78). The notion of multiple pathways for VEGF induction is also supported by findings that hypoxia and PDGF-BB synergizes in VEGF induction (10) and that VEGF regulation is mediated by both protein kinase C activation and cyclic adenosine monophosphate-dependent protein kinase pathways (79).

Summary and conclusions

Acquisition by tumours of the ability to attract and support growth of new blood vessels is thought to result from a genetic switch, i.e. from a stochastic genetic event in the succession of genetic hits that underlie tumour progression. However, recent studies have suggested that tumour cells share with normal tissues the ability to activate angiogenesis in response to an ischaemic stress. Similarly to physiological and developmental processes that represent a feedback response to insufficient vascularity, ischaemia-induced angiogenesis in tumours is mediated by up-regulation of the angiogenic factor VEGF. Thus, when the increase in tumour mass is not matched by neovascularization, VEGF induces compensatory neovascularization. Stress conditions conducive for VEGF induction develop naturally during growth of many tumours and the angiogenic response is manifested in the formation of dense vascular clusters around necrotic regions. Stress-induced angiogenesis is also elicited when the tumour vasculature is impaired, as in certain modes of cancer therapy. Therefore, only a fraction of the angiogenic output is determined by the abnormal genetic programme of the tumour cells and the overall production of angiogenic factors is adjustable and continually modulated in accord with the degree of tissue stress.

Acknowledgement

Research in the laboratory of Eli Keshet is supported by the Mireille & James Levy Foundation (USA).

References

1. Folkman, J., Waston, K., Ingber, D., and Folkman, J. (1989) Induction of angiogenesis during the transition from hyperplasia to neoplasia. *Nature*, **339**, 58–61.
2. Rastinjad, F., Polverini, P., and Bouck, N. P. (1989) Regulation of the activity of a new inhibitor of angiogenesis by a cancer supressor gene. *Cell*, **56**, 345–55.
3. Borowsky, I. W. and Collins R. C. (1989) Metabolic anatomy of brain; a comparison of regional capillary density, glucose metabolism, and enzyme activities. *J. Comp. Neurol.*, **288**, 401–13.
4. Zheng, D., LaMantia, A-S., and Purves, D. (1991) Specialized vascularization of the primate visual cortex. *J. Neurosci.*, **11**, 2522–9.
5. Shweiki, D., Itin, A., Soffer, D., and Keshet, E. (1992). Vascular endothelial growth factor induced by hypoxia may mediate hypoxia-initiated angiogenesis. *Nature*, **359**, 843–5.
6. Kourembanas, S., Hannan, R. L., and Faller, D. V. (1990). Oxygen tension regulates the expression of the platelet-derived growth factor-B chain gene in human endothelial cells. *J. Clin. Invest.*, **86**, 670–4.
7. Banai, S., Shweiki, D., Pinson, A., Chandra, M., Lazarovici, G., and Keshet, E. (1994). Upregulation of vascular endothelial growth factor expression induced by myocardial ischemia: implications for coronary angiogenesis. *Cardiovasc. Res.*, **28**, 1176–9.
8. Shima, D. T., Adamis, A. P., Ferrara, N., Yeo, K. T., Yeo, T. K., Allende, R., *et al.* (1995). Hypoxic induction of endothelial cell growth factors in retinal cells: identification and characterization of vascular endothelial growth factor as a mitogen. *Mol. Med.*, **1**, 182–93.
9. Stone, J., Itin, A., Alon, T., Pe'er, J., Gnessin, H., Chan-Ling, T., and Keshet, E. (1995) Development of retinal vasculature is mediated by hypoxia-induced vascular endothelial growth factor expression by neuroglia. *J. Neurosci.*, **15**, 4738–47.
10. Stavri, G. T., Hong, Y., Zachary, I. C., Breier, G., Baskerville, P. A., Yla-Herttula, S., Risau, W., *et al.* (1995). Hypoxia and platlet-derived growth factor-BB synergistically upregulate the expression of vascular endothelial growth factor in smooth muscle cells. *FEBS Lett.*, **30**, 311–15.
11. Schaper, W., Sharma, H. S., Quinkler, W., Market, T., Wunsch, M., and Schaper, J. (1990). Molecular biological concept of coronary anastomoses. *J. Am. Coll. Cardiol.*, **15**, 513–18.
12. Banai, S., Jaklitsch, M. T., Shou, M., Lazarous, D. F., Scheinowitz, M., Biro, S., *et al.* (1994). Angiogenic-induced enhancement of collateral blood flow to ischemic myocardium by vascular endothelial growth factor in dogs. *Circulation*, **89**, 2183–9.
13. Takeshita, S., Pu, L. Q., Stein, L. A., Sniderman, A. D., Bunting, S., Ferrara, N., *et al.* (1994). Intramuscular administration of vascular endothelial growth factor induces dose-dependent collateral artery augmentation in a rabbit model of chronic limb ischemia. *Circulation*, **90**, 228–34.
14. Miller, J. W., Adamis, A. P., Shima, D. T., D'Amore, P. A., Moulton, R. S., Oneilly, M. S., *et al.* (1994). Vascular endothelial growth factor/vascular permeability factor is temporally and spatially correlated with ocular angiogenesis in a primate model. *Am. J. Pathol.*, **145**, 574–84.
15. Pe'er, J., Shweiki, D., Itin, A., Hemo, I., Gnessin, H., and Keshet, E. Hypoxia-induced expression of vascular endothelial growth factor by retinal cells is a common factor in neovascularizing ocular diseases. *Lab. Invest.*, **72**, 638–45.
16. Pierce, E. A., Avery, R. L., Foley, E. D., Aiello, L. P., and Smith, L. E. (1994). Vascular endothelial growth factor/vascular permeability factor expression in a mouse model of retinal neovascularization. *Proc. Natl Acad. Sci. USA*, **92**, 905–9.
17. Aiello, L. P., Avery, R. L., Arrigg, P. G., Keyt, B. A., Jampel, H. D., Shah, S. T., *et al.* (1994). Vascular endothelial growth factor in ocular fluid of patients with diabetic retinopathy and other retinal disorders. *N. Engl. J. Med.*, **331**, 1480–7.
18. Sutherland, R. M. (1988). Cell and environment interactions in tumour microregions: the multicell spheroid model. *Science*, **240**, 177–83.
19. James, C. D., Caribom, E., Dumanski, J. P., Hansen, M., Nordenskjold, M., Collins, V. P., and Cavenee, W. K. (1988). Clonal genomuc alterations in glioma malignancy stages. *Cancer Res.*, **48**, 5546–51.
20. Plate, K. H., Breier, G., Widch, H. A., and Risau, W. 1992. Vascular endothelial growth factor is a potential tumour angiogenesis factor in human gliomas *in vivo*. *Nature*, **359**, 845–8.

21. Plate, K. H., Breier, G., Weich, H. A., Mennel, H. D., and Risau, W. (1994). Vascular endothelial growth factor and glioma angiogenesis: coordinate induction of VEGF receptors, distribution of VEGF protein and possible *in vivo* regulatory mechanisms. *Int. J. Cancer.*, **15**, 520–9.

22. Senger, D. R., Galli, S. J., Dvorak, A. M., Perruzzi, C. A., Harvey, V. S., and Dvorak, H. F. (1983). Tumor cells secrete a vascular permeability factor that promotes accumulation of ascites fluid. *Science*, **219**, 983–5.

23. Keck, P. J., Hauser, S. D., Krivi, G., Sanzo, K., Warren, T., Feder, J. and Connolly, D. T. (1989). Vascular permeability factor, an endothelial cell mitogen related to PDGF. *Science*, **246**, 1309–12.

24. Brown, L. F., Berse, B., Jackman, R. W., Tognazzi, K., Guidi, A. J., Dvorak, H. F., *et al.* (1995). Expression of vascular permeability factor (vascular endothelial growth factor) and its receptors in breast cancer. *Hum. Pathol.*, **26**, 86–91.

25. Kim, K. J., Li. B., Winer, J., Armanini, M., Gillett, N., Phillips, H. S., and Ferrara, N. (1993). Inhibition of vascular endothelial growth factor-induced angiogenesis suppresses tumour growth *in vivo*. *Nature*, **362**, 841–4.

26. Shweiki, D., Neeman, M., Itin, A. and Keshet, E. (1995). Induction of vascular endothelial growth of factor expression by hypoxia and by glucose deficiency in multicell spheroids: implications for tumour angiogenesis. *Proc. Natl Acad. Sci USA*, **92**, 768–72.

27. Russel, D. S. and Rubinstein, L. J. (1989). *Pathology of tumours of the nervous system.* Edward Arnold, London.

28. Mueller-Klieser, W. (1987). Multicellular spheroids: a review on cellular aggregates in cancer research. *J. Cancer Res. Clin. Oncol.*, **113**, 101–22.

29. Casciari, J. J., Sotirchos, S. V., and Sutherland, R. M. (1992). Mathematical modelling of microenvironment and growth in EMT6/Ro multicellular tumour spheroids. *Cell Prolif.*, **25**, 1–22.

30. Zwi, L. J., Baguley, B. C., Gavin, J. B., and Wilson, W. R. (1990). The use of vascularized spheroids to investigate the action of flavone acetic acid on tumour blood vessels, *Br. J. Cancer*, **62**, 231–7.

31. Abramovitch, R., Meir, G., and Neeman, M. (1995). Neovascularization induced growth of implanted C6 glioma multicellular spheroids: magnetic resonance microimaging. *Cancer Res.*, **55**, 1956–62.

32. Freyer, J. P. and Sutherland, R. M. (1986). Regulation of growth saturation and development of necrosis in EMT6/Ro multicellular spheroids by the oxygen and glucose supply. *Cancer Res.*, **46**, 3504–12.

33. Freyer, J. P. and Schor, P. L. (1989). Automated selective dissociation of cells from different regions of multicellular spheroids. *In Vitro Cell Dev. Biol.*, **25**, 9–19.

34. Rofstad, E. K. and Sutherland, R. M. (1989). Growth and radiation sensitivity of the MLS human ovarian carcinoma cell line grown as multicellular spheroids and xenografted tumours. *Br. J. Cancer*, **59**, 28–35.

35. Bardies, M., Thedrez, P., Gestin, J. F., Marcille, B. M., Guerreau, D., Faivre-Chauvet, A., *et al.* (1992). Use of multicell spheroids of ovarian carcinoma as an intraperitoneal radio-immunotherapy model: uptake, retention kinetics and dosimetric evaluation. *Int. J. Cancer*, **50**, 984–91.

36. Nederman, T. and Twentyman, P. (1984). Spheroids for studies of drug effects. In *Spheroids in cancer research: methods and perspectives* (ed. H. Acker, J. Carlsson, R. Durand, and R. M. Sutherland), pp. 84–102. Springer-Verlags, New York.

37. Schiffenbauer, Y. S., Tempel, C., Abramovitch, R., Meir, G., and Neeman, M. (1995) Cyclocreatine accumulation leads to cellular swelling in C6 glioma multicellular spheroids: diffusion and one dimensional chemical shift nuclear magnetic resonance microscopy. *Cancer Res.*, **55**, 153–8.

38. Kobayashi, H., Man, S., Graham, C. H., Kapitain, S. J., Teicher, B. A., and Kerbel, R. S. (1993). Acquired multicellular-mediated resistance to alkylating agents in cancer. *Proc. Natl Acad. Sci. USA*, **90**, 3294–8.

39. Sillerud, L. O., Freyer, J. P., Neeman, M., and Mattingly, M. A. (1990). Proton NMR microscopy of multicellular tumor spheroid morphology. *Magn. Reson. Med.*, **16**, 380–9.

40. Neeman, M., Jarret, K. A., Sillerud, L. O., and Freyer, J. P. (1991). Self diffusion of water in multicellular spheroids measured by magnetic resonance microimaging. *Cancer Res.*, **51**, 4072–9.

41. Mueller-Klieser, W. (1984). Microelectrode measurements of oxygen tension distributions in multicellular spheroids cultured in spinner flasks. In *Spheroids in cancer research: methods and perspectives* (ed. H. Acker, J. Carlsson, R. Durand, and R. M. Sutherland, pp. 134–9. Springer-Verlag, New York.

42. Vaupel, P., Kallinowski, F., and Okunieff, P. (1989). Blood flow, oxygen and nutrient supply, and metabolic microenvironment of human tumours: a review. *Cancer Res.*, **49**, 6449–65.

43. Walenta, S., Dotsch, J., and Mueller-Klieser, W. (1990). ATP concentrations in multicellular spheroids assessed by single photon imaging and quantitative bioluminescence, *Eur. J. Cell Biol.*, **52**, 389–93.

44. Dobrucki, J. W., Sutherland, R. M., and Swartz, H. M. (1991). Nonperturbing test for cytotoxicity in isolated cells and spheroids, using electron paramagnetic resonance. *Mag. Reson. Med.*, **19**, 42–55.

45. Stein, I., Neeman, M., Shweiki, D., Itin, I., and Keshet, E. (1995). Stabilization of vascular endothelial growth factor (VEGF) mRNA by hypoxia and hypoglycemia and co-regulation with other ischemia-induced genes. *Mol. Cell. Biol.*, **15**, 5363–8.

46. Trotter, M. J., Chaplin, D. J., Durand, R. E., and Olive, P. L. (1989). The use of fluorescent probes to identify regions of transient perfusion in murine tumours. *Int. J. Radiat. Oncol. Biol. Phys.*, **16**, 931–4.

47. Chaplin, D. J., Olive, P. L., and Durand, R. E. (1987). Intermittent blood flow in a murine tumor: radiobiological effects. *Cancer Res.*, **47**, 597–601.

48. Folkman, J. (1990) What is the evidence that tumors are angiogenesis dependent? *J. Natl Cancer Inst.*, **82**, 4–6.

49. Folkman, J. (1995). Angiogenesis in cancer, vascular, rheumatoid, and other disease. *Nature Med.*, **1**, 27–31.

50. O'Reilly, M. S., Holmgren, L., Shing, Y., Chen, C., Rosenthal, R. A., Moses, M., *et al.* (1994). Angiostatin: a novel angiogenesis inhibitor which mediates the suppression of metastasis by a Lewis lung carcinoma. *Cell*, **79**, 315–28.

51. Dameron, J., Volpert, O. V., Tainsky, M. A., and Bouck, N. (1994) Control of angiogenesis in fibroblasts by p53 regulation of thrombospondin-1. *Science*, **265**, 1582–4.

52. Van Meir, E. G., Polverini, P. J., Chazin, V. R., Su Huang, H-J., de Tribolet, N., and Cavenee, W. K. (1994). Release of an inhibitor of angiogenesis upon induction of wild type p53 expression in glioblastoma cells. *Nature Genet.*, **8**, 171–6.

53. Zhang, H. T., Craft, P., Scott, P. A., Ziche, M., Harris, A. L., and Bicknell, R. (1995). Enhancement of tumor growth and

vascular density by transfection of vascular endothelial growth factor into MCF-7 human breast carcinoma. *J. Natl Cancer Inst.*, **87**, 213–19.

54. Wizigmann-Voos, S., Breier, G., Risau, W., and Plate, K. H. (1995) Up-regulation of vascular endothelial growth factor in Von Hippel-Lindau disease-associated and sporadic hemangioblastomas. *Cancer Res.*, **55**, 1358–64.

55. Boocock, C. A., Charnock-Jones, D. S., Sharkey, A. M., McLaren, J. Barker, P. J., Wright, K. A., *et al.* (1995). Expression of vascular endothelial growth factor and its receptors in ovarian carcinoma. *J. Natl Cancer Inst.*, **87**, 506–16.

56. Warren, R. S., Yuan, H., Malti, M. R., Gillett, N. A., and Ferrara, N. (1995). Regulation of vascular endothelial growth factor of human colon cancer tumorigenesis in a mouse model of experimental liver metastasis. *J. Clin. Invest.*, **95**, 1789–97.

57. Brown, L. F., Berse, B., Jackman, R. W., Toghazzi, K., Manseau, E. J., Dvonak, H. F., and Senger, D. R. (1993). Increased expression of vascular permeability factor (vascular endothelial cells and its receptors in kidney and bladder carcinoma. *Am. J. Pathol.*, **143**, 1255–62.

58. Kieser, A., Weich, H. A., Brandner, G., Marme, D., and Kolch, W. (1994). Mutant p53 potentiates protein kinase C induction of vascular endothelial growth factor expression. *Oncogene*, **9**, 963–9.

59. Xu, M., Kumar D., Srinvas, S. *et al.* (1997). *Human Gene Therapy*, **8**, 177–85.

60. Millauer, B., Wizigmann-Voos, S., Schnürch, H., Martinez, R., Moller, N. H. P., Risau, W., and Ullrich, A. (1993). High affinity VEGF binding and developmental expression suggest Flk-1 as a major regulator of vasculogenesis and angiogenesis. *Cell*, **72**, 835–46.

61. Haran, E. F., Maretzek, A. F., Goldberg, I., Horowitz, A., and Degani, H. (1994). Tamoxifen enhances cell death in implanted MCF7 breast cancer by inhibiting endothelial growth. *Cancer Res.*, **54**, 5511–14.

62. Furman, E., Margalit, R., Bendel, P., Horowitz, A., and Degani, H. (1991). *In vivo* studies by magnetic resonance imaging and spectroscopy of the response to tamoxifen of MCF7 human breast cancer implanted in nude mice. *Cancer Commun.*, **9**, 287–97.

63. Hashimoto, E., Kage, K., Ogita, T., Nakaoka, T., Matsuoka, R., and Kira, Y. (1994). Adenosine as an endogenous mediator of hypoxia for induction of vascular endothelial growth factor mRNA in U-937 cells. *Biochem. Biophys. Res. Commun.*, **204**, 318–24.

64. Fischer, S., Sharma, H. S., Karliczek, G. F., and Schaper, W. (1995). Expression of vascular permeability factor/vascular endothelial growth factor in pig cerebral microvascular endothelial cells and its upregulation by adenosine. *Brain Res. Mol. Brain Res.*, **28**, 141–8.

65. Ladoux, A. and Frelin, C. (1994). cobalt stimulates the expression of vascular endothelial growth factor mRNA in rat cardiac cells. *Biochem. Biophys. Res. Commun.*, **28**, 794–8.

66. Ikeda, E., Achen, M., Breier, G., and Risau, W. (1995). Hypoxia-induced transcriptional activation and increased mRNA stability of vascular endothelial growth factor (VEGF) in C6 glioma cells. *J. Biol. Chem.*, **270**, 19761–6.

67. Greenberg, M. E. and Bealasco, J. G. (1993). Control of the decay of labile protooncogene and cytokine mRNAs. In *Control of messenger RNA stability*, (ed. J. Belasco, and G. Brawerman), pp. 199–218. Academic Press, New York.

68. Goldberg, M. A., Gaut, C. C., and Bunn, H. F. (1991). Erythropoietin mRNA levels are governed by both the rate of the gene transcription and post transcriptional events. *Blood*, **77**, 271–7.

69. Goldberg, M. A. and Schneider, T. J. (1994). Similarities between the oxygen-sensing mechanisms regulating the expression of vascular endothelial growth factor and erythropoietin. *J. Biol. Chem.*, **269**, 4355–69.

70. Wertheimer, E., Sasson, S., Gerasi, E., and Ben-Neriah, Y. (1991). The ubiquitous glucose transporter GLUT-1 belongs to the glucose-regulated protein family of stress-inducible proteins. *Proc. Natl Acad. Sci. USA*, **88**, 2525–9.

71. Murphy, B. J., Laderoute, K. R., Short, S. M., and Sutherland, R. M. (1991). The identification of hemeoxygenase as a major hypoxic stress protein in Chinese hamster ovary cells. *Br. J. Cancer*, **64**, 69–73.

72. Minchenko, A., Salceda, S., Bauer, T., and Caro, J. (1994). Hypoxia regulatory elements of the human vascular endothelial growth factor gene. *Cell Mol. Biol. Res.*, **40**, 35–9.

73. Ferrara, N. and Dans-Smyth, T. (1997). *Endocrine Revs*, **18**, 4–23.

74. Huang, L. E., Arany, Z., Livingston, D. M., and Bunn, H. F. (1996). *J. of Biol. Chem.*, **271**, 32253–9.

75. Tian, H., McKnight, S. L., and Russell, D. W. (1997). *Genes and Develop.*, **11**, 72–82.

76. Shweiki, D., Itin, A., Neufeld, G., Gitay-Goren, H., and Keshet, E. (1993). Patterns of expression of vascular endothelial growth factor (VEGF) and VEGF receptors in mice suggest a role in hormonally regulated angiogenesis. *J. Clin. Invest.*, **91**, 2235–43.

77. Cullinan-Bove, K. and Koos, R. D. (1993). Vascular endothelial growth factor/vascular permeability factor expression in the uterus: rapid stimulation by estrogen correlates with estrogen-induced increases in uterine capillary permeability and growth. *Endocrinology*, **93**, 829–37.

78. Li, J., Perrela, M. A., Tsai, J. C., Yet, S. F., Hsieh, C. M., Yoshizumi, M., *et al.* (1995). Induction of vascular endothelial growth factor expression by interleukin-1 beta in rat aortic smooth muscle cells. *J. Biol. Chem.*, **270**, 308–12.

79. Claffey, K. P., Wilkinson, W. O., and Spiegelman, B. M. (1992). Vascular endothelial growth factor regulation by cell differentiation and activated second messenger pathways. *J. Biol. Chem.*, **267**, 16317–22.

8. The role of macrophages in tumour angiogenesis

Russell D. Leek, Claire E. Lewis, and Adrian L. Harris

Introduction

Solid tumours do not consist of neoplastic cells in isolation, rather, they comprise of a range of cellular types, which often outnumber the tumour cell population (1,2). The tumour cells are usually surrounded by a supportive stroma consisting of a fibrous extracellular matrix (ECM) laid down by fibroblasts. Insinuating into this environment are blood vessel endothelial cells, which provide nutritional and respiratory support for the tumour. Often, there is also an infiltrate of inflammatory cells such as lymphocytes, natural killer cells, neutrophils, and macrophages. These cells communicate by a complex network of intercellular signalling pathways mediated by surface adhesion molecules and soluble polypeptides called cytokines and their receptors (3,4).

Many recent studies have demonstrated the production of various cytokines by both the malignant and non-malignant cell populations present in solid human tumours (1,3,4), and that they regulate such intratumoral processes as:

1. The proliferation, progression, and metastatic activity of the neoplastic cell population.

2. The tumoricidal activity of the inflammatory cell infiltrate.

3. The establishment of the stromal compartment by the deposition of the ECM and the stimulation of angiogenesis.

Until recently, it was assumed that the source of angiogenic growth factors was the malignant cell population itself. However, macrophages account for a large percentage of the tumour mass in a number of solid tumours, sometimes comprising up to 50% of the total cellular mass in some breast carcinomas (1,2,4). This has led to increased interest in the possibility that tumour-associated macrophages are involved in the angiogenic process (4,5). Macrophages are versatile multifunctional cells, capable of influencing a large number of physiological and pathological processes via their secreted products. Evidence is now accumulating that they can directly influence angiogenesis. For example, implanted syngeneic fibrosarcomas in mice were markedly less vascularized when their hosts were depleted of monocytes (5) and Polverini and Leibovitch demonstrated that tumour-associated macrophage (TAM) derived conditioned medium was capable of inducing angiogenesis in a number of *in vivo* assays (6). Moreover, Kobayashi *et al.* demonstrated that interferon (IFN) γ-activated macrophages are capable of enhancing angiogenesis in cultured endothelial cells or rat aorta (7). Inhibition of macrophage infiltration by interleukin 10 (IL-10) is correlated with reduced tumour growth (8) and the degree of vascularization has been correlated with macrophage infiltration in transplanted human tumour cell lines (5). Recently, in this laboratory, we have found a direct correlation between vascularization and focally increased macrophage infiltration in human carcinomas of the breast. We have also identified focal macrophage infiltration as an important prognostic factor in these tumours (see the section on 'Macrophages and tumour angiogenesis,' p. 86). These findings, and others, suggest that TAMs may be important regulators of angiogenesis in tumours, and that they may be stimulated in hypoxic, avascular areas to secrete a range of angiogenic factors such as ECM degrading enzymes, and angiogenic cytokines such as vascular endothelial growth factor (VEGF), basic fibroblast growth factor (bFGF), tumour necrosis factor (TNF) α, insulin growth-like factor (IGF)-α and -β, interferons, and endothelial growth factor (EGF). They also demonstrate that the TAM population of tumours could be a useful target for future anti-angiogenic therapies.

The origin of macrophages

Macrophage development

The macrophage is the major terminally differentiated cell type of the mononuclear phagocyte system. Its origins lie in the bone marrow, where its progenitor cell is located. Macrophages and neutrophils share a common progenitor

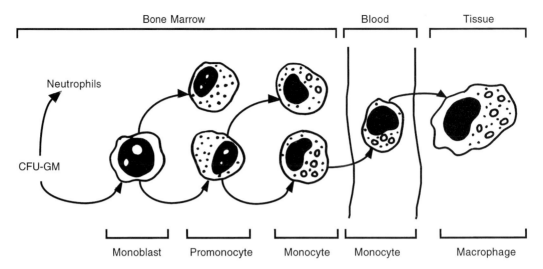

Figure 8.1. Macrophage development. The precursor cell of the macrophage is the colony forming unit/granulocyte–macrophage (CFU–GM) which differentiates into a monoblast which divides to form promonocytes, further division produces monocytes which migrate into the bloodstream before migrating into the tissues where they mature into fully differentiated macrophages.

cell called the colony-forming unit, granulocyte–macrophage (CFU-GM), which becomes committed to one or other differentiation pathway at a very early stage (Fig. 8.1). This progenitor differentiates into either a promyelocyte leading to eventual maturity as a neutrophil, or into a monoblast, which is the most immature cell type of the mononuclear phagocyte lineage. At this stage, however, the potential still exists to follow the granulocyte differentiation pathway, giving rise eventually to maturation as a neutrophil. If the monoblast is destined to follow the monocytic pathway of differentiation, its division will produce two promonocytes. It is now that the macrophage progenitors are committed to this maturation pathway. Promonocytes exhibit some of the functions of mature macrophages of which the monoblasts are incapable, most notably the ability to pinocytose, like the monoblast they have immunoglobulin (Ig) G receptors and have limited phagocytic abilities. Division of a promonocyte gives rise to two monocytes which remain in the bone marrow for about 24 h before entering the peripheral bloodstream where they have a circulating half-time of up to 70 h in the normal human adult.

The next stage in the normal life cycle of a monocyte is to migrate from the blood circulation into the extravascular tissues. This is achieved by the adherence of the circulating monocyte to the endothelium utilizing high molecular weight surface glycoproteins such as LFA-1 (lymphocyte function-associated molecule 1, CD11a/CD18) expressed by the monocyte, interacting with ICAM-1 (intercellular adhesion molecule-1, CD54) which is present on the luminal surface of vascular endothelial cells (9). This interaction anchors the monocyte to the luminal surface of the blood vessel prior to its extravasation into the surrounding tissue. Monocytes share expression of a number of different adhesion molecules and adhesion receptors with other circulating myelocytic and lymphocytic cell lineages, for example, in common with monocytes, lymphocytes also express LFA-1 as well as VLA-4 (very late antigen-4, CD49d/CD29), and like neutrophils, monocytes express CR3 (complement receptor-3, CD11b/CD18) and the PADGEM/GMP140 ligand (CD62) (10). This indicates that similar migration mechanisms are used by these cell types.

In sites of inflammation, expression of adhesion molecules by blood vessels can be up-regulated by cytokines such as interleukin (IL) 1 IFN-γ, and TNF-α (11), which serves to facilitate monocyte migration into these areas.

In healthy tissues the migration of monocytes into various organ systems appears to be random. Once there, the monocytes terminally differentiate into tissue macrophages, and remain resident in their organ sites for several months, their eventual fate remaining unclear. Although it is thought that they may still be able to undergo further divisions in some cases, such as the alveolar macrophages of the lung, eventually they probably either undergo apoptosis *in situ* or leave the tissue via the efferent lymph channels to the local lymph nodes, where they remain until they die (for review see reference 12).

Macrophage heterogeneity

The tissue destination of monocytes appears to be random and no evidence has been produced to contest this. All circulating monocytes would appear to exhibit the same potential to differentiate into their mature macrophage forms. The final form of the macrophage, is however, highly heterogeneous and dependent on a number of factors, including the final destination of the monocyte, where local factors will determine differentiation (in the case of resident macrophages), and involvement in pathological processes where additional modulating factors will be present (in the case of elicited macrophages).

A number of histological subtypes of resident macrophages have been identified with distinct morphological and functional characteristics dependent on the organ in which they are to be found. They include alveolar macrophages which are found in the lung, where they are involved in local defence against particulate contamination which they phagocytose and destroy with a battery of degradative enzymes, and have an early role in inflammation directed against pathogenic organisms. Similarly, the Kuppfer cells of the liver are involved in clearance of particulate and soluble substances as well as micro-organisms. The liver, as an organ of detoxification, is exposed to a wide array of toxic compounds in high concentrations, some of which are highly carcinogenic. Stress induced by these compounds can cause hepatocyte cell death and neoplastic transformation, the role of the Kuppfer cells in these situations may well involve clearance of dead cells and tumoricidal activity towards neoplastic cells. The macrophages of the spleen are heterogeneous in themselves, with variations in phenotype and appearance probably reflecting functional differences. In the marginal zone of the spleen they are involved in the trapping and processing of foreign antigens, in the lymphoid areas they interact with T and B lymphocytes, and in the red pulp they phagocytose redundant erythrocytes. In the bone marrow, macrophages appear to act as supporting cells where they are found in intimate contact with haemopoietic cells, and are essential for the maintenance of growth and differentiation of these maturing cells. Macrophages are also found in the specialized gut-associated lymphoid tissues (GALT), such as the tonsils and Peyer's patches, where they are thought to be involved in antigen processing and presentation. In addition to these very specialized macrophage populations, resident macrophages are found in all the tissues of the body including the brain and skin. There is also some debate as to whether macrophages are the precursors to the antigen-presenting cells, such as the Langerhans cells (13–15) of the skin and the dendritic cells of the lymph nodes. It is theorized that the terminally differentiated form of the macrophage is the multinucleated giant cell, the function of which is uncertain, but they are often found in granulomatous lesions and are a feature of many tumours (for review see reference 12).

Macrophage functions

Broadly speaking, the cellular functions of the macrophage can be categorized into four main areas: phagocytosis, antigen processing, secretion, and chemotaxis.

Phagocytosis

Phagocytosis is the process by which macrophages can engulf foreign bodies and pathogenic micro-organisms, or defective or dead host cells. Macrophages are an important factor in the destruction of numerous micro-organisms including bacteria, viruses, fungi, and protozoan parasites. They migrate towards the xenobiotic object following a trail of chemoattractants emanating from it (16). Once in position the macrophages are prevented from leaving the area by the migration inhibition factor (MIF) secreted by T cells (17). The xenobiotic objects are coated with opsonins, generally IgG and complement fragments (18), which the macrophage recognizes as labelling the object for destruction, although opsonization is not always necessary for phagocytosis to occur (19). In the case of defective or senescent host cells the recognition mechanism is unknown, although it is hypothesized that, in senescent cells, progressive loss of membrane sialic acid or progressive accumulation of non-specifically bound IgG on the cellular membrane act as triggers for phagocytosis (20). In some instances, neoplastic cells may be recognized by expression of oncogene products on the cell surface in association with MHC class I (major histocompatibility complex, CD8) molecules (21). Once the object has been engulfed and is within the phagosomal vacuole, granules forming at the base of the vacuole, exocytose their contents into it. The contents of these granules or lysosomes are responsible for the killing and degradation of the organism or object and their contents are dependent on the nature of the engulfed material (22). Reactive oxygen species, such as superoxide, hydroxyl radicals, and hydrogen peroxide (23), or enzymes such as elastase collagenases, deoxyribonucleases, lipases, and polysaccharidases (24) can be secreted into the phagosomal vacuole. The pH of the phagosomal vacuole can also be acidified rapidly to aid in the destruction of its contents (25).

Antigen presentation

In order for the host's immune system to be able to mount a cell-mediated immune response against a 'foreign' pathogen by cytotoxic T cells, the antigen has to be presented to the T-cell population so that they can recognize and mount an attack against any cell expressing the antigen. Presentation of antigen is performed by a number cell types including the dedicated antigen-presenting cells, such as dendritic cells and Langerhans cells, and other cells such as the macrophage. Once a macrophage has phagocytosed a 'foreign' cell its antigens are processed by the macrophage and expressed on the cell membrane in association with class II MHC molecules for recognition by class II restricted (CD4 expressing) T cells. Non-phagocytosed antigen present in the cytoplasm of the macrophage is processed in a different manner. The antigen is expressed in association with a class I MHC molecule for recognition by a class I restricted (CD8 expressing) cytotoxic T cell. In this case the macrophage is destroyed (10).

Chemotaxis

Chemotaxis involves the migration of the macrophage along a concentration gradient. The macrophage must have have receptors for the chemoattractant and these can be up- or down-regulated in response to a variety of other factors (26). A vast array of cytokines, cell surface markers, and other factors, including oxygen gradients have been shown to be chemotactic to macrophages. Many of these factors are also important in the process of activation (for review see reference 12).

Secretion

Macrophages can secrete an enormous repertoire of biologically active substances depending upon their state of activation. These include enzymes, enzyme inhibitors, complement components, reactive oxygen intermediates, arachidonic acid intermediates, coagulation factors, and cytokines. With regards to tumour angiogenesis, the most interesting secretory products of macrophages are angiogenic cytokines and ECM-degrading enzymes, many of which have pronounced modulatory effects on angiogenesis and will be discussed at length later. Some cytokines secreted by macrophages have been reported as having anti-tumour effects, specifically IL-1 (27,28), TNF-α (29), IL-6 (30), and the prostaglandins (31), which are able to inhibit tumour cell division. In addition, macrophages are able to lyse tumour cells directly in a non-phagocytic, contact-dependent, process known as macrophage-mediated tumour toxicity. Following recognition and binding of a macrophage to a tumour cell, the macrophage secretes cytotoxic substances directly on to the target cell. These substance are thought to include TNF-alpha, serine proteases, and reactive oxygen species (32).

Macrophage activation

Macrophages have a bewildering array of functions, and can be said to be truly multipurpose cells. However, macrophages only perform specific functions, as, and when, they are activated. This provides a robust multiple redundant system which does not rely on a specific terminally differentiated cell type for any one essential function. The process of activation is complex, and is dependent on the nature of the activation signal, be it a cytokine, adhesion molecule, or other factor, the signals can also be inhibitory as well as stimulatory. In addition, the mechanisms regulating the genes responsible for the various activation states can be modulated in a variety of ways depending on the balance of inhibitory and stimulatory signals, and this balance is further effected by the particular activation pathway, toward which, the cell is being driven.

In summary, a newly elicited macrophage is activated to perform a specific function or range of functions, the nature of which are dependent upon factors present in the cell's microenvironment. In tumours the macrophage population within the tumour mass is generally not derived from the local resident macrophages, but from newly arrived (or exudate) macrophages which have been recruited from the circulating monocyte population (33,34). Resident macrophages seem to be resistant to activation, but exudate macrophages are extremely responsive to activation cues (18). The process of activation was first described in TAMs as the acquisition of tumoricidal activity (18); however, it would now appear that activation can occur in a number of different ways at differing levels, resulting in a wide range of macrophage functions. In short, activation is the process of acquisition by a macrophage of the ability to perform a variety of different tasks. In the case of TAMs, these functions may include tumoricidal activity, or, perhaps more importantly, the ability to induce angiogenesis (35).

Tumour-associated macrophages in neoplasia

In recent years more emphasis has been placed on the study of the stromal compartment of the tumour, and it has been realized that these associated cells are important, not only as a source of potential anti-tumour molecules (in the form of inflammatory cells of the immune system) but also as regulators of the growth and continued survival of malignant cells (36). An important cell type commonly found in the stroma of tumours is, of course, the TAM. These cells were originally thought to be part of the host's immune defence against the neoplastic cells. However, recent evidence suggests that this may not be so, and that TAMs are, in fact, supportive of the development of tumours, most notably of tumour angiogenesis.

Attraction of macrophages to tumours

A range of factors are known to be chemotactic towards macrophages, some of which are produced by tumour cells (Table 8.1). Both mouse and human tumours have been shown to produce tumour-derived chemotactic factors capable of stimulating monocyte migration (37–39). Monocyte chemotactic protein-1 (MCP-1) is 76 amino acids long and belongs to the C-C family of chemokines which have four cys residues, the first two of which are in tandem (40,41). In addition to tumour cells, it is also produced by fibroblasts, smooth muscle cells and macrophages can produce it themselves (36). Expression of MCP-1 has been correlated with mononuclear cell infiltration in human melanoma (37) and MCP-1 derived from transplanted murine tumours has been shown to induce tumour infiltration of monocyte derived-macrophages. It is also expressed in Kaposi sarcoma cell lines (36), and has also been observed in human tumour cell lines of epithelial origin such as breast, colon, and ovary (39,42,43), but knowledge of its expression *in vivo*

is still limited. MCP-2 and MCP-3 are two additional members of the C-C family of chemokines which are chemotactic toward macrophages, and have recently been identified in tumour cell lines, and it is likely that they are important factors in macrophage migration into tumours (36,44). Macrophage colony-stimulating factor (M-CSF) and granulocyte–macrophage colony-stimulating factor (GM-CSF) are commonly produced in a range of different tumour types (39,45), and are also chemotactic for macrophages *in vitro* (46,47). Transplanted mouse tumours transfected with the G-CSF gene exhibit increased TAM infiltration (48,49). VEGF is a potent angiogenic cytokine produced by tumour cells, macrophages, and T cells in many human tumours (4). It too has been found to be chemotactic for macrophages *in vitro* (50), and a correlation has been observed between the macrophage and VEGF content of human tumour ascites (51). This illustrates a mechanism whereby angiogenesis may be potentiated by secretion of additional angiogenic factors by TAMs drawn to sites of active angiogenesis by VEGF.

Anti-tumour effects of macrophages

The anti-tumour effects of macrophages can be broadly divided into two categories. Direct cytotoxic activity whereby the macrophage itself kills tumour cells, and indirectly by the secretion of tumour inhibitory factors.

Direct cytotoxicity is manifested in two forms (Fig. 8.2), macrophage-mediated tumour cytotoxicity (MTC) and antibody-dependent cellular cytotoxicity (ADCC); both mechanisms are thought to require activa-

Table 8.1. Multiple factors involved with macrophage-mediated angiogenesis.

Monotactic factors produced by tumour cells	Angiogenic cytokines produced by TAMs	Macrophage-derived ECM modulators	
		Enzymes and inhibitors	Cytokines
MCP-1	VEGF		
MCP-2	bFGF	Collagenase	bFGF
MCP-3	EGF	tPA	TGF-β
GMCSF	TNF-α	uPA	TNF-α
GCSF	TP	PAI-1	Angiotropin
MCSF	HGF/SF		PDGF
VEGF	IGF-1		IL-6
	IL-8		

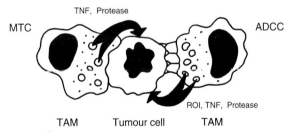

Figure 8.2. Direct tumour cell cytotoxicity by tumour-associated macrophages (TAMs). Macrophage-mediated tumour cytotoxicity (MTC) involves direct cellular contact and is antibody independent, it is a slow process requiring 72 h to complete. Antibody-dependent cellular cytotoxicity (ADCC) also requires intimate cell contact but is much faster than MTC, taking only 6 h to complete. TNF, tumour necrosis factor; ROI, reactive oxygen intermediates.

tion. MTC involves the direct binding of a macrophage to a tumour cell and is antibody independent, the mechanism of recognition is not fully understood. Following cell contact, the macrophage secretes cytotoxic factors directly on to the neoplastic cell resulting in its lysis. This process is very slow, taking up to 3 days to complete. The toxic factors thought to be involved in this process are TNF-α and serine proteases (32). ADCC is a similar process requiring intimate cell contact, it is generally faster than MTC, taking about 6 h to complete, and resulting in the lysis of the target cell (18,32). This process, however, is dependent on the presence of antibody on the tumour cell, and may therefore be affected by human leucocyte antigen (HLA) class 1 loss by the tumour. The Fab portion of the immunoglobulin is bound to the tumour cell surface antigen, the Fc portion of the antibody then binds the Fc receptors of a passing TAM, the cross-linking of which stimulates the macrophage to kill the tumour cell. The killing mechanism is similar to that described for MTC, with secretion of TNF-alpha and reactive oxygen intermediates such as hydrogen peroxide causing lysis of the target cell.

Some cytokines secreted by TAMs are growth inhibitory for tumour cells. They include IL-1 (30,36), IL-6 (30), IL-8 (36), and TNF-α (52). IL-1 increases the binding efficiency of natural killer (NK) cells, IL-6 and IL-8 are also immunomodulatory cytokines affecting B- and T-cell activation and proliferation, and neutrophil activation, respectively. TNF-α also has some immunomodulatory functions, in addition to being directly toxic to tumour cells.

Tumour-promoting effects of macrophages

As has been mentioned earlier, macrophages and TAMs are capable of secreting a wide array of cytokines, many of which have direct growth-promoting properties on tumour cells. They include cytokines such as platelet-derived growth factor (PDGF), (TGF β, and EGF (5,53). EGF is a good example of a tumour-promoting cytokine produced by macrophages involved in a paracrine loop with tumour cells. In breast cancer high expression of EGF receptors (EGFR) is a major prognostic factor, indicating reduced overall and relapse-free survival (54). It was originally thought that that the ligand for this receptor, EGF or TGF-α, was produced by the tumour cells themselves, stimulation resulting from an autocrine loop. Many studies show breast cancers make TGF-α. However, our recent evidence suggests that the secretion of EGF is also due to a subpopulation of TAMs, thereby implying that tumour growth is regulated in a paracrine rather than an autocrine manner (53).

As angiogenesis is important in tumour progression, a great deal of effort has gone into isolating cytokines which are angiogenic. Some angiogenic cytokines such as bFGF have been known for some time to have angiogenic properties as well as various other functions. Others such as VEGF are newly discovered and act specifically on endothelial cells to stimulate growth. It is now apparent that a number of these angiogenic cytokines are in fact produced by TAMs, and so the importance of the TAM as a stimulator of tumour angiogenesis has been realized (55).

Macrophages and tumour angiogenesis: effect on prognosis

Angiogenesis is a complex process involving several steps. First, there is dissolution of the ECM surrounding the blood vessel, permitting extension of vascular buds from the existing vasculature to penetrate the stroma. The buds elongate initially and migrate, they are then replaced by newly divided endothelial cells, the cells of the neovascularized network then differentiate and mature into capillaries with deposition of a basement membrane. All the phases of this process can be influenced by the secretory products of macrophages either by direct action on endothelial cells, or indirectly via effects on the local ECM.

Macrophages and angiogenesis

Given that macrophages produce of angiogenic factors, recent work in this laboratory has attempted to assess whether there is a measurable relationship between macrophage infiltration and angiogenesis in human breast carcinoma. Several studies have shown a relationship between angiogenesis and prognosis in a number of tumour types, and we have developed a morphometric analysis method of enumerating the number of vessels, immunohistochemically stained with an anti-CD31-monoclonal antibody, in three vascular 'hotspots' using a Chalkley point eyepiece graticule. This method has shown an association between higher vascular count and worsened prognosis in cases of the top third Chalkley vascular count group (56). Using the same methodology, with a monoclonal anti-CD68 macrophage marker, we enumerated the degree of focal macrophage infiltration in the same tumours and compare this with the degree of angiogenesis. Figure 8.3 illustrates that the mean macrophage count is significantly higher in the top third, poor prognosis vascular count group.

With double staining it is possible to assess the spatial relationships between areas of angiogenesis and focal

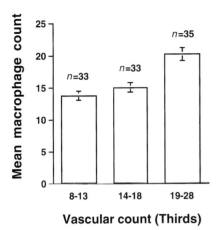

Figure 8.3. Association of tumour-associated macrophage infiltration with tumour angiogenesis. When tumour vascular count is ennumerated, the highest third are found to have a significantly worsened prognosis as a result. The high vascular grade group also has a significantly higher mean macrophage count (P = 0.03, bar—SEM).

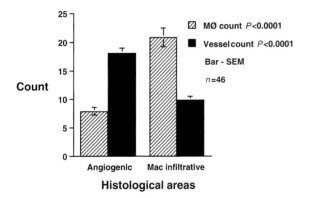

Figure 8.4. Inverse relationship between areas of angiogenesis and areas of tumour-associated macrophage (TAM) infiltration. In carcinomas of the breast there is relationship between the distribution of blood vessel hotspots and TAM hotspots with highly angiogenic areas having a lower degree of macrophage infiltration, while areas with high TAM concentrations are poorly vascularized. This could mean that TAMs are attracted to poorly vascularized regions and once there become angiogenically active. Once the area is re-vascularized the TAMs migrate out of the region.

macrophage infiltration. We have double stained a number of breast carcinomas in this way using a mouse mono-

clonal anti-CD68 macrophage marker, and a rabbit poly-clonal anti-von Willebrand factor endothelial cell marker. First, the three densest vascular fields were enumerated for vascularisation and macrophage infiltration, followed by the three densest areas of macrophage infiltration being enumerated for vessels and macrophages (Fig. 8.4). This shows that the highest areas of macrophage infiltration are situated away from the vessel 'hotspot' areas. In summary, higher numbers of macrophages are found in angiogenic breast tumours, but they are found in focal concentrations away from the most vascular areas of these tumours.

It is possible that areas situated away from vascular areas are hypoxic, and it is thought that tumour angiogenesis may be driven in part by reduced oxygen tension. Some cell types are capable of sensing falling oxygen levels by an as yet unknown mechanism, and responding with the secretion of VEGF (57). Hypoxia is also capable of inducing angiogenic activity in macrophages *in vitro*, for example the secretion of TNF-alpha (58). Thus, rapidly growing tumours may outstrip their blood supply resulting in focal areas of hypoxia. This could then lead to the attraction of TAMs into the area, either by following a falling oxygen gradient or a trail of chemoattractant molecules released by stressed or necrotic tumour cells. Once in position, the TAMs may then express an angiogenic phenotype, stimulating vascularization of the area and enhancing local tumour growth. The tumour cells may then enter the systemic blood circulation via gaps between the immature endothelial cells of the adjacent neovasculature.

Macrophages and prognosis

Breast cancer account for 20% of all cancer deaths in the Western world, and in the United Kingdom, which has the highest mortality rates, the estimated lifetime risk that a woman will develop breast cancer is 1:12. The cause of breast cancer is unknown, and its biological behaviour is complex. This has led to an interest in predicting its possible future behaviour, so that alternative therapeutic strategies can be tailored to the severity of the tumour. The most important prognostic indicator is the number of involved lymph nodes, with prognosis worsening with increased numbers involved. The histological grade of the tumour is also important, as is its size and also the age of the patient at presentation and the presence of tumour infiltration of blood vessels and lymphatics. Other significant molecular markers of prognosis in common clinical usage include oestrogen, progesterone (59), and epidermal growth factor receptors (54). There is a great deal of interest in establishing new prognostic factors because of their possible relevance as future targets for therapy. It is now well established that vascular grade, as measured by various vessel counting procedures, is a good marker of prognosis, with highly vascularized tumours having a worsened prognosis as a result (60,61). In 1989, Rosen *et al.* reviewed the prognostic significance of a range of markers in a large series of 644 patients with a median follow-up time of 18.2 years (62). This study showed that an intense lymphoplasmacytic reaction around the tumour was an unfavourable clinicopathological feature. The infiltration of inflammatory cells into tumours is a common feature of many tumour types, and the correlation of macrophage infiltration with angiogenesis suggests that TAMs could play a major part in tumour angiogenesis. Indeed, work in this laboratory has shown that the degree of macrophage infiltration into breast tumours is not only associated with angiogenesis, but is an independent prognostic factor in itself.

In a recent study we showed increased macrophage density in so-called 'hotspot' areas was associated with a worsened prognosis (Figs 8.5 and 8.6). Where the macrophage index (MØI) was higher than the median cut-point of 12, there was a significant worsening of prognosis for both relapse-free and overall survival. For relapse-free survival, there was an increased hazard ratio of 3.32 in the high MØI patients, whilst for overall survival, the high MØI group of patients were 11.19 times more at risk of dying from their disease than patients from the lower group. In the case of breast cancer, it would appear that vascularization and macrophage infiltration are closely related, while both being independent prognostic factors (63), in rather the same manner as nodal involvement and tumour size. This suggests that macrophages do play an

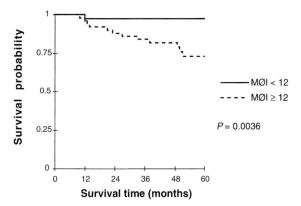

Figure 8.6. Association of high macrophage index with poor overall survival. Breast cancer patients with a high macrophage index (MØI = >12) have a significantly reduced overall survival when compared with those in the lower MØI group (hazard ratio = 11.19, $P = 0.0036$).

important part in the stimulation of tumour vascularization in breast cancer, but that they are also able to promote the tumours progression in other ways, probably via the secretion of tumour cell promoting factors such as EGF.

Angiogenic growth factors secreted by tumour-associated macrophages

Tumour-associated macrophages and tumour angiogenesis

Until recently it had been assumed that tumour angiogenesis was induced by the tumour cells themselves. However, this assumption has been challenged by the fact that TAMs have been shown to be capable of producing a broad spectrum of angiogenesis-modulating factors including cytokines and ECM-degrading enzymes. The implanted fibrosarcomas of mice depleted of monocytes are markedly less vascularized as a result (5). Also, macrophages isolated from tumours are able to induce vascularization in the rat corneal assay (64,65). There is now an increasing body of evidence indicating a primary role for TAMs in tumour angiogenesis.

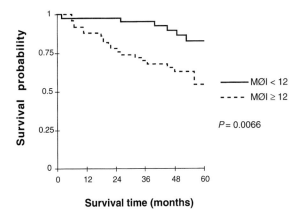

Figure 8.5. Association of high macrophage index with reduced relapse free survival. Breast cancer patients with a macrophage index (MØI) of more than 12 have a significantly increased risk of recurrence than those in the lower MØI group (hazard ratio = 3.32, $P = 0.0066$).

Activation and stimulation of angiogenic activity in tumour-associated macrophages

Activation is necessary for macrophages to become angiogenic (35), several studies have shown that monocytes are incapable of promoting neovascularization unless they are treated with activators such as concavalin A or endotoxin (66,67). However, the specific mechanism of angiogenic activation *in vivo* has yet to be elaborated, although the conditions found within the environment of wounds such as elevated concentrations of lactic acid, pyruvic acid, and hydrogen ions promote angiogenic activity in macrophages (68). Macrophages also become angiogenic in hypoxic conditions, a situation which is thought to be common in tumours (69). It could also be possible that TAMs are angiogenically activated by cytokines secreted by the tumour such as IFN-gamma and GM-CSF, or by endothelial cell derived factors, such as platelet-activating factor (PAF) and monocyte chemotactic protein (MCP), during the extravasation process. Specific markers of angiogenic activation in macrophages remain unknown at this time. However, macrophages with an angiogenic phenotype have been shown to upregulate MHC class II molecules on their cell surface (70), although this is also found on macrophages activated for antigen presentation and other functions. The urokinase receptor could be one potential candidate for a specific angiogenic activation marker, and importantly, cell adhesion molecules such as E-selectin, P-selectin, and ICAM-3 which are up-regulated on the tumour vasculature may be important mechanisms involved the entry of macrophages into tumours (71).

Tumour-associated macrophage-derived angiogenic cytokines

A number of angiogenic cytokines are known to be produced by macrophages (Table 8.1) and the evidence for this is reviewed below.

Vascular endothelial growth factor

VEGF is a heparin-binding growth factor existing as four splice variants having 121, 165, 189, and 206 amino acid chains. Also known as vascular permeability factor (VPF), it is a potent endothelial cell specific mitogen and can be sequestered by the ECM by virtue of its heparin-binding qualities (72). It is expressed strongly in human glioblastoma, a highly malignant brain tumour which is characteristically highly vascularized (73). Up-regulation of VEGF is seen in a number of human cancers including adenocarcinoma of the stomach, colon, and pancreas, renal cell carcinoma, ovarian and breast carcinoma (4), and an association has been found between microvessel density and VEGF expression in invasive carcinoma of the breast (74). VEGF expression has been localized to the malignant cell population of many tumours, but it has also been found in macrophages in breast carcinoma (4). Further evidence

implicating macrophages in VEGF production comes from the finding that a growth factor, secreted by macrophages isolated from the ascitic fluid aspirates of ovarian carcinoma, had a direct angiogenic effect both in *in vitro* and *in vivo* systems (75). Further studies indicated that this factor was probably VEGF (76). VEGF mRNA has been detected in tumour and stromal cells in areas adjacent to necrosis in some solid tumours. In glioblastoma, VEGF has been observed to be up-regulated in the tumour cells of hypoxic regions close to areas of necrosis (57). Necrosis is a significant feature of tumours with an aggressive phenotype, and, as has been mentioned earlier, VEGF is a strong chemoattractant for macrophages. As mentioned earlier, VEGF may not only stimulate angiogenesis directly, but also attract TAMs to areas of hypoxia, in order assist in the promotion of vascular in growth into theses areas.

Basic fibroblast growth factor

bFGF is a direct endothelial cell mitogen that has been detected in mouse peritoneal macrophages and human monocytes (77–79). It has been observed to be produced by TAMs in carcinomas of the liver and gastrointestinal tract (80,81). It is also produced by other cell types including neoplastic cells (4). Like VEGF, it is a heparin-binding growth factor and is therefore able to be sequestered by the ECM. Its mode of action is interesting as it lacks the signal peptide necessary for active secretion, this has led to the view that its release is dependent upon cellular damage (82). During the inflammatory process in tumours there is a high turnover of macrophages, which may be the mechanism of delivery of bFGF by this cell type.

Epidermal growth factor/transforming growth factor alpha

EGF and TGF-alpha are significant growth factors in the development of several human tumours, where they are potent promoters of neoplastic cell growth, in many carcinomas. They are also mitogenic for endothelial cells in a range of experimental systems (83). TGF-α has been shown to be released by macrophages following activation (84,85) and we have recently described EGF secretion by a subpopulation of TAMs in ductal carcinoma of the breast; however, no correlation was observed between EGF secretion and EGFR expression by tumour cells (53).

Tumour necrosis factor alpha

TNF-α is cytotoxic toward tumour cells (86). In addition, *in vitro* and *in vivo* studies have implied that TNF-α can both stimulate and inhibit angiogenesis in a dose-dependent manner (87). With the use of a disc angiogenesis system and an osmotic millipump in mice, it has been found that high doses of TNF-α (1–5 μg) are inhibitory, whereas, low doses (0.01–1 ng) are stimulatory for angiogenesis. This suggests that in *in vivo* tissues, where the concentration of TNF-α is unlikely to reach the microgram range, the overall effect of TNF-α is stimulatory towards angiogenesis. In breast and ovarian carcinomas, macrophages are a major source of TNF-α and TNF-α receptors are expressed on the tumour endothelium (52,88). In fact some TAMs, along with neoplastic and endothelial cells, are capable of making both p55 and p75 (52,88), the soluble receptors for TNF-α (TNF-αR). These soluble receptors could intercept TNF-α before it is able to interact with the receptors on the target cell. This would reduce the local concentrations of TNF-α to levels where they could become stimulatory to nearby endothelial cells. Hypoxia has been shown to stimulate a human macrophage cell line in culture to up-regulate the release of TNF-α and its receptors (58).

Platelet-derived endothelial cell growth factor/thymidine phosphorylase

Platelet-derived endothelial cell growth factor (PDECGF) is mitogenic for endothelial cells and was originally isolated from platelets. It is now becoming more commonly known as thymidine phosphorylase (TP), an enzyme involved in pyrimidine nucleoside metabolism (89). TP lacks a signal peptide and acts intracellularly (90). It is thought not to act directly in the manner of a cytokine to exert its angiogenic activity, but rather is angiogenic as a

consequence of its enzymatic activity (91,92). Furthermore, it has been observed in many tumour types including thyroid as well as squamous (93), breast, lung, and bladder carcinomas. We have identified TP expression immunocytochemically in a number of cell types in breast carcinoma, including neoplastic cells and stromal fibroblasts and macrophages (4). It has been observed in TAMs in glioblastoma (92). TP is most highly expressed in normal tissue macrophages in most organs and may represent a way of controlling angiogenesis in response to injury (Fig. 8.7). DNA released from dying cells and engulfed from apoptotic cells may be degraded to thymidine intracellularly or extracellularly. Thymidine may freely enter cells and macrophages attracted to injured areas then metabolize thymidine via TP to angiogenically active metabolities. Cytokines such as TNF-α, IL-1, and IFN-gamma further up-regulate TP to amplify this process.

Insulin-like growth factor I and II (IGF-I and -II)

IGF-I increases DNA synthesis in endothelial cells *in vitro* and promotes tube formation and endothelial cell migration (94). IGF-I expression has not been reported in TAMs, but it is secreted by macrophages after they have been activated (95,96), and a role in inflammatory angiogenesis has been suggested. Therefore a possible role in angiogenesis following the inflammatory response to neoplasia cannot be ruled out. Indeed, Singer *et al.* have recently shown that IGF-II is up-regulated in breast tumour-derived fibroblasts (97).

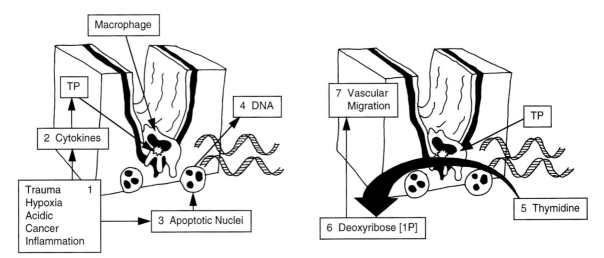

Figure 8.7. Angiogenic pathway of thymidine phosphorylase (TP). Thymidine released from dying cells passes freely into macrophages and other cells, or it is engulfed with apoptotic cells by macrophages. Macrophage-derived TP then metabolizes thymidine into 6 deoxyribose [1P] an angiogenically active metabolite either intra- or extracellulary.

Interleukin 8

IL-8 has yet to be shown to be produced by TAMs, but is produced by activated macrophages (98,99). IL-8 is mitogenic in *in vitro* assays and stimulates angiogenesis in the rat corneal assay (100,101). The same effects have been observed when the supernatants from activated macrophages were used on the same assays, these effects were markedly down-regulated in the presence of anti-Il-8 antibodies (99).

Extracellular matrix modulating factors produced by tumour-associated macrophage

The importance of the extracellular matrix in tumour angiogenesis

When considering angiogenesis, it is important not to forget the role of the ECM in the process. The ECM is both a barrier to migrating endothelial cells, and an extracellular source of angiogenic growth factors. The ECM is degraded by proteolytic enzymes, after which growth factors are released, while simultaneously providing a route for endothelial cell infiltration into the tumour mass, and a route for invasive tumour cells to enter the vasculature. The macrophage is able to modulate events in the ECM, either by the direct secretion of degradative enzymes or by ECM modulating cytokines. Many angiogenic cytokines are heparin binding, and as a consequence are sequestered by the ECM by binding to heparin-like glycosaminoglycans. Examples of heparin-binding angiogenic growth factors are VEGF, bFGF, TGF-β, and pleiotrophin, which can all be released from the ECM following proteolysis, and are then able to exert their angiogenic effects. In addition, some ECM molecules become angiogenic following hydrolytic cleavage (102). Fragments of hyaluronic acid are angiogenic in the chorioallantoic membrane (CAM) assay (103), and fibrin, following plasmin digestion, also stimulates neovascularization in this assay (104,105).

Tumour-associated macrophage-derived extracellular matrix modulators

Macrophages are a rich source of enzymes and cytokines that effect the mechanical and molecular structure of the ECM see Table 8.1, p. 85). They are capable of secreting an array of ECM degradative enzymes, and are major sources of metaloproteases such as collagenase (106,107), and serine proteases, such as tissue type and urokinase plasminogen activator (tPA, uPA) (107,108). It has been found that TAMs derived from human colonic adenocarcinomas produce type IV collagenase (109), and it has also been observed that the chemokine MCP-1 is capable of up-regulating uPA and uPA receptor (uPAR) expression in murine TAMs (36). In human invasive ductal carcinoma of the breast, uPAR is located partly in the TAM population (110). When uPA binds to uPAR, uPA catalysed plasminogen activation is greatly enhanced, and so in this instance the TAM population may be directing ECM proteolysis to the sites of tumour and vascular invasion. Studies have shown that expression of uPA by macrophages leads to the release of ECM bound bFGF (111,112). Cathepsin D is able to release ECM bound bFGF (113) and has been observed in macrophages of invasive breast carcinomas where its presence was associated with a worse prognosis (114).

The proteolysis of the ECM does not go unchecked and a range of inhibitors are in evidence, many of which are produced by macrophages. Macrophage-derived inhibitors of ECM degradation include tissue inhibitor of metalloproteases (TIMP) and plasminogen activator inhibitor 1 (PAI-1) (115). Simultaneous expression of enzyme and inhibitor stimulates neovascularization, while protecting newly vascularized tissues. Endothelial cells also produce proteolytic enzymes enabling them to penetrate the basement membrane and migrate into surrounding tissues (116). Macrophages can modulate this behaviour by the secretion of enzyme inhibitors, and the production of cytokines which alter enzyme secretion by endothelial cells. Such cytokines include bFGF, TGF-β, TNF-α, and granulocyte colony-stimulating factor (G-CSF). bFGF and G-CSF increase, while TGF-β decreases plasminogen activation in endothelial cells (117).

The role of TGF-β in ECM proteolysis is interesting. In bovine endothelial cells in culture it can up-regulate both uPA and its inhibitor, with the overall balance favouring anti-proteolysis (118). However, TGF-β can also stimulate macrophages to produce u-PA leading to the release of bFGF in a three-dimensional collagen gel experimental system (112,119). This suggests that the regional balance of proteolytic factors within a tumour may be regulated, in part, by local concentrations of TGF-β.

In summary, TAMs could effect the ECM of tumours in three different ways:

1. Direct secretion of ECM-degrading enzymes, releasing bound angiogenic growth factors, and promoting endothelial cell migration.

2. proteolytic cleavage of the ECM yielding angiogenic fragments.

3. Secretion of cytokines which modulate ECM composition by acting on other cell types in a paracrine

fashion, or alternatively on the TAM itself through an autocrine pathway.

Angiogenic cytokine networks involving the macrophage

Macrophages have the potential to be involved in all areas of tumour angiogenesis, acting on a range of cell types, in a number of different ways. It is useful to summarize these activities by looking at the system as a whole, and locating the position of the macrophage within the broader context of the tumour environment (Fig. 8.8). Angiogenic cytokines and other factors can be produced by a wide range of cell types, including neoplastic cells, fibroblasts, endo-

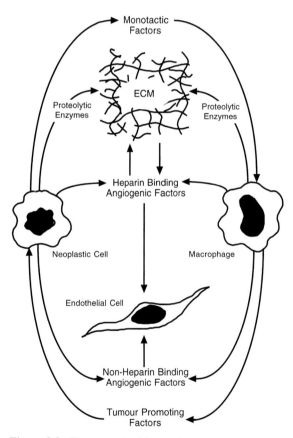

Figure 8.8. The network of factors involved in tumour angiogenesis. Tumour angiogenesis may be regulated by a complex network of interacting cell types producing extracellular matrix (ECM) modulating factors, tumour promoting factors, chemotactic factors, and angiogenic factors.

thelial cells, and macrophages. These cells, and their products, have complex interrelationships which are both stimulatory and inhibitory towards angiogenesis. Therefore the net balance of these factors at any one site in a tumour regulates angiogenesis at that site.

Hypoxia is an interesting element of tumour biology. As small tumours grow they develop hypoxic areas which act as a stimulus for production of angiogenic cytokines. Hypoxia stimulates VEGF production in tumour cells (57), and is also an attractant for macrophages (50). Necrosis, often induced by hypoxia, is a feature of many tumours with an aggressive phenotype, and may also be a source of release of factors such as bFGF (120) and pleiotrophin (4). In this way, tumour cells and/or macrophages could release angiogenic factors at sites of hypoxia and necrosis to stimulate the development of new blood vessels and the infiltration of angiogenic macrophages to such sites.

Cytokines in the tumour microenvironment can also interact to regulate their own expression as well as that of ECM-modulating enzymes. VEGF is sequestered by the ECM and can be released by proteolytic enzymes derived from a number of cellular sources including macrophages, endothelial cells, and neoplastic cells (121). In capillary cells in culture VEGF can also up-regulate uPA and tPA, which can then release further growth factors from the ECM (122). This illustrates how the balance of macrophage-derived factors such as VEGF can be effected by factors secreted by both macrophages and other cell types. In addition, VEGF and bFGF, when present together, act synergistically on angiogenesis (123). bFGF can be derived from TAMs in addition to neoplastic cells and fibroblasts (80,81,90), and is also sequestered by the ECM and may be released from it proteolytically via a number of cell types (113). In addition, breast cancer cell lines have been shown to express bFGF receptors, stimulation of which induces the ECM-degrading enzyme, cathepsin D. So the potential feedback loops modulating angiogenesis, involving various factors and cellular sources are quite complex. EGF can stimulate VEGF secretion in glioma cell lines (124), it can also induce t-PA production in vascular cultures, as can TGF-α (125). Both tumour cells and macrophages produce TGF-α in solid tumours (83,126).

TNF-α is able to induce prostaglandin production in a number of tumour cell lines (127), and macrophage production of TNF-α is inhibited by prostaglandin E_2 (128), thus producing a negative feedback loop. TNF-α is also able to stimulate uPA production by the human umbilical vein endothelial cell (HUVEC) culture (129), which could potentially lead to the release of other factors from the ECM.

TGF-β1 has the capability to induce both macrophages and cultured bovine endothelial cells to synthesize uPA

(118). In tumours of the gastrointestinal system (130) and breast (131,132), TGF-β has been localized immunohisto-chemically to neoplastic cells, undefined stromal cells, and the ECM. At high concentration, TGF-β inhibits VEGF- and bFGF-induced endothelial cell migration and tube for-mation, while at low concentrations it potentiates these effects (119,133).

It appears that no one cell type or factor is wholly responsible for the control of angiogenesis, but rather that regulation of angiogenesis is brought about by the balance of factors in the local environment. In the tumour, the fine balance seen in normal systems may be tipped in favour of the tumour by virtue of the neoplastic cells themselves and the inflammatory cells that they directly or indirectly attract.

In the tumour a process of evolution is constantly occurring, with survival of the fittest for that environment. The genetic instability that characterizes cancer provides a potent source of clonal variation. Presumably tumour cells sensitive to the tumoricidal or growth inhibitory effects of macrophages will die, while those that are not will become the dominant population. Thus, by the time a tumour is detectable, a macrophage population may have interacted with the tumour in this way, and the tumour evolved to work in synergy with its infiltrating macrophages. Therefore this macrophage population provides a novel host target for anti-cancer therapy.

Summary and conclusions

The tumour-associated macrophage as mediator of tumour angiogenesis

The macrophage is a sophisticated cell type capable of functioning in a wide variety of ways. In the tumour context, it would appear that the TAM is specifically capable of influencing every stage of tumour progression, from tumour cell proliferation, to the induction of angio-genesis. Many *in vivo* and *in vitro* experiments have shown that TAMs influence tumour development in this way, that they are readily drawn towards tumours tumour sites by chemokines released by malignant and other cell types, as well as other chemotactic factors. Once in posi-tion in the tumours, a subpopulation at least, are activated to exhibit an angiogenic phenotype. TAMs can influence angiogenesis by releasing angiogenic cytokines directly, or indirectly by secreting ECM-degrading enzymes which release angiogenic factor which have been sequestered by the matrix. The TAM population of a tumour is, however, heterogeneous, and they can be expressing a range of dif-ferent phenotypes dependent upon their state of activation.

But even in their cytotoxic mode they can have an effect on angiogenesis by the release of cellular non-secreted factors, such as bFGF, from target cells.

TAMs are found in abundance in many tumour types, including carcinoma of the breast, where their presence focally in large numbers correlates with angiogenesis and is an indicator of poor prognosis with reduction of overall and relapse-free survival times. The nature of the signals responsible for the angiogenic activation of TAMs is cur-rently not understood, but enough is known to formulate some hypotheses about the mechanisms involved in macrophage stimulation of tumour angiogenesis. One such theory, presently under investigation in this laboratory, is that reduced oxygen tension in rapidly proliferating tumours, brings about focal cell death in the hypoxic areas of the tumour. The factors subsequently released by these dead and dying cells, which may even be undergoing hypoxia-induced apoptosis, serve to stimulate extra-vasation of monocytes from the blood vessels closest to these areas. Once the monocytes have entered the tumour environment they are activated by factors peculiar to the tumour microenvironment and migrate towards the areas of hypoxia, perhaps following an oxygen gradient, lactic acid produced by hypoxic cells, or chemokines released by surrounding tumour cells or other inflammatory cells which have passed previously. Once in the hypoxic areas the macrophages begin to debride the area in much the same manner as when they are present at wound sites. In this situation they then release factors which both stimu-late growth of surrounding epithelial cells, and initiate re-endothelialization and angiogenesis into the area. As the vessels grow into the area the macrophages may disperse and the nutritional and respiratory needs of the otherwise highly proliferative tumour are restored. The previously quiescent surrounding tumour cells are then the subject of an increased growth stimulus and have a ready supply of nutrients and oxygen supplied by an immature vasculature, which is easily penetrable as it is incomplete and lacks a basement membrane, thus providing an easy route for the metastatic dissemination of the tumour cells into the sys-temic circulation. The macrophages may even play a part in this context, whereby their production of ECM-degrad-ing enzymes facilitates the growth of endothelial cells and loosens the fibrous network of the ECM sufficiently thus allowing potentially metastatic tumour cells increased mobility. There is even some evidence that macrophages themselves may drag tumour cells into the circulation (134,135) perhaps by virtue of sialoadhesin molecules on their surface binding to sialic acid residues on the surface of the tumour cells (136). Macrophages at distant sites may also capture circulating tumour cells with the same mechanism.

Thus it would appear that the macrophage is potentially an extremely important cell type in tumour biology, especially tumour angiogenesis. The next logical step that many researchers are taking is the investigation of the TAM as a target for tumour therapy.

The tumour-associated macrophage as a target for future anti-angiogenic therapies

Many of the anti-angiogenic drugs currently in the clinical trial stage, exert their effects by blocking the interaction of angiogenic cytokines with their receptors on the endothelial cell (137), and a great deal of effort is being concentrated on elucidating the nature of the receptors to VEGF and other cytokines, with a view to producing compounds which can compete with and suppress the receptor/ ligand interaction. Many of these therapies would obviously be effective in the inhibition of angiogenic stimuli produced by cytokines secreted by TAMs; however, with the seemingly central role that the macrophage could play in tumour angiogenesis, the macrophage itself becomes an appealing target for future therapeutic strategies which could probably be used in conjunction with other therapies.

Presently compounds being studied with regards to their macrophage modulating effects fall broadly into two categories: (i) those that suppress secretion of angiogenic substances by macrophages, and (ii) those that inhibit macrophage infiltration into the tumour mass. IFN-γ and chloroquine fall into the first category of compounds. IFN-gamma in low doses has been shown to inhibit secretion of TNF-α by macrophages (138), and similarly chloroquine inhibits TNF-α gene transcription in macrophages (139). Thiol-containing compounds such as gold sodium thiomalate, which have been used in the treatment of rheumatoid arthritis, are potent inhibitors of macrophage-derived angiogenic activity (140), and may exert their effects by the inhibition of macrophage production of reactive oxygen species (141), such as nitric oxide.

Another strategy may include inhibition of macrophage-derived collagenases by compounds, such as tetracycline and its derivatives such as minocycline, which are potent inhibitors of angiogenesis. In the second category of compounds, those that inhibit macrophage migration, IL-10 and linomide are the most studied. In mice, transplantable tumours transfected with IL-10 show markedly less macrophage infiltration than their non-transfected counterparts (8). Linomide has anti-tumour activity when given in vivo but lacks this effect in vitro studies, and is able to inhibit angiogenesis in vivo (142,143). However, treatment of tumour-bearing rats with linomide reduces the number of tumour infiltrative macrophages by over 50% (144).

Work on drugs capable of inhibiting macrophage-mediated angiogenesis is at a comparatively early stage. One point worth making in summary, is that tumours are composed of more than just malignant cells. They are, in effect, complex micro-ecosystems whose progression is dependent upon the interaction of many cellular types, including the fibroblasts of the supporting stromal matrix, the endothelial cells of the vascular supply, and the tumour-associated macrophages with their tumour-promoting activities. It appears that neoplastic cells alone are incapable of generating a viable tumour, and that they require support in order to do this from other non-neoplastic cells. Without this support they will quickly regress and disappear, and it might well be that this happens undetectably with very high frequency. In recent years more scientists have begun to examine tumours in this broader context and it seems likely that, as the underlying mechanisms of these cellular interactions are revealed, new and novel anti-tumour strategies will evolve.

References

1. O'Sullivan, C. and Lewis, C. E. (1994). Tumour-associated leucocytes: friends or foes in breast carcinoma. *J. Pathol.*, **172**, 229–35.
2. Kelly, P. M., Davison, R. S., Bliss, E. and McGee, J. O'D. (1988). Macrophages in human breast disease: a quantitative immunohistochemical study. *Br J Cancer*, **57**, 174–7.
3. Lewis, C. E. (1992). Cytokines in neoplasia. In *The Oxford textbook of pathology* (ed. N. Wright, P. G. Isaacson, and J. O'D. Mcgee), pp. 709–15. Oxford University Press.
4. Leek, R. D., Harris, A. L., and Lewis, C. E. (1994). Cytokine networks in solid human tumors: regulation of angiogenesis. *J. Leukoc. Biol.*, **56**, 423–35.
5. Sunderkotter, C., Steinbrink, K. Goebeler, M. Bhardwaj, R. and Sorg C (1994). Macrophages and angiogenesis. *J. Leukoc. Biol.*, **55**, 410–22.
6. Polverini, P. J. and Leibovich, S. J. (1984). Induction of neovascularization *in vivo* and endothelial proliferation *in vitro* by tumor-associated macrophages. *Lab. Invest.*, **51**, 635–42.
7. Kobayashi, S., Nagaura, T., Kimura, I., and Kimura, M. (1994). Interferon-gamma-activated macrophages enhance angiogenesis from endothelial cells of rat aorta. *Immunopharmacology*, **27**, 23–30.
8. Richter, G., Kruger, K. S., Hein, G., Huls, C., Schmitt, E., Diamantstein, T., *et al.* (1993). Interleukin 10 transfected into Chinese hamster ovary cells prevents tumor growth and macrophage infiltration. *Cancer Res.*, **53**, 4134–7.
9. Rothlein, R., Dustin, M. L., Marlin, S. D., and Springer, T. A. (1986). A human intercellular adhesion molecule (ICAM-1) distinct from LFA-1. *J. Immunol.*, **137**, 1270–4.
10. Auger, M. J. and Ross, J. A. (1992). The biology of the macrophage. In *The macrophage* (ed. C. E. Lewis and J. O'D. McGee), pp. 23–5. Oxford University Press.
11. Dustin, M. L., Rothlein, R., Bhan, A. K., Dinarello, C. A., and Springer, T. A. (1986). Induction by IL 1 and inter-

feron-gamma: tissue distribution, biochemistry, and function of a natural adherence molecule (ICAM-1). *J. Immunol.*, **137**, 245–54.

12. Lewis, C. E. and McGee, J. O'D. (1992). *The macrophage*, Oxford University Press.
13. Murphy, G. F., Messadi, D., Fonferko, E., and Hancock, W. W. (1986). Phenotypic transformation of macrophages to Langerhans cells in the skin. *Am. J. Pathol.*, **123**, 401–6.
14. Groh, V., Gadner, H., Radaszkiewicz, T., Rappersberger, K., Konrad, K., Wolff, K., *et al.* (1988). The phenotypic spectrum of histiocytosis X cells. *J. Invest. Dermatol.*, **90**, 441–7.
15. Franklin, W. A., Mason, D. Y., Pulford, K., Falini, B., Bliss, E., Gatter, K. C., *et al.* (1986). Immunohistological analysis of human mononuclear phagocytes and dendritic cells by using monoclonal antibodies. *Lab. Invest.*, **54**, 322–35.
16. Metchnikoff, E. (1905). *Immunity in infective disease*. Cambridge University Press.
17. Rocklin, R. E., Bendtzen, K., and Greineder, D. (1980). Mediators of immunity: lymphokines and monokines. *Adv. Immunol.*, **29** 55–136.
18. Adams, D. O. and Hamilton, T. A. (1984). The cell biology of macrophage activation. *Annu. Rev. Immunol.*, **2**, 283–318.
19. Sung, S. S., Nelson, R. S., and Silverstein, S. C. (1983). Yeast mannans inhibit binding and phagocytosis of zymosan by mouse peritoneal macrophages. *J. Cell Biol.*, **96**, 160–6.
20. Kay, M. M. (1975). Mechanism of removal of senescent cells by human macrophages *in situ*. *Proc. Natl. Acad. Sci. USA*, **72**, 3521–5.
21. Kaklamanis, L., Gatter, K. C., Hill, A. B., Mortensen, N., Harris, A. L., Krausa, P., *et al.* (1992). Loss of HLA class-1 alleles, heavy chains and beta-2-microglobulin in colorectal cancer. *Int. J. Cancer*, **51**, 379–85.
22. Hirsch, J. G. (1962). Cinemicrophotographic observations on granule lysis in polymorphonuclear leucocytes during phagocytosis. *J. Exp. Med.*, **116**, 827–33.
23. Klebanoff, S. J. (1988). Phagocytic cells: products of oxygen metabolism. In *Inflammation: basic principles and clinical correlates* (ed. J. I. Gallin, I. M. Goldstein, and R. Snyderman), pp. 325–40. Raven, New York.
24. Elsbach, P. and Weiss, J. (1988). Phagocytic cells: oxygen independent antimicrobial systems. In *Inflammation: basic principles and clinical correlates* (ed. J. I. Gallin, I. M. Goldstein, and R. Snyderman), pp. 341–54. Raven, New York.
25. Gabig, T. G. and Babior, B. M. (1981). The killing of pathogenes by phagocytes. *Annu. Rev. Med.*, **32**, 313–26.
26. Brown, C. C. and Gallin, J. I. (1988). Chemotactic disorders. In *Haematology/oncology clinics of North America. Phagocytic defects*, Vol. 1, *Abnormalities outside of the respiratory burst* (ed. J. T. Curnette), pp. 162–76. W. B. Saunders, Philadelphia.
27. Sisson, S. D. and Dinarello, C. A. (1989). Interleukin 1. In *Human monocytes* (ed. M. Zembela and G. L. Asherson), pp. 183–94. Academic Press, London.
28. Ben, A. M., Leroy, E., Lantz, O., Metivier, D., Autran, B., Charpentier, B., *et al.* (1987). rIL 2-induced proliferation of human circulating NK cells and T lymphocytes: synergistic effects of IL 1 and IL 2. *J. Immunol.*, **139**, 443–51.
29. Sugarman, B. J., Aggarwal, B. B., Hass, P. E., Figari, I. S., Palladino, M. J., and Shepard, H. M. (1985). Recombinant human tumor necrosis factor-alpha: effects on proliferation of normal and transformed cells *in vitro*. *Science*, **230**, 943–5.

30. Erroi, A., Sironi, M., Chiaffarino, F., Chen, Z. G., Mengozzi, M., and Mantovani, A. (1989). IL-1 and IL-6 release by tumor-associated macrophages from human ovarian carcinoma. *Int. J. Cancer*, **44**, 795–801.
31. Malick, A. P., Elgert, K. D., Garner, R. E., and Adkinson, N. J. (1987). Prostaglandin E2 production by Mac-2+ macrophages: tumor-induced population shift. *J. Leukoc. Biol.*, **42**, 673–81.
32. Adams, D. O. and Hamilton, T. A. (1988). Phagocytic cells: Cytotoxic activities of macrophages. In *Inflammation: basic principles and clinical correlates* (ed. J. I. Gallin, I. M. Goldstein, and R. Snyderman), pp. 471–92. Raven, New York.
33. Wood, G. W. and Gollahon, K. A. (1977). Detection and quantitation of macrophage infiltration into primary human tumors with the use of cell-surface markers. *J. Natl Cancer Inst.*, **59**, 1081–7.
34. Eccles, S. A. and Alexander, P. (1974). Macrophage content of tumours in relation to metastatic spread and host immune reaction. *Nature*, **250**, 667–9.
35. Steinman, R. M. (1988). Cytokines amplify the function of accessory cells. *Immunol. Lett.*, **17**, 197–202.
36. Mantovani, A. (1994). Tumor-associated macrophages in neoplastic progression: a paradigm for the *in vivo* function of chemokines. *Lab. Invest.*, **71**, 5–16.
37. Benomar, A., Ming, W. J., Taraboletti, G., Ghezzi, P., Balotta, C., Cianciolo, G. J., *et al.* (1987). Chemotactic factor and P15E-related chemotaxis inhibitor in human melanoma cell lines with different macrophage content and tumorigenicity in nude mice. *J. Immunol.*, **138**, 2372–9.
38. Graves, D. T. and Valente, A. J. (1991). Monocyte chemotactic proteins from human tumor cells. *Biochem. Pharmacol.*, **41**, 333–7.
39. Bottazzi, B., Ghezzi, P., Taraboletti, G., Salmona, M., Colombo, N., Bonazzi,, C., *et al.* (1985). Tumor-derived chemotactic factor(s) from human ovarian carcinoma: evidence for a role in the regulation of macrophage content of neoplastic tissues. *Int. J. Cancer*, **36**, 167–73.
40. Oppenheim, J. J., Zachariae, C. O., Mukaida, N., and Matsushima, K. (1991). Properties of the novel proinflammatory supergene 'intercrine' cytokine family. *Annu. Rev. Immunol.*, **9**, 617–48.
41. Schall, T. J. (1991). Biology of the RANTES/SIS cytokine family. *Cytokine*, **3**, 165–83.
42. Bottazzi, B., Polentarutti, N., Acero, R., Balsari, A., Boraschi, D., Ghezzi, P., *et al.* (1983). Regulation of the macrophage content of neoplasms by chemoattractants. *Science*, **220**, 210–2.
43. Mahe, Y., Hirose, K., Clausse, B., Chouaib, S., Tursz, T. and Mariame, B. (1992). Heterogeneity among human nasopharyngeal carcinoma cell lines for inflammatory cytokines mRNA expression levels. *Biochem. Biophys. Res. Commun.*, **187**, 121–6.
44. Van, D. J., Proost, P., Lenaerts, J. P., and Opdenakker, G. (1992). Structural and functional identification of two human, tumor-derived monocyte chemotactic proteins (MCP-2 and MCP-3) belonging to the chemokine family. *J. Exp. Med.* **176**, 59–65.
45. Fu, Y. X., Cai, J. P., Chin, Y. H., Watson, G. A., and Lopez, D. M. (1992). Regulation of leukocyte binding to

endothelial tissues by tumor-derived GM-CSF. *Int. J. Cancer*, **50**, 585–8.

46. Wu, S., Boyer, C. M., Whitaker, R. S., *et al.* (1993). Tumor necrosis factor alpha as an autocrine and paracrine growth factor for ovarian cancer: monokine induction of tumor cell proliferation and tumor necrosis factor alpha expression. *Cancer Res.*, **53**, 1939–44.

47. Pyke, C., Kristensen, P., Ralfkiaer, E., Grondahl-Hansen, J., Eriksen, J., *et al.* (1991). Urokinase-type plasminogen activator is expressed in stromal cells and its receptor in cancer cells at invasive foci in human colon adenocarcinomas. *Am. J. Pathol.*, **138**, 1059–67.

48. Heike, Y., Sone, S., Yano, S., Seimiya, H., Tsuruo, T., and Ogura, T. (1993). M-CSF gene transduction in multidrug-resistant human cancer cells to enhance anti-P-glycoprotein antibody-dependent macrophage-mediated cytotoxicity. *Int. J. Cancer*, **54**, 851–7.

49. Dorsch, M., Hock, H., Kunzendorf, U., Diamantstein, T., and Blankenstein, T. (1993). Macrophage colony-stimulating factor gene transfer into tumor cells induces macrophage infiltration but not tumor suppression. *Eur. J. Immunol.*, **23**, 186–90.

50. Clauss, M., Gerlach, M., Gerlach, H., Brett, J., Wang, F., Familletti, P. C., *et al.* (1990). Vascular permeability factor: a tumor-derived polypeptide that induces endothelial cell and monocyte procoagulant activity, and promotes monocyte migration. *J. Exp. Med.*, **172**, 1535–45.

51. Yeo, K. T., Wang, H. H., Nagy, J. A., Sioussat, T. M., Ledbetter, S. R., Hoogewerf, A. J., *et al.* (1993). Vascular permeability factor (vascular endothelial growth factor) in guinea pig and human tumor and inflammatory effusions. *Cancer Res.*, **53**, 2912–8.

52. Pusztai, L., Clover, L. M., Cooper, K., Starkey, P. M., Lewis, C. E., and McGee, JO'D. (1994). Expression of tumour necrosis factor alpha and its receptors in carcinoma of the breast. *Br. J. Cancer*, **70**, 289–92.

53. O'Sullivan, C., Lewis, C. E., Harris, A. L., and McGee, JO'D. (1993). Secretion of epidermal growth factor by macrophages associated with breast carcinoma. *Lancet*, **342**, 148–9.

54. Sainsbury, J. R., Farndon, J. R., Needham, G. K., Malcolm, A. J., and Harris, A. L. (1987). Epidermal-growth-factor receptor status as predictor of early recurrence of and death from breast cancer. *Lancet*, **i**, 1398–402.

55. Lewis, C. E., Leek, R., Harris, A. L., and McGee, JO'D. (1995). Cytokine regulation of angiogenesis in breast cancer: the role of tumor-associated macrophages. *J. Leukoc. Biol.*, **57**, 747–51.

56. Fox, S. B., Leek, R. D., Weekes, M. P., Whitehouse, R. M., Gatter, K. C., and Harris, A. L. (1995). Quantitation and prognostic value of breast cancer angiogenesis: comparison of microvessel density, Chalkley count, and computer image analysis. *J. Pathol.*, **177**, 275–83.

57. Shweiki, D., Itin, A., Soffer, D., and Keshet, E. (1992). Vascular endothelial growth factor induced by hypoxia may mediate hypoxia initiated angiogenesis. *Nature*, **359**, 843–5.

58. Scannell, G., Waxman, K., Kaml, G. J., Ioli, G., Gatanaga, T., Yamamoto, R., *et al.* (1993). Hypoxia induces a human macrophage cell line to release tumor necrosis factor-alpha and its soluble receptors *in vitro*. *J. Surg. Res.*, **54**, 281–5.

59. Howell, A., Barnes, D. M., Harland R. N. L., Redford, J., Bramwell, V. H. C., Wilkinson, M. J. S., *et al.* (1984). Steroid-hormone receptors and survival after first relapse in breast cancer. *Lancet*, **i**, 588–91.

60. Craft, P. S. and Harris, A. L. (1994). Clinical prognostic significance of tumour angiogenesis. *Ann. Oncol.*, **5**, 305–11.

61. Gasparini, G. and Harris, A. L. (1995). Clinical importance of the determination of tumour angiogenesis in breast carcinoma: much more than a new prognostic tool. *J. Clin. Oncol.*, **13**, 765–82.

62. Rosen, P. P., Groshen, S., Saigo, P. E., Kinne, D. W., and Hellman, S. (1989). Pathological prognostic factors in stage I (T1NOMO) and stage II (T1N1MO) breast carcinoma: a study of 644 patients with median follow-up of 18 years. *J. Clin. Oncol.*, **7**, 1239–51.

63. Leek, R. D., Lewis, C. E., Whitehouse, R., Greenall, M., Clarke, J. and Harris, A. L. (1996). Association of macrophage infiltration with angiogenesis and prognosis in invasive breast carcinoma. *Cancer Res.*, **56**, 4625–9.

64. Clark, R. A., Stone, R. D., Leung, D. Y., Silver, I., Hohn, D. C., and Hunt, T. K. (1976). Role of macrophages in wound healing. *Surg. Forum*, **27**, 16–8.

65. Hunt, T. K., Knighton, D. R., Thakral, K. K., Goodson, W3, and Andrews, W. S. (1984). Studies on inflammation and wound healing: angiogenesis and collagen synthesis stimulated *in vivo* by resident and activated wound macrophages. *Surgery*, **96**, 48–54.

66. Koch, A. E., Polverini, P. J., and Leibovich, S. J. (1986). Induction of neovascularization by activated human monocytes. *J. Leukoc. Biol.*, **39**, 233–8.

67. Meyer, K. C., Kaminski, M. J., Calhoun, W. J., and Auerbach, R. (1989). Studies of bronchoalveolar lavage cells and fluids in pulmonary sarcoidosis. I. Enhanced capacity of bronchoalveolar lavage cells from patients with pulmonary sarcoidosis to induce angiogenesis *in vivo*. *Am. Rev. Respir. Dis.*, **140**, 1446–9.

68. Jensen, J. A., Hunt, T. K., Scheuenstuhl, H., and Banda, M. J. (1986). Effect of lactate, pyruvate, and pH on secretion of angiogenesis and mitogenesis factors by macrophages. *Lab. Invest.*, **54**, 574–8.

69. Knighton, D. R., Hunt, T. K., Scheuenstuhl, H., Halliday, B. J., Werb, Z., and Banda, M. J. (1983). Oxygen tension regulates the expression of angiogenesis factor by macrophages. *Science*, **221**, 1283–5.

70. Warren, M. K. and Vogel, S. N. (1985). Bone marrow-derived macrophages: development and regulation of differentiation markers by colony-stimulating factor and interferons. *J. Immunol.*, **134**, 982–9.

71. Fox, S. B., Turner, G. D. H., Gatter, K. C., and Harris, A. L. (1995). The increased expression of adhesion molecules ICAM-3 and e- and p-selectins on breast cancer epithelium. *J. Pathol.*, **177**, 369–76.

72. Ferrara, N., Houck, K., Jakeman, L., and Leung, D. W. (1992). Molecular and biological properties of the vascular endothelial growth factor family of proteins. *Endocr. Rev.*, **13**, 18–32.

73. Plate, K. H., Breier, G., Weich, H. A., and Risau, W. (1992). Vascular endothelial growth factor is a potential tumour angiogenesis factor in human gliomas *in vivo*. *Nature*, **359**, 845–8.

74. Toi, M., Hoshina, S., Takayanagi, T., and Tominaga, T. (1994). Association of vascular endothelial growth factor expression with tumor angiogenesis and with early relapse in primary breast cancer. *Jpn. J. Cancer Res.*, **85**, 1045–9.

75. Sheid, B. (1992). Angiogenic effects of macrophages isolated from ascitic fluid aspirated from women with advanced ovarian cancer. *Cancer Lett.*, **62**, 153–8.

76. Yeo, K. T., Wang, H. H., Nagy, J. A., Sioussat, T. M., Ledbetter, S. R., Hoogewerf, A. J., *et al.* (1993). Vascular permeability factor (vascular endothelial growth factor) in guinea pig and human tumor and inflammatory effusions. *Cancer Res.*, **53**, 2912–18.

77. Baird, A., Mormede, P., and Bohlen, P. (1985). Immunoreactive fibroblast growth factor in cells of peritoneal exudate suggests its identity with macrophage-derived growth factor. *Biochem. Biophys. Res. Commun.*, **126**, 358–64.

78. Joseph, S. J., Moscatelli, D., and Rifkin, D. B. (1988). The development of a quantitative RIA for basic fibroblast growth factor using polyclonal antibodies against the 157 amino acid form of human bFGF. The identification of bFGF in adherent elicited murine peritoneal macrophages. *J. Immunol. Methods*, **110**, 183–92.

79. Schulze, O. K., Risau, E., Vollmer, E., and Sorg, C. (1990). *In situ* detection of basic fibroblast growth factor by highly specific antibodies. *Am. J. Pathol.*, **137**, 85–92.

80. Alvarez, J. A., Baird, A., Tatum, A., Daucher, J., Chorsky, R., Gonzalez, A. M., *et al.* (1992). Localization of basic fibroblast growth factor and vascular endothelial growth factor in human glial neoplasms. *Mod. Pathol.*, **5**, 303–7.

81. Motoo, Y., Sawabu, N., Yamaguchi, Y., Terada, T., and Nakanuma, Y. (1993). Sinusoidal capillarization of human hepatocellular carcinoma: possible promotion by fibroblast growth factor. *Oncology*, **50**, 270–4.

82. Rifkin, D. B. and Moscatelli, D. (1989). Recent developments in the cell biology of basic fibroblast growth factor. *J. Cell Biol.*, **109**, 1–6.

83. Bicknell, R. and Harris, A. L. (1991). Novel growth regulatory factors and tumour angiogenesis. *Eur. J. Cancer*, **27**, 781–5.

84. Madtes, D. K., Raines, E. W., Sakariassen, K. S., Assoian, R. K., Sporn, M. B., Bell, G. I., *et al.* (1988). Induction of transforming growth factor-alpha in activated human alveolar macrophages. *Cell*, **53**, 285–93.0

85. Rappolee, D. A., Mark, D., Banda, M. J., and Werb, Z. (1988). Wound macrophages express TGF-alpha and other growth factors *in vivo*: analysis by mRNA phenotyping. *Science*, **241**, 708–12.

86. Cerami, A. and Beutler, B. (1988). The role of cachetin/TNF in endotoxic shock and cachexia. *Immunol. Today*, **9**, 28–31.

87. Fajardo, L. F., Kwan, H. H., Kowalski, J., Prionas, S. D., and Allison, A. C. (1992). Dual role of tumour necrosis factor-alpha in angiogenesis. *Am. J. Pathol.*, **140**, 539–44.

88. Naylor, M. S., Stamp, G. W., Foulkes, W. D., Eccles, D. Balkwill, F. R. (1993). Tumor necrosis factor and its receptors in human ovarian cancer. Potential role in disease progression. *J. Clin. Invest.*, **91**, 2194–206.

89. Moghaddam, A., Zhang, H. T., Fan, T. P., Hu, D. E., Lees, V. C., Turley, H., *et al.* (1995). Thymidine phosphorylase is angiogenic and promotes tumor growth. *Proc. Natl Acad. Sci. USA*, **92**, 998–1002.

90. Christofori, G. and Hanahan, D. (1994). Molecular dissection of multi-stage tumorigenesis in transgenic mice. *Semin. Cancer Biol.*, **5**, 3–12.

91. Finnis, C., Dodsworth, N., Pollitt, C. E., Carr, G., and Sleep, D. (1993). Thymidine phosphorylase activity of platelet-derived endothelial cell growth factor is responsible for endothelial cell mitogenicity. *Eur. J. Biochem.*, **212**, 201–10.

92. Haraguchi, M., Miyadera, K., Uemura, K., Sumizawa, T., Furukawa, T., Yamada, K., *et al.* (1994). Angiogenic activity of enzymes (letter). *Nature*, **368**, 198.

93. Klagsbrun, M. (1991). Angiogenic factors: regulators of blood supply-side biology. FGF, endothelial cell growth factors and angiogenesis: a keystone symposium, Keystone, CO, USA, April 1–7, 1991. *New Biol.*, **3**, 745–9.

94. Nakao, H. J., Ito, H., Kanayasu, T., Morita, I., and Murota, S. (1992). Stimulatory effects of insulin and insulin-like growth factor I on migration and tube formation by vascular endothelial cells. *Atherosclerosis*, **92**, 141–9.

95. Filkins, J. P. (1980). Endotoxin-enhanced secretion of macrophage insulin-like activity. *J. Reticuloendothel. Soc.*, **27**, 507–11.

96. Rom, W. N., Basset, P., Fells, G. A., Nukiwa, T., Trapnell, B. C., and Crysal, R. G. (1988). Alveolar macrophages release an insulin-like growth factor I-type molecule. *J. Clin. Invest.*, **82**, 1685–93.

97. Singer, C., Rasmussen, A., Smith, H. S., Lippman, M. E., Lynch, H. T., and Cullen, K. J. (1995). Malignant breast epithelium selects for insulin-like growth factor II expression in breast stroma: evidence for paracrine function. *Cancer Res.*, **55**, 2448–54.

98. Yoshimura, T., Matsushima, K., Tanaka, S., Robinson, E. A., Appella, E., Oppenheim, J. J., *et al.* (1987). Purification of a human monocyte-derived neutrophil chemotactic factor that has peptide sequence similarity to other host defense cytokines. *Proc. Natl Acad. Sci. USA*, **84**, 9233–7.

99. Koch, A. E., Polverini, P. J., Kunkel, S. L., Harlow, L. A., DiPietro, L. A., Elner, V. M., *et al.* (1992). Interleukin-8 as a macrophage-derived mediator of angiogenesis. *Science*, **258**, 1798–801.

100. Strieter, R. M., Kunkel, S. L., Elner, V. M., Martonyi, C. L., Koch, A. E., Polverini, P. J., *et al.* (1992). Interleukin-8. A corneal factor that induces neovascularization. *Am. J. Pathol.*, **141**, 1279–84.

101. Hu, D. E., Hori, Y., and Fan, T. P. (1993). Interleukin-8 stimulates angiogenesis in rats. *Inflammation*, **17**, 135–43.

102. West, D. C. and Kumar, S. (1989). The effect of hyaluronate and its oligosaccharides on endothelial cell proliferation and monolayer integrity. *Exp. Cell Res.*, **183**, 179–96.

103. West, D. C., Hampson, I. N., Arnold, F., and Kumar, S. (1985). Angiogenesis induced by degradation products of hyaluronic acid. *Science*, **228**, 1324–6.

104. Thompson, W. D., Campbell, R., and Evans, T. (1985). Fibrin degradation and angiogenesis: quantitative analysis of the angiogenic response in the chick chorioallantoic membrane. *J. Pathol.*, **145**, 27–37.

105. Thompson, W. D., Smith, E. B., Stirk, C. M., Marshall, F. I., Stout, A. J., and Kocchar, A. (1992). Angiogenic activity of fibrin degradation products is located in fibrin fragment E. *J. Pathol.*, **168**, 47–53.

106. Nathan, C. F. (1987). Secretory products of macrophages. *J. Clin. Invest.*, **79**, 319–26.

107. Adams, D. O. and Hamilton, T. A. (1992). Macrophages as destructive cells in host defense. In *Inflammation: basic principles and clinical correlates* (ed. J. I. Gallin, I. M.

Goldstein, and R. Snyderman pp. 325–40. Raven Press, New York.

108. Klimetzek, V. and Sorg, C. (1977). Lymphokine-induced secretion of plasminogen activator by murine macrophages. *Eur. J. Immunol.*, **7**, 185–7.

109. Pyke, C., Ralfkiaer, E., Tryggvason, K., and Dano, K. (1993). Messenger RNA for two type IV collagenases is located in stromal cells in human colon cancer. *Am. J. Pathol.*, **142**, 359–65.

110. Pyke, C., Graem, N., Ralfkiaer, E., Ronne, E., Hoyer-Hansen, G., *et al.* (1993). Receptor for urokinase is present in tumor-associated macrophages in ductal breast carcinoma. *Cancer Res.*, **53**, 1911–5.

111. Falcone, D. J., McCaffrey, T. A., Haimovitz, F. A., Vergilio, J. A., and Nicholson, A. C. (1993). Macrophage and foam cell release of matrix-bound growth factors. Role of plasminogen activation. *J. Biol. Chem.*, **268**, 11951–8.

112. Falcone, D. J., McCaffrey, T. A., Haimovitz, F. A., and Garcia, M. (1993). Transforming growth factor-beta 1 stimulates macrophage urokinase expression and release of matrix-bound basic fibroblast growth factor. *J. Cell Physiol.*, **155**, 595–605.

113. Briozzo, P., Badet, J., Capony, F., Pieri, I., Montcourrier, P., Barritault, D., *et al.* (1991). MCF7 mammary cancer cells respond to bFGF and internalize it following its release from extracellular matrix: a permissive role of cathepsin D. *Exp. Cell Res.*, **194**, 252–9.

114. Joensuu, H., Toikkanen, S., and Isola, J. (1995). Stromal cell cathepsin, D. expression and long-term survival in breast cancer. *Br. J. Cancer*, **71**, 155–9.

115. Wohlwend, A., Belin, D., and Vassalli, J. D. (1987). Plasminogen activator-specific inhibitors produced by human monocytes/macrophages. *J. Exp. Med.*, **165**, 320–39.

116. van, H. V., Kooistra, T., Emeis, J. J., and Koolwijk, P. (1991). Regulation of plasminogen activator production by endothelial cells: role in fibrinolysis and local proteolysis. *Int. J. Radiat. Biol.*, **60**, 261–72.

117. Flaumenhaft, R., Abe, M., Mignatti, P., and Rifkin, D. B., (1992). Basic fibroblast growth factor-induced activation of latent transforming growth factor beta in endothelial cells: regulation of plasminogen activator activity. *J. Cell. Biol.*, **118**, 901–9.

118. Pepper, M. S., Montesano, R., Orci, L., and Vassalli, J. D. (1991). Plasminogen activator inhibitor-1 is induced in microvascular endothelial cells by a chondrocyte-derived transforming growth factor-beta. *Biochem. Biophys. Res. Commun.*, **176**, 633–8.

119. Pepper, M. S., Belin, D., Montesano, R., Orci, L., and Vassalli, J. D. (1990). Transforming growth factor-beta 1 modulates basic fibroblast growth factor-induced proteolytic and angiogenic properties of endothelial cells *in vitro*. *J. Cell Biol.*, **111**, 743–55.

120. Klagsbrun, M. (1989). The fibroblast growth factor family: structural and biological properties. *Prog. Growth Factor Res.*, **1**, 207–35.

121. Houck, K. A., Leung, D. W., Rowland, A. M., Winer, J., and Ferrara, N. (1992). Dual regulation of vascular endothelial growth factor bioavailability by genetic and proteolytic mechanisms. *J. Biol. Chem.*, **267**, 26031–7.

122. Pepper, M. S., Ferrara, N., Orci, L., and Montesano, R. (1991). Vascular endothelial growth factor (VEGF) induces plasminogen activators and plasminogen activator inhibitor-

1 in microvascular endothelial cells. *Biochem. Biophys. Res. Commun.*, **181**, 902–6.

123. Pepper, M. S., Ferrara, N., Orci, L., and Montesano, R., (1992). Potent synergism between vascular endothelial growth factor and basic fibroblast growth factor in the induction of angiogenesis *in vitro*. *Biochem. Biophys. Res. Commun.*, **189**, 824–31.

124. Goldman, C. K., Kim, J., Wong, W. L., King, V., Brock, T., and Gillespie, G. Y. (1993). Epidermal growth factor stimulates vascular endothelial growth factor production by human malignant glioma cells: a model of glioblastoma multiforme pathophysiology. *Mol. Biol. Cell.*, **4**, 121–33.

125. Sato, Y., Okamura, K., Morimoto, A., Hamanaka, R., Hamaguchi, K., Shimada, T., *et al.* (1993). Indispensable role of tissue-type plasminogen activator in growth factor-dependent tube formation of human microvascular endothelial cells *in vitro*. *Exp. Cell Res.*, **204**, 223–9.

126. Blood, C. H. and Zetter, B. R. (1990). Tumor interactions with the vasculature: angiogenesis and tumor metastasis. *Biochim. Biophys. Acta*, **1032**, 89–118.

127. Hayakawa, M., Oku, N., Takagi, T., Hori, T., Shibamoto, S., Yamanaka, Y., *et al.* (1991). Involvement of prostaglandin- producing pathway in the cytotoxic action of tumor necrosis factor. *Cell Struct. Funct.*, **16**, 333–40.

128. Fieren, M. W., van den Bemd, G., Ben, E. S., and Bonta, I. L. (1992). Prostaglandin E2 inhibits the release of tumor necrosis factor-alpha, rather than interleukin 1 beta, from human macrophages. *Immunol. Lett.*, **31**, 85–90.

129. Niedbala, M. J. and Stein, M. (1991). Tumor necrosis factor induction of urokinase-type plasminogen activator in human endothelial cells. *Biomed. Biochim. Acta*, **50**, 427–36.

130. Mizoi, T., Ohtani, H., Miyazono, K., Miyazawa, M., Matsuno, S., and Nagura, H. (1993). Immunoelectron microscopic localization of transforming growth factor beta 1 and latent transforming growth factor beta 1 binding protein in human gastrointestinal carcinomas: qualitative difference between cancer cells and stromal cells. *Cancer Res.*, **53**, 183–90.

131. Dalal, B. I., Keown, P. A., and Greenberg, A. H. (1993). Immunocytochemical localization of secreted transforming growth factor-beta 1 to the advancing edges of primary tumors and to lymph node metastases of human mammary carcinoma. *Am. J. Pathol.*, **143**, 381–9.

132. Tsutsui, J., Kadomatsu, K., Matsubara, S., Nakagawara, A., Hamanone, M., Takao, S., *et al.* (1993). A new family of heparin-binding growth/differentiation factors: increased midkine expression in Wilms' tumor and other human carcinomas. *Cancer Res.*, **53**, 1281–5.

133. Pepper, M. S., Vassalli, J. D., Orci, L., and Montesano, R. (1993). Biphasic effect of transforming growth factor-beta 1 on *in vitro* angiogenesis. *Exp. Cell Res.*, **204**, 356–63.

134. Van Netten, J., Ashmead B. J., Parker, R. L., Thornton, I. G., Fletcher, C., Cavers, D., *et al.* (1993). Macrophage-tumor cell associations: a factor in metastasis of breast cancer? *J. Leukoc. Biol.*, **54**, 360–2.

135. Weir, D. M., Grahame, L. M., and Ogmundsdottir, H. M. (1979). Binding of mouse peritoneal macrophages to tumour cells by a 'lectin-like' macrophage receptor. *J. Clin. Lab. Immunol.*, **2**, 51–4.

136. Crocker, P. R., Mucklow, S., Bouckson, V., McWilliam, A., Willis, A. C., Gorden, S., *et al.* (1994). Sialoadhesin, a

macrophage sialic acid binding receptor for haemopoietic cells with 17 immunoglobulin-like domains. *EMBO J.*, **13**, 4490–503.

137. Kim, K. J., Li B. Winer, J., Armanini, M., Gillett, N., Phillips, H. S., *et al.* (1993). Inhibition of vascular endothelial growth factor-induced angiogenesis suppresses tumour growth *in vivo*. *Nature*, **362**, 841–4.

138. Pighetti, G. M. and Sordillo, L. M. (1994). Regulation of mammary gland macrophage tumour necrosis factor-alpha production with interferon-gamma. *Res. Vet. Sci.*, **56**, 252–5.

139. Zhu, X., Ertel, W., Ayala, A., Morrison, M. H., Perrin, M. M., and Chaudry, I. H. (1993). Chloroquine inhibits macrophage tumour necrosis factor-alpha mRNA transcription. *Immunology*, **80**, 122–6.

140. Koch, A. E., Burrows, J. C., Polverini, P. J., Cho, M., and Leibovich, S. J. (1991). Thiol-containing compounds inhibit the production of monocyte/macrophage-derived angiogenic activity. *Agents Actions*, **34**, 350–7.

141. Koch, A. E., Cho, M., Burrows, J. C., Polverini, P. J., and Leibovich, S. J. (1992). Inhibition of production of monocyte/macrophage-derived angiogenic activity by oxygen free-radical scavengers. *Cell Biol. Int. Rep.*, **16**, 415–25.

142. Borgstrom, P., Torres, F. I., Vajkoczy, P., Strandgarden, K., Polacek, J., and Hartley, A. B. (1994). The quinoline-3-carboxamide linomide inhibits angiogenesis *in vivo*. *Cancer Chemother. Pharmacol.*, **34**, 280–6.

143. Vukanovic, J., Passaniti, A., Hirata, T., Traystman, R. J., Hartley, A. B., and Isaacs, J. T. (1993). Antiangiogenic effects of the quinoline-3-carboxamide linomide. *Cancer Res.*, **53**, 1833–7.

144. Vukanovic, J. and Isaacs, J. T. (1995). Linomide inhibits angiogenesis, growth, metastasis, and macrophage infiltration within rat prostatic cancers. *Cancer Res.*, **55**, 1499–504.

9. Oncogenes and tumour suppressor genes in the regulation of angiogenesis

Farzan Rastinejad and Noël Bouck

Introduction

The cells that comprise a successful solid tumour have developed two distinct new capabilities that are not possessed by the normal cells from which they arose. They proliferate without internal constraints and they create an environment *in vivo* where their growth potential can be realized. The ability to induce angiogenesis is a major component of this permissive *in vivo* environment. Without neovascularization, even cells that are perfectly capable of growing without constraint cannot form tumours of a clinically relevant size (1–3).

Although all tumours are angiogenic and able to induce the formation of new vasculature, the normal cells from which these tumours arise are commonly antiangiogenic. They frequently secrete low levels of inducers that are masked by high levels of inhibitors of angiogenesis. As these normal cells progress to malignancy they become potently angiogenic. Evidence now accumulating suggests that cells in a developing tumour acquire their hyper-angiogenic phenotype in the same way that they acquire the ability to grow without restraint, namely as a result of the sequential activation of oncogenes and inactivation of tumour suppressor genes (4). For, in addition to the well documented effects of these oncogenes and tumour suppressor genes on cell growth, many of them also control the production of a variety of secreted molecules that regulate angiogenesis.

Progressive development of the angiogenic phenotype

The normal cells from which tumours arise are not angiogenic. When conditioned media are collected from normal human or mouse keratinocytes (4,5,6), or human fibroblast (7), glial (8,9) or retinal (10) cells, they do not induce angiogenesis in either *in vitro* or *in vivo* assays. In fact such media are usually inhibitory and able to block the stimulation of endothelial cell migration and corneal angiogenesis induced by known angiogenic agents. In contrast, media conditioned by tumour cells always give a potently positive angiogenic response.

When cultured cells progressing towards malignancy are examined, they become angiogenic in what seems at first to be a single discrete step both *in vitro* (7,11) and *in vivo* (6,12,13). But when the development of the angiogenic phenotype was examined quantitatively in one system it was found to develop in a series of steps involving both a decrease in the secretion of inhibitors and increases in the production of several inducers (14). Media were collected from normal human fibroblasts and from fibroblasts cultured from Li-Fraumeni patients and their derivatives which had spontaneously immortalized and subsequently become tumorigenic as a result of transfection with oncogenic H-*ras* (15). The overall angiogenic and anti-angiogenic activity secreted by these cells at the various times during their progression to malignancy was quantitated by determining the amount of total secreted protein required to induce or inhibit the migration of capillary endothelial cells by 50%. Where necessary, inducers were measured in the presence of antibodies that blocked the activity of inhibitors. The results, illustrated in Fig. 9.1, showed that inhibitory activity fell precipitously upon immortalization (7) and that inducing activity increased in a step-wise fashion both when cells immortalized (16) and when they were transfected with oncogenic *ras* (14). These data suggest that angiogenic activity may be acquired incrementally in steps that coincide with oncogene activation and tumour suppressor gene loss.

Oncogenes can be positive regulators of angiogenesis

A number of oncogenes and proto-oncogenes play a key role in the multistep induction of tumour angiogenesis.

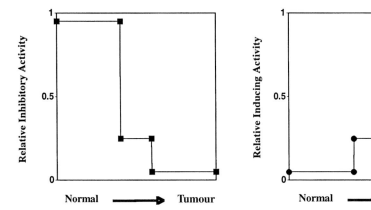

Figure 9.1. Changes in the total amount of angiogenic inducing and inhibitory activity elaborated by human fibroblasts during their progression to tumorigenicity *in vitro*. Normal fibroblasts are anti-angiogenic, secreting low amounts of inducing activity and high amounts of inhibitory activity. As they become immortal and lose p53, inhibitory activity falls and inducing activity increases slightly. Upon subsequent transfection with activated ras, inducing activity increases further and remains high in clones that also become tumorigenic (7,14,16).

The rapid rate of angiogenesis observed during early development is coincident with the time when many proto-oncogenes are activated in expanding tissues. Like developmental angiogenesis, tumour angiogenesis requires that endothelial cells receive angiogenic signals from their environment. Oncogenes enable tumours to provide these signals by enhancing the secretion of angiogenic factors, by limiting the production of inhibitors, and by stimulating the degradation of the extracellular matrix. These stimuli activate proto-oncogenes within endothelial cells as they respond to form new blood vessels. The involvement of oncogenes and cellular proto-oncogenes in mediating angiogenesis is depicted in Fig. 9.2.

Proto-oncogenes and oncogenes in endothelial cells

Both tumour angiogenesis and developmental angiogenesis are dependent on the responsiveness of endothelial cells to environmental stimuli. Endothelial cells can detect exogenous stimuli through proto-oncogenes that function as signal transducing receptor kinases. The timing of expression of vascular endothelial cell growth factor (VEGF) receptors FLK-1/KDR and FLT-1, and other tyrosine kinase receptors, Tek, Tie, and flt-related protein, in the developing embryonic vascular endothelium suggest that these kinases may play an important part in proliferation and differentiation of endothelial cells (17,18). Gene knockout studies in mice also support the essential role of some of these receptors in vessel formation (19–21). Tie expression is minimal in the mature vasculature, however,

expression levels are elevated in the growing blood vessels associated with metastatic melanoma (22). Recent results demonstrate that Tek is required for recruitment of smooth muscle cells and pericytes into the growing vessel walls. Absence of Tek ligand, angiopoietin, or mutation of the receptor lead to abnormal vessel formation (23–25).

Receptors for the endothelial cell-specific mitogen VEGF are induced to high levels in endothelial cells within and near growing glioma tumours, but are much less abundant in the normal vasculature (26–30). FLK-1 kinase activity can also be induced by secreted HIV Tat protein (31). Suppression of the VEGF effect on endothelial cells by neutralizing antibodies or by expression of a dominant negative receptor suppresses tumour-induced angiogenesis as does lavendustin A, a tyrosine kinase inhibitor (32–34).

Other members of the kinase family of oncogenes can contribute to angiogenesis by activating endothelial cells. The Fps oncogene is a cytoplasmic kinase that can be constitutively activated by mutations that localize it to the cell membrane. Such localization is sufficient to stimulate blood vessel growth as mutant Fps induces widespread hypervascularization leading to multifocal haemangiomas in transgenic animals (35). Certain mutations in the erb B oncogene which encodes the receptor for endothelial growth factor EGF cause angiosarcomas (36). The mos proto-oncogene is a serine/threonine kinase that has been implicated in maturation of germ cells (37). If expressed ectopically, mos can immortalize endothelial cells *in vitro* (38). *In vivo*, mos promotes Kaposi sarcoma-like lesions which contain replicating endothelial cells (39).

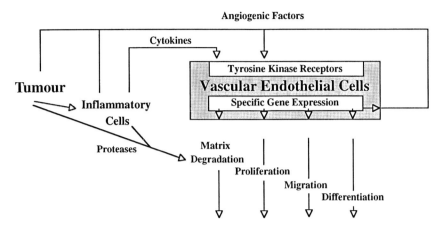

Figure 9.2. Specific steps in the process of tumour angiogenesis which are regulated proto-oncogenes and oncogenes. Angiogenic factors belonging to the growth factor class of oncogenes can simultaneously support tumour cell growth and sustain angiogenesis. In some instances, tumour cells stimulate vascular endothelial cells indirectly through recruitment of inflammatory cells that release angiogenic cytokines and growth factors. In addition, oncogenes promote protease production by tumour cells which facilitates vessel growth by supplementing the matrix-degrading function of activated endothelial cells. Upon activation, endothelial cells express proto-oncogenes of the transcription factor class which in turn activate the expression of both growth factor and growth factor receptor classes of cellular proto-oncogenes. Together, this network of proto-oncogenes provides endothelial cells the means to receive and respond to angiogenic stimuli.

The *ras* oncogene, a guanosine triphosphate (GTP)-binding protein with a well-established role in signal transduction, appears to play an important part in endothelial cell activation. *Ras* function appears to be necessary for endothelial cell motility. Introduction of activated Ha-*ras* promotes random movement of endothelial cells (40). Inactivation of normal *ras* function by injection of neutralizing antibodies or introduction of dominant-negative *ras* into normal endothelial cells can suppress directed cell migration (40,41). Time-course studies suggest that *ras* is not only required to initiate signalling for cell migration, but also essential for persistence of the migratory phenotype. The prominant role of *ras* in endothelial cell activation is further demonstrated by its ability to immortalize cultured endothelial cells (38). These *in vitro* data are supplemented by organ culture of reconstituted prostate where expression of activated *ras* significantly increases the number of new blood vessels and by the ability of mutant H-*ras* to cause frequent haemangiomas when introduced into the mouse skin (42–44).

In activated endothelial cells, the oncogenic transcription factors c-ets-1 and c-*rel*/NF-κB function to induce specific gene expression (45). In these endothelial cells c-ets-1 regulates the expression of a number of genes involved in matrix degradation including collagenase, stromelysin, and urokinase-type plasminogen activator (46,47).

Transcriptional activation of these target genes suggests that c-ets-1 promotes endothelial cell invasion of the stroma surrounding tumours. The c-*rel* family of transcription factors appears to influence the expression of adhesion proteins such as E-selection that allow endothelial cells to migrate toward angiogenic stimuli (48). IκB-α is an inhibitor of the NF-κB/c-*rel* transcription factors that is expressed in endothelial cells and is degraded upon their activation (49). This degradation involves phosphorylation which may be mediated by one or more of the endothelial cell kinases.

While endothelial cells are primed to utilize proto oncogenes of receptor, signal transducer, and transcription factor classes to respond to angiogenic signals, they require signals in the form of angiogenic growth factors to initiate their angiogenic programme. Constitutive activation of this programme by introduction of dominant oncogenes such as the polyoma middle T antigen into endothelial cells can lead to tumours of endothelial cell origin known as haemangiomas (50). Haemangiomas represent an interesting situation where endothelial cells constitutively produce and secrete high levels of proteases and other proteins that support endothelial cell growth (51,52). The release of these factors by implanted transformed endothelial cells can be sufficient to recruit normal host endothelial cells into developing haemangiomas (53).

Oncogenes expressed in tumour cells

Oncogenes expressed by a variety of tumour types can stimulate the proliferation and migration of surrounding normal endothelial cells. Oncogenes may encode angiogenic factors or act indirectly to stimulate the production of angiogenic factors from tumour cells. There are also occasional examples of cells in which oncogene expression is pro-angiogenic because it decreases the elaboration of angiogenesis inhibitors. Inhibitory thrombospondin can be down-regulated by v-*myc* (54), c-*jun* (55), and PDGF (56). TIMP expression is negatively regulated by the *ras* oncogene (57). The expression of oncogenic *ras* in tumour cells can further induce angiogenesis by stimulating the expression of the angiogenic factor insulin-like growth factor (IGF) (42,43) and VEGF (60,61), and by enhancing the hypoxia-mediated VEGF production from tumours (62). Similarly, erb-A stimulates platelet-derived growth factor (PDGF) expression in glioma cells which can contribute to their angiogenic phenotype (63).

Elevated expression of a number of secreted proto-oncogene growth factors can initiate and sustain angiogenesis. PDGF, granulocyte colony-stimulating factor (G-CSF), EGF, and transforming growth factor (TGF) α have been shown to induce angiogenesis (64–66). Transfection of VEGF into Chinese hamster ovary (CHO) or HeLa cells provides a tumorigenic growth advantage which is associated with enhanced vascularization of tumours growing in nude mice (67,68). VEGF is produced by a large variety of tumours. Hypoxia, a condition encountered by growing tumour stimulates VEGF production via the activation of the *src* oncogene (69–72). Tumours that do not express VEGF may still utilize this growth factor to induce angiogenesis through the recruitment of inflammatory cells. Inflammatory cells secrete tumour necrosis factor (TNF)-α, a cytokine which has been shown to induce VEGF production by normal cells (73).

VEGF appears to be one of the most commonly expressed tumour angiogenic factors that acts both as a mitogen and an attractant for endothelial cells. The *fos* protooncogene stimulates the angiogenic process in papillomas by stimulating VEGF production (74). The v-*src* oncogene promotes VEGF production in a variety of tumour types (75). The inactivation of even a single VEGF allele in transgenic mice is embryonically lethal, and the abnormalities observed in the embryos are consistent with a critical role for VEGF in developmental vascularization (76).

The role of scatter factor (SF) in tumour angiogenesis is also well documented. Although SF is expressed in both normal and tumour tissues, its production is elevated in a number of tumours including prostate and Kaposi sarcoma

(77,78). SF is a potent angiogenic factor *in vivo* and stimulates endothelial cell protease production, motility, proliferation, and differentiation *in vitro* (79,80). SF activity is mediated through the proto-oncogene receptor tyrosine kinase, c-*met*. *Met* kinase activity is sufficient to stimulate angiogenesis in endothelial cells as a chimeric protein composed of the nerve growth factor (NGF) ligand binding domain and the *met* kinase domain allows the stimulation of endothelial cells with NGF (81). c-*met* expression is not restricted to endothelial cells, consistent with the observation that SF can induce the differentiation-associated, lumen-forming phenotype in liver, kidney, and breast as well as in newly forming blood vessels (82,83).

The basic fibroblast growth factor (bFGF) family of angiogenic factors and their receptors are also widely expressed throughout different tissues while playing a significant part in tumour-induced angiogenesis. The bFGF family includes the oncogenes int-2 (FGF-3), hst, and FGF-5 which are often expressed at high levels in tumour cells. All three contain signal peptides that facilitate their export from producing cells (84). A non-secreted form of bFGF can act as an oncogene upon addition of a signal peptide suggesting that the oncogenic activity is dependent on efficient secretion of the product (85). Int-2 expression is strongly linked to vascularization in human tumours. It is overexpressed in over 50% of Kaposi sarcomas, and when introduced into immortalized breast epithelial cells it enhances angiogenesis (86,87).

Proteases stimulated by oncogenes in tumour cells contribute to the establishment and maintenance of the angiogenic phenotype. Activated endothelial cells mediate the proteolytic degradation of matrix proteins, an essential step in the budding of new blood vessels into tumours and the existing connective tissues (88,89). Tumour cells driven by oncogenes secrete enzymes that supplement this activity. Two of the most potent oncogenes, *ras* and *src*, each induce the release of metalloproteinases and activators of latent proteases (90–93). The release of proteolytic enzymes together with angiogenic factors are the means by which oncogenes drive tumours to overcome the checks and balances on neovascularization which limit this normally transient process.

Several tumour suppressor genes are negative regulators of angiogenesis

When tumour suppressor genes exert an influence on angiogenesis they seem to do so most often by stimulating the cells in which they are expressed to secrete high levels

Table 9.1. Human tumour suppressor genes that influence angiogenesis

Cell origin	Added tumour suppressor gene or chromosome	Effect	Reference
Immortal fibroblast	P53	↑ TSP-1	7, 16
Neuroblastoma	Chromosome 17	↑ Inhibitory activity*	†
Glioblastoma	p53	↑ Inhibitory activity*	97
		↓ VEGF	14, 75
	Chromosome 10	↑ TSP-1	6
Retinoblastoma	Retinoblastoma	↑ Inhibitory activity*	101
Osteosarcoma	Retinoblastoma	↑ Inhibitory activity*	101
Renal cell carcinoma	von Hippelo–Lindau	↓ VEGF	102–104

* Angioinhibitory activity not due to TSP-1 (thrombospondin 1).
† Tolsma *et al.* unpublished data.

of inhibitors of angiogenesis (Table 9.1 and Fig. 9.3). This has been demonstrated both by inactivating tumour suppressor genes in premalignant cells and by reintroducing them into malignant tumour cell lines.

A variety of cells expressing tumour suppressor genes switch their phenotype from anti-angiogenic to angiogenic when a tumour suppressor gene is inactivated. This was first seen using a fibroblastic line of baby hamster kidney cells that has progressed towards tumorigenicity to the point that only loss of a single additional tumour suppressor gene allele is required to make it tumorigenic (94). The inactivation of this genetically defined tumour sup-

pressor gene by any one of a variety of means caused the phenotype of the cells to switch from anti-angiogenic to angiogenic (11). This switch was the result of decreased synthesis and secretion of an inhibitor of angiogenesis, thrombospondin 1 (11,95).

A similar phenomenon has been observed in a unique *in vivo/in vitro* model of tumour progression in hamster epithelial cells. Moroco *et al.* (6) treated the buccal pouch of Syrian hamsters with carcinogen and then cultured transformed keratinocytes from the treated tissue at various stages during the progression towards tumorigenicity. The longer the time that elapsed between carcinogen treatment and the time the keratinocytes were put into culture, the more *in vitro* characteristics of transformation they exhibited. The cultured keratinocytes became angiogenic midway in this progression and this phenotype was shown by cell fusions to be under the control of a tumour suppressor gene (6) and to be accompanied by the loss of angioinhibitory activity (96). Neither the inhibitor nor the suppressor gene have yet been identified in this system.

Suppressor control of angiogenesis via regulation of an inhibitor has also been demonstrated in human cells. Loss of wild-type p53 tumour suppressor gene causes a decrease in the secretion of the inhibitor thrombospondin by human fibroblasts and, as a result, the cells switch from an anti-angiogenic to an angiogenic phenotype (7,16). These data describe a new function for the wild-type p53 tumour suppressor gene, one that is apparently fully active when the p53 protein is expressed at normal ambient levels in the cell and does not depend on overexpression of the tumour suppressor protein. The *in vitro* data on the relevance of the loss of the p53 tumour suppressor gene to tumour angiogenesis in fibrosarcomas is supported by a transgenic mouse model. In developing fibrosarcomas initiated by bovine papilloma virus, the inactivation of the p53 gene has been observed to coincide with the acquisition of an angiogenic phenotype *in vivo* (13).

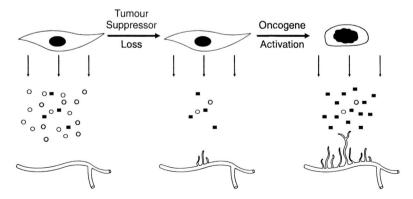

Figure 9.3. Generalized role of oncogenes and tumour suppressor genes in the development of the angiogenic phenotype during tumour progression.

A second way to demonstrate control of the angiogenic phenotype by a tumour suppressor gene is to return a suppressor gene to an angiogenic tumour cell line. This strategy has resulted in expression of angio-inhibitory activity in a number of instances. Elevated expression of wild-type p53 in a human glioblastoma tumour line results in the production of an inhibitor of angiogenesis (97). Although not yet identified, this inhibitor is not thrombospondin. Reversion to a non-transformed and anti-angiogenic phenotype was observed upon infection of a breast carcinoma line with a retrovirus encoding wild-type p53. These cells became anti-angiogenic due to the secretion of the inhibitor thrombospondin (98). The return of the retinoblastoma tumour suppressor gene to retinoblastoma or osteosarcoma cells simultaneously reduced tumorigenicity (99,100) and caused the cells to become anti-angiogenic (101).

A number of human tumour lines can lose their tumorigenic potential as a result of the introduction of a normal human chromosome bearing one or more tumour suppressor genes. Several of such revertants simultaneously return to an anti-angiogenic phenotype and begin to secrete angio-inhibitory activity. This has been shown in neuroblastomas reverted by chromosome 17 (Tolsma, Bader, Stanbridge, Polverini, and Bouck, unpublished data) and in several human glioblastoma lines reverted by chromosome 10 (8).

Suppressor control of inhibitors of angiogenesis seems to be cell context dependent. The same suppressor gene can have different effects in different cell lineages. Whereas p53 induces thrombospondin in fibroblasts (7) it induces a different inhibitor in glioblastoma (97). In other contexts p53 may be irrelevant to angiogenesis. In a transgenic mouse model, the inactivation of p53 by Simian Virus 40 large T antigen in the beta cells of the pancreas does not seem to be sufficient to cause these cells to become angiogenic (12). The return of the retinoblastoma tumour suppressor gene to osteosarcoma and retinoblastoma cells that have lost it seems to induce angio-inhibitory activity, along with suppression of tumorigenicity. This same gene does not induce an inhibitory activity when introduced into a human prostate line, although tumorigenicity is inhibited (105). Tumour suppressor control of angiogenesis can at times resemble a tangled web. A single suppressor gene can stimulate different inhibitors of angiogenesis, as described above for p53, and a single inhibitor of angiogenesis can be stimulated by different tumour suppressor genes. Thrombospondin can be induced by p53 in fibroblasts, but its secretion from glioblastoma cells is stimulated not by p53, but by an unidentified gene on chromosome 10q (8).

Although a variety of different inhibitors seem to be under the control of various tumour suppressor genes, only one of them has been identified so far. Thrombospondin is induced by an unidentified tumour suppressor gene in hamster fibroblasts (11,95), by the p53 tumour suppressor gene in human fibroblasts (7,16) and human breast carcinoma cells (98) and by a suppressor gene on chromosome 10 in human glioblastomas (8). Regulation seems to be at the level of transcription in the fibroblasts, but primarily post-transcriptional in the glial cells (Hsu and Bouck, unpublished data). Thrombospondin is an effective inhibitor of corneal and inflammatory neovascularization in vivo (106). It can also depress in vivo tumorigenicity when it is overexpressed in human breast carcinoma cells (107) or in transformed mouse endothelial cells (108).

Tumour suppressor genes returned to tumour cells can also influence angiogenesis by blocking the production of inducers, although it is not clear how meaningful such changes are in the context of overall angiogenic phenotype of the cells. Wild-type p53 returned to immortal fibroblasts (14) decreases VEGF mRNA and protein by about 3-fold, and increases inhibitory thrombospondin. At least in vitro, it is the reduction in the inhibitor that is most critical to the angiogenic phenotype of the cells. Wild-type p53 can also depress the VEGF promoter transiently in a variety of tumour cells (72). Re expression of the von Hippel-Lindau tumour suppressor gene in a human renal cell carcinoma line suppressed VEGF production (102), restoring its hypoxia inducibility (103). Finally transgenic mouse models suggest the possibility that loss of the APC tumour suppressor gene may mediate the increased expression of prostaglandin H synthase-2 during progression of polyps to adenomas in the colon (109,110). As prostaglandins can be potent angiogenic agents, the APC tumour suppressor gene may be at least in part responsible for development of angiogenic phenotype in colon cancer.

Inhibitors of angiogenesis released by cells carrying tumour suppressor genes seem to form a significant impediment to the development of tumour angiogenesis. They are produced at a level that is high enough to block the angiogenesis inducers from tumour cells. When media conditioned by hamster keratinocytes or fibroblasts producing suppressor-dependent inhibitors is mixed one to one with tumour conditioned media, the mixture suppresses angiogenesis (11; Lingen and Polverini, unpublished data). Inhibitory thrombospondin is produced by fibroblasts expressing p53 and by glioblastoma cells suppressed with chromosome 10 at a level that is sufficient to suppress angiogenesis induced by a variety of tumour lines (7,8,16). These data suggest that the loss of inhibitory activity mediated by loss of a tumour suppressor gene may often be essential in order for the developing tumour cells to become angiogenic.

Summary and conclusions

Oncogene activation and tumour suppressor gene loss are well known as events that are responsible for the dramatic cell–autonomous deregulation of growth that characterizes all malignant cells. Data accumulating more recently indicate that these same genes are also responsible for the development of a second essential characteristic of all malignant cells, the ability to induce the neovascularization on which their progressive growth *in vivo* depends. Oncogene activation and tumour suppressor gene loss often appear to make distinctly different contributions to the angiogenic phenotype of developing tumours (Fig. 9.3). Cells that lose a tumour suppressor gene become more angiogenic usually because they secrete decreased amounts of inhibitors of angiogenesis. Cells in which an oncogene is activated also become more angiogenic, but in this case it is usually because they increase their secretion of inducers of angiogenesis. Both inhibitor loss and inducer enhancement seem to be essential if a normal cell is to develop into a tumour cell able to grow and metastasize *in vivo*.

References

1. Gimbrone, M. A., Leapman, S. B., Cotran, R. S., and Folkman, J. (1972). Tumor dormancy *in vivo* by prevention of neovascularization. *J. Exp. Med.*, **136**, 261–76.
2. O'Reilly, M. S., Holmgren, L., Shing, Y., Chen, C., Rosenthal, R. A., Moses, M., *et al.* (1994). Angiostatin: a novel angiogenesis inhibitor that mediates the suppression of metastases by a Lewis lung carcinoma. *Cell*, **79**, 315–28.
3. Folkman, J. (1995). Tumor angiogenesis. In *The molecular basis of cancer* (ed. J. Mendelsohn, P. M. Howley, M. A. Israel, and L. A. Liotta), pp. 206–32. W. B. Saunders.
4. Bouck, N., Stellmach, V., and Hsu, S. (1996). How tumors become angiogenic. *Adv. in Cancer Res.*, **69**, 135–74.
5. Lingen, M., Polverini, P., and Bouck, N. (1996). Retinoic acid induces cells cultured from oral squamous cell carcinomas to become anti-angiogenic. *Am J. Pathology*, **149**, 247–58.
6. Moroco, J. R., Solt, D. B., and Polverini, P. J. (1990). Sequential loss of suppressor genes for three specific functions during *in vivo* carcinogenesis. *Lab. Invest.*, **63**, 298–306.
7. Dameron, K. M., Volpert, O. V., Tainsky, M. A., and Bouck, N. (1994). Control of angiogenesis in fibroblasts by p53 regulation of thrombospondin-1. *Science*, **265**, 1582–4.
8. Hsu, S. C., Volpert, O. V., Steck, P. A., Mikkelsen, T., Polverini, P. J., Cavenee, W. K., and Bouck, N. P. (1994). Chromosome 10 regulates the angiogenic phenotype in glioblastoma cells by modulating thrombospondin. *Proc. Am. Assoc. Cancer Res.*, **35**, 67.
9. Hsu, S., Volpert, O., Steck, P., Mikkelsen, T., Polverini, P., Rao, S., Chou, P., and Bouck, N. (1996). Inhibition of angiogenesis in human glioblastomas by chromosome 10 induction of thrombospondin-1. *Cancer Res.*, **56**, 5684–91.
10. Glaser, B. M., Campochiaro, P. A., Davis, J. L., and Sato, M. (1985). Retinal pigment epithelial cells release an inhibitor of neovascularization. *Arch. Ophthalmol.*, **103**, 1870–5.
11. Rastinejad, F., Polverini, P. J., and Bouck, N. P. (1989). Regulation of the activity of a new inhibitor of angiogenesis by a cancer suppressor gene. *Cell*, **56**, 345–55.
12. Folkman, J., Watson, K., Ingber, D., and Hanahan, D. (1989). Induction of angiogenesis during the transition from hyperplasia to neoplasia. *Nature*, **339**, 58–61.
13. Christofori, G. and Hanahan, D. (1994). Molecular dissection of multi-stage tumorigenesis in transgenic mice. *Cancer Biol.*, **5**, 3–12.
14. Volpert, O., Dameron, K., and Bouck, N. (1997). Sequential development of an angiogenic phenotype by human fibroblasts progressing to tumorigenicity. *Oncogene*, in press.
15. Bischoff, F. Z., Strong, L. C., Yim, S. O., Pratt, D. R., Siciliano, M. J., Giovanella, B. C. and Tainsky, M. A. (1991). Tumorigenic transformation of spontaneously immortalized fibroblasts from patients with familial cancer syndrome. *Oncogene*, **6**, 183–6.
16. Dameron, K. M., Volpert, O. V., Tainsky, M. A., and Bouck, N. (1994). The p53 tumor suppressor gene inhibits angiogenesis by stimulating the production of thrombospondin. *Cold Spring Harbor Symp. Quant. Biol.* **LIX** 483–9.
17. Kaipainen, A., Korhonen, J., Pajusola, K., Aprelikova, O., Persico, M., Terman, B., and Alitalo, K. The related FLT4, FLT1, and KDR receptor tyrosine kinases show distinct expression patterns in human fetal endothelial cells. *J. Exp. Med.*, **178**, 2077–88.
18. Yamaguchi, T., Dumont, D., Conlon, R., Breitman, M., and Rossant, J. (1993). flk-1, an flt-related receptor tyrosine kinase is an early marker for endothelial cell precursors. *Development*, **118**, 489–98.
19. Shalaby, F., Rossant, J., Yamaguchi, T., Gertsenstein, M., Wu, X., Breitman, M., and Schuh, A. (1995). Failure of blood-island formation and vasculogenesis in Flk-1-deficient mice. *Nature*, **376**, 62–6.
20. Fong, G., Rossant, J., Gertsenstein, M., and Breitman, M. (1995). Role of the Flt-1 receptor tyrosine kinase in regulating the assembly of vascular endothelium. *Nature*, **376**, 66–70.
21. Puri, M., Rossant, K., Bernstein, A., and Partanen, J. (1995). The receptor tyrosine kinase TIE is required for integrity and survival of vascular endothelial cells. *EMBO J.*, **14**, 5884–91.
22. Kaipainen, A., Vlaykova, T., Hatva, E., Bohling, T., Jekunen, A., Pyrhonen, S., and Alitalo, K. (1994). Enhanced expression of the tie receptor tyrosine kinase messenger RNA in the vascular endothelium of metastatic melanomas. *Cancer Res.*, **54**, 6571–7.
23. Davis, S., Aldrich, T., Jones, P., Acheson, A., Compton, D., Jain, V., Ryan, T., Bruno, J., Radziejewski, C., Maisonpierre, P., and Yancopoulos, G. (1996). Isolation of angiopoietin-1, a ligand for the TIE2 receptor, by serectiontrap expression cloning. *Cell*, **87**, 1161–9.
24. Suri, C., Jones, P., Patan, S., Bartunkova, S., Maisonpierre, P., Davis, S., Sato, T., and Yancopoulos, G. (1996). Requisite role of angiopoietin-1, a ligand for the TIE2 receptor, during embryonic angiogenesis. *Cell*, **87**, 1171–80.
25. Vikkula, M., Boon, L., Carraway, K., Calvert, J., Diamonti, A., Goumnerov, B., Pasyk, K., Marchuk, D., Warman, M.,

Cantley, L., Mulliken, J., and Olsen, B. (1996). Vascular dysmorphogenesis caused by an activating mutation in the receptor tyrosine kinase TIE2. *Cell*, **87**, 1181–90.

26. Plate, K., Breier, G., Millauer, B., Ullrich, A., and Risau, W. (1993). Up-regulation of vascular endothelial growth factor and its cognate receptors in a rat glioma model of tumor angiogenesis. *Cancer Res.*, **53**, 5822–7.
27. Plate, K., Breier, G., Weich, H., Mennel, H., and Risau, W. (1994). Vascular endothelial growth factor and glioma angiogenesis: coordinate induction of VEGF receptors, distribution of VEGF protein and possible *in vivo* regulatory mechanisms. *Int. J. Cancer*, **59**, 520–9.
28. Hatva, E., Kaipainen, A., Mentula, P., Jaaskelainen, J., Paetau, A., Haltia, M., and Alitalo, K. (1995). Expression of endothelial cell-specific receptor tyrosine kinases and growth factors in human brain tumors. *Am. J. Pathol.*, **146**, 368–78.
29. Barleon, B., Hauser, S., Schollmann, C., Weindel, K., Marme, D., Yayon, A., and Weich, H. (1994). Differential expression of the two VEGF receptors flt and KDR in placenta and vascular endothelial cells. *J. Cell. Biochem.*, **54**, 56–66.
30. Peters, K., De Vries, C., and Williams, L. (1993). Vascular endothelial growth factor receptor expression during embryogenesis and tissue repair suggests a role in endothelial differentiation and blood vessel growth. *Proc. Natl Acad. Sci. USA*, **90**, 8915–9.
31. Albini, A., Soldi, R., Giunciuglio, D., Giraudo, E., Benelli, R., Primo, L., Moonan, D., Salio, M., Caussi, G., Rockl, W., and Bussolino, F. (1996). The angiogenesis induced by HIV-1 tat protein is mediated by the FLK-1/KDR receptor in vascular endothelial cells. *Nature Medicine*, **2**, 1371–4.
32. Kim, K., Li, B., Winer, J., Armanini, M., Gillett, N., Phillips, H., and Ferrara, N. (1993). Inhibition of vascular endothelial growth factor-induced angiogenesis suppresses tumour growth *in vivo*. *Nature*, **362**, 841–4.
33. Millauer, B., Shawver, L., Plate, K., Risau, W., and Ullrich, A. (1994). Glioblastoma growth inhibited *in vivo* by a dominant-negative Flk-1 mutant. *Nature*, **367**, 576–9.
34. Hu, D. and Fan, T. (1995). Suppression of VEGF-induced angiogenesis by the protein tyrosine kinase inhibitor, lavendustin A. *Br. J. Pharmacol.*, **114**, 262–8.
35. Greer, P., Haigh, J., Mbamalu, G., Khoo, W., Bernstein, A., and Pawson, T. (1994). The Fps/Fes protein-tyrosine kinase promotes angiogenesis in transgenic mice. *Mol. Cell. Biol.*, **14**, 6755–63.
36. Robinson, H., Tracy, S., Nair, N., Taglienti-Sian, C., and Gamett, D. (1992). Characterization of an angiosarcoma-inducing mutation in the erbB oncogene. *Oncogene*, **7**, 2025–30.
37. Yew, N., Strobel, M., and Vande Woude, G. (1993). Mos and the cell cycle: the molecular basis of the transformed phenotype. *Curr. Opin. Genet. Dev.*, **3**, 19–25.
38. Faller, D., Kourembanas, S., Ginsberg, D., Hannan, R., Collins, T., Ewenstein, B., *et al.* (1988). Immortalization of human endothelial cells by murine sarcoma viruses, without morphologic transformation. *J. Cell. Physiol.*, **134**, 47–56.
39. Stoica, G. (1994). Sarcoma viruses containing the mos oncogene induce lesions resembling Kaposi's sarcoma. *In Vivo*, **8**, 43–7.
40. Fox, P., Sa, G., Dobrowolski, S., and Stacey, D. (1994). The regulation of endothelial cell motility by p21 ras. *Oncogene*, **9**, 3519–26.

41. Sosnowski, R., Feldman, S., and Feramisco, J. (1993). Interference with endogenous ras function inhibits cellular responses to wounding. *J. Cell Biol.*, **121**, 113–9.
42. Thompson, T., Southgate, J., Kitchener, G., and Land, H. (1989). Multistage carcinogenesis induced by ras and myc oncogenes in a reconstituted organ. *Cell*, **56**, 917–30.
43. Burns, P., Jack, A., Neilson, F., Haddow, S., and Balmain, A. (1991). Transformation of mouse skin endothelial cells *in vivo* by direct application of plasmid DNA encoding the human T24 H-ras oncogene. *Oncogene*, **6**, 1973–8.
44. Weinberg, W., Morgan, D., George, C., and Yuspa, S. (1991). A comparison of interfollicular and hair follicle derived cells as targets for the v-rasHa oncogene in mouse skin carcinogenesis. *Carcinogenesis*, **12**, 1119–24.
45. Iwasaka, C., Tanaka, K., Abe, M., and Sato, Y. (1996). Ets-1 regulates angiogenesis by inducing the expression of urokinase-type plasminogen activator and matrix metalloproteinase-1 and the migration of vascular endothelial cells. *J. Cell. Physiology*, **169**, 522–31.
46. Vandenbunder, B., Wernert, N., and Stehelin, D. (1994). Comment les tumeurs abusent leur hote: le facteur de transcription c-Ets1 et la regulation de l'angiogenese ou de l'invasion tumorale. *Contracept. Fertil. Sex*, **22**, 656–60.
47. Vandenbunder, B., Wernert, N., and Stehelin, D. (1993). L'oncogene c-ets 1 participe-t-il a la regulation de l'angiogenese tumorale? *Bull. Cancer*, **80**, 38–49.
48. Kaszubska, W., van Huijsduijnen, R., Ghersa, P., DeRaemy-Schenk, A., Chen, B., Hai, T., *et al.* (1993). Cyclic AMP-independent ATF family members interact with NF-kappa B and function in the activation of the E-selectin promoter in response to cytokines. *Mol. Cell. Biol.*, **13**, 7180–90.
49. Read, M., Whitley, M., Williams, A., and Collins, T. (1994). NF-kappa B and I kappa B alpha: an inducible regulatory system in endothelial activation. *J. Exp. Med.*, **179**, 503–12.
60. Wagner, E. and Risau, W. (1994). Oncogenes in the study of endothelial cell growth and differentiation. *Semin. Cancer Biol.*, **5**, 137–45.
51. Montesano, R., Pepper, M., Mohle-Steinlein, U., Risau, W., Wagner, E., and Orci, L. (1990). Increased proteolytic activity is responsible for the aberrant morphogenetic behavior of endothelial cells expressing the middle T oncogene. *Cell*, **62**, 435–45.
52. Taraboletti, G., Belotti, D., Dejana, E., Mantovani, A., and Giavazzi, R. (1993). Endothelial cell migration and invasiveness are induced by a soluble factor produced by murine endothelioma cells transformed by polyoma virus middle T oncogene. *Cancer Res.*, **53**, 3812–6.
53. Williams, R., Risau, W., Zerwes, H., Drexler, H., Aguzzi, A., and Wagner, E. (1989). Endothelioma cells expressing the polyoma middle T oncogene induce hemangiomas by host cell recruitment. *Cell*, **57**, 1053–63.
54. Tikhonenko, A., Black, D., and Linial, M. (1996). Viral myc oncoprotein in infected fibroblasts down-modulates thrombospondin-1, a possible tumor supresor gene. *J. Biol. Chemistry*, **271**, 30741–7.
55. Mettouchi, A., Cabon, F., Montreau, N., Vernier, P., Mercier, G., Blangy, D., Tricoire, H., Vigier P., and Binetruy, B. (1994). SPARC and thrombospondin genes are repressed by the c-jun oncogene in rat embryo fibroblasts. *EMBO J.*, **13**, 5668–78.
56. Majack, R., Midlbrandt, J., and Dixit, V. (1987). Induction of thrombospondin messenger RNA levels occurs as an

immediate primary response to platelet-derived growth factor. *J. Biol. Chemistry*, **262**, 8821–25.

57. Ponton, A., Coulombe, B., and Skup, D. (1991). Decreased expression of tissue inhibitor of metalloproteinases in metastatic tumor cells leading to increased levels of collagenase activity. *Cancer Res.*, **51**, 2138–43.

58. Dawson, T., Radulescu, A., and Wynford-Thomas, D. (1995). Expression of mutant p21 ras induces insulin-like growth factor 1 secretion in thyroid epithelial cells. *Cancer Res.*, **55**, 915–20.

59. Grant, M., Mames, R., Fitzgerald, C., Ellis, E., Caballero, S., Chegini, N., and Guy, J. (1993). Insulin-like growth factor I as an angiogenic agent. *In vivo* and *in vitro* studies. *Ann. N.Y. Acad. Sci.*, **692**, 230–42.

60. Mitsuhashi, R., Bayko, L., Shirasawa, S., Sasazuki, T., and Kerbel, R., (1995). Mutant ras upregulates VEGF/VPF expression: implications for induction and inhibition of tumor angiogenesis. *Cancer Res.*, **55**, 4575–80.

61. Grugel, S., Finkenzeller, G., Weindel, K., Barleon, B. and Marme, D. (1995). Both v-Ha-ras and v-raf stimulate expression of the vascular endothelial growth factor in NIH 3T3 cells. *J. Biol. Chemistry*, **270**, 25915–19.

62. Mazure, N., Chen, E., Yeh, P., Laderoute, K., and Giaccia, A. (1996). Oncogenic transformation and hypoxia synergistically act to modulate vascular endothelial growth factor expression. *Cancer Res.*, **56**, 3436–40.

63. Inglesias, T., Llanos, S., Lopez-Barahona, M., Seliger, B., Rodriguez-Pena, A., Bernal, J., and Munoz, A. (1995). Induction of platelet-derived growth factor B/c-sis by the v-erbA oncogene in glial cells. *Oncogene*, **10**, 1103–10.

64. Risau, W., Drexler, H., Mironov, V., Smits, A., Siegbahn, A., Funa, K., and Heldin, C. (1992). Platelet-derived growth factor is angiogenic *in vivo*. *Growth Factors*, **7**, 261–6.

65. Bussolino, F., Ziche, M., Wanf, J. M., Alessi, D., Morbidelli, L., Dremona, O., et al. (1991). *In vitro* and *in vivo* activation of endothelial cells by colony-stimulaing factors. *J. Clin. Invest.*, **87**, 986–95.

66. Schreiber, A., Winkler, M., and Derynck, R. (1986). Transforming growth factor-alpha: a more potent angiogenic mediator than epidermal growth factor. *Science*, **232**, 1250–3.

67. Ferrara, N., Winer, J., Burton, T., Rowland, A., Siegel, M., Phillips, H., et al. (1993). Expression of vascular endothelial growth factor does not promote transformation but confers a growth advantage *in vivo* to Chinese hamster ovary cells. *J. Clin. Invest.*, **91**, 160–70.

68. Kondo, S., Asano, M., and Suzuki, H. (1993). Significance of vascular endothelial growth factor/vascular permeability factor for solid tumor growth, and its inhibition by the antibody. *Biochem. Biophys. Res. Commun.*, **194**, 1234–41.

69. Shweiki, D., Itin, A., Neufeld, G., Gitay-Goren, H., and Keshet, E. (1993). Patterns of expression of vascular endothelial growth factor (VEGF) and VEGF receptors in mice suggest a role in hormonally regulated angiogenesis. *J. Clin. Invest.*, **91**, 2235–43.

70. Ladoux, A., and Frelin, C. (1993). Hypoxia is a strong inducer of vascular endothelial growth factor mRNA expression in the heart. *Biochem. Biophys. Res. Commun.*, **195**, 1005–10.

71. Minchenko, A., Bauer, T., Salceda, S., and Caro, J. (1994). Hypoxic stimulation of vascular endothelial growth factor expression *in vitro* and *in vivo*. *Lab. Invest.*, **71**, 374–9.

72. Mukhopadhyay, D., Tsiokas, L., Zhou, X., Foster, D., Brugge, J., and Sukhatme, V. (1995). Hypoxic induction of human vascular endothelial growth factor expression through c-src activation. *Nature*, **375**, 577–9.

73. Detmar, M., Brown, L., Claffey, K., Yeo, K., Kocher, O., Jackman, R., et al. (1994). Overexpression of vascular permeability factor/vascular endothelial growth factor and its receptors in psoriasis. *J. Exp. Med.*, **180**, 1141–6.

74. Saez, E., Rutberg, S., Mueller, E., Oppenheim, H., Smoluk, J., Yuspa, S., and Spiegelman, B. (1995). c-fos is required for malignant progression of skin tumors. *Cell*, **82**, 721–32.

75. Mukhopadhyay, D., Tsiokas, L., and Sukhatme, V. (1996). Wild-type p53 and v-Src exert opposing influences on human vascular endothelial growth factor gene expression. *Cancer Res.*, **55**, 6161–5.

76. Ferrara, N., Carver-Moore, K., Chen, H., Dowd, M., Lu, L., O'Shea, K., Powell-Braxton, L., Hillan, K., and Moore, M. (1996). Heterozygous embryonic lethality induced by targeted inactivation of the VEGF gene. *Nature*, **380**, 439–42.

77. Zhau, H., Pisters, L., Hall, M., Zhao, L., Troncoso, P., Pollack, A., and Chung, L. (1994). Biomarkers associated with prostate cancer progression. *J. Cell. Biochem. Suppl.*, **19**, 208–16.

78. Naidu, Y., Rosen, E., Zitnick, R., Goldberg, I., Park, M., Naujokas, M., et al. (1994). Role of scatter factor in the pathogenesis of AIDS-related Kaposi sarcoma. *Proc. Natl Acad. Sci. USA*, **91**, 5281–5.

79. Grant, D., Kleinman, H., Goldberg, I., Bhargava, M., Nickoloff, B., Kinsella, J., et al. (1993). Scatter factor induces blood vessel formation *in vivo*. *Proc. Natl Acad. Sci. USA*, **90**, 1937–41.

80. Rosen, E., Grant, D., Kleinman, H., Goldberg, I., Bhargava, M., Nickoloff, B., et al. (1993). Scatter factor (hepatocyte growth factor) is a potent angiogenesis factor *in vivo*. *Symp. Soc. Exp. Biol.*, **47**, 227–34.

81. Weidner, K. M., Sachs, M., and Dirchmeier, W. (1993). The met receptor tyrosine kinase transduces motility, proliferation, and morphogenic signals of scatter factor/ hepatocyte growth factor in epithelial cells. *J. Cell Biol.*, **121**, 145–54.

82. Montesano, R., Matsumoto, K., Nakamura, T., and Orci, L. (1991). Identification of a fibroblast-derived epithelial morphogen as hepatocyte growth factor. *Cell*, **67**, 901–8.

83. Tsarfaty, I., Resau, J., Rulong, S., Keydar, I., Faletto, D., and Vande Woude, G. (1992). The met proto-oncogene receptor and lumen formation. *Science*, **257**, 1258–61.

84. Thomas, K. (1988). Transforming potential of fibroblast growth factor genes. *TIBS*, **13**, 327–8.

85. Rogelj, S., Weinberg, R., Fanning, P., and Klagsbrun, M. (1988). Basic fibroblast growth factor fused to a signal peptide transforms cells. *Nature*, **331**, 173–5.

86. Huang, Y., Li, J., Moscatelli, D., Basilico, C., Nicolaides, A., Zhang, W., et al. (1993). Expression of Int-2 oncogene in Kaposi's sarcoma lesions. *J. Clin. Invest.*, **91**, 1191–7.

87. Costa, M., Danesi, R., Agen, C., Di Paolo, A., Basolo, F., Del Bianchi, S., and Del Tacca, M. (1994). IMCF-10A cells infected with the int-2 oncogene induce angiogenesis in the chick chorioallantoic membrane and in the rat mesentery. *Cancer Res.*, **54**, 9–11.

88. Taraboletti, G., Garofalo, A., Belotti, D., Drudis, T., Borosotti, P., Scanziani, E., et al. (1995). Inhibition of angiogenesis and murine hemangioma growth by batimastat, a synthetic inhibitor of matrix metalloproteinases. *J. Natl Cancer Inst.*, **87**, 293–8.

89. Pepper, M., Ferrara, N., Orci, L., and Montesano, R. (1995). Leukemia inhibitory factor (LIF) inhibits angiogenesis *in vitro*. *J. Cell Sci.*, **108**, 73–83.

90. Ballin, M., Gomez, D., Sinha, C., and Thorgeirsson, U. (1988). Ras oncogene mediated induction of a 92 kDa metalloproteinase; strong correlation with the malignant phenotype. *Biochem. Biophys. Res. Commun.*, **154**, 832–8.

91. Hamaguchi, M., Yamagata, S., Thant, A., Xiao, H., Iwata, H., Mazaki, T., and Hanafusa, H. (1995). Augmentation of metalloproteinase (gelatinase) activity secreted from Rous sarcoma virus-infected cells correlates with transforming activity of src. *Oncogene*, **10**, 1037–43.

92. Zhang, J., and Schultz, R. (1992). Fibroblasts transformed by different ras oncogenes show dissimilar patterns of protease gene expression and regulation. *Cancer Res.*, **52**, 6682–9.

93. Berkenpas, M., and Quigley, J. (1991). Transformation-dependent activation of urokinase-type plasminogen activator by a plasmin-independent mechanism: involvement of cell surface membranes. *Proc. Natl Acad. Sci. USA*, **88**, 7768–72.

94. Bouck, N. P., and di Mayorca, G. (1982). Chemical carcinogens transform BHK cells by inducing a recessive mutation. *Mol. Cell. Biol.*, **2**, 97–105.

95. Good, D. J., Polverini, P. J., Rastinejad, F., Le Beau, M. M., Lemons, R. S., Frazier, W. A., and Bouck, N. P. (1990). A tumor suppressor-dependent inhibitor of angiogenesis is immunologically and functionally indistinguishable from a fragment of thrombospondin. *Proc. Natl Acad. Sci. USA*, **87**, 6624–8.

96. Lingen, M., Dipietro, L., Solt, D., Bouck, N., and Polverini, P. (1997). The angiogenic switch in hamster buccal pouch keratinocytes is dependent on TGFB-1 and is unaffected by ras activation. *Carcinogenesis*, **18**, 329–38.

97. Van Meir, E. G., Polverini, P. J., Chazin, V. R., Su Huang, H-J., de Tribolet, N., and Cavenee, W. K. (1994). Release of an inhibitor of angiogenesis upon induction of wild type p53 expression in glioblastoma cells. *Nature Genet.*, **8**, 171–6.

98. Volpert, O. V., Stellmach, V., and Bouck, N. (1995). The modulation of thrombospondin and other naturally occurring inhibitors of angiogenesis during tumor progression. *Breast Cancer Res. Treatment* **36**, 119–26.

99. Huang, H-J. S., Yee, J-K., Shew, J-Y., Chen, P-L., Bookstein, R., Friedmann, T., *et al.* (1988). Suppression of the neoplastic phenotype by replacement of the RB gene in human cancer cells. *Science*, **242**, 1563–6.

100. Sumegi, J., Uzvolgy, E., and Klein, G. (1990). Expression of the RB gene under the control of MuLVLTR suppresses tumorigenicity of WERI-RB-27 retinoblastoma cells in immunodefective mice. *Cell Growth Differ.*, **1**, 247–50.

101. Dawson, D. W., Tolsma, S. S., Volpert, O. V., Polverini, P. J., Bouck, N. P. (1995). Retinoblastoma gene expression alters angiogenic phenotype. *Proc. Am. Soc. Cancer Res.*, **63**, 88.

102. Siemeister, G., Weindel, K., Mohrs, K., Barleon, B., Martiny-Baron, G., and Marme, D. (1996). Reversion of deregulated expression of vascular endothelial growth factor in human renal carcinoma cells by von Hippel-Lindau tumor suppressor protein. *Cancer Res.*, **56**, 2299–301.

103. Gnarra, J., Zhou, S., Merrill, M., Wagner, J., Krumm, A., Papavassiliou, E., Oldfield, E., Klausner, R., and Linehan, W. (1996). Post-transcriptional regulation of vascular endothelial growth factor mRNA by the product of the VHL tumor suppressor gene. *Proc. Natl. Acad. Sci.*, **93**, 10589–94.

104. Iliopoulos, O., Levy, A., Jiang, C., Kaelin, W., and Goldberg, M. (1996). Negative regulation of hypoxia-inducible genes by the von Hippel-Lindau protein. *Proc. Natl. Acad. Sci.*, **93**, 10595–9.

105. Bookstein, R., Shew, J-Y., Chen, P-L., Scully, P., and Lee, W-H. (1990). Suppression of tumorigenicity of human prostate carcinoma cells by replacing a mutated RB gene. *Science*, **247**, 712–5.

106. Tolsma, S. S., Volpert, O. V., Good, D. J., Frazier, W. F., Polverini, P. J., and Bouck, N. (1993). Peptides derived from two separate domains of the matrix protein thrombospondin-1 have anti-angiogenic activity. *J. Cell Biol.*, **122**, 497–511.

107. Weinstat-Saslow, D. L., Zabrenetzky, V. S., VanHoutte, K., Frazier, W. A., Roberts, D. D. and Steeg, P. S. (1994). Transfection of thrombospondin 1 complementary DNA into a human breast carcinoma cell line reduces primary tumor growth, metastatic potential, and angiogenesis. *Cancer Res.*, **54**, 6504–11.

108. Sheibani, N. and Frazier, W. A. (1995). Thrombospondin-1 expression in transformed endothelial cells restores a normal phenotype and suppresses their tumorigenesis. *Proc. Natl Acad. Sci. USA*, **92**, 6788–92.

109. Prescott, S. and White, R. (1996). Self-promotion? Intimate connections between APC and prostaglandin H synthase-2. *Cell*, **87**, 783–6.

110. Masanobu, O., Dinchuk, J., Kargman, S., Oshima, H., Hancock, B., Kwong, E., Trzaskos, J., Evans, J., and Taketo, M. (1996). Suppression of intestinal polyposis in APC knockout mice by inhibition of cyclooxygenase 2 (COX-2). *Cell*, **87**, 803–9.

10. The complex molecular network regulating tumour angiogenesis: the importance of context

Claire E. Lewis and Frances R. Balkwill

Since the early descriptions of angiogenesis in malignant tumours some 25 years ago (1,2), over 3000 papers have been published describing the involvement of myriad individual factors in the various cellular steps of the angiogenic pathway. These include cytokines, enzymes, and other macromolecules which regulate the dissolution of the basement membrane around existing vessels, and the orientation, motility, proliferation, and differentiation of endothelial cells to form new ones (3).

Many of the following chapters in this volume bear testimony to the enormous quantity of work performed on the angiogenic function(s) of a wide range of such effector molecules. The ever increasing list of these include: (i) the polypeptide cytokines: vascular endothelial growth factor (VEGF), basic fibroblast growth factor (bFGF), tumour necrosis factor alpha (TNF-α), transforming growth factors alpha and beta (TGF-α and -β), epidermal growth factor (EGF), pleitrophin, midkine, angiogenin, hepatocyte growth factor, angiostatin, and thrombospondin 1; (ii) the enzymes: plasmin, thrombin, thymidine phosphorylase, hyaluronidase, and various collagenases and matrix metalloproteinases; (iii) components of the extracellular matrix: laminin, vitronectin, fibronectin as well as various collagens, proteoglycans, and glycoaminoglycans; and (iv) the cell surface molecules, urokinase-type plasminogen activator receptor (uPAR), various selectins, tissue factor, and the integrin heterodimers, $\alpha_2\beta_1$, $\alpha_5\beta_1$, and $\alpha_v\beta_3$ integrins (also reviewed by us in reference 4).

Although we have a much better understanding of the potential of some of these factors to regulate angiogenesis in both *in vitro* angiogenesis assays and *in vivo* animal models, the complex interrelationship between them in the tumour microenvironment is becoming increasingly apparent. The presence of such a complex network of factors reflects, in part, the considerable heterogeneity of cell types present in most solid tumours, including not only malignant cells themselves but also such stromal cells as macrophages, lymphocytes, natural killer (NK) cells, fibroblasts, and endothelial cells (5–7). Each of these is capable of releasing a number of pro- or anti-angiogenic

factors in a highly regulated, dynamic fashion, which means that, at a given site in the tumour, the level of expression of each factor depends on the number of producer cells present as well as the local balance of stimulatory and inhibitory cues regulating their secretory activity.

This can result in what appears to be a focal pattern of expression of angiogenic substances, sometimes called cytokine 'hotspots' (8,9). However, these may not actually mirror a high level of angiogenic activity as this depends on whether, once released, the cytokine is free to diffuse across the extracellular space to act on target cells or becomes rapidly bound to insoluble components of the extracellular matrix (ECM). In the latter case, the factors (*e.g.* VEGF, bFGF, TGF) become temporarily inactivated until the necessary enzymes are released by neighbouring cells to cause their release from the ECM. Recent reports indicate that fragments of macromolecules liberated from the ECM itself can also exert enzymatic activity on the ECM to play a part in this phenomenon (10).

Even if a given cytokine is actually liberated as a free entity into the extracellular space its ability to alter endothelial cell function then depends on such parameters as: (i) the concentration of the factor present; (ii) how long it is maintained at a certain level in the extracellular space (which reflects both producer cell activity, target cell or ECM uptake and/or enzyme breakdown); (iii) the presence of other soluble factors or ECM components which block its access to receptors on endothelial cells (*e.g.* soluble cytokine receptors); and (iv) the presence of other soluble mediators in the network which prime or inhibit the responsiveness of endothelial cells to the cytokine. Furthermore, many of these factors have indirect effects on tumour angiogenesis by regulating the expression of other factors in the network (4–6) and/or the expression/responsiveness of their receptors on target cells (11).

Other agents with the capacity to modulate the secretion of angiogenic cytokines in solid tumours include oxygen, glucose, pyruvate, pH, and lactate. For example, VEGF, bFGF, and TNF-α are up-regulated by exposure of producer cells (whether tumour cells or stromal cell such as macrophages) to a deficiency in oxygen (hypoxia) or glucose (hypoglycaemia) (12–15). These signs of tissue 'stress' occur at sites where tumour expansion temporarily outstrips the development of the vasculature or the existing vasculature collapses, resulting in insufficient perfusion and the development of transient ischaemia. As many of these cytokines have pleiotrophic actions on different cell types in solid tumours, it is interesting to note that a number of recent reports have indicated that hypoxia down-regulates many of their anti-tumour (*e.g.* cytotoxic or cytostatic) effects (16,17). This raises the possibility that rapid tumour expansion and/or differences in blood flow in distinct tumour areas (both of which are capable of generating in hypoxia, hyperglycaemia, etc.) (see Chapter 6) not only switches on angiogenic factor production by tumour and stromal cells in such areas, but also streamlines the actions of these cytokines so that they are maximally effective in tumour angiogenesis and relatively ineffective in various anti-tumour mechanisms.

Taken together, these findings indicate that the action of cytokines in tumour angiogenesis is a complex, *context-specific* phenomenon, in which they work together with other factors present in the tumour microenvironment in a dynamic, reciprocal fashion. Only at certain tumour sites is this likely to be sufficiently co-ordinated to lead to the appropriate temporal sequence of multiple endothelial cell changes which take place in the formation, rearrangement, function, or destruction of tumour blood vessels in tumour angiogenesis.

Dellian and his co-workers have recently used novel quantitative angiogenesis assays in mice to show the importance of *microenvironmental factors* on the rate and type of new blood vessel formation (18). The rate of growth and the properties of new blood vessels was seen to depend as much upon their location as the presence/levels of such pro-angiogenic cytokines as VEGF or bFGF. Indeed, in some instances the rate of angiogenesis and the level of hyperpermeability of the vessels formed was dictated by the *site* at which angiogenesis was provoked and was largely independent of the original angiogenic stimulus. This means that many such 'pro-angiogenic' factors may be mainly responsible for triggering or halting the angiogenic process, whereas the speed and exact nature of the endothelial cell changes involved in angiogenesis are controlled primarily by other site-specific, tumour microenvironmental factors.

Implications for the development of effective anti-cancer therapies

Over the past 20 years, there has been considerable emphasis placed on the research and development of cytokine therapies to slow the growth of, or stimulate the immune response to, solid tumours (reviewed by us in reference 19). These have led to regimens involving exogenously applied cytokines. Clinical trials of systematically administered cytokines have met with some success, most notably interferon α in haematological malignancies (20) and interteukin (IL) 2 in a small minority of patients with renal cell carcinoma and melanoma (21). Aside from these few examples, cytokines have not fulfilled the predictions of pre-clinical studies. The reasons are complex, and may be attributed to optimistic interpretation of animal model and tissue culture data, inappropriate methods of administration, and/or unexpected sometimes severe, toxicities.

There may also be an additional explanation for the failure of cytokine therapy, the presence of such an abnormal, complex cytokine/enzyme network in the tumour microenvironment. The role of multiple endogenous factors in influencing the net effect of exogenously applied cytokines in tumours has received little attention to date and generally not been considered when designing cytokine-based therapies for cancer.

This has been evident most recently in the rapid proliferation of new anti-angiogenic therapies based on the blockade of such individual factors as VEGF. Little expense has been spared, for example, in the hunt for specific kinase inhibitors to block the pro-angiogenic action of this cytokine via one of its receptors, *flk*-1, on endothelial cells (22,23). Although such agents may prove to be highly specific and non-toxic in pre-clinical or early clinical trials, it is quite feasible that such a complex, dynamic network of interrelated factors as that present in solid tumours, may be more than capable of compensating for the loss of one factor by increasing the production or effect of alternative pro-angiogenic molecule (*e.g.* bFGF).

Future studies defining the complex molecular context in which cytokines act in tumours will not only enhance our understanding of tumour biology, but may lead to novel and more effective cytokine therapies. Indeed, it may even fall to mathematical biologists to generate complex, multifactorial, computer-driven mathematical models to simulate the complex interplay of factors involved in the molecular regulation of tumour angiogenesis (24–26). It may then prove possible to test the net effect of various doses or different types of administration of a given factor (*e.g.* therapeutic cytokine or enzyme inhibitor) in such computer simulation a tumour before committing it to pre-clinical or clinical testing. Whether even these advanced forms of biological analysis are capable of achieving such an ambitious goal remains to be seen.

References

1. Greenblatt, M. and Shubi, P. (1968). Tumour angiogenesis: transfilter diffusion studies in the hamster by the transport chamber technique. *J. Natl Cancer Inst.*, **41**, 111–24.
2. Folkman, J. (1971). Tumour angiogenesis. *N. Engl. J. Med.*, **285**, 1182–6.
3. Paweletz, N. and Knierim, M. (1989). Tumour-related angiogenesis. *Crit. Rev. Oncol. Heamatol.*, **9**, 197–42.
4. Leek, R. D., Harris, A. I., and Lewis, C. E. (1994). Cytokine networks in solid human tumours: regulation of angiogenesis. *J. Leuk. Biol.*, **56**, 423–35.
5. Lewis, C. E. and McGee, JO'D. (1996). Growth factors in breast cancer. The role of TNF alpha: implications for prognosis and possible strategies for intervention. *Horizons Med.* (in press).
6. Senger, D. R. (1996). Molecular framework for angiogenesis. *Am J. Pathol.* **149**, 1–8.
7. Balkwill, F. R. (1994). Cytokine therapy of cancer. The importance of knowing the context. *Eur. Cytokine Network*, **5**, 379–85.
8. Pusztai, L, Clover, L. M., Cooper K, Starkey, P. M., Lewis, C. E., and McGee, JO'D. (1994). Expression of TNFα and it's receptors in breast carcinoma. *Br. J. Cancer*, **70**, 289–292.
9. Plate, K. H., Breier, G., Weich, H. A., Mennel, H. D., and Risau W. (1994). Vascular endothelial growth factor and glioma angiogenesis: coordinate induction of VEGF receptors, distribution of VEGF protein and possible *in vivo* mechanisms. *Int. J. Cancer*, **15**, 520–9.
10. Boudjennah, L., Daletfumeron, V., Ylatupa, S., and Pagano, M. (1996). Immunopurification and characterization of a collagenase/gelatinase domain issued from basement membrane fibronectin. *FEBS Lett.*, **391**, 52–6.
11. Patterson, C., Perrella, M. A., Endege, W. O., Yoshizumi, M., Lee, M. E., and Haber, E. (1996). Down regulation of vascular endothelial growth factor receptors by tumour necrosis factor alpha in cultured human vascular endothelial cells. *J. Clin. Invest.*, **98**, 490–6.
12. Schweiki, D., Itin, A., Soffer, D., and Keshet, E. (1992). Vascular endotheial growth factor induced by hypoxia may mediate hypoxia-initiated angiogenesis. *Nature*, **359**, 843–5.
13. Scannell, G., Waxman, K., and Kaml, G. J. (1993). Hypoxia induces a human macrophage cell line to release tumour necrosis factor alpha and its soluble receptors. *J. Surg. Res.*, **54**, 281–5.
14. Knighton, D. R. and Hunt, T. K. (1983). Oxygen tension regulates the expression of angiogenesis factor by macrophages. *Science*, **221**, 1283–5.
15. Jensen, J. A., Hunt, T. K., Scheuenstuhl, H., and Banda, M. J. (1986). Effect of lactate, pyruvate and pH on the secretion of angiogenesis and mitogenesis factors by macrophages. *Lab. Invest.*, **54**, 574–8.
16. Lynch, E. M., Sampson, L. E., Khalil, A. A., Horsman, M. R., and Chaplin, D. J. (1995). Cytotoxic effect of tumour necrosis factor alpha on sarcoma F cells at tumour relevant oxygen tensions. *Acta Oncol.*, **34**, 423–7.
17. Loeffler, D. A., Juneau, P. L., and Masserant (1992). Influence of tumour physico-chemical conditions in IL-2-stimulated lymphocyte proliferation. *Brit. J. Cancer*, **66**, 619–22.
18. Dellian, M., Witwer, B. P., Salehi, H. A., Yuan, F., and Jain, R. K. (1996). Quantitation and physiological characterzation of angiogenic vessels in mice: effect of basic fibroblast growth factor, vascular endothelial growth factor/vascular permeability factor and host environment. *Am. J. Pathol.*, **149**, 59–71.
19. Gutterman, J. U. (1994). Cytokine therapeutics: lessons from interferon-alpha. *Proc. Natl Acad. Sci. USA*, **91**, 1198–205.
20. Vedantham, S., Gamliel, H., and Golomb, H. M. (1992). Mechanism of interferon action in hairy cell leukemia: a model of effective cancer biotherapy. *Cancer Res.*, **52**, 1056–9.
21. Dillman, R. O., Church, C., Oldham, R. K., West, W. H., Schwartzberg, L., and Birch, R. (1993). Inpatient continuous-infusion interleukin 2 in 788 patients with cancer. The national biotherapy study group experience. *Cancer*, **71**, 2358–62.
22. Rak, J. W., Bradley, D. St. C., and Kerbel, R. S. (1995). Consequences of angiogenesis for tumour progression, metastasis and cancer therapy. *Anti-cancer Drugs*, **6**, 3–18.
23. Strawn, L. M., McMahon, G., App, H., Schreck, R., Kuchler, W. R., Longhi, M. P., *et al.* Flk-1 as a target for tumour growth inhibition. *Cancer Res.*, **56**, 3540–5.
24. Stokes, C. L. and Lauffenburger, D. A. (1991). Analysis of the roles of microvessel endothelial random motility and chemotaxis in angiogenesis. *J. Theor. Biol.*, **152**, 377–403.
25. Chaplain, M. A. J., Giles, S. M., Sleeman, B. D., and Jarvis, R. J. (1995). A mathematical analysis of a model for tumour angiogenesis. *J. Math. Biol.*, **33**, 744–70.
26. Chaplain, M. A. J. and Stuart, A. M. (1993). A model mechanism for the chemotactic response of endothelial cells to tumour angiogenesis factor. *IMA J. Math. Appl. Med. Biol.*, **10**, 149–68.

11. The role of proteases in angiogenesis

Andreas Bikfalvi, Sharon Klein, Giuseppe Pintucci, and Daniel B. Rifkin

Introduction

Angiogenesis is defined as the process of vascular neoformation that occurs during development, menstruation, and several pathological conditions such as neoplasia. Angiogenesis requires the co-ordinate activation of a series of molecular events that are responsible for endothelial cell migration, proliferation, and differentiation into capillary structures. Proteolytic activity is critical for migration and invasion of endothelial cells into the neighbouring tissue (1,2). Several protease systems have been identified as being involved in angiogenesis including the plasminogen activator (PA) system and the matrix metalloproteinases (1,2). Urokinase-type PA (uPA) not only converts plasminogen into plasmin to allow matrix degradation, but may also provide signals for endothelial cell movement (3,4). These protease systems are controlled by a variety of soluble angiogenic factors such as fibroblast growth factors (FGFs), transforming growth factor (TGF)-β or vascular endothelial growth factor (VEGF) (1,2,5–7).

The roles of two participants in the control of neovascularization and protease production, (FGF) 2 (bFGF) and TGF-β, have been extensively investigated. In this chapter we will not review all the protease systems potentially involved in angiogenesis. Instead, we will focus on the PA system and summarize our views about molecules involved in the regulation of PA activity during angiogenesis by illustrating the roles of FGF-2 and TGF-β.

The plasminogen activator/inhibitor system

Structure and spectrum of activities

The best characterized protease system involved in angiogenesis is the PA system (1,2,6,7). uPA and tissue-type PA (tPA) convert plasminogen into plasmin. Plasmin has a wide spectrum of activities and can degrade fibrin as well as extracellular matrix (ECM) compounds such as laminin or fibronectin. Besides this role, plasmin can activate metalloproteases and elastases. Whereas tPA is associated with fibrinolysis, uPA plays an important part in physiological or pathological tissue remodelling (1,2). uPA has a molecular weight of 55 kDa and consists of two polypeptides chains. The A chain contains one 'kringle' structure and an NH$_2$-terminal epidermal growth factor (EGF)-like domain. Residues 13–30 of this EGF-like domain mediate enzyme binding to the uPA receptor. The B chain contains the catalytic site encompassing the catalytic triad His, Asp, and Ser residues. uPA is secreted as a single chain proenzyme (pro-uPA) and is converted into the two chain form by limited proteolysis. uPA interacts at the cell surface with the uPA receptor, a 35–60 kDa glycosylated protein linked to the plasma membrane by a glycosyl-phosphatidylinositol anchor (8–11). After secretion, pro-uPA binds the uPA receptor. Pro-uPA is then activated by trace amounts of plasmin. The interaction of uPA with its receptor focalizes the enzyme activity on the surface, accelerates plasmin generation and stimulates signal transduction through the uPA receptor. As discussed below, signal transduction through the uPA receptor can also occur upon receptor occupancy by pro-uPA. Pro-uPA is not only converted into active uPA by plasmin but may also be cleaved by a serine protease associated with Rous sarcoma transformed chicken fibroblasts and by cathepsin B (12).

PA inhibitors and PAs are coexpressed in endothelial cells. Endothelial cells express PA inhibitor 1 (PAI-1) (13). PAI-1 is a single chain molecule that binds the active two chain form of uPA and tPA with a molar ratio of 1:1. PAI-1 is released from the ECM of human umbilical vein endothelial cells by proteases such as thrombin, which inactivates PAI-1 (14), and cathepsin G, which results in an increase in PAI-1 activity (15). PAI-1 has an important role in the turnover of uPA. Internalization of uPA by its receptor is stimulated when PAI-1 is bound to uPA. Thus, PAI-1 participates in the clearance of inactivated uPA from the cell surface.

Role of the plasminogen activator system in angiogenesis

Multiple roles have been attributed to the PA system in modulating the endothelial cell phenotype. uPA induces cell migration and invasion in endothelial cells as well as epithelial cells and fibroblasts (3,4,16). For example, anti-uPA antibodies inhibit endothelial cell migration (3). NIH 3T3 cells that are transfected with the uPA cDNA acquire the ability to migrate and to invade (16). This demonstrates that endogenous uPA triggers migration and invasion. In addition, pro-uPA is able to induce cell movement (3,4). The presence of the uPA receptor appears to be critical for the induction of migration (17,18) as little migration or invasion are observed in uPA receptor negative cells (18). However, after transfection of uPA receptor cDNA into these cells, migration and invasion are induced (18). In agreement with the latter experiments, transfection of invasive cells with uPA anti-sense cDNA inhibits their invasive potential (18).

The mechanism by which migration is induced by uPA has been characterized in the epithelial cell line WISH. Indeed, Busso et al. (4) have shown that pro-uPA activates the uPA receptor, induces migration, and induces the phosphorylation of a 47 and a 55 kDa protein on serine residues. Partial sequence analysis of these proteins showed homology to cytokeratins 8 and 18. This phosphorylation of cytokeratins 8 and 18 is mediated by protein kinase C type ε (PKC ε). However, the cascade by which PKC ε is activated is not yet known.

uPA must be focalized on the cell surface in order to promote migration (19). Indeed, Pepper et al. (19) have demonstrated that endothelial cells derived from haemangiomas of transgenic mice expressing polyoma-middle T antigen did not form capillary cord structures in in vitro angiogenic assays using fibrin gels but grew into cyst-like structures. These cells have deregulated uPA expression. In the presence of protease inhibitors such as bovine pancreatic trypsin inhibitor, the cyst-like structures are converted into endothelial cords. In addition, Dubois-Stringfellow et al. (20) compared the ability of transformed endothelial cells and normal endothelial cells to differentiate in fibrin gels and matrigel. Transformed endothelial cells but not normal endothelial cells grew into cystic structures. This behaviour correlated with excessive PA production by the transformed cells. Inhibition of plasminogen activation by neutralizing anti-uPA antibodies prevented cyst formation and allowed capillary cord formation. Normal endothelial cells always grew into cord-like structures. The manipulation of the PA system did not affect the morphogenic behaviour of normal endothelial cells. These data need to be reinforced by additional experiments designed to block specifically the interaction of uPA with its cell surface receptor. Dubois-Stringfellow et al. (20) also observed that on Matrigel, transformed endothelial cells did not form cysts but only cords and that the manipulation of the PA system did not have any effect on this substrate. They concluded that cord formation in

Matrigel is independent of the PA system. However, in vitro angiogenic assays using matrigel may not be an ideal model for in vitro angiogenesis because other cell types form cord structures on this substratum (21).

What are the molecular mechanisms regulating PA production and activity by endothelial cells? Growth factors interact with cell surface receptors and other molecules present at the cell surface to stimulate uPA expression. The putative mechanisms by which FGF is able to achieve this will be reviewed later in this chapter. The proto-oncogene c-ets-1 activates transcription of uPA by interaction with the PEA3 motif present in the promoter region (22). It has been postulated that paracrine factors such as FGF-2 might regulate uPA expression by stimulating the interaction of c-ets or another transcription factor with the PEA3 motif.

The in vivo pattern of uPA and PAI-1 expression has been compared during angiogenesis of ovarian follicles, the corpus luteum, and the maternal decidua (23). uPA was detected in the ovary along the route of capillary extensions. Following ovulation, uPA was expressed in capillary sprouts within the developing corpus luteum. During decidual neovascularization, uPA was detected in endothelial cell cords. PAI-1 was also observed in areas where endothelial cells expressed uPA. These results suggest that uPA and PAI-1 expression are coordinately involved in physiological neovascularization.

The phenotypes of uPA, tPA, or PAI-1 knockout mice have demonstrated no abnormality in vasculo- or angiogenesis (24). However, careful examination of the phenotypes of these knockout mice has revealed striking differences in smooth muscle cell proliferation and migration after balloon injury (Carmeliet et al., personal communication). It is likely that additional abnormalities including endothelial cell dysfunction may be found in response to pharmacological or experimental manipulations of these mice.

Besides its role in promoting angiogenesis, the PA system may control two inhibitory signals. The first is the generation of TGF-β, which will be discussed later in this chapter. The second is the formation of a fragment of plasminogen that functions as a specific angiogenic inhibitor. Recently, it was reported that a 32 kDa plasminogen fragment named angiostatin is a specific inhibitor of angiogenesis (25). Angiostatin has been identified in the urine of mice with Lewis lung carcinomas. The removal of the primary tumour is followed by a rapid onset of metastasis. It was suggested that the primary tumour produces angiostatin to inhibit angiogenesis. Therefore, the removal of the source of angiostatin, the primary tumour, allows angiogenesis to occur supporting tumour growth and metastasis. The inhibitor is present in tumour-bearing mice, but not in control mice. The inhibitory activity is specific for endothelial cells and blocks neovascularization *in vivo*. Thus plasminogen, besides its role in matrix degradation, may generate, when processed, an angiogenesis inhibitor.

Factors regulating protease or protease inhibition in endothelial cells

Fibroblast growth factors

FGFs represent a family comprising nine members, designated FGF-1 to FGF-9 (26,27). The interaction of FGF-2 with protease systems has been characterized extensively (1,6). Several forms of FGF-2 have been described, including an 18 kDa FGF-2 and higher molecular weight forms (26) (Fig. 11.1).

Exogenous 18 kDa fibroblast growth factor 2

FGF-2 was initially identified and cloned as an 18 kDa molecule found in the brain, in the vasculature, and in several cell lines (26,28). This molecule stimulates endothelial cell proliferation, migration, and *in vitro* differentiation (26). Different FGF receptor families have also been identified. These include FGF-R1 (flg), FGF-R2 (bek), FGF-R3, FGF-R4, and FGF-R5 (26,29). Although the first four receptor types are classical tyrosine kinase receptors, the fifth receptor is a cysteine-rich protein and is devoid of a tyrosine kinase domain (29). Endothelial cells express FGF-R1 and FGF-R2 (27). FGF-2 stimulates protease production in endothelial cells (1,5,6,7). uPA and PAI-I expression are also modulated by FGF-2 (1,5,6,7). In addition to its effect on uPA expression, FGF-2 regulates uPA receptor levels. Indeed, Mignatti *et al.* (30) demonstrated that FGF-2 up-regulates uPA receptor levels in human umbilical vein endothelial cells (HUVECs). Thus, FGF-2 exhibits a double stimulatory effect on the

PA system by stimulating the expression of both the ligand and its receptor.

FGF-2 is concentrated in the ECM because of its high affinity for heparan sulphate proteoglycans (1,5,26,31). The ECM and cell surface-associated heparan sulphates protect FGF-2 from proteolytic degradation. The interaction with proteoglycan is important for FGF-2 binding and signalling through high-affinity receptors (32–36). Recently, it has been reported that perlecan but not syndecan or other proteoheparan sulphates binds FGF-2 at the cell surface (37). Plasmin and PAI-1 are also present in the ECM (38,39). Thus, FGF-2 and components of the PA system are located in the ECM. FGF-2 may be released from ECM and cell surface heparan sulfates not only by plasmin but also by heparinase, phospholipase C (PLC), phospholipase D (PLD), and thrombin (40–44). When plasmin activity is increased, FGF-2 is mobilized from the ECM into the medium. Conversely, when PA activity is decreased, FGF-2 is mostly associated with the ECM. PLC and PLD mobilize FGF-2–heparan-sulphate complexes in an active form. However, it is more likely that PLD, not PLC, is involved under physiological conditions as PLD but not PLC is found extracellularly (43). Activated polymorphonuclear cells were also found to release FGF-like molecules from cultured endothelial cells (45). The proteases elastase and cathepsin G seem to be responsible for this activity. Thus, proteases and heparanases may constitute a regulatory system that allows mobilization of cell surface or ECM-associated FGF-2.

What are the structural requirements at the cellular level for FGF-2 stimulation of the PA system? In the current paradigm a growth factor must interact with its cell surface receptor to generate intracellular signalling. However, it has recently been proposed that PA may be induced in cells lacking FGF receptors and that this is mediated through interaction with heparan sulphates. Quarto and Amalric (46) have recently reported that FGF induces PA in FGF receptor negative rat L6 myoblasts. In support of this view, Isacchi *et al.* (47) have reported that a mutated

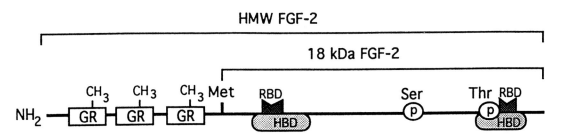

Figure 11.1. Structure of 18 kDa FGF-2 and HMW FGF-2. RBD, receptor binding domain; HBD, heparin binding domain; GR, glycine/arginine-rich box; P, potential phosphorylation sites on serine or threonine residues.

form of FGF-2 that did not induce signalling at the cell surface is able to induce PA. How FGF induces PA in this model is speculative. Either FGF-2 might stimulate signalling through heparan sulphates or it might be internalized and induce PA at a nuclear site. An intracellular signal transduction cascade by which FGFs stimulate uPA production has not been described. It has been reported that uPA induction by FGF-2 is independent of PKC activation (48). The target of the FGF-stimulated signal pathway for uPA induction may be the PEA3 motif. As already mentioned, this motif is involved in the activation of transcription by the c-ets proto-oncogene that interacts with the PEA3 motif (22). The PEA3 sequence also plays a part in the stimulation of transcription of uPA by c-ets. Perhaps, FGFs induce uPA by stimulating the interaction of transcription factors like c-ets with the PEA3 motif. FGF-2 may regulate uPA expression at both transcriptional and post-transcriptional levels. This is suggested by an experiment in which a mutant FGF-2 protein added to aortic endothelial cells was shown to up-regulate uPA mRNA production but not uPA activity. Only when heparin was added was uPA activity increased by the mutant FGF-2 (49). A putative scheme for FGF-2 action on uPA production is depicted in Fig. 11.2.

Is migration induced by FGF-2 dependent upon the induction of pro-uPA and a subsequent stimulation of the signal transduction through the uPA receptor? Recent data from our laboratory indicate that this might be the case. Odekon *et al.* (3) have demonstrated that pro-uPA is

induced by FGF-2 in bovine endothelial cells and that FGF-2-dependent cell migration is blocked by anti-FGF-2 antibodies. This indicates that uPA production and release is the general trigger for FGF-2-induced cell movement. It remains to be demonstrated whether this is valid only for a specific cell type or has general significance for FGF-2-induced cell migration.

The effect of FGF-2 on the PA system can be pharmacologically modulated. Angiostatic steroids inhibit PA activity induced by FGF-2 (50). The angiostatic steroid medroxyprogesterone at maximum inhibitory concentrations decreased PA levels by approximately 80%. This decrease was mediated by an induction of PAI-1. Thus, steroids may inhibit angiogenesis by increasing PAI-1 expression which, in turn, blocks PA activity.

Endogenous 18 kDa and high molecular weight fibroblast growth factor (FGF) 2

In addition to the 18 kDa FGF-2 form, high molecular weight FGF-2 (HMW FGF-2) forms were described in the placenta, guinea-pig brain, and in endothelial cells (51–54). Additional experiments revealed that the cloned FGF-2 RNA encoded additional 22, 22.5, and 24 kDa forms (HMW bFGF), whose translation initiates at CUG codons (55,56). HMW bFGF is primarily nuclear and 18 kDa bFGF cytoplasmic (57–59). Endothelial cells express all four forms of FGF-2. The level of expression of FGF-2 varies according to the origin of the endothelial cells; i.e. microvascular endothelial cells usually express more FGF-2 than macrovascular endothelial cells.

Because FGF-2 exists in high and low molecular weight forms, it is important to identify which form induces a given phenotype. HMW FGF-2 and 18 kDa FGF-2 both induce proliferation, migration, and PA production when added to cells (51,60,61). Endogenous FGF-2 forms, however, differentially affect the cell phenotype. This view derives from several experiments. First, the movement of bovine capillary endothelial cells is blocked with anti-FGF-2 antibodies (52). This suggests a role for endogenous FGF-2 in migration as well as an extracellular localization of FGF-2. Second, NIH 3T3 cells expressing all FGF-2 forms display enhanced migration that is abrogated with anti-FGF-2 antibodies (62). We have recently examined which FGF-2 form is responsible for a given phenotype, i.e. migration or proliferation, by establishing transfected cell lines expressing different FGF-2 isoforms and subsequently supertransfected with cDNAs expressing a truncated FGF receptor (60). Cells expressing 18 kDa bFGF demonstrated enhanced migration whereas cells expressing HMW FGF-2 did not. Cells expressing HMW FGF-2 grew in low serum, whereas cells expressing 18

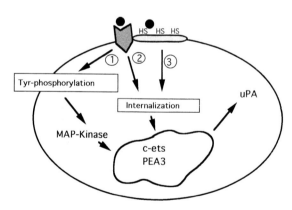

Figure 11.2. Potential mechanisms of action of fibroblast growth factor (FGF)-2 on urokinase plasminogen activator (uPA) production. 1, receptor-mediated activation at the cell surface; 2, internalization of FGF-2 by FGF receptors and possible intracellular (nuclear) stimulation of uPA production; 3, internalization of FGF-2 by heparin sulphate proteoglycans and intracellular (nuclear) stimulation of uPA production.

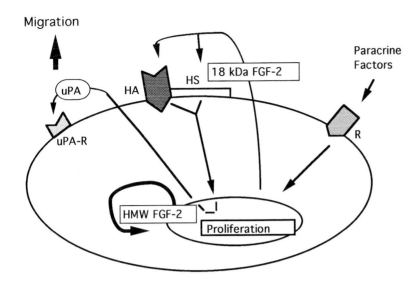

Figure 11.3. Model of the effect of endogenous fibroblast growth factor (FGF)-2 on cell phenotype and plasminogen activator production. HA, high-affinity FGF receptor; HS, heparan sulphates, R, receptor of paracrine growth factors.

kDa FGF-2 did not. Cells expressing HMW FGF-2 transfected with a cDNA encoding the 18 kDa FGF-2 form displayed an increase in migration. The properties related to 18 kDa FGF-2 could be reverted by the supertransfection with a dominant negative FGF receptor cDNA but those properties related to HMW FGF-2 expression could not. These results indicate that 18 kDa FGF-2 and HMW FGF-2 have different properties when expressed in cells and act through different pathways, i.e. receptor-dependent for 18 kDa FGF-2 and receptor-independent for HMW FGF-2. In our view it is unlikely that endogenous HMW FGF-2 will induce PA as cell movement is not affected by overexpression of HMW FGF-2 and anti-FGF-2 antibodies will inhibit endogenous PA production. The model of action of endogenous FGF-2 is depicted in Fig. 11.3.

FGF-2 must be released in order to interact with its cell surface receptor or heparan sulphates and to stimulate protease production. FGF-2 does not contain a signal sequence and is not released through the classical signal sequence pathway (62,63). Two models of FGF release have been proposed. In the first model, FGF is released after cell damage or wounding (64). Several tumours undergo cell death and necrosis at a certain stage of their development, and this might be a way by which FGF-2 reaches neighbouring endothelial cells. Another mechanism, the release by an alternative secretory pathway, has also been proposed (63). This hypothesis is based on the fact that, as stated above, the migration of single cells transfected with the cDNA encoding 18 kDa FGF-2 is inhibited by anti-FGF-2 antibodies (62). In addition, it has been shown that FGF-1 is released by heat shock from cells transfected with the FGF-1 cDNA (65). Dimerization has been postulated to be important for this release.

Fibrosarcoma cells release high amounts of FGF-2 at the onset of the angiogenic switch (66). Taken together, these data suggest that FGF-2 is possibly released as a paracrine or autocrine (endothelial cell-derived) growth factor and might then interact with the FGF receptor and heparan sulphates to induce migration and protease production.

Transforming growth factor -β

Another autocrine and paracrine growth regulator for endothelial cells is TGF-β. Endothelial cells express TGF-β as an inactive precursor consisting of the active homodimer plus the two propetides (latent TGF-β: LTGF-β) (Fig. 11.4). This high molecular weight complex is unable to interact with its receptor. In addition, another protein, named the latent TGF-β binding protein (LTBP), is covalently bound to the LTGF-β propeptide forming a complex of about 210 kDa. In order to be active, TGF-β must be released in the extracellular milieu. The mechanism of this activation has been extensively studied in our laboratory (for review see reference 67). Co-cultures of bovine endothelial cells and either pericytes or smooth muscle cells convert LTGF-β to TGF-β. Activation is species specific, requires cell to cell contact, proteases, and interaction of LTBP with the cell surface. TGF-β activation can be divided into two mechanisms, one plasmin-dependent, the other plasmin-independent. The plasmin-dependent pathway involves binding of TGF-β to mannose 6-phosphate receptors, cross-linking by tissue transglutaminase and cleavage by plasmin. Plasmin is generated by cell surface associated uPA from plasminogen. This activation occurs only in heterotypic cultures when endothelial cells

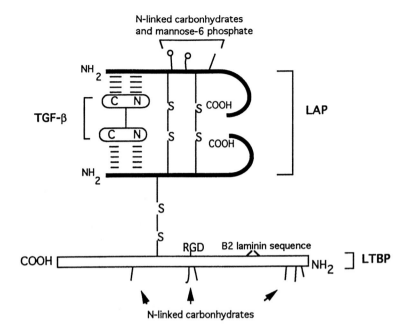

Figure 11.4. Structure of transforming growth factor (TGF) β. LAP, latency associated protein; LTBP, latent TGF-β binding protein.

are co-cultured with smooth muscle cells or pericytes. The second mechanism involves activation of TGF-β by thrombospondin (68). This activation does not require plasmin.

The effect of TGF-β on angiogenesis is controversial. Our laboratory has reported that TGF-β inhibits cell migration and stimulates PAI-1 production (69). In agreement with these data, Pepper *et al.* (70) have reported that TGF-β exhibits mainly anti-angiogenic effects *in vitro*, because the balance of uPA to PAI-1 favours an anti-proteolytic response. This finding correlates with an inhibition of tube-like structure formation, resulting in the formation of superficial cords devoid of a capillary lumen. In opposition, Iruela-Arispe and Sage (71) have reported that TGF-β induces capillary cord formation *in vitro*. These authors demonstrated that TGF-β induces proliferation of endothelial cells during cord formation. The population of cells within the cord was the selective target for TGF-β. In addition, active TGF-β was generated during cord formation. These different data may be reconciled by postulating that TGF-β plays either a stimulatory or inhibitory role on capillary cord formation under specific conditions but that TGF-β is certainly not required for intracapillary lumen formation.

Upon its formation, TGF-β may counteract the stimulatory effect of angiogenic molecules such as FGF-2. TGF-β1 antagonizes the stimulatory effects of FGF-2 by down-regulating uPA expression and by stimulating PAI-1 synthesis. This blocks extracellular proteolysis and the

plasmin-induced activation of TGF-β. However, when no TGF-β is generated, the effect of FGF-2 becomes predominant and protease production subsequently increases. This represents a self-regulatory system at two levels: (i) alternate cycles of activation or inhibition of extracellular proteolysis, and (ii) alternate cycles of release and/or activation of growth factors or growth inhibitors (Fig. 11.5).

Vascular endothelial growth factor

VEGF is a growth factor having high specificity for endothelial cells (for review see reference 72). Pepper *et al.* (73) have reported that VEGF stimulates uPA, tPA, and PAI-I expression in cultures of bovine capillary endothelial cells., However, PA production was not stimulated in human umbilical vein endothelial cells by VEGF (74). The reason for this difference probably lies in the clonal heterogeneity of endothelial cells. Pepper *et al.* (73) used bovine capillary endothelial cells that have been preselected with angiogenic growth factors, whereas Bikfalvi *et al.* (74) used primary cultures only grown in human serum and on fibronectin. The former cells are possibly enriched in VEGF-responsive cells, whereas the latter are a mixture of responsive and non-responsive cells.

It has been demonstrated that plasmin cleaves the large form of VEGF and releases it from its cell surface binding site into the medium (75). The cleavage is thought to occur

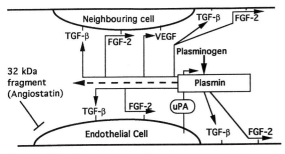

Figure 11.5. Plasmin-dependent cleavage and release of angiogenic growth factors. Plasmin generated by endothelial cell-derived urokinase-type plasminogen activator (uPA) may cleave-off cell surface or matrix-associated fibroblast growth factor (FGF)-2 or vascular endothelial growth factor (VEGF). FGF-2 will be cleaved-off as a proteoheparan sulphate/FGF complex, whereas a small VEGF form not associated with proteoheparan sulphate, is cleaved from the large VEGF form. Cleavage might occur at the surface or in the matrix of endothelial cells or neighbouring cells. FGF-2 or VEGF released from the cell surface or matrix will provide a positive angiogenic stimulus. Angiogenesis is negatively controlled by the generation of active transforming growth factor (TGF) β released by plasmin from its latent complex. Activation may occur at the cell surface or in the extracellular matrix.

at the site of the VEGF-producing cell and activates the molecule. Activated VEGF may then interact with neighbouring endothelial cells and stimulate angiogenesis.

Hepatocyte growth factor

Another angiogenic factor and modulator of PA production is hepatocyte growth factor (HGF), also known as scatter factor. Cultured microvascular endothelial cells accumulate and secrete significant quantities of uPA upon HGF stimulation (76). In combination with other growth factors such as TGF-β and FGF-2, HGF may act to maximize the angiogenic stimulus. uPA may also activate the inactive precursor of HGF.

Summary and conclusions

We have summarized recent findings about the role of the PA system and of proteases activating growth factors in angiogenesis. The following conclusions may be derived from these studies.

First, there are many converging data indicating a central role for the PA system in angiogenesis. The PA system modulates angiogenesis by acting on migration, invasion, and possibly lumen formation. Migration may be triggered by pro-uPA and this might be achieved by signal transduction through the uPA receptor. In epithelial cells, phosphorylation of intermediate filaments through PKC ε activation has been shown to be important. It is possible that an analogous activation cascade operates in endothelial cells. Plasmin generated by the action of uPA will degrade matrix and will allow invasion to occur. In in vitro angiogenic systems using fibrin gels, lumen formation is dependent on the balance between uPA and PAI-1.

Second, the factors regulating PA or its inhibitor expression by endothelial cells include FGFs, TGF-β, and VEGF. Several FGF-2 isoforms have been described. Migration and PA can be induced by 18 kDa FGF-2 and HMW FGF-2 when added to cells. Endogenous FGF-2 isoforms affect the cell phenotype differentially; the 18 kDa form induces migration, whereas the HMW form affects proliferation. Several mechanisms for the induction of uPA by FGF-2 have been proposed. These are activation of the FGF receptor and signalling at the cell surface, nuclear translocation of the FGF receptor/FGF-2 complex, and signalling through heparan sulphates. Further experiments will decide which of these possibilities is valid. TGF-β induces predominantly PAI-1. The extent of induction is dependent on the extracellular TGF-β concentrations.

Third, several feedback loops dependent on the PA system exist. These are: (i) liberation of matrix or cell surface bound FGF-2; (ii) cleavage of the large form of cell surface bound VEGF and its release; (iii) activation of TGF-β from the large latent complex; and (iv) generation of a 32 kDa plasmin fragment that functions as an angiogenic inhibitor. Whereas the two former loops provide positive angiogenic control, the two latter provide negative controls. Cell surface or matrix bound FGF-2 may be liberated by plasmin in an active form and subsequently be associated with the high-affinity receptor. The high molecular weight cell surface bound form of VEGF is active once liberated from the ECM by the action of plasmin and may stimulate endothelial cells by a paracrine mechanism. The plasminogen fragment, angiostatin, is a potent inhibitor of endothelial cell proliferation and differentiation. This fragment may control suppression of angiogenesis in several tumours before the onset of the angiogenic switch. Tumour angiogenesis in metastatic foci may be initiated by the loss of this inhibitor. How this fragment is generated in vivo is at present unclear. It is possible that a not yet identified tumour-derived protease may be released from the primary tumour to generate angiostatin by proteolytic cleavage of plasminogen. The activation of TGF-β requires co-culture conditions, binding to mannose 6-phosphate receptors and cross-linking to the cell surface by transglutaminase. Activated TGF-β will negatively influence PA and will balance the ratio of uPA/PAI-1 in favour of the inhibitor.

Fourth, angiogenic growth factors and proteases are integrated in self-regulatory systems. Protease production may be sequentially switched on or off by the protease-dependent release or activation of FGF-2 and TGF-β. On the other hand, FGF-2 and TGF-β activity is controlled by proteases. This will not only allow feedback regulation of protease activity but also control other properties induced by these growth factors.

Acknowledgements

This work was supported by grants from the National Institutes of Health (NOS CA29753 and CA34282) and the Juvenile Diabetes Foundation (194169) to D.B.R., and the International Agency for Cancer Research (WHO) to A.B. S.K. was supported by NIH grant (No. 5T32GM07238–19) and a Berlex student fellowship. G.P. was a recipient of a fellowship from the Regional Council of Abruzzo (Italy) and the Commission of the European Communities (CEE/Abruzzo).

References

1. Mignatti, P. and Rifkin, D. B. (1993). Biology and biochemistry of proteinases in tumor invasion. *Physiol. Rev.*, **73**, 161–95.
2. Vassalli, J. D., Sappino, A-P., and Belin, D. (1991). The plasminogen activator/plasmin system. *J. Clin. Invest.*, **88**, 1067–72.
3. Odekon, L. E., Sato, Y., and Rifkin, D. B. (1992). Urokinase-type plasminogen activator mediates basic fibroblast growth factor-induced bovine endothelial cell migration independent of its proteolytic activity. *J. Cell. Physiol.*, **150**, 258–63.
4. Busso, N., Masur, S. K., Lazega, D., Waxman, S., and Ossowski, L. (1994). Induction of cell migration by pro-urokinase binding to its receptor: possible mechanism for signal transduction in human epithelial cells. *J. Cell. Biol.*, **126**, 259–70.
5. Flaumenhaft, R., Abe, M., Mignatti, P., and Rifkin, D. B. (1992). Basic fibroblast growth factor-induced activation of latent transforming growth factor beta in endothelial cells: regulation of plasminogen activator activity. *J. Cell Biol.*, **118**, 901–9.
6. Montesano, R., Pepper, M. S., Vassalli, J. D., and Orci, L. (1992). Modulation of angiogenesis *in vitro*. *EXS*, **61**, 129–36.
7. Pepper, M. S. and Montesano, R. (1990). Proteolytic balance and capillary morphogenesis. *Cell Differ. Dev.*, **32**, 319–27.
8. Behrendt, N., Ronne, E., Ploug, M., Petri, T., Lober, D., Nielsen, L. S., *et al.* (1990). The human receptor for urokinase plasminogen activator. NH₂-terminal amino acid sequence and glycosylation variants. *J. Biol. Chem.*, **265**, 6453–60.
9. Estreicher, A., Muhlhauser, J., Carpentier, J. L., Orci, L., and Vassalli, J-D. (1990). The receptor for urokinase type plasminogen activator polarizes expression of the protease to the leading edge of migrating monocytes and promotes degradation of enzyme-inhibitor complexes. *J. Cell Biol.*, **111**, 783–92.
10. Roldan, A. L., Cubellis, M. V., Masucci, M. T., Behrendt, N., Lund, L. R., Dano, K., *et al.* (1990). Cloning and expression of the receptor for human urokinase plasminogen activator, a central molecule in cell surface, plasmin-dependent proteolysis. *EMBO J.*, **9**, 467–74.
11. Appella, E., Robinson, E. A., Ullrich, S. J., Stoppelli, M. P., Corti, A., Cassani, G., and Blasi, F. (1987). The receptor-binding sequence of urokinase. A biological function for the growth-factor module of proteases. *J. Biol. Chem.*, **262**, 4437–40.
12. Kobayashi, H., Schmitt, M., Goretzki, L., Chucholowski, N., Calvete, J., Kramer M., *et al.* (1991). Cathepsin B efficiently activates the soluble and the tumor cell receptor-bound form of the proenzyme urokinase-type plasminogen activator (Pro-uPA). *J. Biol. Chem.*, **266**, 5147–52.
13. Pepper, M. S., Sappinio, A. P., Montesano, R., Orci, L., and Vassalli, J-D. (1992). Plasminogen activator inhibitor-1 is induced in migrating endothelial cells. *J. Cell. Physiol.*, **153**, 129–39.
14. Ehrlich, H. J., Klein Gebbink, R., Preissner, K. T, Keijer, J., Esmon, N. L., Mertens, K., and Pannekoek, H. (1991). Thrombin neutralizes plasminogen activator inhibitor 1 (PAI-1) that is complexed with vitronectin in the endothelial cell matrix. *J. Cell Biol.*, **115**, 1773–81.
15. Pintucci, G., Iacoviello, L., Castelli, M. P., Amore, C., Evangelista, V., Cerletti, C., and Donati, M. B. (1993). Cathepsin G-induced release of PAI-1 in the culture medium of endothelial cells: a new thrombogenic role for polymorphonuclear leukocytes? *J. Lab. Clin. Med.*, **122**, 69–79.
16. Axelrod, J. H., Reich, R., and Miskin, R. (1989). Expression of the human recombinant plasminogen activators enhances invasion and experimental metastasis of H-ras-transformed NIH 3T3 cells. *Mol. Cell. Biol.*, **9**, 2133–41.
17. Ossowski, L., Clunie, G., Masucci, M. T., and Blasi, F. (1991). *In vivo* paracrine interaction between urokinase and its receptor: effect on tumor cell invasion. *J. Cell Biol.*, **115**, 1107–12.
18. Kook, Y. H., Adamski, J., Zelent, A., and Ossowski, L. (1994). The effect of antisense inhibition of urokinase receptor in human squamous cell carcinoma on malignancy. *EMBO J.*, **13**, 3983–91.
19. Pepper, M. S., Belin, D., Montesano, R., Orci, L., Vassalli, J. D. (1990). Transforming growth factor β1 modulates basic fibroblast growth factor -induced proteolytic and angiogenic properties of endothelial cells *in vitro*. *J. Cell Biol.*, **111**, 743–55.
20. Dubois-Stringfellow, N., Jonczyk, A., and Bautch, V. L. (1994). Perturbations in the fibrinolytic pathway abolish cyst formation but not capillary-like organization of cultured murine endothelial cells. *Blood*, **83**, 3206–17.
21. Bikfalvi, A., Cramer, E. M., Tenza, D., and Tobelem, G. (1991). Phenotypic modulation of human umbilical vein endothelial cells and human dermal fibroblasts using two angiogenic assays. *Biol. Cell*, **72**, 275–8.
22. Wernert, N., Raes, M. B., Lassalle, P., Dehouck, M. P., Gosselin, B., Vandenbunder, B., and Stehelin, D. (1992). C-ets1 proto-oncogene is a transcription factor expressed in endothelial cells during tumor vascularization and other

forms of angiogenesis in humans. *Am. J. Pathol.*, **140**, 119–27.

23. Bacharach, E., Itin, A., and Keshet, E. (1992). *In vivo* patterns of expression of urokinase and its inhibitor PAI-1 suggest a concerted role in regulating physiological angiogenesis. *Proc. Natl Acad. Sci. USA*, **89**, 10686–90.

24. Carmeliet, P., Schoonjans, L., Kieckens, L., Ream, B., Degen, J., Bronson, R., *et al.* (1994). Physiological consequences of loss of plasminogen activator gene function in mice. *Nature*, **368**, 419–24.

25. O'Reilly, M. S., Holmgren, L., Shin, Y., Chen, C., Rosenthal, R. A., Moses, M., *et al.* (1994). Angiostatin: a novel angiogenesis inhibitor that mediates the suppression of metastasis by a Lewis lung carcinoma. *Cell*, **79**, 315–28.

26. Basilico, C. and Moscatelli, D. (1992). The FGF family of growth factors and oncogenes. *Adv. Cancer Res.*, **59**, 115–65.

27. Miyamoto, M., Naruo, K., Seko, C., Matsumoto, S., Kondo, T., and Kurokawa, T. (1993). Molecular cloning of a novel cytokine cDNA encoding the ninth member of the fibroblast growth factor family, which has a unique secretion property. *Mol. Cell. Biol.*, **13**, 4251–9.

28. Abraham, J. A., Mergia, A., Whang, J. L., Tumolo, A., Friedman, J., Hjerrild, K. A., *et al.* (1986). Nucleotide sequence of a bovine clone encoding the angiogenic protein, basic fibroblast growth factor. *Science*, **233**, 545–8.

29. Burrus, L. W., Zuber, M. E., Lueddecke, B. A., and Olwin, B. B. (1992). Identification of a cysteine-rich receptor for fibroblast growth factors. *Mol. Cell. Biol.*, **12**, 5600–9.

30. Mignatti, P., Mazzieri, R., and Rifkin, D. B. (1991). Expression of the urokinase receptor in vascular endothelial cells is stimulated by basic fibroblast growth factor. *J. Cell Biol.*, **113**, 1193–1201.

31. Vlodavsky, I., Folkman, J., Sullivan, R., Fridman, R., Ishai-Michaeli, R., Sasse, J., and Klagsbrun, M. (1987). Endothelial cell-derived basic fibroblast growth factor: synthesis and deposition into the subendothelial extracellular matrix. *Proc. Natl Acad. Sci. USA*, **84**, 2292–6.

32. Yayon, A., Klagsbrun, M., Esko, J. D., Leder, P., and Ornitz, D. M. (1991). Cell surface, heparin-like molecules are required for binding of basic fibroblast growth factor to its high affinity receptor. *Cell*, **64**, 841–8.

33. Ornitz, D. M., Yayon, A., Flanagan, J. G., Svahn, C. M., Levi, E., and Leder, P. (1992). Heparin is required for cell-free binding of basic fibroblast growth factor to a soluble receptor and for mitogenesis in whole cells. *Mol. Cell. Biol.*, **12**, 240–7.

34. Roghani, M., Mansukhani, A., Dell'Era, P., Bellosta, P., Basilico, C., Rifkin D. B., and Moscatelli, D. (1994). Heparin increases the affinity of basic fibroblast growth factor for its receptor but is not required for binding. *J. Biol. Chem.*, **269**, 3976–84.

35. Rapraeger, A. C., Krufka, A., and Olwin, B. B. (1991). Requirement of heparan sulfate for basic fibroblast growth factor-mediated fibroblast growth and myoblast differentiation. *Science*, **252**, 1705–8.

36. Spivak-Kroizmann, T., Lemmon, M. A., Dikic, I., Ladbury, J. E., Pinchasi, D., Huang, J., *et al.* (1994). Heparin-induced oligomerization of FGF molecules is responsible for FGF receptor dimerization, activation, and proliferation. *Cell*, **79**, 1015–24.

37. Aviezer, D., Hecht, D., Safran, M., Eisinger, M., David, G., and Yayon, A. (1994). Perlecan, basal lamina proteoglycan, promotes basic fibroblast growth factor-receptor binding, mitogenesis, and angiogenesis. *Cell*, **79**, 1005–13.

38. Knudsen, B. S., Silverstein, R. L., Leung, L. L., Harpel, P. C., and Nachman, R. L. (1986). Binding of plasminogen to extracellular matrix. *J. Biol. Chem.*, **261**, 10765–71.

39. Mimuro, J. and Loskutoff, D. J. (1989). Binding of type 1 plasminogen activator inhibitor to the extracellular matrix of cultured bovine endothelial cells. *J. Biol. Chem.*, **264**, 5058–63.

40. Saksela, O. and Rifkin, D. B. (1990). Release of basic fibroblast growth factor — heparan sulfate complexes from endothelial cells by plasminogen activator-mediated proteolytic activity. *J. Cell Biol.*, **110**, 767–75.

41. Vlodavsky, I., Fuks, Z., Bar-Ner, M., Ariav, Y., and Schirrmacher, V. (1983). Lymphoma cell-mediated degradation of sulfated proteoglycans in the subendothelial extracellular matrix: relationship to tumor cell metastases. *Cancer Res.*, **43**, 2704–11.

42. Brunner, G., Gabrilove, J., Rifkin, D. B., and Wilson, E. L. (1991). Phospholipase C release of basic fibroblast growth factor from human bone marrow cultures as a biologically active complex with a phosphatidylinositol anchored heparan sulfate proteoglycan. *J. Cell Biol.*, **114**, 1275–83.

43. Brunner, G., Metz, C. N., Nguyen, H., Gabrilove, J., Patel, S. R., Davitz, M. A., *et al.* (1994). An endogenous glycosylphosphatidylinositol-specific phospholipase D releases basic fibroblast growth factor–heparan sulfate proteoglycan complexes from human bone marrow cultures. *Blood*, **83**, 2115–25.

44. Benezra, M., Vlodavsky, I., Ishai-Michaeli, R., Neufeld, G., and Bar-Shavit, R. (1993). Thrombin-induced release of active basic fibroblast growth factor–heparan sulfate complexes from subendothelial extracellular matrix. *Blood*, **81**, 3324–31.

45. Totani, L., Piccoli, A., Pellegrini, G., Di Santo, A., and Lorenzet, R. (1994). Polymorphonuclear leukocytes enhance release of growth factors by cultured endothelial cells. *Arterioscler. Thromb.*, **14**, 125–32.

46. Quarto, N. and Amalric, F. (1994). Heparan sulfate proteoglycans (HSPGs) as transducers of FGF-2 signalling. *J. Cell Sci.*, **107**, 3201–12.

47. Isacchi, A., Statuto, M., Chiesa, R., Bergonzoni, L., Rusnati, M., Sarmientos, P., *et al.* (1991). A six-amino acid deletion in basic fibroblast growth factor dissociates its mitogenic activity from its plasminogen activator-inducing capacity. *Proc. Natl Acad. Sci. USA*, **88**, 2628–32.

48. Presta, M., Maier, J. A. M., and Ragnotti, G. (1989). The mitogenic signaling pathway but not the plasminogen activator-inducing pathway of basic fibroblast growth factor is mediated through protein kinase C in fetal bovine aortic endothelial cells. *J. Cell Biol.*, **109**, 1877–84.

49. Gualandis, A. and Presta, M. (1995). Transcriptional and posttranscriptional regulation of urokinase-type plasminogen activator expression in endothelial cells by basic fibroblast growth factor. *J. Cell. Physiol.*, **162**, 400–9.

50. Blei, F., Wilson, E. L., Mignatti, P., and Rifkin, D. B. (1993). Mechanism of action of angiostatic steroids: suppression of plasminogen activator activity via stimulation of plasminogen activator inhibitor synthesis. *J. Cell. Physiol.*, **155**, 568–78.

51. Moscatelli, D., Joseph-Silverstein, J., Manejias, R., and Rifkin, D. B. (1987). Mr 25 000 heparin-binding protein from guinea pig brain is a high molecular weight form of basic fibroblast growth factor. *Proc. Natl Acad. Sci. USA*, **84**, 5778–82.

52. Sato, Y. and Rifkin, D. B. (1988). Autocrine activities of basic fibroblast growth factor: regulation of endothelial cell movement, plasminogen activator synthesis, and DNA synthesis. *J. Cell Biol.*, **107**, 1199–205.

53. Bikfalvi, A., Alterio, J., Inyang, A. L., Dupuy, E., Laurent, M., Hartmann, M. P., *et al.* (1990). Basic fibroblast growth factor expression in human omental microvascular endothelial cells and the effect of phorbol ester. *J. Cell. Physiol.*, **144**, 151–8.

54. Moscatelli, D., Presta, M., and Rifkin, D. B. (1986). Purification of a factor from human placenta that stimulates capillary endothelial cell protease production, DNA synthesis, and migration. *Proc. Natl Acad. Sci. USA*, **83**, 2091–5.

55. Florkiewicz, R. Z. and Sommer, A. (1989). Human basic fibroblast growth factor gene encodes four polypeptides: three initiate translation from non-AUG codons. *Proc. Natl Acad. Sci. USA*, **86**, 3978–81.

56. Prats, H., Kaghad, M., Prats, A. C., Klagsbrun, M., Lelias, J. M., Liauzun, P., *et al.* (1989). High molecular mass forms of basic fibroblast growth factor are initiated by alternative CUG codons. *Proc. Natl Acad. Sci. USA*, **86**, 1836–40.

57. Quarto, N., Finger, F. P., and Rifkin, D. B. (1991). The NH2-terminal extension of high molecular weight bFGF is a nuclear targeting signal. *J. Cell. Physiol.*, **147**, 311–18.

58. Renko, M., Quarto, N., Marimoto, T., and Rifkin, D. B. (1990). Nuclear and cytoplasmic localization of different basic fibroblast growth factor species. *J. Cell. Physiol.*, **144**, 108–14.

59. Florkiewicz, R. Z., Baird, A., and Gonzalez, A-M. (1991). Multiple forms of bFGF: differential nuclear and cell surface localization. *Growth Factors*, **4**, 265–75.

60. Bikfalvi, A., Klein, S., Pintucci, G., Quarto, N., Mignatti, P., and Rifkin, D. B. (1995). Differential modulation of cell phenotype by different molecular weight forms of basic fibroblast growth factor: possible intracellular signaling by the high molecular weight forms. *J. Cell Biol.*, **129**, 233–43.

61. Rifkin, D. B., Moscatelli, D., Roghani, M., Nagano, Y., Quarto, N., Klein, S., and Bikfalvi, A. (1994). Studies on FGF-2: Nuclear localization and function of high molecular weight forms and receptor binding in the absence of heparin. *Mol. Reprod. Dev.*, **39**, 102–5.

62. Mignatti, P., Morimoto, T., and Rifkin, D. B. (1991). Basic fibroblast growth factor released by single, isolated cells stimulates their migration in an autocrine manner. *Proc. Natl Acad. Sci. USA*, **88**, 11007–11.

63. Mignatti, P., Morimoto, T., and Rifkin, D. B. (1992). Basic fibroblast growth factor, a protein devoid of secretory signal sequence, is released by cells via a pathway independent of the endoplasmic reticulum–Golgi complex. *J. Cell. Physiol.*, **151**, 81–93.

64. McNeil, P. L., Muthukrishnan, L., Warder, E., and D'Amore, P. A. (1989). Growth factors are released by mechanically wounded endothelial cells. *J. Cell Biol.*, **109**, 811–22.

65. Maciag, T., Zhan, X., Garfinkel, S., Friedman, S., Prudovsky, I., Jackson, A., *et al.* (1994). Novel mechanism of fibroblast growth factor 1 function. *Recent Prog. Horm. Res.* **49**, 105–23.

66. Kandel, J., Bossy-Wetzel, E., Radvanyi, F., Klagsbrun, M., Folkman, J., and Hanahan, D. (1991). Neovascularization is associated with a switch to the export of bFGF in the multistep development of fibrosarcoma. *Cell*, **66**, 1095–104.

67. Rifkin, D. B., Kojima, S., Abe, M., Harpel, J. G. (1993). TGF-β: structure, function, and formation. *Thromb. Haemost.*, **70**, 177–9.

68. Schultz-Cherry, S. and Murphy-Ullrich, J. E. (1993). Thrombospondin causes activation of latent transforming growth factor-β secreted by endothelial cells by a novel mechanism. *J. Cell Biol.*, **122**, 923–32.

69. Sato, Y., Tsuboi, R., Lyons, R., Moses, H., and Rifkin, D. B. (1990). Characterization of the activation of latent TGF-β by co-cultures of endothelial cells and pericytes or smooth muscle cells: a self-regulatory system. *J. Cell Biol.*, **111**, 757–63.

70. Pepper, M. S., Belin, D., Montesano, R., Orci, L., and Vassalli, J-D. (1990). Transforming growth factor-β1 modulates basic fibroblast growth factor-induced proteolytic and angiogenic properties of endothelial cells *in vitro*. *J. Cell Biol.*, **111**, 743–55.

71. Iruela-Arispe, M. L. and Sage, E. H. (1993). Endothelial cells exhibiting angiogenesis *in vitro* proliferate in response to TGF-β1. *J. Cell. Biochem.*, **52**, 414–30.

72. Ferrara, N., Houck, K., Jakeman, L., and Leung, D. W. (1992). Molecular and biological properties of the vascular endothelial growth factor family of proteins. *Endocr. Rev.*, **13**, 18–32.

73. Pepper, M. S., Ferrara, N., Orci, L., and Montesano, R. (1991). Vascular endothelial growth factor (VEGF) induces plasminogen activators and plasminogen activator inhibitor type 1 in microvascular endothelial cells. *Biochem. Biophys. Res. Commun.*, **181**, 902–8.

74. Bikfalvi, A., Sauzeau, C., Moukadiri, H., Maclouf, J., Busso, N., Bryckaert, M., *et al.* (1991). Interaction of vasculotropin/vascular endothelial cell growth factor with human umbilical vein endothelial cells: binding, internalization, degradation, and biological effects. *J. Cell. Physiol.*, **149**, 50–9.

75. Houck, K. A., Leung, D. W., Rowland, A. M., Winer, J., and Ferrara, N. (1992). Dual regulation of vascular endothelial growth factor bioavailability by genetic and proteolytic mechanisms. *J. Biol. Chem.*, **267**, 26031–7.

76. Grant, D. S., Kleinman, H. K., Goldberg, I. D., Bhargava, M. M., Nickoloff, B. J., Kinsella, J. L., *et al.* (1993). Scatter factor induces blood vessel formation *in vivo*. *Proc. Natl Acad. Sci. USA*, **90**, 1937–41.

12. Involvement of the extracellular matrix, heparan sulphate proteoglycans, and heparan sulphate degrading enzymes in angiogenesis and metastasis

Israel Vlodavsky, Hua-Quan Miao, Miriam Benezra, Ofer Lider, Rachel Bar-Shavit, Annette Schmidt, and Tamar Peretz

Introduction

Basement membranes (BM) and extracellular matrices (ECMs) are the natural substrates upon which cells migrate, proliferate, and differentiate *in vivo*. Historically, the ECM was regarded as a relatively inert scaffolding which stabilizes the physical structure of tissues. Subsequent studies aimed to elucidate the mode of cellular responses to ECM indicated that the ability of cells to respond to various growth and differentiation factors is determined to a large extent by their shape and orientation and that these are modulated by components of the ECM through interaction with specific transmembrane cell surface integrin receptors (1–4). Studies with mammary gland epithelial cells led to the identification of genes that are dependent upon the ECM for their transcription and to the discovery of 'ECM-response elements' (5). It was demonstrated, for example, that ECM-induced expression of β-casein involves an 'ECM response element' in the promoter of the casein gene that is activated by integrin-mediated signalling (5,6). Studies by Ingber and colleagues (7) postulated that mechanical forces generated through cell–ECM interaction could produce an altered cytoskeleton and nuclear morphology and ultimately changes in the pattern of gene expression. Based on these and other observations, it is recognized that the ECM plays an active and complex part in regulating the morphogenesis of cells that contact it, influencing their development, migration, proliferation, and metabolic functions. It appears that cellular responses to ECM are mediated by the combined action of BM macromolecules (i.e. collagen IV, laminin, nidogen/entactin, proteoglycans) and active molecules (i.e.

growth factors, enzymes) that are immobilized and stored in the ECM by means of binding to its macromolecular constituents, primarily to heparan sulphate proteoglycans (HSPG) (8–11). Heparan sulphate (HS) also contributes to the assembly and integrity of the ECM through binding to various ECM molecules including the fibrillar interstitial collagens (types I, III, and V), fibronectin, laminin, thrombospondin, and tenascin. The ability of HSPG to interact with ECM macromolecules such as collagen, laminin, and fibronectin and with different attachment sites on plasma membranes suggests a key role for this proteoglycan in the self-assembly and insolubility of ECM components, as well as in cell adhesion and locomotion. HSPG are prominent components of blood vessels (12). In large blood vessels they are concentrated mostly in the intima and inner media whereas in capillaries they are found mainly in the subendothelial BM where they support proliferating and migrating endothelial cells and stabilize the structure of the capillary wall. Cleavage of HS may therefore result in disassembly of the subendothelial ECM and hence may play a decisive part in extravasation of blood-borne cells. HSPGs such as syndecan, glypican, and ryudocan are abundant on the luminal surface of endothelial cells (ECs) (12) and have multiple functions there. They interact with plasma protease inhibitors to maintain a non-thrombogenic lining to the vascular system (13). They also interact with heparin-binding angiogenic factors (8,14,15) and are believed to contribute to lipid metabolism by interacting with lipoproteins and lipoprotein lipase (16).

In the present review, we discuss the roles of ECM adhesive interactions, ECM-degrading enzymes and ECM-resident growth factors and enzymes in tumour progression. More specifically, we focus primarily on the involvement of HSPG, HS-degrading enzymes, heparin-like molecules, and heparin/HS-binding growth factors in tumour cell metastasis and angiogenesis.

Modulation of angiogenesis by extracellular matrix constituents and cell matrix interactions

Extracellular matrix constituents

Degradation and remodelling of the ECM are essential processes for angiogenesis. The existing matrix around the vessel must be degraded to allow EC migration into the perivascular space. This degradation is achieved at least in part by collagenases and other metalloendoproteinases. Their activity is regulated by gene expression levels, conversion from latent to active forms, and inhibition by tissue inhibitors of metalloproteinases (TIMPs) (17,18). In addition, ECM components synthesized by endothelial cells [i.e. collagens, laminin, thrombospondin, fibronectin, and SPARC (secreted protein, acidic and rich in cysteine)] function to regulate endothelial cell growth, migration, and shape (19).

The role of fibronectin in vessel growth has been investigated using the rat aortic explant assay. Endothelial sprouts growing out of the aortic ring were found to be surrounded by a sheath of fibronectin that appeared to provide a rudimentary matrix. As the cultures aged, laminin and type IV collagen were detected (20). Peptides containing the Arg-Gly-Asp (RGD) motif inhibited microvessel growth (21), consistent with a role for fibronectin and other RGD-containing molecules in angiogenesis. SPARC is a transiently expressed ECM glycoprotein that differs from typical ECM proteins in that it is anti-adhesive and can disrupt focal adhesions (22,23). A fragment of SPARC (amino acids 113–130) and the Cu^{2+}-binding peptide KGHK contained within this fragment was found to stimulate the growth of microvessels in the chorioallantoic membrane (CAM) assay (23), suggesting that degradation of SPARC by proteases releases angiogenic fragments that then direct the reorganization of endothelial cells into new vessels.

ECM constituents may also inhibit angiogenesis. Thrombospondin, a 450 kDa trimeric glycoprotein secreted into the ECM by various cell types including ECs, inhibits both neovascularization in the rat cornea and migration of capillary endothelial cells *in vitro* (22). Specific domains of thrombospondin with anti-angiogenic activity have been identified by *in vitro* and *in vivo* assays (25).

Cell adhesion molecules in angiogenesis

Interactions between plasma membranes of adjacent ECs as well as intracellular adhesion between regions of plasma membrane must occur in order to extend a capillary blood vessel and enable lumen formation (19). Likewise, inter-actions must occur between ECs and the surrounding matrix molecules, which provide a scaffold for the ECs of the new vessel (19). Both selectins and integrins are involved in these interactions. Antibodies against bovine E-selectin, but not P-selectin, were found to inhibit tube formation, suggesting that E-selectin and a ligand containing sialyl Lewis X/A participate in capillary formation (19,26). Integrin expression and function in human umbilical ECs has been investigated by several laboratories. The integrin heterodimers, $\alpha_2\beta_1$, a receptor for collagens and laminin, and $\alpha_5\beta_1$, a receptor for fibronectin, have been detected at sites of intercellular contact and were found to regulate the integrity and permeability of the monolayer, but are not involved in cell attachment to the substratum (27). It has also been demonstrated that strong adhesion to ECM promotes growth by restraining the cells in a monolayer configuration while less adhesive surfaces allow differentiation into capillary tubes (2,28). Integrins have also been shown to function *in vivo* in vasculogenesis and angiogenesis. Injection of a neutralizing antibody against the β_1 subunit blocked formation of an aortic lumen in quail embryos (29). The angioblasts assembled into a cord-like structure but failed to develop into a patent vessel. Using the CAM assay for avian angiogenesis, Cheresh and colleagues have provided evidence suggesting that $\alpha_v\beta_3$ is required for blood vessel growth (30). An antibody against the $\alpha_v\beta_3$ integrin complex inhibited normal vessel growth and also basic fibroblast growth factor (bFGF)-stimulated or tumour-induced angiogenesis in the CAM assay, but did not disrupt pre-existing vessels. It was found that $\alpha_v\beta_3$ integrin is expressed in growing vessels and participates in angiogenesis but is not present in mature vessels. In a subsequent study, a single intravascular injection of a cyclic RGD peptide or monoclonal antibody antagonist of integrin $\alpha_v\beta_3$ lead to the rapid regression of histologically distinct human tumours transplanted into the CAM (31). Induction of angiogenesis by a tumour or cytokine was found to promote vascular cell entry into the cell cycle and expression of integrin $\alpha_v\beta_3$. After angiogenesis is initiated, antagonists of this integrin induce apoptosis of the proliferative angiogenic vascular cells, leaving pre-existing quiescent blood vessels unaffected. Antagonists of intergrin $\alpha_v\beta_3$ may thus provide a therapeutic approach for the treatment of neoplasia or other diseases characterized by angiogenesis (31).

Extracellular matrix-resident growth factors, cytokines, and growth-factor-binding proteins

Fibroblast growth factors

Fibroblast growth factors (FGFs) comprise a family of ten structurally related polypeptides characterized by high affinity to heparin. They are highly mitogenic for meso-derm- and neuroectoderm-derived cells and are among the most potent inducers of neovascularization and mesenchyme formation (32–34). This gene family includes the prototypes acidic fibroblast growth factor (aFGF) and bFGF which, unlike most other polypeptide growth factors, are primarily cell-associated proteins consistent with the lack of a conventional signal sequence for secretion. Four high-affinity cell surface FGF receptors with intrinsic tyrosine kinase activities were identified, as were low-affinity receptors that consist of HSPG (32–34). Species of heparin and HS promote dimerization and receptor binding of bFGF (35,36) as well as bFGF-mediated mitogenesis in HS-deficient lymphoid cells (36), suggesting that bFGF–HSPG complexes serve as the biologically active form of this growth factor. Cell surface heparin-like molecules are also involved in binding of vascular endothelial growth factor (VEGF) (15) and heparin-binding EGF (HB-EGF) (37) to its high-affinity receptor sites. Despite the ubiquitous presence of bFGF in normal tissues, EC proliferation in these tissues is usually very low, with turnover time measured in years. This raises the question of how these EC growth factors are prevented from acting on the vascular endothelium continuously and in response to what signals do they become available for stimulation of capillary EC proliferation. One possibility is that intracellular FGF may be released in response to a mild cell damage and certain stress conditions associated with tissue injury, irradiation, inflammation, shear force, and tumour necrosis. The released factor may then be sequestered from its site of action by means of binding to HS (14,38) and bFGF receptor proteins (39) in the ECM and saved for emergencies, such as wound repair and neovascularization (Fig. 12.1) (9).

Basic fibroblast growth factor is stored within basement membranes and extracellular matrices

Our studies on the control of cell proliferation and tumour progression by its local environment, focused on the interaction of cells with the ECM produced by cultured corneal and vascular ECs (40,41). This ECM closely resembles the subendothelium *in vivo* in its morphology and molecular composition. It contains primarily collagens (mostly types III and IV, with smaller amounts of types I and V), proteoglycans (mostly HS and dermatan sulphate proteoglycans, with smaller amounts of chondroitin sulphate proteoglycans), laminin, fibronectin, entactin, and elastin. Vascular ECs and other cell types plated in contact with the subendothelial ECM, no longer require the addition of soluble FGF and/or other growth-promoting factors in order to proliferate and express their differentiated functions (42). The presence of HS as a major glycosaminoglycan (GAG) in the subendothelial ECM raised the possibility that ECM

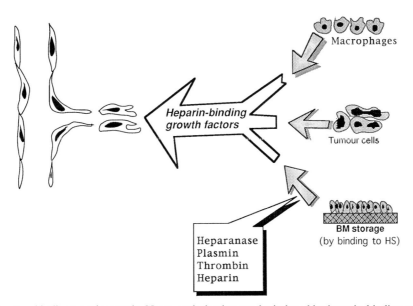

Figure 12.1. Direct and indirect angiogenesis. Neovascularization can be induced by heparin-binding growth factors produced by tumour cells and cells of the immune system (i.e. macrophages) and/or released from basement membrane (BM) and extracellular matrix by various enzymes (i.e. heparanase, collagenase, plasmin, thrombin) and heparin-like molecules. HS, heparan sulphate.

contains heparin-binding EC growth factors that are tightly bound and stabilized by the ECM-HS. In subsequent studies, bFGF was extracted from the subendothelial ECM produced *in vitro* (41) and from BM of the cornea (43), suggesting that ECM may serve as a reservoir for bFGF. Moreover, we have demonstrated that bFGF is an ECM component required for supporting EC proliferation (44), neuronal differentiation, and protection of the vascular endothelium from radiation-induced apoptosis. Antisera directed against the internal and amino terminal portions of bFGF were used to localize bFGF within frozen sections of whole bovine cornea. bFGF appeared to be concentrated in a fine line delineating the outer aspect of Bowman's membrane and throughout the entire thickness of Descemet's membrane (43). Next, we characterized the distribution of bFGF in normal human tissues by immunohistochemical staining of unprocessed fresh frozen sections of various organs (45). Expression of bFGF in normal human tissues was ubiquitously detected in the BM of all size blood vessels. Intensity and patterns of localization in blood vessels were consistent in various tissues, but varied among different regions of the vascular bed. Heterogeneity of expression was found in capillaries, with the most intense immunoreactivity observed at the anastamosing sites of branching regions of capillary beds (45). Strong staining for bFGF was also found in cardiac muscle fibres, smooth muscle cells of mid-size blood vessels, the gut, and the myometrium. bFGF was also found in a subset of central nervous system neurons and in cerebellar Purkinje cells (but not in glial cells), and on epithelial cells of the bronchi, colon, endometrium, and sweat gland ducts of the skin (45). Immunohistochemical methods were applied to study the distribution of bFGF in the 18-day rat fetus (46). Immunoreactive bFGF was associated with tissues of mesodermal and ectodermal origin and was predominantly localized in BM and areas where the epithelium and mesenchyme are in juxtaposition with the ECM (46).

Extracellular matrix sequestration and release of basic fibroblast growth factors

Scatchard analysis of ^{125}I-bFGF binding to ECM revealed that bFGF binds to ECM with an affinity lower than that reported for binding of bFGF to low affinity, presumably heparin-like sites on cell surfaces (38). It appears that bFGF binds specifically to HS in ECM and BM, as up to 90% of the bound growth factor was displaced by heparin, HS, or HS-degrading enzymes (i.e. heparanase), but not by unrelated GAGs or enzymes (38). Oligosaccharides derived from depolymerized heparin and containing as few as 8–10 sugar units, were equivalent to whole heparin in

their ability to release the ECM-bound bFGF (47). These oligosaccharides also supported bFGF-receptor binding and mitogenic activity (36,48). N-desulphation or substitution of N-sulphate groups of heparin by acetyl or hexanoyl residues resulted in inhibition of bFGF release, indicating that N-sulphate groups of heparin are required for binding and release of bFGF (47). Similar results were obtained with bFGF bound to HS on the surface of vascular EC (47). bFGF sequestered by the cell surface is likely to be bound to glycosylphosphatidylinositol anchored HSPG (glypican) (49,50) and to a transmembrane HSPG (syndecan) (51) that binds bFGF. The intriguing pattern of syndecan expression in development may find its rationale in the ability of syndecan to regulate FGF activities. It was suggested that the cell surface-HSPG and ECM-HSPG may act in concert to regulate the availability of otherwise diffusable biological effector molecules to their signal transducing receptor (51).

Heparanase, an endoglycosidase that specifically degrades HS was found to be a most efficient specific releaser of active bFGF from ECM (52). Regardless of the source of heparanase and of whether release of bFGF was brought about by a pure enzyme, intact cells (i.e. platelets, neutrophils, lymphoma cells) or cell lysates, inhibition of bFGF-release correlated with inhibition of heparanase activity, measured by release from ECM of sulphate labelled, HS degradation products (52). These results suggest that heparanase activity expressed by tumour cells may not only function in cell migration and invasion, but at the same time may also elicit an indirect neovascular response by means of releasing the ECM-resident FGF (9,14,53) (Fig. 12.1). Alterations in BM structure and turnover that are associated with tumour progression may thus be responsible for the onset of angiogenic activity upon the transition of an *in situ* carcinoma from the prevascular to the vascularized state. Likewise, platelets, mast cells, and activated cells of the immune system (i.e. macrophages, neutrophils, T lymphocytes) that are often attracted by tumour cells, may indirectly stimulate tumour angiogenesis by means of their heparanase activity (54). These cells may also elicit an angiogenic response in the process of inflammation and wound healing. Apart from HS degrading enzymes, active bFGF is released from ECM by thrombin (55) and plasmin (56) as a non-covalent complex with HSPG or GAGs (Fig. 12.1).

Studies performed by us and other investigators indicate that microgram quantities of heparin and HS inhibit the mitogenic activity of bFGF, but at the same time stabilize and protect the molecule from inactivation and proteolytic degradation (57). It is therefore conceivable that bFGF is stored in ECM in a highly stable but less active form as compared with bFGF in a fluid phase. Release from ECM of bFGF as a complex with HS fragment is likely to yield a form of bFGF that is more stable than free bFGF and yet capable of binding to high-affinity plasma membrane receptors. Moreover, as discussed above, heparin and HS facilitate binding of bFGF to high-affinity cell surface receptors and are directly involved in bFGF-receptor dimerization and signalling (36,58,59).

High-affinity basic fibroblast growth factor receptors associated with the subendothelial extracellular matrix

Soluble forms of the extracellular domains of the high-affinity FGF receptors were characterized (39,61). These FGF-binding proteins circulate in blood (61) and have been proposed to modulate the biological activity of the FGF family of proteins. Immunohistochemical studies revealed that these soluble, truncated FGF receptors are also present in the retinal vascular endothelial cells (39). Although low-affinity receptors for bFGF and TGF-β as well as binding proteins for other growth factors (i.e. insulin) have been identified in BM (8,43,62), the presence of a high-affinity growth factor receptor in the ECM is rather unique. The presence of high-affinity FGF receptors in the ECM may help explain, for example, why the proliferation of FGF target cells is so low *in vivo* despite the presence of bFGF in the adjacent BM (39). It appears that the matrix stores of bFGF are sequestered by both low-affinity HSPG and truncated high-affinity FGF receptors. In order for matrix stores of bFGF to bind to the FGF receptors on adjacent cells, they must be released from these high-affinity receptors in the matrix. It is conceivable that restriction of FGFs in ECM and BM prevents their systemic action on the vascular endothelium, thus maintaining a very low rate of EC turnover and vessel growth. On the other hand, release of bFGF from storage in ECM may elicit a localized EC proliferation and neovascularization in processes such as wound healing, inflammation, and tumour development (9).

Other heparin-binding growth factors and cytokines

The list of growth factors that bind to heparin and HS is growing all the time. Some of the members of this group are not related to the FGF family. These include the hepatocyte growth factor, VEGF, Schwann cell mitogen, members of the EGF family such as amphiregulin and HB-EGF, as well as neurite promoting factors such as pleiotropin and the heparin-binding neurotrophic factor (9). Some of these growth factors appear to be associated

with the ECM. For example, the heparin-binding neurotrophic factor has been localized within chick BM (63). At least one growth factor, TGF-β, binds to proteoglycans through the core protein rather then the GAG moieties. One of three receptors to TGF-β is a cell surface proteoglycan termed betaglycan. Unlike the other two receptors, betaglycan apparently does not function in signal transduction, but rather delivers the bound factor to signal transduction receptors (64). TGF-β also binds to an ECM proteoglycan. This proteoglycan, decorin, is a member of a family of leucine-rich proteins and is associated with type I collagen fibrils in tissues (8). Decorin not only binds TGF-β, but can also neutralize its mitogenic activity (8). These results further emphasize the significance of proteoglycans as binders of growth factors and their function as modulators of growth factor activities. HS, the major GAG of mouse marrow stroma, also binds interleukin (IL) 7, interferon (IFN) γ, IL-3, and granulocyte–macrophage colony-stimulating factor (GM-CSF) (9,10). These growth factors, once bound, can be presented in a biologically active form to haematopoietic cells, thereby providing a mechanistic explanation for the total dependence of haematopoietic cells on intimate contact with stromal cells. Likewise, primary human bone marrow cultures produce bFGF, which is sequestered by HSPG of the stromal matrix and cell surface. This HSPG may serve as a reservoir for bFGF, from which it is released in an active form, primarily by the enzyme phosphatidylinositol phospholipase C (PI-PLC) (50). The ability of HS in the marrow microenvironment to accumulate haematopoietic growth factors mirrors an important function of the ECM, namely, to compartmentalize growth factors synthesized locally by stromal cells or produced elsewhere and to 'present' them in a biologically active form to haematopoietic progenitor cells (65). Likewise, proteoglycans on EC can capture pro-adhesive cytokines (i.e. IL-8, MIP-1β) and 'present' them to passing leucocytes that have come into contact with the endothelium after the initial tethering step of the adhesion cascade (66). These chemokines provide the adhesion-inducing signal to particular leucocyte subsets which initiates their transmigration.

Modulation of basic fibroblast growth factor receptor binding and signalling

HSPG are ubiquitous macromolecules associated with the cell surface and ECM of a wide range of cells of vertebrate and invertebrate tissues (11–13,67). The basic HSPG structure consists of a protein core to which several linear

HS chains are covalently attached. The polysaccharide chains are typically composed of repeating hexuronic and D-glucosamine disaccharide units that are substituted to a varying extent with N- and O-linked sulphate moieties and N-linked acetyl groups (13,67). We applied both cellular and cell-free systems in order to characterize the structural properties of heparin/HS required for stimulation of bFGF-receptor binding, dimerization, and subsequent signal transduction. For this purpose, a series of heparin fragments differing in their molecular size, sulphate content, and distribution of sulphate groups were tested for their capacity to bind and promote receptor binding of bFGF. We have also studied the effect of HSPG isolated from cell surfaces, ECM and arterial tissue on bFGF-receptor interaction in order to identify possible candidate molecules that may potentate or inhibit bFGF-receptor binding and response *in vivo* (48). The involvement of HS in bFGF-receptor binding and growth-promoting activity was investigated by applying HS-deficient cell mutants (35), HS-degrading enzymes, soluble xyloside primers of HS synthesis (68), metabolic inhibitors of sulphation, and various species of HS, heparin, and synthetic polyanionic heparin-mimicking compounds (69–71).

Heparan sulphate primed on β-D-xylosides restores binding of basic fibroblast growth factor to cell surface receptors

GAG biosynthesis normally occurs on proteoglycan core proteins and initiates through the transfer of D-xylose from UDP-xylose to specific serine residues. GAG biosynthesis can also occur on exogenous β-D-xylosides, but most xylosides preferentially stimulate chondroitin sulphate synthesis and only weakly prime HS synthesis (72). Efficient priming of HS was, however, achieved by certain lipophilic β-D-xylosides such as oestradiol-β-D-xyloside (EDX) and naphthyl-β-D-xyloside (NX) (72). We tested whether these novel xyloside primers can restore the binding of bFGF to GAG-deficient Chinese hamster ovary (CHO) cells transfected with the high affinity tyrosine kinase receptor for bFGF. For this purpose, GAG-deficient CHO cell mutants expressing the ectodomain of bFGF receptor-1 (745-*flg* cells) were exposed to increasing concentrations of EDX, NX or *cis/trans*-decahydro-2-naphthyl-β-D-xyloside (DX), washed free of xylosides and tested for their bFGF-binding capacity. High restoration of bFGF binding to low- and high-affinity receptor sites was observed in 745-*flg* cells treated with relatively low concentrations of NX and EDX as compared with DX (68). A similar dose dependence was revealed when the synthesis of HS on the NX, EDX, and DX primers was

measured (68). GAG produced on β-D-xylosides are mostly secreted from cells (Fig. 12.2). To test if the secreted material would restore bFGF binding, 745-*flg* cells were treated with NX or EDX and the medium was collected and transferred on to untreated 745-*flg* cells. Low- and high-affinity binding of bFGF to untreated cells was restored by medium taken from EDX- and NX-treated cells, but there was no restoration when the medium was pretreated with bacterial heparinase. These and other results indicate that soluble HS chains synthesized on xyloside primers act as low-affinity receptor sites for bFGF in a manner similar to that fulfilled by HS chains attached to cellular core proteins (Fig. 12.2) (68).

Sulphate moieties in the subendothelial extracellular matrix are involved in basic fibroblast growth factor sequestration, dimerization and mitogenic stimulation

The essential involvement of sulphate groups in bFGF-receptor binding and activation was demonstrated by applying soluble FGF-receptor constructs, HS-deficient cell mutants and both undersulphated and oversulphated species of heparin. Best results were achieved in the presence of oversulphated heparin fragments, regardless of whether the N-position was sulphated or acetylated (48). Chlorate (73), an inhibitor of adenosine triphosphate sulphurylase and hence of the production of phosphoadenosine phosphosulphate (PAPS), the active sulphate donor for sulphotransferases, was applied to investigate the involvement of sulphate groups in the growth promoting activity of the subendothelial ECM. Measurements of bFGF binding revealed a 50–60% reduction in bFGF binding to ECM produced by chlorate-treated corneal EC, as compared with untreated cells. The amount of HS-bound, heparin/heparinase releasable bFGF was reduced by 70–80%, suggesting that bFGF may bind also to sulphate-depleted GAG side chains, ECM components other than HS (i.e. fibronectin), and possibly ECM-bound bFGF receptors (39).

ECM produced in the absence and presence of chlorate was tested for mitogenic activity toward vascular EC and 3T3 fibroblasts. Sulphate depleted ECM exerted a greatly reduced mitogenic activity towards vascular EC and was devoid of mitogenic activity toward 3T3 fibroblasts, indicating that sulphation is critical for the growth promoting activity of the ECM. Direct immunoquantitation of bFGF in solubilized ECM revealed a nearly 10-fold reduction in the amount of endogenous bFGF in ECM produced in the presence of chlorate as compared with native ECM, suggesting that sulphate-deficient ECM exhibit little or no

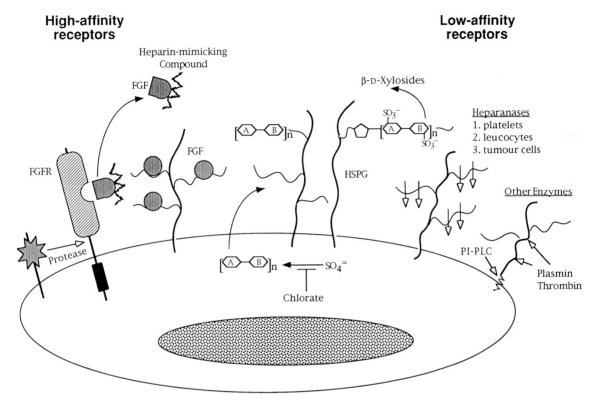

Figure 12.2. Modulation of basic fibroblast growth factor (bFGF) receptor binding and activation by metabolic inhibitors of heparan sulphate (HS) synthesis and sulphation, HS-degrading enzymes and heparin-mimicking compounds. Modulation of bFGF binding to low affinity cell surface receptor sites can be brought about by: (i) enzymes which degrade the HS side chains (i.e. heparanase enzymes expressed by platelets, neutrophils, mast cells, tumour cells) or HSPG core protein (i.e., plasmin, thrombin, PI-PLC) (right), and (ii) soluble primers (β-D-xylosides) of HS synthesis, and metabolic inhibitors (i.e., chlorate) of sulphation (centre). Binding of bFGF to high-affinity cell surface receptor sites can be modulated by: (i) heparin-mimicking compounds (i.e. compound RG-13577) which bind the growth factor and prevent receptor binding and/or dimerization, and (ii) proteolytic enzymes (i.e. MMP-2), which cleave the extracellular domain of the receptor and thus release soluble forms of the receptor (74) (left).

growth promoting activity simply because its HS chains fail to sequester bFGF (75).

Binding of aFGF and bFGF to low-affinity accessory heparin/HS receptor sites induces oligomerization of the FGF molecules (36), thereby indirectly cross-linking and activating the high-affinity receptors, resulting in transmembrane signalling and cell proliferation (58). Intact ECM was found to induce dimerization of ^{125}I-bFGF to a much higher extent as compared with sulphate depleted ECM (75). This result was attributed primarily to the decrease in bFGF binding and sequestration by HSPG in the sulphate deficient ECM. It appears that the highly reduced ability of sulphate depleted ECM to sequester and dimerize bFGF is responsible for the impaired mitogenic activity of this ECM. Oligomerization of ECM-bound bFGF and

possibly other heparin-binding growth factors may contribute to the potent growth- and differentiation- promoting activities of the ECM. This oligomerization is induced by properly sulfated HSPG found in native, but not sulphate-depleted ECM.

Mitogenic response of chlorate-treated endothelial cells plated on extracellular matrix

Heparin was found to restore the ability of chlorate-treated 3T3 fibroblasts to proliferate in response to bFGF (73). We investigated whether native ECM can similarly restore the proliferation of chlorate-treated EC in the absence and presence of added heparin. For this purpose, chlorate-treated vascular ECs were seeded in the presence of chlorate on either regular tissue culture plastic, sulphate-depleted ECM, or native ECM. Heparin was added to some of the cultures. Chlorate-treated ECs exhibited little or no proliferative response to heparin when seeded on regular tissue culture plastic, or sulphate-depleted ECM. A significant mitogenic response was obtained when the chlorate-treated ECs were seeded in contact with native ECM, and best results were obtained when heparin was added to the culture medium (75). Under these conditions there was little or no further stimulation of cell proliferation in response to exogenously added bFGF. These results suggest that sulphate moieties on cell surfaces play an active part in the presentation of ECM-resident bFGF to its high-affinity cell surface receptors and that soluble heparin may exert a similar effect on chlorate-treated, undersulphated endothelial cells (Fig. 12.2).

Previous studies revealed that the K_d value for interaction of bFGF with the cell surface HS is lower $(1 \times 10^{-9} \text{ M})$ (34) than for interaction with HS in the ECM $(1 \times 10^{-7} \text{ M})$ (47), suggesting that ECM-bound bFGF interacts first with HS on the cell surface and then is presented to high-affinity cell surface receptors. Because the cell surface HSPG, unlike that of the ECM, is mobile in the plane of the membrane and can turnover more rapidly by shedding and internalization, it may readily replenish its bFGF from the ECM reservoir, which appears to serve more as an efficient large capacity bFGF storage depot in

the vicinity of cells (51) (Fig. 12.3). It appears that sequestration and subsequent presentation of bFGF to high-affinity receptor sites is not fulfilled by non-sulphated HS present in the ECM and surface of chlorate-treated ECs, respectively (Fig. 12.2). A difference between cell surface- and ECM-derived species of HS in their ability to promote the mitogenic activity of bFGF was also demonstrated in our studies on the growth promoting activity of HS degradation fragments released by bacterial heparinase III from ECM and cell surfaces. In these experiments we applied a cytokine-dependent, HS-deficient lymphoid cell line engineered to express the mouse FGF receptor 1 (36). It was found that HS fragments released from the surface of vascular endothelial and smooth muscle cells by heparinase III were capable of serving as accessory receptors participating in a dual receptor mechanism characteristic of bFGF. In contrast, little or no such activity was associated with HS fragments released by heparinase from the subendothelial ECM. It is conceivable that species of HS derived from vascular endothelial and smooth muscle cells contain the appropriate saccharide sequence capable of promoting bFGF-receptor binding and activation that are not found in HS degradation fragments released from ECM (Fig. 12.3).

A highly sulphated bFGF-binding fragment of HS was isolated from cell surface HSPG of fibroblasts (76). Sulphation in critical positions along the polysaccharide chain, particularly 2-O-sulphation, seems necessary to generate a specific bFGF binding motif that can support

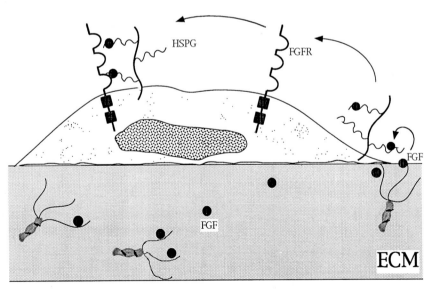

Figure 12.3. Preferential involvement of: (i) extracellular matrix–heparan sulphate proteoglycans (HSPG), and (ii) cell surface-HSPG, in (i) sequestration, storage and stabilization of basic fibroblast growth factor (bFGF), and (ii) bFGF receptor binding, activation, and mitogenic activity, respectively.

high-affinity bFGF-receptor binding and activation (76). In a recent study, small synthetic heparin-derived oligosaccharides were found, when applied at relatively high concentrations, to activate bFGF-receptor binding and activation (59). Several of these saccharides are non-sulphated, suggesting that interactions with the carbohydrate backbone of heparin/HS is sufficient for biological activity. Altogether, these studies demonstrate that properly sulphated HSPG associated with the cell surface and ECM act in concert to regulate the bio-availability of active bFGF and possibly other effector molecules to their signal transducing receptors.

Species of heparan sulphate and heparin-mimicking compounds as potential inhibitors of heparin-induced basic fibroblast growth factor-receptor binding and dimerization

Perlecan, the large basal lamina proteoglycan was suggested as a potential low-affinity accessory receptor for bFGF (77). Affinity-purified perlecan from both soluble and ECM fractions of human fetal lung fibroblasts was found to potentiate, at exceedingly low concentrations, high-affinity binding of bFGF to HS-deficient cells and to soluble FGF receptors (77). In the rabbit ear model for *in vivo* angiogenesis, perlecan was found to be a potent inducer of bFGF-mediated neovascularization (77). Under certain conditions, FGF-receptor binding and signalling was supported also by syndecans and glypican (78). The marked difference in the capacity of various defined heparin fragments and of naturally occurring species of HSPG to potentiate receptor binding of bFGF led us to investigate the possible role of 'non-active' HSPG preparations as potential inhibitors of bFGF-receptor interactions. To address this possibility, we tested the effect of different species of arterial-derived HS on bFGF-receptor binding in the presence of sub-saturating concentrations of heparin. Anti-proliferative, sulphate-rich HS-derived oligosaccharide enriched with 2-O-sulphate uronic acid residues and isolated from arterial tissue (79), was found to be a potent inhibitor of heparin induced bFGF-receptor binding (48). In contrast, sulphate-poor arterial-derived HS oligosaccharides with no anti-proliferative activity, were ineffective in inhibiting heparin-stimulated bFGF-receptor binding (48). Such a clear inverse relation between the capacity of heparin to promote receptor binding and the ability of certain species of HS to suppress this specific interaction, strongly suggests that species of cell surface- and ECM-derived HSPG may function as bFGF growth suppressers by direct interference with the interaction

between bFGF and receptor promoting species of HS and heparin (48).

In recent studies we have identified a series of negatively charged, non-sulphated aromatic compounds that mimic many of the effects of heparin (69–71). These non-toxic compounds, among which are commercially available synthetic dyes (i.e. aurin tricarboxylic acid) compete with bFGF binding to HS on the cell surface and ECM (Fig. 12.2). Aurin tricarboxylic acid and compound RG-13577 (polymer of 4-hydroxyphenoxy acetic acid and formaldehyde ammonium salt, M_r~5800) were found to inhibit the proliferation of vascular smooth muscle cells (70) and to revert the transformed phenotype of bFGF-transfected cells in terms of proliferation rate, morphological appearance, and adhesive properties (69). Two correctly spaced chemical components, a substituted aromatic ring system and a negatively charged acidic residue, were required for these activities. Direct interaction between compound RG-13577 and bFGF was suggested by the ability of the former to compete with heparin on binding to bFGF. RG-13577 binding to bFGF may inhibit subsequent binding of bFGF to low-and high-affinity receptor sites on the cell surface, leading to inhibition of bFGF mitogenic activity (Fig. 12.2). Such inhibition of bFGF receptor binding was revealed in cross-linking experiments between vascular smooth muscle cells and ^{125}I-bFGF, performed in the absence and presence of compound RG-13577 (71). In subsequent experiments we investigated whether heparin-mediated dimerization of bFGF is inhibited by the above described heparin-mimicking compounds. For this purpose, ^{125}I-bFGF was incubated with heparin in the absence or presence of the polyanionic compound RG-13577. Disuccinyimidyl suberate (DSS) was then added and the formation of ^{125}I-bFGF dimers analysed by sodium dodecyl-sulphate poly-acrylamide gel electrophoresis (SDS–PAGE) and auto-radiography. Compound RG-13577 alone, failed to induce dimerization of bFGF. Moreover, it abrogated the di-merizing effect of heparin (71), in a manner similar to that ascribed to sucrose octasulphate (58). It also inhibited FGF-receptor dimerization, signalling and growth-promoting activity. This property may contribute to the anti-proliferative effect of compound RG-13577 and related heparin-mimicking molecules.

The above described studies further emphasize the role of properly sulphated HS present on cell surfaces and ECM in bFGF deposition, dimerization, receptor binding, and growth-promoting activity (Fig. 12.2). Species of heparin, HS, and heparin-mimicking compounds may alter these properties and hence are expected to modulate the involvement of heparin-binding growth factors in processes such as wound healing, restenosis, neovascularization, and tumour progression. The development of defined, non-toxic anionic compounds is therefore of increasing importance for the development of therapeutic agents of widespread utility.

Mammalian heparanases: dual function as chemokines and heparan sulphate degrading enzymes

HS catabolism is observed in inflammation, wound repair, diabetes, and cancer metastasis, suggesting that enzymes which degrade HS play important parts in pathological processes. Heparanase activity has been described in activated immune system cells and highly metastatic cancer cells, but research has been handicapped by the lack of biological tools to explore potential causative roles of heparanase in disease.

A HS-degrading enzyme has recently been purified from activated platelet supernatants (80). N-terminal sequence analysis revealed that the enzymatic activity resides in neutrophil activating peptide-2 (NAP-2) and connective tissue activating peptide-III (CTAP-III), two truncated forms of the CXC chemokine 'platelet basic protein (PBP)' (80). SDS–PAGE analysis of the purified heparanase yielded a single broad band of 8–10 kDa, the known molecular weight of PBP and its truncated derivatives. Gel filtration chromatography of the purified heparanase resulted in peaks of activity corresponding to monomers, dimers, and tetramers. Antisera against a C-terminal synthetic peptide of PBP inhibited heparanase activity by 95%. In contrast, N-terminal peptide antisera bound specifically to the purified platelet heparanase, but failed to neutralize its activity (80). The dual function of CTAPIII/NAP-2 as heparanase and neutrophil chemoattractant suggests that a complex relationship may exist where each activity could complement and/or alter the bioavailability or activity of the other function in various pathological situations such as rheumatoid arthritis, atherosclerosis, restenosis, and tumour metastasis. The possible relation between heparanase and the chemokine family of proinflammatory cytokines prompted us to elucidate the dual involvement of heparanase as a T-cell adhesion molecule (chemokine) and ECM-degrading enzyme in leucocyte-mediated inflammatory reactions and immune surveillance (81).

Human hepatoma and placental heparanases were purified and analysed for their activity at different pH values (81). The ability of cells to degrade HS in the ECM was studied by allowing cells to interact with a naturally produced sulphate-labelled ECM, followed by gel filtration analysis of degradation products released into the culture medium (52). At pH values higher than 6.8, the

heparanase exhibited little or no activity. Maximal release of low M_r HS degradation fragments from ECM occurred at pH values ranging from 5.4 to 6.8. Thus, heparanase-mediated cleavage of the HS scaffold of ECM is a pH-dependent process, which may occur in vivo at the sites of inflammation and tumour growth, where relatively acidic pH values have been detected. Direct binding of heparanase to ECM vs. bovine serum albumin (BSA) was examined by adding ^{125}I-heparanase to microtiter wells coated with either ECM or BSA. At pH 7.2 and 37°C, heparanase bound to ECM in a saturable and specific manner. However, over a 24 h period, most of the ECM-bound heparanase spontaneously dissociated from the ECM. The high spontaneous dissociation could be attributed in part to the activity at 37°C of ECM-associated enzymes, such as collagenase type IV (82) and plasminogen activators (83). In subsequent experiments, heparanase was allowed to bind to ECM at pH not permissive to its enzymatic activity (pH 7.2, 37°C), and the unbound enzyme removed. The pH of the incubation medium was then maintained at 7.2 or decreased to 6.4, and the ensuing release of degraded HS was assessed. Minimal release of HS-degradation fragments occurred if the pH was kept at 7.2. However, at pH 6.4, the enzymatic activity of heparanase was restored, as indicated by release of HS degradation fragments from the ECM (81). Hence, at a physiological pH, the ECM can retain heparanase in an inactive form, but if the pH decreases, the temporarily stored enzyme regained its catalytic activity.

Human placental heparanase was diluted at different pH values, added to ECM-coated microtitre wells, and the unbound heparanase was removed. ^{51}Cr-labelled, resting human CD4+ T cells were then added to the pre-coated wells, and their binding to the substrate was assessed. The T cells adhered well to ECM which had been preincubated with heparanase at pH 7.2–7.4, and only slightly to ECM exposed to heparanase at pH 6.4–6.8. The binding of T cells to heparanase-bound ECM was inhibited by heparin, which competes with HS for heparanase recognition (81). Thus, analogous to proteoglycan-bound chemokines (66), non-enzymatically active heparanase can act as a proteoglycan-associated pro-adhesive molecule for resting T cells. Our results suggest that at relatively low pH values, heparanase, as a pivotal element of the ECM-specific enzymatic repertoire of highly invasive cells, can actively participate in ECM degradation, and thereby facilitates cell migration (81). At a physiological pH, the relatively quiescent enzyme appears to act as a lectin-like, pro-adhesive molecule that can organize the recruitment of resting T cells and possibly blood-borne tumour cells, toward an extravascular loci (81). Besides the particular relevance of these findings for interactions between cells and ECM, the pH-dependent modification of heparanase function may illustrate a general principle that biologically important molecules can adopt their behaviour to context. Thus, the local state of a tissue can regulate the activities of heparanase and can determine whether the molecule will function as an enzyme or as a pro-adhesive molecule.

Involvement of heparanase in tumour cell invasion and metastasis

Circulating tumour cells arrested in the capillary beds of different organs must invade the endothelial cell lining and degrade its underlying BM in order to escape into the extravascular tissue(s) where they establish metastasis (84). Metastatic tumour cells often attach at or near the intercellular junctions between adjacent ECs followed by rupture of the junctions, retraction of the EC borders and migration through the breach in the endothelium toward the exposed underlying basal lamina (84). Once enveloped between EC and the basal lamina, the invading cells must degrade the subendothelial glycoproteins and proteoglycans in order to migrate out of the vascular compartment. Several cellular enzymes (i.e. collagenase IV, plasminogen activator, cathepsin B, elastase) are thought to be involved in degradation of BM (85). Among these enzymes is an endo-β-D-glucuronidase (heparanase) that cleaves HS at specific intrachain sites (53,86,87). Expression of a HS-degrading heparanase was found to correlate with the metastatic potential of mouse lymphoma (86), fibrosarcoma, and melanoma (87) cells. Moreover, elevated levels of heparanase were detected in sera from metastatic tumour-bearing animals and melanoma patients (87) and in tumour biopsies of cancer patients. Heparanase activity is also correlated with the ability of activated cells of the immune system to leave the circulation and elicit both inflammatory and autoimmune responses (81). Among the breakdown products of the ECM generated by heparanase is a tri-sulphated disaccharide that can inhibit T-cell mediated inflammation *in vivo* (88). This inhibition was associated with an inhibitory effect of the disaccharide on the production of biologically active tumour necrosis factor-α by activated T cells *in vitro* (88). Thus, the disaccharide, a natural product of inflammation, can regulate the functional nature of the T cell's response to activation. This feedback control mechanism could enable the T cell to assess the extent of tissue degradation and adjust its behaviour accordingly (88).

Structural requirements for inhibition of melanoma lung colonization by heparanase-inhibiting species of heparin

We and other investigators have shown that heparanase activity derived from either normal or neoplastic cells can be effectively inhibited by heparin, several modified non-anticoagulant species of heparin, and other sulphated polysaccharides (87,89). Moreover, there was a reasonable good correlation between the heparanase-inhibiting activity of these compounds and their ability to inhibit tumour metastasis in experimental animals (87,90–92).

A number of studies have shown that sulphated polysaccharides (i.e. heparin, dextran sulphate, pentosan polysulphate, laminarin sulphate, xylose sulphate) can inhibit tumour growth and metastasis (90,91). Although all of the inhibitory polysaccharides were anticoagulants, the anti-metastatic potential of the molecules did not correlate with their anticoagulant activity (87,91,92). Inhibitory polysaccharides did not affect adhesion of tumour cells to the vascular endothelium (90). Parish *et al.* (91) have demonstrated that sulphated polysaccharides inhibit metastatic dissemination of rat mammary adenocarcinoma cells by inhibiting their heparanase activity (90). This conclusion was strengthened in our studies by applying both chemically modified species of heparin and size homogeneous oligosaccharides derived from depolymerized heparin. Species of heparin that inhibited heparanase-mediated degradation of HS in intact ECM were also potent inhibitors of B16 melanoma extravasation and lung colonization (92).

Although heparin is best known for its anticoagulant and anti-thrombotic properties, it affects various physiological processes such as vascular endothelial and smooth muscle cell proliferation, angiogenesis, inflammation, and autoimmunity (12,79,93). It is, however, virtually impossible to assign structure–function relationships based on studies with native heparin due to variations in the size of the polysaccharide chains and the degree and distribution of sulphate groups. The availability of a large collection of chemically modified and low M_r species of heparin enabled us to determine structural requirements for inhibition of heparanase activity and tumour metastasis, in comparison with other effects of heparin such as release of ECM-bound bFGF (47) and stimulation of bFGF binding to high-affinity cell surface receptors (48). Inhibition of heparanase and tumour metastasis was achieved by heparin species containing 16 sugar units or more and having sulphate groups at both the N and O positions. Low sulphate oligosaccharides were less effective heparanase inhibitors than medium and high sulphate fractions of the same size (92). While O-desulphation abolished the heparanase inhibiting and anti-metastatic effect of heparin, N-acetyl- or N-hexonylheparin retained a high inhibitory activity, provided that the N-substituted molecules had a molecular size of about 4000 daltons or more. Efficient inhibition of melanoma lung colonization by N-acetylated heparin was also reported by Nakajima *et al.* (87). No correlation was found between the anti-thrombotic activity (anti-factor Xa activity) of heparin and its anti-metastatic and bFGF-releasing activities.

Release of extracellular matrix-bound basic fibroblast growth factor

We investigated structural requirements for release of ECM-bound and cell surface-bound bFGF by heparin and heparin-like molecules. For this purpose the subendothelial ECM was incubated with ^{125}I-bFGF, washed free of unbound bFGF and exposed to various chemically modified species of heparin and to homogenously sized oligosaccharides derived from depolymerized heparin. Unlike the inhibition of heparanase activity and lung colonization, the presence of N-sulphates was necessary for release of ECM-bound bFGF by species of heparin (47). Thus, total substitution of N-sulphates with acetyl or hexanoyl groups resulted in an almost complete inhibition of the bFGF-releasing activity of heparin, despite a normal content of O-sulphate groups. O-sulphation facilitated bFGF release, but was not an absolute requirement, as indicated by the relatively high bFGF-releasing activity of totally N/O-desulphated, N-resulphated heparin fragment (47). A nearly maximal release of ECM-bound bFGF was obtained already by the octasaccharide, while the hexasaccharide exhibited about 60% of the activity of intact heparin. The ability of a given compound to release bFGF from ECM was dependent primarily on the position of the sulphate group rather than on the total level of sulphation (47).

Basic fibroblast growth factor-receptor binding

The capacity of various species of heparin and HS to promote bFGF-receptor binding was investigated using CHO mutant cells deficient in cell surface HSPG and a soluble bFGF receptor–alkaline phosphatase fusion protein (36,48). bFGF-receptor binding was induced by heparin-derived oligosaccharides containing as little as 8–10 sugar units (36,48). Oligosaccharides containing 14 sugar units or more were comparable with intact heparin in their ability to restore binding of bFGF to high-affinity receptors in HS-deficient CHO cells (36,48). A low sulphate fraction of a given oligosaccharide was less efficient in restoring bFGF binding than medium and high sulphate fraction of the same oligosaccharide. Both N- and O-sulphates of heparin were required for restoration of bFGF-receptor binding as

there was little or no effect to either totally N-desulphated heparin or to N-/O-desulphated, N-resulphated heparin (48). Substitution of the N-sulphates with acetyl or hexanoyl residues resulted in an almost complete inhibition of the capacity of heparin to restore the binding of bFGF to high-affinity cell surface receptor sites. The highest level of bFGF-receptor binding was achieved in the presence of over-sulphated heparin, regardless of whether the N position was sulphated or acetylated. Thus, there was an absolute requirement for O-sulphation and a synergistic effect of N-linked sulphates (48).

Our results indicate that different effects of heparin are mediated by different sugar sequences and that unique heparin-like molecules can be designed to elicit or inhibit a specific function. For example, N-substituted species of heparin and in particularly N-hexanoyl heparin fragment could be applied to inhibit tumour metastasis, as their efficient inhibition of heparanase activity was not associated with a significant ability to release active bFGF from cells and ECM, resulting in potential induction of tumour angiogenesis. On the other hand, oligosaccharides derived from depolymerized heparin and containing 8–10 sugar units, or N-sulphated, O-desulphated species of heparin can possibly be applied to stimulate neovascularization and wound healing by virtue of their efficient bFGF releasing activity. These molecules may not interfere, for example, with the normal function of the immune system as they do not inhibit the heparanase enzyme expressed by activated lymphocytes, neutrophils, and mast cells (54,92,93).

Heparanase activity in the urine of cancer patients

In an attempt to elucidate further the involvement of heparanase in tumour progression and its relevance to human cancer, we screened urine samples for heparanase activity. Heparanase activity was detected in the urine of some, but not all, cancer patients. High levels of heparanase activity were determined in the urine of patients with an aggressive metastatic disease and there was no detectable activity in the urine of healthy donors. In many, but not all of the heparanase-positive urine samples there were also high levels of bFGF (94), suggesting the formation of strongly bound heparanase–bFGF complexes. In fact, heparanase and bFGF were co-purified when tissue extracts were subjected to cation exchange-, heparin-, and ConA-Sepharose chromatographies and our purified preparations of human placenta and hepatoma heparanases always contained bFGF as detected by immunoblot analysis and mitogenic activity. The physiological significance of heparanase–bFGF complexes is not clear, but it may well be that heparanase activity provides a means for secretion of a positively charged molecule, such as bFGF, through the polyanionic HS network of the glomerular BM. We propose that heparanase may overcome the filtration barrier of BM and ECMs simply by virtue of its ability to degrade the HS moieties that are held responsible for their permeaselective properties.

Summary and conclusions

Cellular activities depend on multifactorial events involving soluble-phase molecules, such as cytokines and growth factors, and solid phase ECM macromolecules. Numerous studies indicate that the ECM provides a storage depot for growth factors, enzymes and plasma proteins and that some of the effects of ECM can be attributed to the combined action of structural components and ECM-immobilized molecules that are thereby protected and stabilized. This may allow a more localized, regulated and persistent mode of action, as compared with the same molecules in a fluid phase. Proteoglycans have been found to function as the principal binders of growth factors and cytokines and more than 20 known heparin-binding proteins contain a consensus structural motif which participates in this binding. Because proteoglycans are abundant and ubiquitous components of ECM, BM, and cell surfaces, they are likely to be able to capture most of those growth factors and cytokines that have affinity for the GAG or protein part of proteoglycans. Cell surface HSPG may function as a key regulator of cell interaction with heparin-binding growth factors, cytokines, enzymes, and plasma proteins because it can bind a wide variety of polypeptides and can turn over rapidly by shedding or internalization. Because it is mobile in the plane of the membrane, it may replenish its ligand from the ECM which may thus serve as a backup reservoir system. Of particular significance are members of the chemokine family of cytokines that are presented to leucocytes in a controlled fashion by HS on cell surfaces and ECM, triggering leucocyte recruitment and cell migration in a haptotactic and/or chemotactic fashion. Under certain conditions, some of these cytokines (i.e. CTAPIII, NAP-2) may degrade HS and hence may participate in the actual extravasation of circulating metastatic tumour cells and activated cells of the immune system.

The mode of action, biological significance, and clinical applications of heparin-binding growth factors (i.e. bFGF, aFGF, HB-EGF, VEGF, KGF), HS-degrading enzymes, and polyanionic heparin-mimicking compounds in normal and pathological situations are being studied extensively. As new members of the heparin-binding family of growth factors and the respective cell surface receptors are being discovered, it appears that the effect of heparin and HS is quite complex, resulting in stimulation or inhibition of receptor binding and signalling. The question of how the interaction of FGFs with the same high affinity receptor is coordinated has not been elucidated. For example, heparin/HS potentiates the mitogenic activity of acidic FGF but inhibits that of keratinocyte growth factor (KCF), although both growth factors bind the KGF receptor with high affinity (95). Thus, a cell associated HS, depending on its local concentration, can either promote or restrict the binding of a certain FGF to its high affinity receptor. This suggests a regulatory role for HS as coordinators of the interaction of FGFs, KGF and other heparin-binding growth factors with their signalling receptors and of the related cellular responses (95). Future studies are expected to better define the exact mode of interaction and complex formation between the growth factor and its high affinity (tyrosine kinase) and low-affinity (HS) cell surface receptor sites. Future studies are also expected to elucidate how certain heparin-binding growth factors (i.e. bFGF, aFGF) lacking a signal peptide are deposited into the ECM and secreted into the blood and urine of cancer patients. Molecules that modulate the activity of heparin-binding growth factors via interaction with the growth factor itself and/or its low- and high-affinity cell surface receptors are expected to be identified, synthesized, and applied to stimulate or inhibit cell proliferation and neovascularization in processes such as tissue repair, collateral formation, restenosis, diabetic retinopathy, and tumour progression. Define species of heparin and heparin-mimicking compounds may also be applied to inhibit extravasation of blood-borne cells associated with tumour metastasis inflammation and autoimmune disorders.

Acknowledgements

The excellent assistance of Ruth Atzmon and Rivka Ishai-Michaeli is greatly appreciated. This work was supported by grants from G. I. F., The German-Israeli Foundation for Scientific Research and Development, the USA–Israel Binational Science Foundation; the Israel Science Foundation administered by the Israel Academy of Sciences and Humanities; and the GSF (German Forschungzentrum für Umwelt and Gesundheit).

References

1. Gospodarawicz, D., Greenberg, G., and Birdwell, C. R. (1978). Determination of cellular shape by the extracellular matrix and its correlation with control of cellular growth. *Cancer Res.*, **38**, 4155–71.

2. Ingber, D. E. (1990). Fibronectin controls capillary endot-helial cell growth by modulating cell shape. *Proc. Natl Acad. Sci. USA*, **87**, 3579–83.

3. Hynes, R. O. (1992). Versatility, modulation and signaling in cell adhesion. *Cell*, **69**, 11–25.

4. Boudrean, N., Myers, C., and Bissell, M. J. (1995). From laminin to lamin: regulation of tissue-specific gene expression by the ECM. *Trends Cell Biol.*, **5**, 1–4.

5. Damsky, C. H. and Werb, Z. (1992). Signal transduction by integrin receptors for extracellular matrix. Cooperative processing of extracellular information. *Curr. Opin. Cell Biol.*, **4**, 772–81.

6. Roskelley, C. D., Desprez, P. Y., and Bissell, M. J. (1994). Extracellular matrix-dependent tissue-specific gene expression in mammary epithelial cells requires both physical and biochemical signal transduction. *Proc. Natl Acad. Sci. USA*, **91**, 12378–82.

7. Ingber, D. E. (1993). The riddle of morphogenesis: A question of solution chemistry or molecular cell engineering? *Cell*, **75**, 1249–1252.

8. Ruoslahti, E. and Yamaguchi, Y. (1991). Proteoglycans as modulators of growth factor activities. *Cell*, **64**, 867–9.

9. Vlodavsky, I., Bar-Shavit, R., Korner, G., and Fuks, Z. (1993). Extracellular matrix-bound growth factors, enzymes and plasma proteins. In *Basement membranes: cellular and molecular aspects* (ed. D. H. Rohrbach and R. Timpl), pp. 327–43. Academic Press, Orlando, Fl.

10. Roberts, R., Gallagher, J., Spooncer, S., Allen, T. D., Bloomdield, F., and Dexter, T. M. (1988). Heparan sulphate bound growth factors: a mechanism for stromal cell mediated haemopoiesis. *Nature*, **332**, 376–8.

11. Wight, T. N., Kinsella, M. G., and Qwarnstromn, E. E. (1992). The role of proteoglycans in cell adhesion, migration and proliferation. *Curr. Opin. Cell Biol.*, **4**, 793–801.

12. Jackson, R. L., Busch, S. J., and Cardin, A. L. (1991). Glycosaminoglycans: Molecular properties, protein interactions and role in physiological processes. *Physiol. Rev.*, **71**, 481–539.

13. Wight, T. N. (1989). Cell biology of arterial proteoglycans. *Arteriosclerosis*, **9**, 1–20.

14. Vlodavsky, I., Bar-Shavit, R., Ishai-Michaeli, R., Bashkin, P., and Fuks, Z. (1991). Extracellular sequestration and release of fibroblast growth factor: a regulatory mechanism? *Trends Biochem. Sci.*, **16**, 268–71.

15. Gitay-Goren, H., Soker, S., Vlodavsky, I., and Neufeld, G. (1992). Cell surface associated heparin-like molecules are required for the binding of vascular endothelial growth factor (VEGF) to its cell surface receptors. *J. Biol. Chem.*, **267**, 6093–8.

16. Eisenberg, S., Sehayek, E., Olivecrona, T., and Vlodavsky, I. (1992). Lipoprotein lipase enhances binding of lipoproteins to heparan sulfate on cell surfaces and extracellular matrix. *J. Clin. Invest.*, **90**, 2013–21.

17. Liotta, L. A., Steeg, P. A., and Stetler-Stevenson, W. G. (1991). Cancer metastasis and angiogenesis in an imbalance of positive and negative regulation. *Cell*, **64**, 327–36.

18. Kleiner, D. E. and Stetler-Stevenson, W. G. (1993). Structural biochemistry and activation of matrix metalloproteases. *Curr. Opin. Cell Biol.*, **5**, 891–7.

19. Bischoff, J. (1995). Approaches to studying cell adhesion molecules in angiogenesis. *Trends Cell Biol.*, **5**, 69–74.

20. Nicosia, R. F. and Madri, J. A. (1987). The microvascular extracellular matrix. Developmental changes during angiogenesis in the aortic ring–plasma clot model. *Am. J. Pathol.*, **128**, 78–90.

21. Nicosia, R. F., Bonanno, E., and Smith, M. (1993). Fibronectin promotes the elongation of microvessels during angiogenesis *in vitro*. *J. Cell. Physiol.*, **154**, 654–61.

22. Iruela-Arispe, M. L., Hasselaar, P., and Sage, H. (1991). Differential expression of extracellular proteins is correlated with angiogenesis *in vitro*. *Lab. Invest.*, **64**, 174–86.

23. Lane, T. F. and Sage, E. H. (1994). The biology of SPARC, a protein that modulates cell-matrix interactions. *FASEB J.*, **8**, 163–73.

24. Good, D. J., Polverini, P. J., Rastinejad, F., Le-Beau, M. M., Lemons, R. S., and Frazier, W. A. (1990). A tumor suppressor-dependent inhibitor of angiogenesis is immunologically and functionally indistinguishable from a fragment of thrombospondin. *Proc. Natl Acad. Sci. USA*, **87**, 6624–8.

25. Tolsma, S. S., Volpert, O. V., Good, D. J., Frazier, W. A., Polverini, P. J., and Bouck, N. (1993). Peptides derived from two separate domains of the matrix protein thrombospondin-1 have anti-angiogenic activity. *J. Cell Biol.*, **122**, 497–511.

26. Nguyen, M., Strubel, N. A., and Bischoff, J. (1993). A role for sialyl Lewis-X/A glycoconjugates in capillary morphogenesis. *Nature*, **365**, 267–9.

27. Lampugnani, M. G., Resnati, M., Dejana, E., and Marchisio, P. C. (1991). The role of integrins in the maintenance of endothelial monolayer integrity. *J. Cell Biol.*, **112**, 479–90.

28. Gamble, J. R., Mattias, L. J., Meyer, G., Kaur, P., Russ, G., Faull, R., and Berndt, M. C. (1993). Regulation of *in vitro* capillary tube formation by anti-integrin antibodies. *J. Cell Biol.*, **121**, 931–43.

29. Drake, C. J., Davis, L. A., and Little, C. D. (1992). Antibodies to beta 1-integrins cause alterations of aortic vasculogenesis, *in vivo*. *Dev. Dyn.*, **193**, 83–91.

30. Brooks, P. C., Clark, R. A., and Cheresh, D. A. (1994). Requirement of vascular integrin alpha v beta 3 for angiogenesis. *Science*, **264**, 569–71.

31. Brook, P. C., Montgomery, A. M. P., Rosenfeld, M., Reisfeld, R. A., Hu, T., Klier, G., and Cheresh, D. A. (1994). Integrin alpha v beta 3 antagonists promote tumor regression by inducing apoptosis on angiogenic blood vessels. *Cell*, **79**, 1157–64.

32. Burgess, W. H. and Maciag, T. (1989). The heparin-binding (fibroblast) growth factor family of proteins. *Annu. Rev. Biochem.*, **58**, 575–606.

33. Folkman, J. and Klagsbrun, M. (1987). Angiogenic factors. *Science*, **235**, 442–7.

34. Rifkin, D. B. and Moscatelli, D. (1989). Recent developments in the cell biology of basic fibroblast growth factor. *J. Cell Biol.*, **109**, 1–6.

35. Yayon, A., Klagsbrun, M., Esko, J. D., Leder, P., and Ornitz, D. M. (1991). Cell surface, heparin-like molecules are required for binding of basic fibroblast growth factor to its high affinity receptor. *Cell*, **64**, 841–8.

36. Ornitz, D. M., Yayon, A., Flanagan, J. G., Svahn, C. M., Levi, E., and Leder, P. (1992). Heparin is required for cell-free binding of basic fibroblast growth factor to a soluble receptor and for mitogenesis in whole cells. *Mol. Cell. Biol.*, **12**, 240–7.

37. Aviezer, D. and Yayon, A. (1994). Heparin-dependent binding and autophosphorylation of epidermal growth factor (EGF) receptor by heparin-binding EGF-like growth factor but not by EGF. *Proc. Natl Acad. Sci. USA*, **91**, 12173–7.

38. Bashkin, P., Doctrow, S., Klagsbrun, M., Svahn, C. M., Folkman, J., and Vlodavsky, I. (1989). Basic fibroblast growth factor binds to subendothelial extracellular matrix and

is released by heparitinase and heparin-like molecules. *Biochemistry*, **28**, 1737–43.

39. Hanneken, A., Maher, P. A., and Baird, A. (1995). High affinity immunoreactive FGF receptors in the extracellular matrix of vascular endothelial cells — implications for the modulation of FGF-2. *J. Cell Biol.*, **128**, 1221–8.

40. Vlodavsky, I., Liu, G. M., and Gospodarowicz, D. (1980). Morphological appearance, growth behavior and migratory activity of human tumor cells maintained on extracellular matrix vs. plastic. *Cell*, **19**, 607–16.

41. Vlodavsky, I., Folkman, J., Sullivan, R., Fridman, R., Ishai-Michaelli, R., Sasse, J., and Klagsbrun, M. (1987). Endothelial cell-derived basic fibroblast growth factor: synthesis and deposition into subendothelial extracellular matrix. *Proc. Natl Acad. Sci. USA*, **84**, 2292–6.

42. Gospodarowicz, D., Delgado, D., and Vlodavsky, I. (1980). Permissive effect of the extracellular matrix on cell proliferation *in vitro*. *Proc. Natl Acad. Sci. USA*, **77**, 4094–8.

43. Folkman, J., Klagsbrun, M., Sasse, J., Wadzinski, M., Ingber, D., and Vlodavsky, I. (1980). A heparin-binding angiogenic protein — basic fibroblast growth factor — is stored within basement membrane. *Am. J. Pathol.*, **130**, 393–400.

44. Rogelj, S., Klagsbrun, M., Atzmon, R., Kurokawa, M., Haimovitz, A., Fuks, Z., and Vlodavsky, I. (1989). Basic fibroblast growth factor is an extracellular matrix component required for supporting the proliferation of vascular endothelial cells and the differentiation of PC12 cells. *J. Cell Biol.*, **109**, 823–31.

45. Cardon-Cardo, C., Vlodavsky, I., Haimovitz-Friedman, A., Hicklin, D., and Fuks, Z. (1990). Expression of basic fibroblast growth factor in normal human tissues. *Lab. Invest.*, **63**, 832–40.

46. Gonzalez, A. M., Buscaglia, M., Ong, M., and Baird, A. (1990). Distribution of basic fibroblast growth factor in the 18-day rat fetus: localization in the basement membranes of diverse tissues. *J. Cell. Biol.*, **110**, 753–65.

47. Ishai-Michaeli, R., Svahn, C-M., Chajek-Shaul, T., Korner, G., Ekre, H-P., and Vlodavsky, I. (1992). Importance of size and sulfation of heparin in release of basic fibroblast factor from the vascular endothelium and extracellular matrix. *Biochemistry*, **31**, 2080–8.

48. Aviezer, D., Levy, E., Safran, M., Svahn, C., Buddecke, E., Schmidt, A., *et al.* (1994). Differential structural requirements of heparin and heparan sulfate proteoglycans that promote basic fibroblast growth factor binding to its receptor. *J. Biol. Chem.*, **269**, 114–21.

49. Bashkin, P., Neufeld, G., Gitay, G. H., and Vlodavsky, I. (1992). Release of cell surface-associated basic fibroblast growth factor by glycosylphosphatidylinositol-specific phospholipase C. *J. Cell Physiol.*, **151**, 126–37.

50. Brunner, G., Gabrilove, J., Rifkin, D. B., and Wilson, E. L. (1991). Phospholipase C release of basic fibroblast growth factor from human bone marrow cultures as a biologically active complex with a phosphatidylinositol–anchored heparan sulfate proteoglycan. *J. Cell Biol.*, **114**, 1275–83.

51. Bernfield, M. and Hooper, K. C. (1991). Possible regulation of FGF activity by syndecan, an integral membrane heparan sulfate proteoglycan. *Ann. N. Y. Acad. Sci.*, **638**, 182–94.

52. Ishai-Michaeli, R., Eldor, A., and Vlodavsky, I. (1990). Heparanase activity expressed by platelets, neutrophils and lymphoma cells releases active fibroblast growth factor from extracellular matrix. *Cell Reg.*, **1**, 833–42.

53. Vlodavsky, I., Korner, G., Ishai-Michaeli, R., Bashkin, P., Bar-Shavit, R., and Fuks, Z. (1990). Extracellular matrix-resident growth factors and enzymes: possible involvement in tumor metastasis and angiogenesis. *Cancer Met. Rev.*, **9**, 203–26.

54. Vlodavsky, I., Eldor, A., Haimovitz-Friedman, A., Matzner, Y., Ishai-Michaeli, R., Levi, E., *et al.* (1992). Expression of heparanase by platelets and circulating cells of the immune system: Possible involvement in diapedesis and extravasation. *Invasion Metastasis*, **12**, 112–27.

55. Benezra, M., Vlodavsky, I., Ishai-Michaeli, R., Neufeld, G., and Bar-Shavit, R. (1993). Thrombin-induced release of active basic fibroblast growth factor–heparan sulfate complexes from subendothelial extracellular matrix. *Blood*, **81**, 3324–31.

56. Saksela, O. and Rifkin, D. B. (1990). Release of basic fibroblast growth factor–heparan sulfate complexes from endothelial cells by plasminogen activator-mediated proteolytic activity. *J. Cell Biol.*, **110**, 767–75.

57. Saksela, O., Moscatelli, D., Sommer, A., and Rifkin, D. B. (1988). Endothelial cell-derived heparan sulfate binds basic fibroblast growth factor and protects it from proteolytic degradation. *J. Cell Biol.*, **107**, 743–51.

58. Spivak-Kroizman, T., Lemmon, M. A., Dikic, I., Ladbury, J. E., Pinchasi, D., Huang, J., *et al.* (1994). Heparin-induced oligomerization of FGF molecules is responsible for FGF receptor dimerization, activation, and cell proliferation. *Cell*, **79**, 1015–24.

59. Ornitz, D. M., Herr, A. B., Nilsson, M., Westman, J., Svahn, C-M., and Waksman, G. (1995). FGF binding and FGF receptor activation by synthetic heparan-derived di- and trisaccharides. *Science*, **268**, 432–6.

60. Baird, A. and Walicke, P. A. (1989). Fibroblast growth factors. *Br. Med. Bull.*, **45**, 438–52.

61. Hanneken, A., Ying, W., Ling, N., and Baird, A. (1994). Identification of soluble forms of the fibroblast growth factor receptor in blood. *Proc. Natl Acad. Sci. USA*, **91**, 9170–4.

62. Jones, J. I., Gockerman, A., Busby, W. H., Camacho-Hubner, C., and Clemmons, D. R. (1993). Extracellular matrix contains insulin-like growth factor binding protein-5: potentiation of the effects of IGF-1. *J. Cell Biol.*, **121**, 679–87.

63. Vigny, M., Raulais, D., Puzenat, N., Duprez, D., Hartmann, M. P., Jeanny, J. C., and Courtois, Y. (1989). Identification of a new heparin-binding protein localized within chick basement membranes. *Eur. J. Biochem.*, **186**, 733–40.

64. Massague, J., Attisano, L., and Wrana, J. L. (1994). The TGF-beta family and its composite receptors. *Trends Cell Biol.*, **4**, 172–8.

65. Gordon, N. Y., Riley, G. P., Watt, S. M., and Greaves, M. F. (1987). Compartmentalization of a haematopoietic growth factor (GM-CSF) by glycosaminoglycans in the bone marrow microenvironment. *Nature*, **326**, 403–5.

66. Tanaka, Y., Adams, D. H., and Shaw, S. (1993). Proteoglycans on endothelial cells present adhesion-inducing cytokines to leukocytes. *Immunol. Today*, **14**, 111–115.

67. Kjellen, L. and Lindahl, U. (1991). Proteoglycans: structures and interactions. *Annu. Rev. Biochem.*, **60**, 443–75.

68. Miao, H-Q., Fritz, T. A., Esko, J. D., Zimmermann, J., Yayon, A., and Vlodavsky, I. (1995). Heparan sulfate primed on beta-D-xylosides restores binding of basic fibroblast growth factor. *J. Cell. Biochem.*, **57**, 173–84.

69. Benezra, M., Vlodavsky, I., Yayon, A., Bar-Shavit, R., Regan, J., Chang, M., and Ben-Sasson, S. (1992). Reversal of basic fibroblast growth factor-mediated autocrine cell transformation by aromatic anionic compounds. *Cancer Res.*, **52**, 5656–62.

70. Benezra, M., Ben-Sasson, S., Regan, J., Chang, M., Bar-Shavit, R., and Vlodavsky, I. (1994). Antiproliferative activity to vascular smooth muscle cells and receptor binding of heparin-mimicking polyaromatic anionic compounds. *Arterioscler. Thromb.*, **14**, 1992–9.

71. Vlodavsky, I., Miao, H. Q., Atzmon, R., Levi, E., Zimmermann, J., Bar-Shavit, R., *et al.*, (1995). Control of cell proliferation by heparan sulfate and heparin-binding growth factors. *Thromb. Haemost.*, **74**, 534–40.

72. Fritz, T. A., Lugemwa, F. N., Sarkar, A. K., and Esko, J. D. (1994). Biosynthesis of heparan sulfate on beta-D-xylosides depends on aglycone structure. *J. Biol. Chem.*, **269**, 300–7.

73. Rapraeger, A., Krufka, A., and Olwin, B. R. (1991). Requirement of heparan sulfate for bFGF-mediated fibroblast growth and myoblast differentiation. *Science*, **252**, 1705–8.

74. Levi, E., Fridman, R., Miao, H. Q., Ma, Y.-C., Yayon, A., and Vlodavsky, I. (1996). Matrix metalloproteinase-2 (MMP-2) releases active soluble ectodomain of fibroblast growth factor receptor-1. *Proc. Natl Acad. Sci. USA*, **96**, 7069–74.

75. Miao, H.-Q., Ishai-Michaeli, R., Atzmon, R., Peretz, T., and Vlodavsky, I. (1996). Sulfate moieties in the subendothelial extracellular matrix are involved in basic fibroblast growth factor sequestration, dimerization, and stimulation of cell proliferation. *J. Biol. Chem.*, **271**, 4879–86.

76. Turnbull, J. E., Femig, D. G., Ke, Y., Wilkinson, M., and Gallagher, J. T. (1992). Identification of basic fibroblast growth factor binding sequence in fibroblast heparan sulfate. *J. Biol. Chem.*, **267**, 10337–41.

77. Aviezer, D., Hecht, D., Safran, M., Eisinger, M., David, G., and Yayon, A. (1994). Perlecan, basal lamina proteoglycan, promotes basic fibroblast growth factor-receptor binding, mitogenesis, and angiogenesis. *Cell*, **79**, 1005–13.

78. Steinfeld, R., Van Den Berghe, H., David, G. (1996). Stimulation of fibroblast growth factor receptor-1 occupancy and signaling by cell surface-associated syndecans and glypican. *J. Cell Biol.*, **133**, 405–16.

79. Schmidt, A., Yoshida, K., and Buddecke, E. (1992). The antiproliferative activity of arterial heparan sulfate resides in domains enriched with 2-*O*-sulfated uronic acid residues. *J. Biol. Chem.*, **267**, 19242–7.

80. Hoogewerf, A. J., Leone, J. W., Reardon, M., Howe, W. J., Asa, D., Heinrikson, R. L., and Ledbetter, S. R. (1995). CXC chemokines connective tissue activating peptide-III and neutrophil activating peptide-2 are heparin/heparan sulfate-degrading enzymes. *J. Biol. Chem.*, **270**, 3268–77.

81. Gilat, D., Hershkoviz, R., Goldkorn, I., Cahalon, L., Korner, G., Vlodavsky, I., and Lider, O. (1995). Molecular behavior adapts to context: heparanase functions as an extracellular matrix-degrading enzyme or as a T cell adhesion molecule, depending on the local pH. *J. Exp. Med.*, **181**, 1929–34.

82. Menashi, S., Vlodavsky, I., Ishai-Michaeli, R., Legrand, Y., and Fridman, R. (1995). The extracellular matrix produced by bovine corneal endothelial cells contains progelatinase A. *FEBS Lett.*, **361**, 61–4.

83. Korner, G., Bjornsson, T., and Vlodavsky, I. (1993). Extracellular matrix produced by cultured corneal and aortic endothelial cells contains active tissue-type and urokinase-type plasminogen activators. *J. Cell Physiol.*, **154**, 456–65.

84. Nicolson, G. L. (1988). Organ specificity of tumor metastasis: role of preferential adhesion, invasion and growth of malignant cells at specific secondary sites. *Cancer Metastasis. Rev.*, **7**, 143–88.

85. Liotta, L. A., Rao, C. N., and Barsky, S. H. (1983). Tumor invasion and the extracellular matrix. *Lab. Invest.*, **49**, 639–49.

86. Vlodavsky, I., Fuks, Z., Bar-Ner, M., Ariav, Y., and Schirrmacher, V. (1983). Lymphoma cell mediated degradation of sulfated proteoglycans in the subendothelial extracellular matrix: relationship to tumor cell metastasis. *Cancer Res.*, **43**, 2704–11.

87. Nakajima, M., Irimura, T., and Nicolson, G. L. (1988). Heparanase and tumor metastasis. *J. Cell. Biochem.*, **36**, 157–67.

88. Lider, O., Cahalon, L., Gilat, D., Hershkovitz, R., Siegel, D., Margalit, R., *et al.* (1995). A disaccharide that inhibits tumor necrosis factor a is formed from the extracellular matrix by the enzyme heparanase. *Proc. Natl Acad. Sci. USA*, **92**, 5037–41.

89. Bar-Ner, M., Eldor, A., Wasserman, L., Matzner, Y., and Vlodavsky, I. (1987). Inhibition of heparanase mediated degradation of extracellular matrix heparan sulfate by modified and non-anticoagulant heparin species. *Blood*, **70**, 551–7.

90. Coombe, D. R., Parish, C. R., Ramshaw, I. A., and Snowden, J. M. (1987). Analysis of the inhibition of tumor metastasis by sulphataed polysaccharides. *Int. J. Cancer*, **39**, 82–88.

91. Parish, C. R., Coombe, D. R., Jakobsen, K. B., and Underwood, P. A. (1987). Evidence that sulphated polysaccharides inhibit tumor metastasis by blocking tumor cell-derived heparanase. *Int. J. Cancer*, **40**, 511–17.

92. Vlodavsky, I., Mohsen, M., Lider, O., Ishai-Michaeli, R., Ekre, H-P., Svahn, C. M., *et al.* (1995). Inhibition of tumor metastasis by heparanase inhibiting species of heparin. *Invasion Metastasis*, **14**, 290–302.

93. Lider, O., Baharav, E., Mekori, Y., Miller, T., Naparstek, Y., Vlodavsky, I., and Cohen, I. R. (1989). Suppression of experimental autoimmune diseases and prolongation of allograft survival by treatment of animals with heparinoid inhibitors of T lymphocyte heparanase. *J. Clin. Invest.*, **83**, 752–6.

94. Nguyen, M., Watanabe, H., Budson, A. E., Richie, J. P., Hayes, D. F., and Folkman, J. (1994). Elevated levels of an angiogenic peptide, basic fibroblast growth factor, in the urine of patients with a wide spectrum of cancers [see comments]. *J. Natl Cancer Inst.*, **86**, 356–61.

95. Reich-Slotky, R., Bonneh-Barkay, D., Shaoul, E., Bluma, B., Svahn, C.-M., and Ron, D. (1994). Differential effect of cell-associated heparan sulfates on the binding of keratinocyte growth factor (KGF) and acidic fibroblast growth factor to the KGF receptor. *J. Biol. Chem.*, **269**, 32279–85.

13. The role of collagens and proteoglycans in tumour angiogenesis

P. Rooney, P. Kumar, J. Ponting, and S. Kumar

Introduction

The natural history of tumour development and growth is well established. A population of cells within a host is exposed to an initiation factor and a new wave of gene expression occurs, removing normal growth constraints from the primary tumour (1,2). The primary tumour can grow to approximately 1–2 mm in diameter but will grow no further unless it is vascularized (3–5). Tumour angiogenesis is a multistep cascade of events which proceeds only when a proportion of cells within the tumour, estimated to be less than 10% (6,7), switches to an angiogenic phenotype, and releases factors which either act directly on endothelial cells of neighbouring blood vessels or stimulate surrounding stromal tissue to release factors which act on the endothelial cells. Once activated, endothelial cells are induced to degrade local extracellular matrix (ECM), migrate through the ECM, proliferate, and reach the tumour. Thus, tumour angiogenesis occurs as a combination of interactions with soluble angiogenic mediators and insoluble ECM macromolecules (4,5,8–13). Tumour angiogenesis is important as it allows a primary tumour to grow beyond 2 mm and is a prerequisite for tumour metastasis (14,15). Metastasis is also a multistep cascade involving two stages of tumour angiogenesis — the primary tumour becomes vascularized, tumour cells migrate to and breach the blood vessel basal lamina. Tumour cells circulating in the blood may adhere to a basal lamina at a distant site, migrate through the blood vessel wall and become lodged in another tissue, cell proliferation occurs and vascularization of a secondary tumour(s) is induced (6,14–16). Secondary tumour angiogenesis appears to involve similar mechanisms to that of primary tumour angiogenesis.

Several reports have linked a high microvessel density in primary tumours with high metastatic potential and a poor prognosis (16,17), e.g. invasive breast carcinoma, melanoma, non-small cell lung carcinoma, prostate carcinoma, and head and neck carcinoma.

A number of soluble angiogenic mediators have been identified, these include the family of fibroblast growth factors (FGFs) (18,19), the family of transforming growth factors (20,21), platelet-derived endothelial cell growth factor (22), vascular endothelial cell growth factor (23,24), tumour necrosis factor α (25), hepatocyte growth factor (scatter factor) (26), angiogenin (27,28), and prostaglandins (29,30). Some insoluble ECM macromolecules, e.g. proteoglycans and glycosaminoglycans (GAGs) also act as angiogenic mediators (31,32).

This chapter will not deal with the production of angiogenic mediators but rather will concentrate on the molecular and cellular events following activation of endothelial cells by exposure to the mediator(s). We will highlight the parts played by ECM macromolecules, particularly collagens and proteoglycans, in directing and regulating angiogenesis and suggest that as these molecules interact directly with endothelial cells, they may be suitable candidates for targets in the inhibition of angiogenesis.

The amount of ECM within tumours varies depending on the type of tumour, e.g. breast carcinomas have a high ECM content while small cell carcinomas of the lung contain little ECM (33). Tumour cells constantly interact with ECM macromolecules to facilitate tumour growth and expansion. The composition of the ECM and its interaction with tumour cells may determine the metastatic potential of tumours (34–36). However, as angiogenesis must involve endothelial cells, we will investigate only interactions between endothelial cells and ECM molecules.

Composition of the extracellular matrix

The main components of the ECM are collagens, proteoglycans, glycoproteins, and elastin (32,37). Of these, the most abundant and possibly the most important are collagens and proteoglycans. Collagens are thought to provide structural strength to the tissue while proteoglycans resist compressive forces and allow diffusion of soluble molecules (38–42).

Collagen molecules have as a central feature one or more triple-helical rod-like structures composed of three α chains either in a homotrimeric or heterotrimeric form. At least 19 different collagen types have been identified and separated into five groups depending on whether they form fibrils and the degree to which the triple helix is interrupted (38,39,43,44). We will mainly examine the roles of collagen types I and VIII in angiogenesis, although collagen types III, IV, and VII will also be discussed.

Proteoglycans are macromolecules composed of a protein core with O- and N-linked polysaccharides and sulphated GAGs attached (41,45). The protein core, showing considerable heterogeneity, can range from 11 to >220 kDa and can have as many as 100 GAG side chains (46,47). Five types of GAG have been identified. Four of these are generally sulphated: chondroitin sulphate, keratan sulphate, dermatan sulphate, and heparan sulphate (41,45,48). The remaining GAG, hyaluronan (HA), is distinct in that it is not sulphated, is considerably larger than the others, is synthesized on the cell membrane and is extruded while still elongating (49,50). HA is composed of a repeating disaccharide unit of D-glucuronic acid and N-acetyl-D-glucosamine (51). It can form the backbone to which aggregating proteoglycans bind via non-covalent bonds or it can exist as a free GAG which may be linked to other proteins (50,52).

HA has been implicated in tumour growth and spread (53), features probably related to its angiogenic properties demonstrated by our group (31,32). Native, high molecular weight HA is anti-angiogenic and may be important for tumour invasion and expansion within a host. However, HA degradation products within a specific size range: 3–10 disaccharide units, are angiogenic both *in vivo* and *in vitro* (31,54–56) (Fig. 13.1).

Binding of angiogenic mediators

The first stage in tumour angiogenesis is activation of endothelial cells by an angiogenic mediator. Several reports have indicated that the onset of angiogenesis is associated with protein phosphorylation and cell surface protein kinase activity (57). If protein kinase C (PKC) is experimentally activated, either *in vitro* using human umbilical vein endothelial cells (HUVEC), or *in vivo* on the chorioallantoic membrane of the chick embryo (CAM), enhanced angiogenesis is observed (58,59). In contrast, if PKC inhibitors are added, angiogenesis is inhibited (58,60). A similar inhibition of angiogenesis is observed if intracellular levels of cyclic adenosine monophosphate (cAMP) are increased, *e.g.* by the addition of forskolin (58). HA binding to the RHAMM protein (receptor for HA mediated motility) on fibroblasts also results in enhanced protein tyrosine phosphorylation and enhanced cell motility (61).

Once activated, HUVEC cells rapidly undergo sprouting within collagen gels, or within Matrigel (a mixture of collagen, laminin, and glycoproteins). This sprouting has

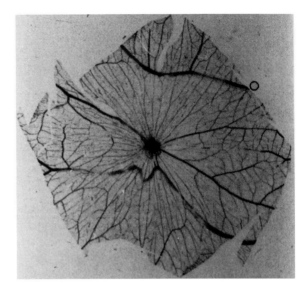

(a)

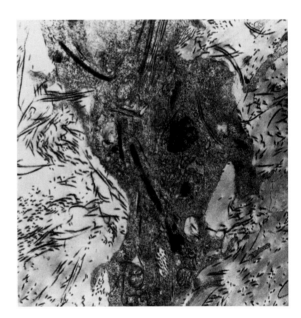

(b)

Figure 13.1. Chicken chorioallantoic membrane assay. Application of angiogenic oligosaccharides of hyaluronan (HA) induces neovascularization (a). Electron microscopy of an HA treated CAM shows abundant collagen fibrils at the site of angiogenesis (b) (For details see West *et al.* (1985). *Science*, **228**, 289 (31) and Rooney *et al.* (1993). *J. Cell Sci.*, **105**, 213 (56).)

been linked to G-protein activation and integrin function (59,62).

The role of integrins in angiogenesis and metastasis is receiving attention and it has been demonstrated that 76% of primary tumours and 82% of secondary tumours express the integrin dimer $\alpha_3\beta_1$ (63). The vascular endothelial cell line EAhy926 forms sprouts within 12–16 h when plated on to Matrigel and, once again, invasion is associated with expression of G-proteins and integrin subunits α_6 and/or β_1 (62). The $\alpha_2\beta_1$ collagen-binding integrin has also been shown to be important in collagen-induced endothelial cell tube formation (64). It is likely that many of the interactions between endothelial cells and the ECM will be regulated by integrins during the migratory phase of angiogenesis (65).

Gene expression

Once an angiogenic mediator has bound to the cell surface, protein phosphorylation and signal transduction pathways are switched on and a wave of gene expression is observed. We have demonstrated that when HA oligosaccharides of 3–10 disaccharide units in length are added to bovine aortic endothelial cells (BAEC) a rapid up-regulation of immediate early response genes (ERGs) is observed (our unpublished data). Within 30 min of the addition of HA oligosaccharides, the ERGs c-*fos*, c-*jun*, Jun-B, *krox*-20 and *krox*-24 are all expressed. In contrast, c-*myc* is not up-regulated. Similarly, during embryonic development and in wound healing, the ERG c-*ets*-1 is also up-regulated at the onset of angiogenesis (66).

Each of these ERGs are transcription factors which bind to DNA and regulate the transcription of genes for matrix metalloproteinases (MMPs), e.g. collagenases, stromelysin, and urokinase plasminogen activator — enzymes responsible for ECM degradation (66–68). Thus, binding of an angiogenic mediator to endothelial cells sets in motion a sequence leading to local ECM degradation. It may be important to note that the addition of angiogenic oligosaccharides of HA to BAEC *in vitro* does not stimulate cell proliferation until at least 48 h after exposure (13,69). It would appear that, as in *in vivo* angiogenesis, cell proliferation is a late phenomenon and the earliest stages in the angiogenic process involve local dissolution of ECM macromolecules and cell migration.

Collagen degradation during angiogenesis

Tumour ECM contains a mixture of collagens and proteoglycans, of which type IV collagen and laminin in the basement membrane have received the greatest attention, as the basal lamina has to be degraded for metastasis to occur (70). Little attention has been paid to the observation that basement membranes in carcinomas also contain type VII collagen (anchoring plaques) whereas normal tissue does not. This lack of attention may need to be rectified as evidence suggests that type VII collagen is often degraded prior to type IV collagen degradation (70).

Owing to the complexity of tumour ECM, many studies have been performed on endothelial cells grown *in vitro* within or on top of a three-dimensional gel. If cells invade the gel and produce a lumen-like structure, this is taken to represent *in vitro* angiogenesis. Care has to be taken in interpreting these data as the type of cell and the type of gel utilized can produce conflicting results. HUVEC will invade a collagen gel composed of type III collagen more quickly than a type I collagen gel (71). Bovine brain endothelial cells, bovine carotid artery endothelial cells, and BAEC all invade Matrigel; however, only brain endothelial cells will invade if plated on top of a type I collagen gel. Carotid artery cells and BAEC require a second layer of collagen gel before invasion proceeds, i.e. these cells will only invade when embedded in type I collagen (72).

Endothelial cell invasion of three-dimensional gels is associated with the production of MMPs. Invasion of gels by HUVEC and EAhy926 causes synthesis of interstitial collagenase, gelatinase A, and gelatinase B but not stromelysin (62,73). Cellular invasion can be inhibited by the addition of tissue inhibitor of metalloproteinases or the synthetic peptide BB-94 (73,74). *In vitro* angiogenesis can be enhanced by the addition of the laminin peptide SIKVAV to Matrigel and once again, invasion is linked to the production of type IV collagenase (75).

Collagen synthesis during tumour angiogenesis

The role of collagens in angiogenesis has recently received much attention. Metabolic inhibition of synthesis of collagen types I and IV inhibits capillary formation on the CAM (76,77). We have demonstrated that the experimentally induced angiogenesis on the CAM is associated with the deposition of large amounts of collagen (56) (Fig. 13.1). Endothelial cell migration from aortic explants within collagen gels is inhibited if grown in the presence of the proline analogue *cis*-hydroxyproline, once again indicating the need for normal collagen synthesis (78).

In vitro studies suggest that co-expression of type I collagen and the calcium-binding protein SPARC (secreted protein, acidic, and rich in cysteine) is initiated when BAEC undergo sprouting angiogenesis (79–81). Type VIII collagen is also synthesized during sprouting and has been localized to proliferating endothelial cells within endothelial cords (81). Histological examination of normal, tumour, and experimentally induced angiogenesis has extended the demonstration that type I and type VIII collagens are localized within endothelial cords and tubes (82,83). Type I collagen is believed to aid endothelial cell migration, while type VIII collagen is considered to be involved in endothelial cell migration and tube formation (56,79–81).

How type VIII collagen aids cell migration has not yet been fully elucidated. Native type VIII collagen is most abundant in the Descemet's membrane of the eye where it forms a hexagonal lattice (84). Type VIII collagen is composed of a heterotrimer of $[\alpha_1 (VIII)]_2, \alpha_2 (VIII)$. It is a short chain collagen with a molecular weight of 60–62 kDa (43,56), similar in size, chemical characteristics and gene structure to type X collagen, a protein produced only by hypertrophic chondrocytes. Both proteins have their triple-helical region encoded by one exon (85–87). Type X collagen also forms a hexagonal lattice and is thought to alter the existing structure of the ECM within cartilage (88). If type VIII collagen secreted during angiogenesis forms a lattice, this could alter the already partially degraded local ECM structure, allowing migration of cells. Type VIII collagen is believed to interact directly with ECM molecules such as HA or another polyanionic GAG (82,85).

We have reported that when BAEC are exposed to angiogenic HA oligosaccharides, type I collagen synthesis is up-regulated 4.5-fold and synthesis of type VIII collagen is enhanced 5.8-fold within 12 h (56).

Although the synthesis of collagens may be important for angiogenesis, it may not necessarily enhance it. When S13 tumour cells are implanted beneath the skin of BALB/c mice, a rapid angiogenic response is observed. If type I collagen is also added, it has no effect on the rate or degree of angiogenesis (89). In contrast, the addition of fibronectin or fibronectin-derived peptides greatly reduces the angiogenic response (89).

Proteoglycans, glycosaminoglycans, and angiogenesis

The role of these ECM macromolecules in tumour angiogenesis has received little attention and what evidence there is in the literature is conflicting. In some instances, most intact proteoglycans and sulphated GAGs have been noted to induce an anti-angiogenic response on the CAM, as seen with native HA and, if used in conjunction with corticosteroids, this anti-angiogenesis is enhanced

(31,90,91). These ECM macromolecules have to become partially degraded to elicit an angiogenic response. Other reports which are in disagreement with these conclusions are discussed in the next section.

Partial degradation of HA may be a physiological occurrence. Daily injections of native HA into the rabbit ear chamber inhibit vascularization of granulation tissue, whereas intermittent injections significantly increase vascularization (92). It was concluded that intermittent injection can allow activation of macrophages and angiogenic mediators, but it is also possible that, between injections, native HA becomes partially degraded into an angiogenic form. HA with angiogenic properties has been extracted from mouse ovaries but the molecular size has not been determined (93,94). A correlation between metastasizing tumours and HA size has been observed in the sera of children with a bone-metastasizing variant of renal tumour compared with Wilms' tumour, which does not normally metastasize. The presence of raised levels of low molecular weight HA signifies a probability of metastasis (95).

The angiogenic action of HA is specific to endothelial cells. HA oligosaccharide binding to BAEC induces cell migration and proliferation but has little effect on smooth muscle cells and fibroblasts. When applied to rat skin, HA oligosaccharides significantly increase the number of blood vessels per unit area (69).

One other proteoglycan which is known to have angiogenic properties is heparan sulphate proteoglycan (HSPG), discussed in greater detail in the next section. HSPG binds to the angiogenic factor, basic fibroblast growth factor (bFGF), in an inactive form within the ECM (96). Upon HSPG degradation, bFGF is released and is free to stimulate angiogenesis. Many tumours are associated with an accumulation of mast cells and as mast cell lysates and granules contain heparanase, it has been suggested that mast cells may facilitate HSPG degradation and thus bFGF release (97,98) (see also next section for more details).

Cell surface HSPG is also believed to be an angiogenic mediator. In HT-29 human colon adenocarcinoma cells, HSPG with a molecular weight in excess of 200 kDa stimulates angiogenesis by binding another angiogenic mediator, angiogenin, thereby initiating the signal transduction pathway outlined above (99).

Mast cells

Friedrich von Recklinghausen, in 1863, noticed mast cells in the unstained mesentery of frogs. Fifteen years later Paul Ehrlich stained these cells and christened them Mastzellen ('well fed cells') (100). Over the years, mast cells have attracted considerable attention, particularly from immunopharmacologists, because of their well-established role in hypersensitivity and inflammatory diseases. Activation of mast cells releases a plethora of potent mediators such as prostaglandins, leukotrienes, histamine, cytokines, neutral proteases, heparin, etc. (101,102). Mast cells are normally present in the connective tissues of most organs, in serosal cavities and mucosal epithelia. They differ in different anatomical situations — skin mast cells contain large amounts of chymase whereas lung mast cells have little or no chymase. A number of observations on their spatial and temporal locations suggest that they are associated with neovascularization and thus may be important in angiogenesis (101–113). Following the original observation of Kessler *et al.* (104) that tumour implants in chick embryo lead to a 40-fold increase in mast cell density, we repeatedly encountered mast cells around and at the apparent 'tip' of budding blood vessels (105–108) (Fig. 13.2). Mast cell-mediated angiogenesis has been demonstrated by the selective activation of autogenous mast cells *in situ* in adult rats (109) and mice (110) using the mesenteric–window angiogenesis assay. Mast cell activation was elicited by intraperitoneal injections of the archetypal histamine liberator compound 48/80, which is highly selective and potent in these species. In guinea-pigs, the mast cells of which are unresponsive to the secretagogue, the same intraperitoneal treatment with compound 48/80 caused no effect (109). As the test tissue

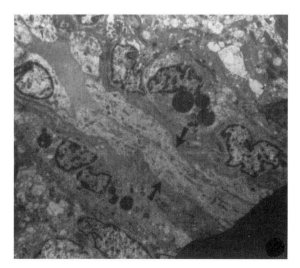

Figure 13.2. Electron micrograph of human rheumatoid joint; mast cells are often found in tissues undergoing angiogenesis particularly in close proximity to blood vessels. Here a mast cell is located at the apparent tip of a sprouting blood vessel. (For details see Kumar *et al.* (1985). *Cancer Res.*, **45**, 4339 (107).)

lacks significant angiogenesis physiologically, *de novo* angiogenesis was induced following mast cell activation. Although the evidence for the involvement of mast cells in tumour growth and spread is strong (reviewed in reference 101), it is important to point out that angiogenesis, albeit at a diminished rate, can proceed in situations where mast cells are scarce, *e.g.* in diabetic retinopathy and in mast cell deficient mice (W/W^{v}). In the latter situation reconstitution of the phenotype with mast cells can almost completely restore tumour angiogenesis (101). How mast cells augment angiogenesis is not known. As mentioned in a previous section, it could be through the interaction of heparin-binding growth factors and other mast cell products such as type VIII collagen and cytokines.

Heparin is a highly sulphated glycosaminoglycan which is produced by and stored in mast cells alone (109). Heparin can stimulate migration and proliferation of endothelial cells *in vitro* (113). While Folkman's group found that heparin was not angiogenic by itself *in vivo*, it did potentiate the angiogenic activity of tumour cell extracts (114). In contrast, Norrby demonstrated that systemic administration of commercial, unfractionated preparations of heparin (UFH) could augment angiogenesis in the rat mesenteric–window assay (Fig. 13.3) (111). He further noticed that the effect of heparin on angiogenesis was size-dependent, i.e. high molecular mass UFH was angiogenic whereas low molecular mass heparin, of a certain size range, present in the same UFH preparation was anti-angiogenic (Table 13.1). There was in fact a clear size-dependent correlation with angiogenesis. This difference was independent of sulphate content, molarity, and anti-coagulant activity (111). Systemic injection of any of these heparin preparations failed to cause local haematoma or ulceration and there was no weight loss. Heparin enhances the mitogenic action of bFGF (115,116).

Heparan sulphate, a GAG structurally related to heparin, is present on the endothelial cell surface and in the basement membrane and can bind bFGF, maybe serving as its reservoir (115). Mast cell heparin can induce both release of bFGF and prolong the half-life of released bFGF by shielding it from enzymatic degradation and heat deactivation. Recently, considerable information has become available to enable speculation on the possible mechanism of induction of angiogenesis by heparin (117–121). bFGF uses a dual receptor system to mediate activation of signal transduction pathways. This consists of a family of five receptor tyrosine kinases and HSPGs (120,121). It was found that the role of HSPGs can be performed by octa- or decasaccharide fragments derived chemically or enzymatically from heparin (117,118). However these preparations contain mixtures of isomers (primarily due to differences in the distribution of SO$_3$ groups) with

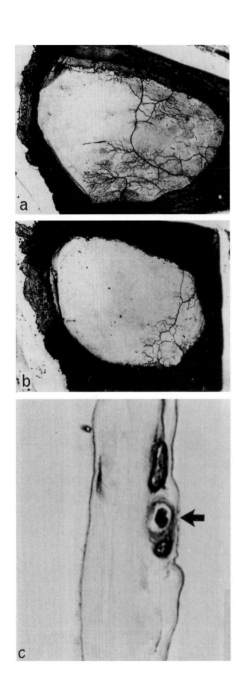

Figure 13.3. Adult rat mesenteric window assay for the quantification of angiogenesis. Low power photomicrographs of treated (a) and control (b) mesentery wherein vasculature has been visualized by an ATPase staining reaction. Bottom figure (c) is a 3 μm tissue section of a mesentery — arrow points to a blood vessel containing a red blood cell. (From Norrby (1993). *Int. J. Microcirc. Clin. Exp.*, **12**, 119.)

modified oligosaccharide ends making the task of determining true structure/function relationships extremely difficult. To overcome these problems, Ornitz and his colleagues have chemically synthesized and determined the function of non-sulphated di-, tri- and tetrasaccharides corresponding to structures found in heparin (120). These synthetic molecules are isometrically pure and do not contain modified sugar residues. Their data show that both non-sulphated di- and trisaccharides can activate the FGF signalling pathway in a F32 cell line which expresses FGF receptor and requires bFGF for its growth. In the light of recent developments in the study of the mechanism of FGF activation it should soon be possible to evaluate the clinical usefulness of synthetic fragments in modulation of angiogenesis and to embark on the design of growth factor antagonists by protein engineering or through structure-based drug design.

The production of type VIII collagen by endothelial cells and its role in angiogenesis has been discussed in the section on 'collagen synthesis during tumour angiogenesis'. Recently, Neale's group in New Zealand, using monoclonal and polyclonal antibodies to type VIII collagen and its α1 (VIII) chain and by *in situ* hybridization, demonstrated that type VIII collagen and its mRNA were localized to a subset of mast cells, especially in fibrotic diseases (122). This is the first report of any ECM component being produced by mast cells in humans or animals. These mast cells did not express interstitial collagens, namely types I, III, and V. This is an intriguing observation and raises some important questions. Why do two cell types (endothelial and mast cells) which are in close proximity during angiogenesis synthesize the same molecule? The production of type VIII collagen by one cell type might precede production by the other cell type and the former might induce its synthesis by the latter. Co-culture studies of these two cell types may be able to resolve this issue. At present almost nothing is known of molecular mechanisms capable of modulating mast cell activation (123).

Temporal sequence of angiogenesis

Upon exposure to and binding by an angiogenic mediator, the initial response of endothelial cells is to up-regulate expression of transcription factors for MMPs (66–68). Local degradation of ECM is known to be an important early factor in the angiogenic cascade. Several pieces of data suggest that angiogenesis cannot proceed without new collagen synthesis (76,77). Indeed, we have shown that synthesis of type I and VIII collagens is a prerequisite for BAEC migration (56). We would suggest that angio-

Table 13.1. Angiogenic response of unfractionated heparin (UFH) and heparin saccharides (mean molecular weights of 2.4, 8, 15, and 22 kDa) using rat mesenteric window assay; details with regard to their molarity, sulphate content and anticoagulant activity are given. The body weights of treated animals are expressed as mean percentage of controls (modified from Norrby, *Haemostasis* 1993; **23**: 141[111])

Source of heparin	Angiogenic response*	Concentration			Sulphate content (%)	Body weight (% controls)
		Weight (mg/ml)	Molarity (nmol/ml)	Activity (IU/ml)		
Unfractionated	100	5	0.40	870	10.6	101.09 ± 1.19
Fractionated saccharides						
2.4 kDa	50	8	3.33	<10	12.0	99.90 ± 1.24
8 kDa	112	5	0.68	630	11.1	102.56 ± 1.11
15 kDa	120	5	0.39	800	10.1	101.63 ± 1.43
22 kDa	225	5	0.21	620	10.2	101.33 ± 0.95

* Unfractionated heparin response was normalized to 100. A linear regression analysis between the mean molecular weight of the fractions and the normalized response showed that $r = 0.97$ ($y = 32.16 + 8.02x$). The response to the 2.4 kDa fraction was significantly lower ($P<0.001$) than UFH, and to the 22 kDa fraction was significantly higher than UFH ($P<0.01$). The differences between the 8 kDa and the 22 kDa fractions and between the 15 kDa and the 22 kDa fractions were also significant ($P<0.005$ and $P<0.02$, respectively[111]).

genesis is not only a well-regulated local event, but that it is also closely regulated in a temporal fashion.

Maximal stimulation of ERG expression occurs within 30 min of exposure to HA oligosaccharides, indicating that MMP production would be very rapid. In contrast, collagen synthesis cannot be detected immunocytochemically until approximately 12 h after stimulation (56). We believe that local degradation of ECM begins and ceases within that time, producing a loose ECM with extracellular spaces. Collagen synthesis is then initiated and endothelial cells migrate into and through the spaces. It is also possible that during the angiogenic process, waves of ECM degradation and collagen synthesis occur along the length of the newly formed endothelial cord. ECM degradation would occur at the tip where the endothelial cells come into contact with an angiogenic mediator such as low molecular weight HA and collagen synthesis would occur in the middle and base of the cord in association with cell proliferation and migration. It is important to note that HA has been localized to the tip of invading capillaries and that an inverse relationship between HA and collagen synthesis occurs in several systems (31,83).

Summary and conclusions

Many reports suggest that anti-angiogenic therapy may be useful in the control of tumour formation and growth (3–5,14,15,124). By the time an invasive tumour has been diagnosed, the primary tumour is already vascularized and has often metastasized, therefore prevention of secondary

angiogenesis may be the most productive target for clinical development (14).

Several lines of research are concentrated on blocking the effect of some angiogenic mediators on tumours, particularly growth factors such as bFGF, with a varying degree of success. The diverse nature of tumours and the range of angiogenic mediators which act on them make it unlikely that any single molecule will be able to prevent tumour metastasis. We would suggest that as angiogenesis cannot occur without local ECM degradation, local endothelial cell migration, and cell proliferation and as these mechanisms cannot occur without ERG expression and collagen synthesis, then prevention of ERG up-regulation and collagen synthesis, particularly type VIII collagen synthesis, may prove highly beneficial in the retardation of tumour angiogenesis.

Acknowledgements

We are grateful to Professor K. Norrby for his helpful suggestions and for allowing us to use his published data. We would like to thank Mrs M. Massey for typing this manuscript. J.P. is in receipt of a Wellcome Trust Fellowship.

References

1. Dameron, K. M., Volpert, O. V., Tainsky, M. A., and Bouck, N. P. (1994). Control of angiogenesis in fibroblasts by p53 regulation of thrombospondin 1. *Science*, **265**, 1582–4.

2. Antoniades, H. (1992). Linking cellular injury to gene expression and human proliferative disorders: examples with PDGF genes. *Mol. Carcinogeresis*, **6**, 175–81.

3. Brem, S., Brem, H., Folkman, J., Finkelstein, D., and Patz, A. (1976). Prolonged tumour dormancy by prevention of neovascularisation in the vitreous. *Cancer Res.*, **36**, 2807–12.

4. Folkman, J. (1985). Tumour angiogenesis. *Adv. Cancer Res.*, **43**, 175–203.

5. Folkman, J. and Shing, Y. (1992). Angiogenesis. *J. Biol. Chem.*, **267**, 10931–4.

6. Folkman, J. (1992). The role of angiogenesis in tumour growth. *Semin. Cancer Biol.*, **3**, 65–71.

7. Folkman, J., Watson, K. Ingber, D. E., and Hanahan, D. (1991). Induction of angiogenesis during the transition from hyperplasia to neoplasia. *Nature*, **339**, 58–61.

8. Schor, A. M. and Schor, S. L. (1983). Tumor angiogenesis. *J. Pathol.*, **141**, 385–91.

9. Furcht, L. T. (1985). Critical factors controlling angiogenesis: cell products, cell matrix, growth factors. *Lab. Invest.*, **55**, 505–9.

10. Madri, J. A. and Pratt, B. M. (1988). Angiogenesis. In *The molecular and cellular biology of wound repair* (ed. R. A. F. Clark and P. M. Henson), pp. 337–54. Plenum Press, New York.

11. Paweletz, N. and Knierim, M. (1989). Tumour-related angiogenesis. *Crit. Rev. Oncol. Hematol.*, **9**, 197–242.

12. Paku, S. and Paweletz, N. (1991). First steps of tumour-related angiogenesis. *Lab. Invest.*, **65**, 334–46.

13. Rooney, P., Kumar, S., Ponting, J., and Wang, M. (1995). The role of hyaluronan in tumour neovascularization. *Int. J. Cancer*, **60**, 632–6.

14. Weinstat-Saslow, D. and Steeg, P. S. (1994). Angiogenesis and colonization in the tumour metastatic process: basic and applied advances. *FASEB J.*, **8**, 401–7.

15. Stracke, M. L. and Liotta, L. A. (1992). Multi-step cascade of tumour cell metastasis. *In Vivo*, **6**, 306–16.

16. Weidner, N. (1993). Tumor angiogenesis: review of current applications in tumor prognostication. *Semin. Diagn. Pathol.*, **10**, 302–13.

17. Craft, P. S. and Harris, A. L. (1994). Clinical prognostic significance of tumour angiogenesis. *Ann. Oncol.*, **5**, 305–11.

18. Montesano, R., Vassalli, J. D., Baird, A., Guillemin, R., and Orci, L. (1986). Basic fibroblast growth factor induces angiogenesis *in vitro*. *Proc. Natl Acad. Sci. USA*, **83**, 7297–301.

19. Nabal, E. G., Yang, Z., Plantz, G., Forough, R., Zhan, X., Haudenschild, C. C., *et al.* (1993). Recombinant fibroblast growth factor-1 promotes intimal hyperplasia and angiogenesis in arteries *in vivo*. *Nature*, **362**, 844–6,

20. Roberts, A. B., Sporn, M. B., and Assoian, R. K. (1986). Transforming growth factor type beta: rapid induction of fibrosis and angiogenesis *in vivo* and stimulation of collagen formation *in vitro*. *Proc. Natl Acad. Sci. USA*, **83**, 4167–71.

21. Schreiber, A. B., Winkler, M. E., and Derynck, R. (1986). Transforming growth factor alpha: a more potent angiogenesis mediator than epidermal growth factor. *Science*, **232**, 1250–3.

22. Ishikawa, F., Miyazono, K., Hellman, U., Drexler, H., Wernstedt, C., Hagiwara, K., *et al.* (1989). Identification of angiogenic activity and the cloning and expression of platelet-derived endothelial-cell growth factor. *Nature*, **338**, 557–62.

23. Plate, K. H., Breier, G., Weich, H. A., and Risau, W. (1992). Vascular endothelial growth factor is a potential tumour angiogenesis factor in human gliomas *in vivo*. *Nature*, **359**, 845–7.

24. Kim, K. J., Li, B., Winer, J., Armanini, M., and Gillet, N. (1993). Inhibition of vascular endothelial growth factor-induced angiogenesis suppresses tumour growth *in vivo*. *Nature*, **362**, 841–4.

25. Frater-Schroeder, M. F., Risau, W., Hallmann, R., Gautschi, P., and Bohlen, P. (1987). Tumour necrosis factor type-alpha, a potent inhibitor of endothelial cell growth *in vitro*, is angiogenic *in vivo*. *Proc. Natl Acad. Sci. USA*, **84**, 5277–81,

26. Grant, D. S., Kleinman, H. K., Goldberg, I. D., Bhargave, M. M., Nickoloff, B. J., Kinsella, J. L., *et al.* (1993). Scatter factor induces blood vessel formation *in vivo*. *Proc. Natl Acad. Sci. USA*, **90**, 1937–41.

27. Fett, J. W., Strydom, D. L., and Lobb, R. R. (1985). Isolation and characterisation of angiogenic protein from human carcinoma cells. *Biochemistry*, **24**, 5480–6.

28. Weiner, H. L., Weiner, L. H., and Swain, J. (1987). The tissue distribution and developmental expression of the messenger RNA encoding angiogenin. *Science*, **237**, 280–2.

29. Form, D. M. and Auerbach, R. (1983). PGE2 and angiogenesis. *Proc. Natl Acad. Sci. USA*, **172**, 214–18.

30. Graeber, J. E., Glaser, B. M., Setty, B. N. Y., Jerdan. J. A., Walega, R. W., and Stuart, M. J. (1990). 15-Hydroxy-eicosatetraenoic acid stimulates migration of human retinal microvessel endothelium *in vitro* and neovascularization *in vivo*. *Prostaglandins*, **39**, 665–73.

31. West, D. C., Hampson, I. N., Arnold, F., and Kumar, S. (1985). Angiogenesis induced by degradation products of hyaluronic acid. *Science*, **228**, 1324–6.

32. Rooney, P. and Kumar, S. (1993). Inverse relationship between hyaluronan and collagens in development and angiogenesis. *Differentiation*, **54**, 1–9.

33. Ponting, J., Rooney, P., and Kumar, S. (1997). Extracellular matrix and tumour growth. In *Current perspectives in molecular and cellular oncology (ed. D. A. Spandidos). Jai Press, London, (in press).*

34. Stracke, M. L., Murata, J., Aznavoorian, S., and Liotta, L. A. (1994). The role of extracellular matrix in tumor cell metastasis. *In Vivo*, **8**, 49–58.

35. Chiquet-Ehrismann, R. (1993). Tenascin and other adhesion modulating proteins in cancer. *Semin. Cancer Biol.*, **4**, 301–10.

36. Ingber, D. E. (1992). Extracellular matrix as a solid-state regulator in angiogenesis: identification of new targets for anti-cancer therapy. *Semin. Cancer Biol.*, **3**, 57–63.

37. Hay, E. D. (ed.) (1991). *Cell biology of extracellular matrix*. Plenum Press, New York.

38. Mayne, R. and Burgeson, R. E. (ed.) (1987). *Structure and function of collagen types*. Academic Press, New York.

39. Linsenmayer, T. F. (1991). Collagen. In *Cell biology of extracellular matrix* (ed. E. D. Hay), pp. 7–44. Plenum Press, New York.

40. Hardingham, T. E. (1986). Structure and biosynthesis of proteoglycans. *Rheumatology*, **10**, 143–83.

41. Wight, T. N., Heinegard, D. K., and Hascall, V. C. (1991). Proteoglycans: structure and function. In *Cell biology of extracellular matrix* (ed. E. D. Hay), pp. 45–78. Plenum Press, New York.

42. Ruoslahti, E. (1990). Extracellular matrix in the regulation of cellular functions. In *Cell to cell interaction* (ed. M. M. Burger, B. Sordat, and R. M. Zinkernagel), pp. 88–98. Karger, Basel.

43. Van der Rest, M. and Garrone, R. (1991). Collagen family of proteins. *FASEB J.*, **5**, 2814–23.

44. Olsen, B. R. (1991). Collagen biosynthesis. In *Cell biology of extracellular matrix* (ed. E. D. Hay), pp. 177–220. Plenum Press, New York.

45. Yanaghista, M. (1993). A brief history of proteoglycans. *Experientia*, **49**, 366–8.

46. Bourdon, M. A., Oldberg, A., Pierschbacher, M., and Ruoslahti, E. (1985). Molecular cloning and sequence analysis of a chondroitin sulfate proteoglycan cDNA. *Proc. Natl Acad. Sci. USA*, **82**, 1321–5.

47. Doege, K., Sasaki, M., Horigan, E., and Hassell, H. S. (1987). Complete primary structure of the rat cartilage proteoglycan core protein deduced from cDNA clones. *J. Biol. Chem.*, **262**, 17757–67.

48. Hascall, V. C., Heinegard, D. K., and Wight, T. N. (1991). Proteoglycans: Metabolism and pathology. In *Cell biology of extracellular matrix* (ed. E. D. Hay), pp. 149–75. Plenum Press, New York.

49. Prehm, P. (1984). Hyaluronate is synthesized at plasma membranes. *Biochem. J.*, **220**, 597–600.

50. Toole, B. P. (1991). Proteoglycans and hyaluronan in morphogenesis and differentiation. In *Cell biology of extracellular matrix* (ed. E. D. Hay), pp. 305–41. Plenum Press, New York.

51. Chakrabarti, B. and Park, J. W. (1980). Glycosaminoglycans: structure and interaction. *CRC Crit. Rev. Biochem.*, **8**, 225–313.

52. Burd, D. A. R., Siebert, J. W., Ehrlich, H. P., and Garg, H. G. (1989). Human skin and post-burn scar hyaluronan: demonstration of the association with collagen and other proteins. *Matrix*, **9**, 322–7.

53. Knudson, W., Biswas, C., Li, X. Q., Nemec, R. E., and Toole, B. P. (1989). The role and regulation of tumour associated hyaluronan. In *The biology of hyaluronan* (ed. D. Evered and J. Whelan), Ciba Foundation Symposium, **143**, pp. 150–69. Wiley, Chichester.

54. Kumar, S., Ponting, J., Rooney, P., Kumar, P., Pye, D., and Wang, M. (1994). Hyaluronan and angiogenesis: molecular mechanisms and clinical applications. In *Angiogenesis: molecular biology, clinical aspects* (ed. M. E. Maragoudakis, P. M. Gullino and P. I. Lelkes), pp. 219–31. Plenum Press, New York.

55. Feinberg, R. N. and Beebe, D. L. (1983). Hyaluronate in vasculogenesis. *Science*, **220**, 1177–9.

56. Rooney, P., Wang, M., Kumar, P., and Kumar, S. (1993). Angiogenic oligosaccharides of hyaluronan enhance the production of type I and type VIII collagens by endothelial cells. *J. Cell Sci.*, **105**, 213–18.

57. Tsopanoglou, N. E., Pipili-Synetos, E., and Maragoudakis, M. E. (1993). Protein kinase C involvement in the regulation of angiogenesis. *J. Vasc. Res.*, **30**, 202–8.

58. Tsopanoglou, N. E., Haralabopoulos, G. C., and Maragoudakis, M. E. (1994). Opposing effects on modulation of angiogenesis by protein kinase C and cAMP-mediated pathways. *J. Vasc. Res.*, **31**, 195–204.

59. Kinsella, J. L., Grant, D. S., Weeks, B. S., and Kleinman, H. K. (1992). Protein kinase C regulates endothelial cell tube formation on basement membrane matrix, Matrigel. *Exp. Cell Res.*, **199**, 56–62.

60. Wright, P. S., Cross-Doerson, D., Miller, J. A., Jones, W. D., and Bitonti, A. J. (1992). Inhibition of angiogenesis *in vitro* and *in vivo* with an inhibitor of cellular protein kinases, MDL 27032. *J. Cell. Physiol.*, **152**, 448–457.

61. Turley, E. A. (1992). Hyaluronan and cell locomotion. *Cancer Metastasis Rev.*, **11**, 21–30.

62. Bauer, J. Margolos, M., Schreiner, C., Edgell, C. J., Azizkhan, J., Lazarowski, E., and Juliano, R. L. (1992). *In vitro* model of angiogenesis using a human endothelium-derived permanent cell line: contribution of induced gene expression, G-proteins and integrins. *J. Cell. Physiol.*, **153**, 437–49.

63. Bartolazzi, A., Cerboni, C., Nicotra, M. R., Mottolese, M., Bigotti, A., and Natali, P. G. (1994). Transformation and tumour progression are frequently associated with expression of the alpha3/beta 1 heterodimer in solid tumors. *Int. J. Cancer*, **58**, 488–91.

64. Elices, M. J. and Hemler, M. E. (1989). The human integrin VLA-2 is a collagen receptor on some cells and a collagen/laminin receptor on others. *Proc. Natl Acad. Sci. USA*, **86**, 9906–10.

65. Schwartz, M. A. and Ingber, D. E. (1994). Integrating with integrins. *Mol. Biol. Cell*, **5**, 389–93.

66. Vandenbunder, B., Wernert, N., and Stehelin, D. (1993). L'oncogene c-ets 1 participe-t-il a la regulation de l'angiogenese tumorale? *Bull. Cancer*, **80**, 38–49.

67. Latchman, D. S. (1991). *Eukaryotic transcription factors*, pp. 153–76. Academic Press, London.

68. Curran, T. and Franza, B. R. (1988). *Fos* and *jun*: the AP-1 connection. *Cell*, **55**, 395–7.

69. Sattar, A., Rooney, P., Kumar, S., Pye, D., West, D. C., Scott, I., and Ledger, P. (1994). Application of angiogenic oligosaccharides of hyaluronan increase blood vessel numbers in rat skin. *J. Invest. Dermatol.*, **103**, 576–9.

70. Bosman, F. T. (1994). The borderline: basement membranes and the transition from pre-malignant to malignant neoplasia. *Microsc. Res. Tech.*, **28**, 216–25.

71. Kanzawa, S., Endo, H., and Shioya, N. (1993). Improved *in vitro* angiogenesis model by collagen density reduction and the use of type III collagen. *Ann. Plast. Surg.*, **30**, 244–51.

72. Kaneko, T., Nagata, I., Miyamoto, S., Kubo, H., Kikuchi, H., Fujisato, T., and Ikada, Y. (1992). Rapid morphological changes in bovine brain microvascular endothelial cells on extracellular matrices. *Neurol. Med-Chir.* **32**, 549–53.

73. Fisher, C., Gilbertson-Beadling, S., Powers, E. A., Petzold, G., Poorman, R., and Mitchell, A. (1994). Interstitial collagenase is required for angiogenesis *in vitro*. *Dev. Biol.*, **162**, 449–510.

74. Passaniti, A., Taylor, R. M., Pili, R., Guo, Y., Long, P. V., Haney, J. A., *et al.* (1992). A simple quantitative method for assessing angiogenesis and antiangiogenic agents using reconstituted basement membrane, heparin and fibroblast growth factor. *Lab. Invest.*, **67**, 519–28.

75. Kibbey, M. C., Grant, D. S., and Kleinman, H. K. (1992). Role of the SIKVAV site of laminin in promotion of angiogenesis and tumour growth: an *in vivo* Matrigel model. *J. Natl Cancer Inst.*, **84**, 1633–8.

76. Ingber, D. E. and Folkman, J. (1988). Inhibition of angiogenesis through modulation of collagen metabolism. *Lab. Invest.*, **59**, 44–51.

77. Maragoudakis, M. E., Missirlis, E., Karakiulakis, G., Bastiki, M., and Isopanoglou, N. (1991). Basement membrane biosynthesis as a target for developing inhibitors of

angiogenesis with anti-tumour activity. *Int. J. Radiat. Biol.*, **60**, 54–9.

78. Nicosia, R. F., Belser, P., Bonanno, E., and Diven, J. (1991). Regulation of angiogenesis *in vitro* by collagen metabolism. *In Vitro Cell Dev. Biol.*, **27A**, 961–6.

79. Iruela-Arispe, M. L., Hasselaar, P., and Sage, E. H. (1991). Differential expression of extracellular proteins is correlated with angiogenesis *in vitro*. *Lab. Invest.*, **64**, 174–6.

80. Jarvelainen, H. T., Iruela-Arispe, M. L., Kinsella, M. G., Sandell, L. J., Sage, E. H., and Wight, T. N. (1992). Expression of decorin by sprouting bovine aortic endothelial cells exhibiting angiogenesis *in vitro*. *Exp. Cell Res.*, **203**, 395–401.

81. Iruela-Arispe, M. L., Diglio, C. A., and Sage, E. H. (1991). Modulation of extracellular matrix proteins by endothelial cells undergoing angiogenesis *in vitro*. *Arterioscler. Thromb.* **11**, 805–15.

82. Sage, E. H. and Iruela-Arispe, M. L. (1990). Type VIII collagen in murine development. Association with capillary formation *in vitro*. In *Structure, molecular biology and pathology of collagens* (ed. R. Fleischmajer, B. R. Olsen, and K. Kuhn), pp. 17–31. New York Academy of Science, New York.

83. Kittelberger, R., Davis, P. F., Flynn, D. W., and Greenhill, N. S. (1990). Distribution of type VIII collagen in tissues: an immunohistochemical study. *Connect. Tissue Res.*, **24**, 303–18.

84. Sawada, H. (1982). The fine structure of the bovine Descemet's membrane with special reference to its biochemical nature. *Cell Tissue Res.*, **226**, 241–55.

85. Yamaguchi, N., Benya, P. D., van der Rest, M., and Ninomiya, Y. (1989). The cloning and sequencing of α1 (VIII) collagen cDNAs demonstrate that type VIII collagen is a short chain collagen and contains triple-helical and carboxyl-terminal non-triple-helical domains similar to those of type X collagen. *J. Biol. Chem.*, **264**, 16022–9.

86. Yamaguchi, N., Mayne, R., and Ninomiya, Y. (1991). The α1 (VIII) collagen gene is homologous to the α1 (X) collagen gene and contains a large exon encoding the entire triple-helical and carboxyl-terminal non-triple-helical domains of the α1 (VIII) polypeptide. *J. Biol. Chem.*, **266**, 4508–13.

87. Kielty, C. M., Kwan, A. P. L., Holmes, D. F., Schor, S. L., and Grant, M. E. (1985). Type X collagen, a product of hypertrophic chondrocytes. *Biochem. J.*, **27**, 545–54.

88. Kwan, A. P. L., Cummings, C. E., Chapman, J. A., and Grant, M. E. (1991). Macromolecular organization of chicken type X collagen *in vitro*. *J. Cell Biol.*, **114**, 597–604.

89. Eijan, A. M., Davel, L., Oisgold-Daga, S., and de Lustig, E. S. (1991). Modulation of tumour-induced angiogenesis by proteins of extracellular matrix. *Mol. Biother.*, **3**, 38–40.

90. Hahnenberger, R. and Jakobson, A. M. (1991). Anti-angiogenic effect of sulphated and non-sulphated glycosaminoglycans and polysaccharides in the chick embryo chorioallantoic membrane. *Glycoconj. J.*, **8**, 350–52.

91. Jakobson, A. M. and Hahnenberger, R. (1991). Anti-angiogenic effect of heparin and other sulphated glycosaminoglycans in the chick embryo chorioallantoic membrane. *Pharmacol. Toxicol.*, **69**, 122–6.

92. Lebel, L. and Gerdin, B. (1991). Sodium hyaluronate increases vascular ingrowth in the rabbit ear. *Int. J. Exp. Pathol.*, **72**, 111–18.

93. Sato, E., Miyamoto, H., and Koide, S. S. (1990). Hyaluronic acid-like substance from mouse ovaries with angiogenic activity. *J. Biosci.*, **45**, 873–80.

94. Sato, E., Tanaka, T., Takeya, T., Miyamoto, H., and Koide, S. S. (1991). Ovarian glycosaminoglycans potentiate angiogenic activity of epidermal growth factor in mice. *Endocrinology*, **128**, 2402–6.

95. Kumar, S., West, D. C., Ponting, J. M., and Gattamaneni, H. R. (1989). Sera of children with renal tumours contain low molecular mass hyaluronic acid. *Int. J. Cancer*, **44**, 445–8.

96. Vlodavsky, I., Kormer, G., Ishai-Michaeli, R., Bashkin, P., Bar-Shevit, R., and Fuks, Z. (1990). Extracellular matrix–resident growth factors and enzymes: possible involvement in tumour metastasis and angiogenesis. *Cancer Metastasis Rev.*, **9**, 203–26.

97. Bashkin, P., Razin, E., Eldor, A., and Vlodavsky, I. (1990). Degranulating mast cells secrete an endoglycosidase that degrades heparan sulfate in subendothelial extracellular matrix. *Blood*, **75**, 2204–12.

98. Meininger, C. J. and Zetter, B. R. (1992). Mast cells and angiogenesis. *Semin. Cancer Biol.*, **3**, 73–9.

99. Soncin, F., Shapiro, R., and Fett, J. W. (1994). A cell-surface proteoglycan mediates human adenocarcinoma HT-29 cell adhesion to human angiogenin. *J. Biol. Chem.*, **269**, 8999–9005.

100. Ehrlich, P. (1879). Beitrage zur kenntniss der granulirten bindegewebszellen und der eosinophilen leukocyten. *Arch. Anat. Physiol.* **3**, 166–9.

101. Meininger, C. J. and Zetter, B. R. (1992). Mast cells and angiogenesis. *Cancer Biol.* **3**, 73–9.

102. Galli, S. J. (1991). New concepts about the mast cell. *N. Engl. J. Med.* **328**, 257–65.

103. Eady, R. A. J., Cowen, T., Marshall, T. F., Plummer, V., and Greaves, M. W. (1979). Mast cell population density, blood vessel density and histamine content in normal skin. *Br. J. Dermatol*, **100**, 635–40.

104. Kessler, D. A., Langer, R. S., Pless, N. A., and Folkman, J. (1976). Mast cells and tumor angiogenesis. *Int. J. Cancer*, **18**, 703–9.

105. Kumar, S. (1980). Angiogenesis and antiangiogenesis. *J. Natl Cancer Inst.* **64**, 683–7.

106. Kumar, S., Marsden, H. B., Lynch, P. G., and Earnshaw, E. (1980). Weibel-Palade bodies in endothelial cells as a marker for angiogenesis in brain tumours. *Cancer Res*, **40**, 2010–19.

107. Kumar, P., Erroi, A., Sattar, A., and Kumar, S. (1985). Weibel-Palade bodies as a marker for neovascularization induced by tumour and rheumatoid angiogenesis factor. *Cancer Res*, **45**, 4339–48.

108. Sattar, A., Kumar, P., and Kumar, S. (1986). Rheumatoid- and osteoarthritis: quantitation of ultrastructural feature of capillary endothelial cells. *J. Pathol.*, **148**, 45–53.

109. Norrby, K., Jakobsson, A., and Sorbo, J. (1986). Mast-cell-mediated angiogenesis: a novel experimental model using the rat mesentery. *Virchows Arch. B Cell Pathol.*, **52**, 195–206.

110. Norrby, K., Jakobsson, A., and Sörbo, J. (1989). Mast-cell secretion and angiogenesis, a quantitative study in rats and mice. *Virchows Arch. Cell Pathol.*, **57**, 251–6.

111. Norrby, K. (1993). Heparin and angiogenesis: a low-molecular-weight fraction inhibits and a high-molecular-weight fraction stimulates angiogenesis systemically. *Haemostasis*, **23** (Suppl. 1), 141–9.

112. Azizkhan, R. G., Azizkhan, J. C., Zetter., B. Z., and Folkman, J. (1980). Mast cell heparin stimulates migration of capillary endothelial cells *in vitro*. *J. Exp. Med.* **152**, 931–44.

113. Fraser, R. A. and Simpson, J. C. (1983). Role of mast cells in experimental tumour angiogenesis. In *Development of the vascular system* (ed. J. Nugent and M. O'Connor), pp. 120–31. Pitman, London.

114. Taylor, S. and Folkman, J. (1982). Protamine is an inhibitor of angiogenesis. *Nature*, **297**, 307–12.

115. Damon, D. H., Lobb, R. R., D'Amore, P. A., and Wagner, J. A. (1989). Heparin potentiates the action of acidic fibroblast growth factor by prolonging its biological half-life. *J. Cell. Physiol.*, **140**, 68–74.

116. Gospodarowicz, D. and Cheng, J. (1986). Heparin protects basic and acidic FGF from inactivation. *J. Cell. Physiol.*, **128**, 475–84.

117. Yayon, A., Klagsbrun, M., Esko, J. D., Leder, P., and Ornitz, D. M. (1991). Cell surface, heparin-like molecules are required for the binding of basic fibroblast growth factor to its high affinity receptor. *Cell*, **64**, 841–8.

118. Ornitz, D. M., Yayon, A., Flanagan, J. G., Svahn, C. M., Levi, E., and Leder, P. (1992). Heparin is required for cell-free binding of basic fibroblast growth factor to a soluble receptor and mitogenesis in whole cells. *Mol. Cell. Biol.*, **12**, 240–7.

119. Ishihara, M., Tyrrell, D. J., Stauber, G. B., Brown, S., Cousens, L. S., and Stack, R. J. (1993). Preparation of affinity-fractionated, heparin-derived oligosaccharides and their effects on selected biological activities mediated by basic fibroblast growth factor. *J. Biol. Chem.* **268**, 4675–83.

120. Ornitz, D. M., Herr, A. B., Nilsson, M., Westman, J., Svahn, C. M., and Waksman, G. (1995). FGF binding and FGF receptor activation by synthetic heparan-derived di and trisaccharides. *Science*, **268**, 432–6.

121. Florkiewicz, R. Z., Majack, R. A., Buechler, R. D., and Florkiewicz, E. (1995). Quantitative export of FGF-2 occurs through an alternative, energy-dependent, non-ER/Golgi pathway. *J. Cell. Physiol.*, **162**, 388–99.

122. Ruger, B. M., Dunbar, P. R., Hasan, Q., Sawada, H., Kittelberger, R., Greenhill, N., and Neale, T. J. (1994). Human mast cells produce type VIII collagen *in vivo*. *Int. J. Exp. Pathol.*, **75**, 397–404.

123. Facci, L., Dal-Toso, R. D., Romanello, S., Buriani, A., Skaper, S. D., and Leon, A. (1995). Mast cells express a peripheral cannabinoid receptor with differential sensitivity to anandamide and palmitoylethanolamide. *Proc. Natl Acad. Sci. USA*, **92**, 3376–80.

124. Folkman, J. (1995). Angiogenesis in cancer, vascular, rheumatoid and other disease. *Nature Med.*, **1**, 27–31.

14. The physiological importance and therapeutic potential of nitric oxide in the tumour-associated vasculature

D. G. Hirst and F. W. Flitney

Introduction

The relationship between malignant tumours and their vascular supply differs in many respects from that of most normal tissues. Tumour vasculature is characterized by rapid proliferation (1,2), increased permeability (3,4), and disorganized architecture (5–8), properties which are both a cause and a consequence of inadequate perfusion and oxygenation (9). We may summarize the condition of tumour vasculature as a system that is maximally stimulated, yet still unable to meet the metabolic demands of the tissue it supplies. The consequences of this for cancer therapy are profound (10,11). An inadequate vascular network leads to a heterogeneous blood supply and to areas within most tumours that are deprived of the limiting metabolic substrate, oxygen (12–14). This in turn creates regions with radiobiologically hypoxic cells which are both resistant to radiotherapy and quiescent. The lack of proliferative activity protects them from many chemotherapeutic drugs which are proliferation-dependent in their cytotoxic action. It should occasion no surprise then, that the influence of vasoactive agents on tumour blood flow has received considerable attention over the last 20 years (15,16) and this approach is still seen as a mechanism through which the action of anti-cancer agents could be enhanced. This review will focus on the importance of one highly topical vasoactive molecule, nitric oxide (NO). While the importance of this molecule in cancer therapy generally has been considered in a recent review (17) we will focus on its role in tumour-associated vasculature and evaluate its potential as a target for cancer therapy in this context.

The biological role of nitric oxide

The discovery that NO is synthesized in the body and that it functions as a ubiquitous intercellular signalling agent (18) is one of the most significant developments in modern biology. NO is an extraordinary biological effector molecule. It is a diatomic radical species with a rich redox chemistry (19,20), whose small size, lipid solubility, diffusibility and propensity to act as a ligand for iron and for tissue thiols (R-SH), underpins a plethora of physiological and pathophysiological actions. Typically, these actions are effected by covalent redox reactions with target molecules inside the cell. This frequently involves NO *per se*, as for example in the activation of guanylate cyclase by nitrosyl-haem formation, considered later. However, the biologically active species may be a redox-related oxide of nitrogen instead, formed by reaction with dissolved molecular oxygen or superoxide anions (O_2^-), or it may be NO^+ (the nitrosonium ion), transferred from pre-existing pools of S-nitrosothiols (RS-NO) or iron-sulphur-nitrosyl clusters (FeS-NO), a process called transnitrosation. Covalent modification of the target molecule by NO generally elicits a cell response directly — the 'receptor' for NO is also the 'effector' — in marked contrast with the more familiar non-covalent, agonist-receptor based signal transduction processes.

Biosynthesis of nitric oxide

NO is synthesized from one of two terminal guanidino nitrogen atoms of the amino acid L-arginine by reaction with dioxygen (21). A 5-electron oxidation results in the formation of L-citrulline (22,23) and NO via a hydroxylated intermediate, N^G-hydroxy-L-arginine (24). The process is catalysed by one of several isoforms of the enzyme NO synthase (NOS). While this biosynthetic pathway appears to be universal, the magnitude and time scale of NO production differs from one cell type to another, reflecting the specific part the molecule plays.

NOS exists in several isoforms, all of which are homodimers containing four tightly bound redox cofactors per monomer — flavin–adenine dinucleotide (FAD), flavin mononucleotide (FMN), tetrahydrobiopterin (H_4B), and iron protoporphyrin IX (haem). They comprise a family of proteins, the products of three genes, which can be subdivided into two groups: constitutive (c) and inducible (i) isoforms. Although closely related, the two groups are regulated differently. The constitutive isoforms provide a 'low-output' pathway, chiefly concerned with the normal homeostatic functions of NO, whereas the inducible isoform provides a 'high-output' pathway, responsible for cell killing by cytotoxic, activated macrophages and a key factor in many pathological processes, for example in septic and cytokine-induced shock.

The constitutive isoforms are found in brain neurons (ncNOS or type I NOS) and in vascular endothelial cells (ecNOS or type III NOS). Both have a requirement for NADPH as a co-substrate and calcium-calmodulin (CaM). NO synthesis by the constitutive isoforms is stimulated by agonist-triggered increases in intracellular $[Ca^{2+}]$s, promoting formation of the active CaM–NOS complex. Inducible NOS (iNOS or type II NOS) is also NADPH-dependent, but unlike its constitutive counterparts, the CaM–NOS complex is formed and functional even at low ('resting') intracellular $[Ca^{2+}]$s (24). Thus, once expressed, iNOS continually synthesizes NO over many hours. Transcription of the iNOS gene is switched on by several proinflammatory cytokines (tumour necrosis factor, interferon γ, interleukins 1 and 2) and also by bacterial lipopolysaccharides (26). Other cytokines and growth factors, including tissue growth factor β, macrophage-deactivating factor and interleukins 4 and 10, inhibit transcription of the iNOS gene. Induction of iNOS is also prevented by the glucocorticoid dexamethasone and by inhibitors of poly adenosine diphosphate ribose polymerase (27,28).

Feedback regulation of nitric oxide production

There is evidence that NO itself exerts a negative feedback control of NOS activity. NOS activity was inhibited by NO in crude cerebellar extracts (29) and in a macrophage-like cell line expressing iNOS activity (30). More recently, it was demonstrated (31) that authentic NO inhibited the formation of ^3H citrulline by bovine aortic endothelial cell (BAEC) homogenates, an effect which could be overcome by addition of oxyhaemoglobin. Oxyhaemoglobin alone also enhanced cNOS activity in cell homogenates. Furthermore, the release of NO from perfused BAECs was impaired after pretreatment with the NO donor S-nitroso-N-acetylpenicillamine (SNAP), as measured using a cascade bioassay system. Acetycholine-induced vasodilation of the perfused rabbit hindquarter was also abolished by SNAP. The mechanism underlying end-

product inhibition of NOS is not known, but reaction of NO with the tightly bound haem cofactor is one possibility.

The action of nitric acid synthase inhibitors

Both constitutive and inducible NOS isoforms can be inhibited by synthetic, guanidino-substituted analogues of L (but not D)-arginine (32), including N$^\omega$-monomethyl-L-arginine (L-NMMA), N^G-nitro-L-arginine methyl ester (L-NAME) and N^G-nitro-L-arginine (L-NARG). These are competitive enzyme inhibitors and their actions are generally reversible on addition of excess L-arginine. NO-mediated physiological and pathophysiological processes, including *inter alia*, endothelium-dependent vasodilation (32) and CaM-mediated cell killing (33), are blocked by NOS inhibitors. The discovery recently of an *endogenous* NOS inhibitor, assymmetric dimethylarginine (34), which is synthesized by endothelial cells (35), has aroused considerable interest, although there is no evidence thus far to link it with the aetiology of specific pathological conditions, for example, in chronic hypertension.

Synthetic NOS inhibitors generally block both constitutive and inducible isoforms, which detracts somewhat from their therapeutic potential. The search for isoform-selective NOS inhibitors, especially for iNOS, is the subject of intensive research at the present time. One promising NOS inhibitor, aminoguanidine, is reported to be equipotent with L-NMMA and L-NARG at suppressing endotoxin-induced NO synthesis, but has little or no effect on basal or agonist-stimulated ecNOS activity (36,37).

Nitric oxide and the regulation of vasomotor tone

Identification of nitric oxide as a potent vasodilator

Endothelial cells mediate the vasodilator effects of acetylcholine via the production of a labile factor which was termed endothelium-derived relaxing factor (EDRF) (38). The unstable nature of EDRF — its biological half-life is variously reported as ranging from a few to several tens of seconds — made chemical identification especially difficult. An important clue came from studies of the stabilizing effect of superoxide dismutase (SOD), the enzyme which converts superoxide anions (O_2^-) to hydrogen peroxide. Destruction of O_2^- by SOD potentiated endothelium-dependent relaxations and extended the half-life of EDRF while Fe^{2+} and pyrogallol, both O_2^- generators, attenuated them (39–41). In addition endothelium-dependent relaxations were inhibited by haemoglobin and by methylene blue (MB) (42).

Taken together, these observations led to the suggestion that EDRF might be NO (43). Pharmacological studies comparing authentic NO with EDRF in a cascade bioassay revealed them to be indistinguishable. The vasodilator effect and stability of NO were found to be equally susceptible to known EDRF inhibitors and to be similarly potentiated by SOD (44,45). The definitive experiment was reported later (44). This group demonstrated that NO was released from cultured endothelial cells stimulated with bradykinin, utilizing a chemical reaction with ozone to produce nitrogen dioxide via a chemiluminescent excited intermediate.

Endothelium-derived NO (EDNO) is continually synthesized and is a major determinant of peripheral vascular resistance *in vivo*. Inhibition of ecNOS by systemic administration of NOS inhibitors, for example L-NAME or L-NMMA, increases blood pressure in laboratory animals (46,47) and reduces brachial blood flow in healthy human subjects (34). Systemic administration of NOS inhibitors has been used in animal models (48) and in humans (49) to overcome the severe hypotension which occurs in septic shock. In contrast, endothelium-dependent relaxation is *attenuated* in other disease states, most notably in hypertension (50,51) and in atherosclerosis (52,53).

Endothelium-dependent vasodilators increase EDNO production above basal levels by elevating intracellular $[Ca^{2+}]$s, an effect which is caused by the gating of receptor-operated calcium channels in the cell membrane. Fluid shear stress, an important stimulator of EDNO synthesis, also increases intracellular $[Ca^{2+}]$s (54). Increased intracellular $[Ca^{2+}]$ promotes the interaction of CaM with ecNOS and enhances enzyme activity.

Other potent vasodilators containing ligated nitrosyl groups, the so-called 'nitrovasodilators', including sodium nitroprusside (SNP), amyl nitrite, molsidomine, and glyceryl trinitrate, exert their effects by releasing NO *in vivo*, either after spontaneous thermal decomposition or after biotransformation, effectively bypassing the endothelium (55). The nitrovasodilators have been used clinically as antihypertensive or hypotensive agents for many years, indeed, long before NO was identified as an endogenous regulator of vascular smooth muscle tone, for example in the treatment of angina, the management of hypertensive emergencies and to reduce wound bleeding and improve visibility during surgery.

The role of guanylate cyclase

Guanylate cyclase (GC) is a polymorphic enzyme which exists in both soluble and membrane-bound (particulate) isoforms. The soluble isoenzyme (sGC), a haem-containing heterodimer, catalyses the hydrolysis and cyclization of guanosine 5′ triphosphate (GTP) to form guanosine 3′, 5′ cyclic monophosphate [or cyclic guanosine monophosphate (cGMP)], an important 'second messenger', and pyrophosphate. cGMP can alter cellular processes directly, for example by acting on cGMP-gated ion channels or on cGMP-regulated cyclic nucleotide phosphodiesterases; or indirectly, by activating cGMP-dependent protein kinase (G-kinase). Activated G-kinase can then phosphorylate key protein substrates which modify cellular function, causing relaxation (vasodilation) in the case of vascular smooth muscle.

Early biochemical studies (see review reference 56) led to the idea that the loosely bound, ferrous haem moeity of sGC *suppresses* enzyme activity and that binding of NO forming nitrosyl-haem activates the enzyme by a process of 'disinhibition' (57). Significantly, haem-deficient enzyme was found to be maximally activated by protoporphyrin IX, the demetallated form of haem. EPR studies indicated that binding of NO to sGC weakens the coordinate bonds which hold iron in the plane of the porphyrin ring (58). It was therefore postulated that this would result in an 'out-of-plane' movement of the central iron atom, simulating a protoporphyrin-IX-like interaction, resulting in activation of the enzyme.

sGC can be inhibited (*in vivo* and *in vitro*) by a variety of agents which have been used to investigate the role of the L-arginine-NO-cGMP pathway in mediating cellular responses. MB has been used extensively for this purpose. Haemoglobin also inhibits sGC indirectly, by scavenging NO. Additionally, both MB and Hb are able to generate O_2^- (59) which could alter the oxidation state of the enzyme directly and/or 'inactivate' NO by reacting to form peroxynitrite (60).

sGC activity *in vivo* can be up- or down-regulated. Supersensitivity of blood vessels to nitrovasodilators following acute periods of NO deprivation (*e.g.* after blockade of NOS with L-NMMA or L-NAME) has been documented (18). This phenomenon appears to be at the level of sGC, although the underlying mechanism has not been studied fully. Conversely, sGC can become desensitized following prolonged treatment with nitrovasodilators (61). This is known as 'tolerance' and is especially important in the clinical context where patients are on long-term nitrovasodilator therapy. Oxidized (but not unoxidized) low-density lipoproteins (LDLox) attenuate the effect of NO donors on sGC from bovine lung without influencing the formation of endothelial NO (62). This appears to be a direct effect of LDLox on sGC and may afford an explanation for the hyporesponsiveness of atherosclerotic vessels to endogenous NO and to NO donors.

Nitric oxide production and tumour blood flow

The use of cytokines or drugs to generate large quantities of NO specifically in tumours may ultimately prove to have some therapeutic value, as it has been known for some time that macrophage-generated NO causes tumour cell death. There is now a considerable amount of evidence, however, that NO production may play a particularly important part in tumour vasculature, raising the possibility of tumour-specific blood flow modification.

Blood flow modification by nitric oxide synthase inhibition *in vivo*

The first report of a tumour-specific dependency of tumour vasculature on NO was of a study utilizing a subcutaneous sponge model in the mouse to induce neovasculature (63). In this model, host blood vessels are allowed to infiltrate the sponge matrix either in the presence or absence of tumour cells. Blood flow was measured using the ^{133}xenon washout method at different times after sponge implantation. The administration of various inhibitors of NO synthesis or activity resulted in a highly significant reduction in blood flow in tumour-containing sponges, but little or no effect in sponges without tumour cells. Investigations

using an implanted rat tumour model have also revealed considerable tumour specificity for the action of a NOS inhibitor (64). This group used the uptake of ^{125}I-iodo-antipyrine as an absolute measure of tumour and normal tissue blood flow (Fig. 14.1). They observed a twofold reduction in blood flow in a subcutaneously implanted carcinosarcoma after administration of 10 mg/kg of the NOS inhibitor L-NMMA. Of the eight normal tissues they investigated, only in muscle and spleen was there any significant effect of the drug. A small reduction in blood flow measured by laser Doppler flowmetry has also been reported both for liver tumours and normal liver parenchyma in a rat model (65); the effect was larger in the tumours but not significantly so.

The effects of dexamethasone on tumour blood flow and iNOS immunoreactivity were investigated in a mouse sponge implant model (66). Daily injections (0.5–1.0 mg/kg) given intramuscularly for >10 days post-implantation significantly reduced blood flow in tumour-bearing sponges but not in control sponge implants. Strong iNOS immunoreactivity was seen in untreated tumour implants but absent from tumours in mice pretreated with dexamethasone for 11 days. Importantly, there was no obvious difference in the degree of vascularization of untreated and treated tumours. Again, the results of this study point to an important part for NO in facilitating blood flow in a tumour-selective manner.

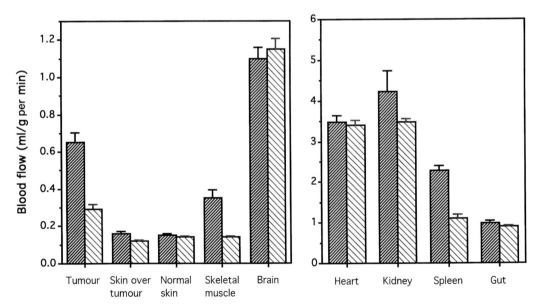

Figure 14.1. Alterations in absolute blood flow in a subcutaneous tumour (P22 carcinosarcoma) and various normal tissues in the rat (BD9) following intravenous injection of 10 mg/kg L-NARG. The dark bars are preinjection, the light bars post injection of L-NARG. There were eight animals per group and the error bars represent ±1 SEM. Replotted from Tozer *et al.* (63).

A method using direct observation of tumour-associated vasculature (67) has also been applied. Tumours (R3230Ac mammary carcinomas) were implanted into subcutaneous window chambers which allowed the tumour vasculature to be viewed directly. The diameter of post-capillary venules and red blood cell flux were measured and the effects of drugs determined. Superfusion with L-NMMA reduced the diameter of these vessels by 13–17% in tumour-bearing chambers, regardless of the location of the vessel in relation to the tumour implant. The venules in control preparations, without tumour, were significantly more sensitive to L-NMMA, constricting by 30%. The diameter changes were reflected in concomitant changes in red blood cell velocity. Interestingly, the addition of an excess of L-arginine completely reversed the effect of L-NMMA in normal chambers, but had little effect in tumour-containing chambers. The authors speculated that this may be due to competition for L-arginine from tumour-associated activated macrophages (68,69). This hypothesis is consistent with our observation (70) that the use of a higher concentration of L-arginine (1000 μmol/l), as opposed to the 200 μmol/l used by Meyer *et al.* (67), completely reversed the effect of L-NMMA (50 μmol/l) in tumour supply vessels (see next section). Furthermore, in our study, the vessels were perfused *ex vivo* and so there were probably fewer macrophages associated with the preparation than when the chamber model was used.

Blood flow modification by nitric oxide synthase inhibition *ex vivo*

We have investigated the effects of NOS inhibitors on tumour-associated vasculature in isolation (70,71). Comparative studies were made of isolated epigastric arteries that had previously supplied either the normal inguinal fat pad of the rat, or a pad that had been largely displaced by the growth of an implanted P22 carcinosarcoma. Arteries were excised, cannulated, and perfused internally at a constant flow rate (0.6 ml/min). Bolus injections (10 μl) of the vasoconstrictor phenylephrine (PE) introduced into the lumen of the artery generated a transient increase in perfusion pressure. Figure 14.2 shows responses of both tumour and normal arteries to a range of PE concentrations. During the initial part of the experiment (<120 min perfusion), normal arteries were significantly more responsive to PE than tumour arteries. Addition of L-NMMA to the perfusate increased the sensitivity of both types of artery to PE so that there was no longer any difference between the two. The effect of L-NMMA was prevented by the addition of a large excess of L-arginine. These results are consistent with enhanced

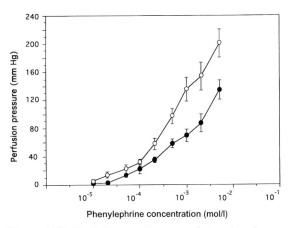

Figure 14.2. The influence of a range of phenylephrine doses on the pressure generated in isolated, perfused rat epigastric arteries that had previously supplied P22 tumours implanted in the inguinal fat pad (closed symbols) or the contralateral normal fat pad (open symbols). Increased pressure indicates increased vascular resistance. Error bars represent ±1 SEM. Replotted from Kennovin *et al.* (70).

NO production by tumour arteries compared with their normal counterpart, presumably as a result of expression of iNOS under the influence of a factor or factors produced by the tumour. This is supported by our observation that the level of NADPH diaphorase staining was significantly higher in tumour arteries (71).

Tumour-associated arteries frequently (24 of a sample of 38) exhibited spontaneous pressure fluctuations (5–15 mmHg every 30 min) which increased in size and frequency (40–85 mmHg every 10 min) with increasing perfusion times and/or after constant infusion of PE (69). Spontaneous oscillations were never observed in normal arteries. However, similar oscillations have been reported in hamster aorta during continuous exposure to PE (72), which the authors attributed to continuous release of NO from the endothelium. The occurrence of spontaneous activity *in vivo* might be a factor contributing to the well documented temporal heterogeneity of blood flow in tumours (73).

During our experiments we observed a marked, time-dependent decrease in sensitivity of normal (but *not* tumour) arteries to PE, so that after ~8 h perfusion the two types of vessel responded similarly. Addition of the protein synthesis inhibitor cycloheximide (10 μM, 2 h) to the internal perfusate prevented this from happening. Surprisingly, we also found that cycloheximide increased the sensitivity of tumour vessels to PE, implying that protein synthesis is required for continued expression and/or activity of iNOS. This result may reflect a rapid turnover of the enzyme itself, or of a protein co-factor essential for its activity. It has been shown that laboratory solutions can become contaminated with trace amounts of bacterial lipopolysaccharide, sufficient to initiate iNOS expression in isolated vascular tissue; enhanced NO production can thus lead to reduced sensitivity to vasoconstrictors (74). It seems probable that this is the explanation for the gradual loss of sensitivity to PE exhibited by normal vessels. The fact that the tumour vessels showed no similar decrease suggests that iNOS is maximally expressed in these arteries.

A similar isolated system was used to perfuse a rat carcinosarcoma complete with its associated vasculature (64). L-NARG (50 μM) caused a twofold or more increase in vascular resistance in these tumour preparations, whereas vessels from the non-tumour-bearing side of the rat responded significantly in only one of the five preparations tested.

All of these studies strongly support the idea that tumour-associated blood vessels are characterized by increased levels of NO production compared with their normal counterparts. The data also indicate that the tumour-associated factor(s) responsible for this difference can exert an influence over a distance of at least several millimetres away from the tumour. The full range of this influence remains to be established.

Expression of nitric oxide synthase in tumours and tumour-associated vasculature

NOS exists in several isoforms which give rise to very different modes of NO production. We need to be aware when considering the production of NO in tumours that several cell types, including macrophages, neutrophils, endothelial cells, smooth muscle cells, and tumour cells, are capable of NOS expression and hence NO production. This can lead to a variety of consequences which will be important for the survival of tumour cells and hence will have therapeutic implications.

Soon after the demonstration that endothelium-derived relaxing factor and NO were identical (45), tumour cells were shown to be capable of expressing iNOS under the influence of cytokines generated by activated macrophages (75). There is now considerable evidence that human cancer cells are capable of expressing NOS genes (76,77), although there is no indication so far to suggest that this phenomenon has any tumour specificity. Expression of iNOS has been demonstrated in rat lung fibroblasts (78),

hepatocytes (79–81), vascular smooth muscle cells (82), glial cells (83), pancreatic islet cells (84,85), and macrophages (86–88). NO production is thought to be an important means by which activated macrophages attack tumour cells (see reference 89 for review). There is also evidence that the release of high levels of NO may be the mechanism by which one class of experimental anti-cancer drug, flavone acetic acid and its analogues, causes tumour necrosis (90).

It is of interest to speculate about the extent to which increased production of NO in tumours compared with normal tissues is a specific, homeostatic response by the tumour to an inadequate supply of nutrients or is simply a consequence of large numbers of infiltrating host cells, mainly macrophages, generating high levels of NO in the course of their phagocytic activity. There is no doubt that cancer cells in tissue culture are capable of expressing NOS genes at the mRNA level (75,76,91) and of generating NO (77,91). A cytokine-induced NOS from human colorectal carcinoma cells has been shown by sequence analysis to be indistinguishable at the genetic level from iNOS obtained from a wide range of normal cells (91). Studies of human colon cancer cells *in vitro* showed that Ca^{2+}-independent iNOS was expressed by three of four cell lines whether they were stimulated with the cytokines tumour necrosis factor α and interferon γ or not (77). One cell line did not express iNOS under any circumstances. Interestingly, all four cell lines expressed mRNA for the Ca^{2+}-dependent cNOS. A similar result was reported for a human cervix carcinoma cell line (92). Thus, the particular isoform of NOS expressed by a tumour tells us little about the cellular origin of any NO production. The level of expression does not even correlate quantitatively with the amount of NO generated, suggesting that post-translational events must influence the NO-generating reaction.

While cancer cells *in vitro* are able to express NOS there is evidence that in some tumours *in vivo* expression of the enzyme may be restricted to the tumour-associated vasculature. A recent immunocytochemical study, using a subcutaneously implanted sponge model in the mouse, stained with antibody to iNOS, revealed that as tumours develop their blood vessels change from being non-immunoreactive to being highly reactive, while parenchymal cells in the tumour remained unreactive (93). iNOS immunoreactivity was detected both in endothelial cells of neovasculature and in the smooth muscle layer of differentiated vessels in well established tumours.

It has been shown, in a study of human tumours *in vivo*, that the levels of iNOS were dependent on the degree of differentiation of the tumour, the less differentiated tumours showing higher levels of expression (94). Whether or not this is related to the rate of growth of the tumours (either potential doubling time or volume doubling time) was not determined.

Cytotoxic action of macrophages

Tumour-infiltrating macrophages are inactive but develop potent tumoricidal activity following induction of iNOS by cytokines known to be present in tumours (95,96). Their cytotoxicity is mediated by NO and is dependent upon L-arginine (97,98). A similar cytotoxic mechanism has been seen in endothelial cells (99). NO produced by cytotoxic-activated macrophages (CAMs) targets several key, non-haem iron containing enzymes in tumour cells, including complexes I and II of the mitochondrial electron transport chain, aconitase, and ribonucleotide reductase (100–102), inhibiting mitochondrial respiration and DNA synthesis. Inactivation of these enzymes by CAM-derived NO involves destruction of iron–sulphur cluster prosthetic groups, resulting in the formation of nitrosylated iron complexes detectable by electron paramagnetic resonance spectroscopy (103). Recent evidence suggests that this process can lead to the induction of apoptosis (104,105).

The ability of tumour cells to generate NO has also been shown to influence their capacity to survive *in vivo* to form metastases (106,107). Metastatic cells showed low levels of NOS activity and were presumably less likely to trigger the cytotoxic action of macrophages and endothelial cells. This observation could have obvious implications for novel forms of cancer therapy.

Therapeutic consequences of nitric oxide synthase inhibition in tumours

Changes in tumour energy metabolism

The development of magnetic resonance spectroscopy (MRS) techniques to measure the ratios of high- to low-energy phosphates *in vivo* has allowed the consequences of altering nutrient availability to tumours to be studied. These methods have been used by one group (81,108,109) to study the effects of altering NO production on the metabolism of a variety of transplanted and spontaneous murine tumours. The intravenous administration of L-NARG caused a two- to fourfold increase in the ratio of inorganic phosphate to total phosphate (P_i total) in tumours, indicative of a reduced energy charge and impaired supply of metabolic substrates, of which the most important is probably oxygen (12,13). The increase in P_i total was linearly dependent on log L-NARG dose over the range 0.2–2.0 mg/kg. Significantly, L-NARG at a dose of 10 mg/kg had no effect on P_i total in normal tissue, predominantly muscle, of the mouse back.

Nitric oxide synthase inhibition and bioreductive drugs

Blood flow reduction following NOS inhibition appears to have considerable specificity for tumour tissue under most circumstances. It follows that NOS inhibitors could be used to enhance hypoxia in tumours, rendering them more susceptible to the effects of bioreductive cytotoxins (110). This hypothesis was tested recently using a transplantable mouse tumour model (109). Administration of L-NARG caused a dose-dependent increase in the radioresistance of RIF-1 tumours in mice and in their sensitivity to the bioreductive pro-drug RB6145 (Fig. 14.3). While this study did not include assays for normal tissue toxicity, investigations of ^{31}P-MRS showed that L-NARG had no effect on the oxygenation of muscle tissue. There is evidence, however, from another recent study (111) that L-NARG administered prior to whole body irradiation in mice acted as a radioprotector, an effect the authors attributed to reduced blood flow to the bone marrow. Definitive experiments in critical normal tissues will be required, however, before this concept can be exploited in the treatment of human cancer.

The effect of nitric oxide synthase inhibitors on tumour growth

There is clear evidence that NOS inhibitors have a detrimental effect on tumour energetics *in vivo* (108,109), so it would not be surprising if prolonged exposure to NOS inhibitors had an impact on tumour growth. Our recent study (71) showed that L-NAME significantly reduced the growth rate of implanted tumours in both rats and mice. From Fig. 14.4 it can be seen that chronic administration of L-NAME in the drinking water reduced tumour growth rates by about 50% in rats. A reduction of about 30% was seen in mouse tumours. A similar effect on growth was seen in two other mouse tumours (Wood *et al.*, personal communication). The effect of L-NAME was significantly greater when the tumours were larger, so that there was little difference in the eventual tumour size between animals that had been fed the drug from the time of tumour implant and those that were given the drug much later when the tumour had already reached 1000 mm^3. This is consistent with the hypothesis that only when tumours exceed a certain size does their growth become severely limited by the inadequacies of their

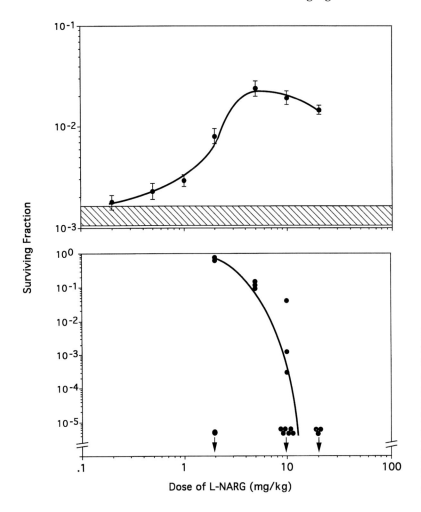

Figure 14.3. The *in vivo* effect of a range of L-NARG doses on the surviving fraction of RIF-1 tumours after a single dose of 20 Gy X-rays (upper panel) or a single intraperitoneal injection of 300 mg/kg of the bioreductive cytotoxin RB6145 (lower panel). Error bars shown ±1 SEM; hatched bar shows surviving fraction after 20 Gy alone. Replotted from Wood *et al.* (108).

vascular supply, such that any further reduction in blood flow significantly affects growth. Furthermore, L-NAME was only effective at slowing tumour growth while it remained in the animal. As seen in Fig. 14.5, tumour growth rate returned to normal as soon as L-NMMA was withdrawn. These two studies (71; Wood *et al.*, personal communication) used L-NAME as the inhibitor of NOS, but L-NARG is equally effective at slowing tumour growth in mice. This is not surprising, as we have shown that L-NAME is completely metabolized to L-NARG in the mouse *in vivo*, within about 10 min (71). A marked decrease in size of tumour sponge implants in dexamethasone treated as compared with untreated mice has also been reported (66), although as dexamethasone is a glucocorticoid which could affect growth directly this effect cannot be attributed to a reduction in blood flow *per se*.

Reduction of tumour blood flow is a plausible explanation for the growth retarding effects of NO synthase inhibition on tumours *in vivo* but we should not rule out the possibility that other mechanisms may be involved, as NO has been shown to play a part in several processes that could influence the rate of tumour growth. It was recently reported (113) that when human adenocarcinoma cells were engineered to generate NO continuously they grew more slowly *in vitro*, an effect that could be reversed by NOS inhibition with *N*-imino-ethyl-L-ornithine. By contrast, the same cell line grew faster in nude mice (113), a result that is consistent with our previous observation (71) that inhibition of NOS slows tumour growth *in vivo*. Thus, the role of NO in the growth of tumours is complex and may not always be predictable.

Regulation of angiogenesis by nitric oxide

There is currently no direct evidence to implicate the L-arginine/NO pathway in determining the angiogenic

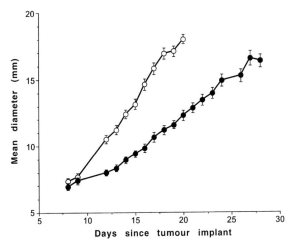

Figure 14.4. Growth curves for P22 carcinosarcomas growing subcutaneously in BD9 rats that were either fed L-NAME at a concentration of 6 mg/ml in the drinking water from the ninth day after tumour implant (filled symbols) or given water without drug (open symbols). Error bars show ±1 SEM. Replotted from Kennovin *et al.* (70).

potential of tumours, though the effects of NOS inhibitors in other models of angiogenesis have recently been investigated. The first report (114) showed that inhibition of NOS by L-NMMA increased vascular density in the chick embryo chorioalantoic membrane (115) while the addition of sodium nitroprusside, an NO donor, reduced it. The authors (114) speculated that NO may act directly to inhibit endothelial cell proliferation, as it does in the case of mesangial cells (116). It was further shown, using an *in vitro* assay (114), that tube formation by endothelial cells could be inhibited by an analogue of cGMP, implying that regulation of angiogenesis by NO operates through the same pathway (via activation of guanylate cyclase) as that involved in smooth muscle relaxation. On the other hand, the angiogenic response to substance P, measured by increased growth and migration of endothelial cells in the rabbit cornea model, was potentiated by sodium nitroprusside (an NO donor) and inhibited by L-NAME (117). Furthermore, pretreatment of endothelial cells with NOS inhibitors abolished cell proliferation and migration in response to substance P, while the angiogenic response to basic fibroblast growth factor (bFGF) was unaffected.

Angiogenic activity can also be mediated through the action of activated macrophages, and there is evidence that this process is dependent on their ability to generate NO via an L-arginine-dependent pathway (118). Thus, the available evidence suggests that NO may affect angio-

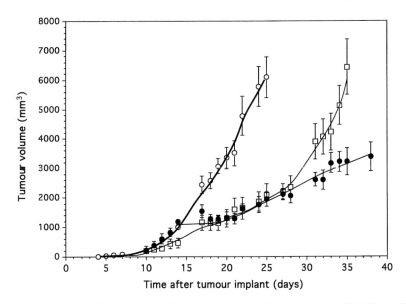

Figure 14.5. Growth curves for P22 tumour growing subcutaneously in three groups of BD9 rats. The control group (open circles) received their normal drinking water. Another group (open squares) were given 3 mg/ml L-NAME in their drinking water from the 10th day after tumour implant and then had the drug withdrawn on day 26. The third group (filled circles) were started on the drug from day 15 and it was maintained until day 36. Error bars show ±1 SEM. Replotted from Kennovin *et al.* (70).

genesis both directly and indirectly. Its direct action on blood vessels appears to be an inhibition of endothelial cell proliferation and tube formation. However, when macrophages are present in an activated condition their ability to generate NO is a requirement for the release of angiogenic stimuli, although NO is not itself the angiogenic molecule. Thus, inhibition of NOS would be expected to modify angiogenesis, although the balance between stimulation and inhibition will depend on a variety of factors, including the number of infiltrating macrophages.

NO has been shown to modulate vascular permeability (119). It is of interest that angiogenic activity and vascular hyperpermeability in tumours are mediated by the same cytokine known as vascular permeability factor (VPF)/ vascular endothelial growth factor (VEGF) (120,121). Two receptors for VPF/VEGF — the *flt* (122) and KDR (123) receptors — have been identified, both of which contain tyrosine kinase domains. VPF/VEGF stimulates the growth of endothelial cells (but not that of other cell types) and it promotes angiogenesis in model systems (124,125). Increased expression of VPF/VEGF has been seen (126) in high-grade (glioblastoma) relative to low-grade (astrocytoma) human gliomas. Glioblastomas typically show enhanced endothelial cell proliferation and increased vascularization as compared with astrocytomas. This study therefore provides circumstantial evidence that VPF/VEGF is involved in angiogenesis in human tumours. VPF/VEGF expression and co-expression of the tyrosine kinase receptors were increased in acute and chronically hypoxic lungs perfused *ex vivo*, an effect which was attenuated by SNP and enhanced by L-NAME (127). This suggests that the *anti*-angiogenic effect of NO may be mediated through suppression of VPF/VEGF expression.

Summary and conclusions

It is 8 years since NO was identified as an intercellular signalling agent in most tissues in the body. Since then there has been a dramatic expansion in our knowledge of its actions, synthesis, and regulation at the molecular level. As a result of its diverse actions, it is not surprising that NO plays an important part in the aetiology of several disease processes and it is now clear that modulation of its production could have important implications for the treatment of malignant disease (Fig. 14.6).

At least four therapeutically significant mechanisms within tumours and their associated vasculature have been identified that are, at least in part, NO dependent.

1. *Tumour blood supply*. The blood vessels that supply malignant tumours express higher than normal levels of an inducible isoform of the enzyme NOS. This may

be a homeostatic mechanism, responding to the inadequate metabolic substrate levels found in tumours, or simply a consequence of the presence of greater numbers of iNOS-expressing macrophages. In any event, tumour blood vessels and normal vessels respond to vasoactive stimuli differently, a characteristic that could be exploited therapeutically. The administration of NOS inhibitors *in vivo* leads to a collapse of tumour blood flow and creates a very hypoxic environment in the tumour, causing cell death and providing conditions which are conducive to the enhanced activation of bioreductive cytotoxins.

2. *Macrophage activation*. It is now known that tumour-infiltrating macrophages are inactive but become cytotoxic following activation by the cytokines present in tumours. This cytotoxicity requires induction of iNOS, is mediated by NO and is L-arginine dependent. There is evidence that this process may involve the NO-dependent induction of apoptosis.

3. *Regulation of angiogenesis*. The role of NO in *tumour* angiogenesis has not yet been investigated. However, studies in other model systems are consistent with the hypothesis that NO *per se* is anti-angiogenic but that it also promotes the release of a pro-angiogenic factor or factors from macrophages. Thus, the balance between pro- and anti-angiogenic influences in a given tumour may depend on the numbers of activated infiltrating macrophages.

4. *Metastatic potential*. There is evidence that the ability of tumour cells to survive *in vivo* is dependent on their level of NOS activity. Low levels were associated with metastatic cells. Cells producing high levels of NO are presumably more likely to stimulate the cytotoxic action of macrophages or endothelial cells.

Acknowledgements

The authors wish to thank Dr G. D. Kennovin and Dr Stuart Bisland for their important contributions to the planning of the contents of this review.

References

1. Denekamp, J. and Hobson, B. (1982). Endothelial cell proliferation in experimental tumours. *Br. J. Cancer*, **46**, 711–20.
2. Hobson, B. and Denekamp, J. (1984). Endothelial proliferation in tumours and normal tissues: continuous labelling studies. *Br. J. Cancer*, **49**, 405–13.

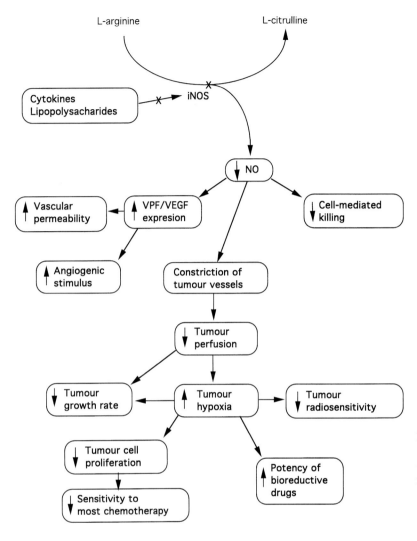

Figure 14.6. Summary of advantageous and deleterious consequences for cancer therapy of reducing the production of nitric oxide (NO) in tumours. VEGF, vascular endothelial growth factor; VPF, vascular permeability factor.

3. Jain, R. K. (1985). Transport of macromolecules in tumour microcirculation. *Biotech. Prog.*, **1**, 81–94.
4. Jain, R. K. (1987). Transport of molecules across tumour vasculature. *Cancer Metastasis Rev.*, **6**, 559–94.
5. Falk, P. (1980). The vascular pattern of the C3H mammary carcinoma and its significance in radiation response. *Eur. J. Cancer*, **26**, 203–13.
6. Falk, P. (1982). Differences in vascular pattern between spontaneous and transplanted C3H mammery carcinoma. *Eur. J. Cancer*, **18**, 155–65.
7. Shubik, P. (1982). Vascularization of tumours: a review. *J. Cancer Res. Clin. Oncol.*, **103**, 211.
8. Warren, B. A. (1979). Vascular morphology of tumours. In *Tumour blood circulation. Angiogenesis, vascular morphology and blood flow of experimental and human tumours* (ed. H-I. Petersson, p. 1. CRC Press, Boca Raton.
9. Jain, R. K. (1988). Determinants of tumour blood flow: a review. *Cancer Res.*, **48**, 3759–64.

10. Jain, R. K. (1989). Delivery of novel therapeutic agents in tumors: physiological Berriers and Strategies *J Natl Cancer Inst.*, **81**, 570–6.
11. Vaupel, P. (1993). Oxygenation of solid tumors. In *Drug resistance in oncology* (ed. B. A. Teicher), pp. 53–85. Marcel Dekker, New York.
12. Tannock, I. F. (1970). Effects of pO₂ on cell proliferation kinetics. In (ed. V. P. Bond, H. D. Suit, and V. Marcial), *Time and dose relationships in radiation biology as applied to therapy* (ed. V. P. Bond, H. D. Suit, and V. Marcial), p. 215. Brookhaven National Laboratory, Upton.
13. Hirst, D. G., Hirst, V. K., Joiner, B., Prise, V., and Shaffi, K. M. (1991). Changes in tumour morphology with alterations in oxygen availability: further evidence for oxygen as a limiting substrate. *Br. J. Cancer*, **64**, 54–8.
14. Hirst, D. G., Joiner, B., and Hirst, V. K. (1994). Is oxygen the limiting substrate for the expansion of cords around blood vessels in tumours. *Adv. Exp. Med. Biol.*, **277**, 431–6.

15. Hirst, D. G. (1994). Blood flow and its modulation in malignant tumors. In *Microspheres and regional cancer therapy* (ed. N. Willmott and, J. Daly), pp. 31–56. CRC Press, Boca Raton.

16. Jirtle, R. L. (1988). Chemical modification of tumour blood flow. *Int. J. Hyperthermia*, **4**, 355–71.

17. Sagar, S. M., Singh, G., Hodson, D. I., and Whitton, A. C. (1995). Nitric oxide and anti-cancer therapy. *Cancer Treatment Rev.*, **21**, 159–81.

18. Moncada, S., Rees, D. D., Schulz, R., and Palmer, R. M. J. (1991). Development and mechanism of a supersensitivity to nitrovasodilators following inhibition of nitric oxide synthesis *in vivo*. *Proc. Natl Acad. Sci. USA*, **88**, 21166–70.

19. Butler, A. R. and Williams, L. H. (1993). The physiological role of nitric oxide. *Chem. Soc. Rev.*, 233–41.

20. Butler, A. R., Flitney, F. W., and Williams, D. L. H. (1995). NO, nitrosium ions, nitroxide ions, nitrosothiols and iron-nitrosyls in biology: a chemist's perspective. *Trends Pharmacol. Sci.*, **16**, 18–22.

21. Leone, A. M., Palmer, R. M. J., Knowles, R. G., Francis, P. L., Ashton, D. S., and Moncada, S. (1992). Molecular oxygen is incorporated into both nitric oxide and citrulline by constitutive and inducible nitric oxide synthases. In *The biology of nitric oxide* (ed. S. Moncada, M. Feelisch, M. R. Busse, and E. A. Higgs), **2**, pp. 7–14. Portland Press, London.

22. Palmer, R. M. J., Ashton, D. D., and Moncada, S. (1988). Vascular endothelial cells synthesize nitric oxide from L-arginine. *Nature*, **333**, 664.

23. Palmer, R. M. J. and Moncada, S. (1989). A novel citrulline forming enzyme implicated in the formation of nitric oxide from L-arginine. *Biochem. Biophys. Res. Commun.*, **158**, 348–52.

24. Steuhr, D. J., Kwon, N. S., Nathan, C. F., Griffith, O. W., and Feldman, P. L. (1991). NG-hydroxy-L-arginine is an intermediate in the biosynthesis of nitric oxide from L-arginine. *J. Biol. Chem.*, **266**, 6259–63.

25. Nathan, C. and Xie, Q. W. (1994). Regulation of biosynthesis of nitric oxide. *J. Biol. Chem.*, **269**, 13725–8.

26. Hibbs, J. B., Vavrin, Z., and Traintor, R. R. (1987). L-arginine is required for expression of the activated macrophage effector mechanism causing selective metabolic inhibition in target cells. *J. Immunol.*, **138**, 550–65.

27. Hauschild, S., Scheipers, P., Bessler, W. B., and Mulsch, A. (1992). Induction of nitric oxide synthase in L929 cells by tumour-necrosis factor α is prevented by inhibitors of poly (ADP-ribose) polymerase. *Biochem. J.*, **288**, 255–60.

28. Pellat-Deceunynck, C., Wietzerbin, J., and Drapier, J-C. (1994). Nicotinamide inhibits nitric oxide synthase mRNA induction in activated macrophages. *Biochem. J.*, **297**, 53–8.

29. Rogers, N. E. and Ignarro, L. J. (1992). Constitutive nitric oxide synthase fromcerebellum is reversibly inhibited by nitric oxide formed from L-arginine. *Biochem. Biophys. Res. Commun.*, **189**, 242–9.

30. Assreuy, J., Cunha, F. Q., Liew, F. Y., and Moncada, S. (1993). A perfusion system for long term study of macrophages. *Br. J. Pharmacol.*, **108**, 833–7.

31. Buga, G. M., Cohen, G. A., Griscavage, J. M., Rodgers, N. E., and Ignarro, L. J. (1994). Negative feedback regulation of nitric oxide synthase and endothelial cell function by nitric oxide. In *The biology of nitric oxide* (ed. S. Moncada, M. Feelisch, M. R. Busse, and E. A. Higgs), **4**, pp. 74–7. Portland Press, London.

32. Rees, D. D., Palmer, R. M. J., Schultz, R., Hudson, H. F., and Moncada, S. (1990). Characterization of three inhibitors of endothelial nitric oxide synthase *in vitro* and *in vivo*. *Br. J. Pharmacol.*, **101**, 746–52.

33. Yim, C.-Y., Bastian, N. R., Smith, R., Hibbs, J. B., and Samlowski, W. E. (1993). Macrophage nitric oxide synthesis delays progression of ultraviolet-light-induced murine skin cancers. *Cancer Res.*, **53**, 5507–11.

34. Vallance, P., Leone, A., Calver, A., Collier, J., and Moncada, S. (1992). Accumulation of an endogenous inhibitor of nitric oxide synthesis in chronic renal failure. *Lancet*, **339**, 572–5.

35. Fickling, S. A., Nussey, S. S., Vallance, P., and Whitley, G. S. J. (1994). Synthesis of NG, NG-dimethylarginine from L-arginine by human vein endothelial cells. In *The biology of nitric oxide* (ed. S. Moncada, M. Feelisch, M. R. Busse, and E. A. Higgs), **4**, pp. 49–52. Portland Press, London.

36. Misko, T. P., Moore, W. M., Kasten, T. P., Nickols, G. A., Corbett, J. A., Tilton, R. G., *et al.* (1993). Selective inhibition of the inducible nitric oxide synthase by aminoguanidine. *Eur. J. Pharmacol.*, **233**, 119–25.

37. Griffiths, M. J. D., Messent, M., MacAllister, R. J., and Evands, T. W. (1993). Aminoguanidine selectively inhibits inducible nitric oxide synthase. *Br. J. Pharmacol.*, **110**, 963–8.

38. Furchgott, R. F. and Zawadski, J. V. (1980). The obligatory role of endothelial cells in the relaxation of arterial smooth muscle by acetylcholine. *Nature*, **288**, 373–6.

39. Gryglewski, R. J., Moncada, S., and Palmer, R. M. J. (1986). Superoxide anion is involved in the breakdown of EDRF. *Nature*, **320**, 454–6.

40. Moncada, S., Palmer, R. M. J., and Gryglewski, R. J. (1986). Mechanism of action of some inhibitors of EDRF. *Proc. Natl Acad. Sci. USA*, **83**, 9164–8.

41. Rubanyi, G. M. and Vanhoute, P. M. (1986). Superoxide anions and hyperoxia inactivate EDRF. *Am. J. Physiol.*, **250**, H822–7.

42. Martin, W., Villani, G. M., Jothianandan, D., and Furchgott, R. F. (1985). Selective blockade of endothelium-dependent and glycyl trinitrate-induced relaxation by haemoglobin and by methylene blue in the rabbit aorta. *J. Pharmacol. Exp. Ther.*, **232**, 708–16.

43. Furchgott, R. F. (1988). Studies on relaxation of rabbit aorta by sodium nitrite: the basis for the proposal that the acid-activatable factor from retractor penis is inorganic nitrite and the endothelium-derived relaxing factor is NO. In *Vasodilation: vascular smooth muscle, peptides, autonomic nerves and the endothelium*. (ed. P. M. van Houte), pp. 401–14. Raven Press, London.

44. Palmer, R. M. J., Ferrige, A. C., and Moncada, S. (1987). Nitric oxide release accounts for the biological activity of EDRF. *Nature*, **327**, 524–6.

45. Ignarro, L. J., Buga, G. M., Wood, K. S., Byrns, R. E., and Chaudhuri, G. (1987). Endothelium-derived relaxing factor produced from artery and vein is nitric oxide. *Proc. Natl Acad. Sci. USA*, **84**, 9265–9.

46. Gardiner, S. M., Compton, A. M., Kemp, P. A., and Bennet, T. (1990). Regional and cardiac haemodynamic effects, NG-nitro-L-arginine methyl ester in conscious Long Evans rats. *Br. J. Pharmacol.*, **101**, 265–7.

47. Aisaka, K., Gross, S. S., Griffith, O. W., and Levi, R. (1989). N^G-nitro methyl arginine, an inhibitor of

endothelium-derived nitric oxide synthase is a potent pressor agent in the guinea pig: does nitric oxide regulate blood pressure *in vivo*? *Biochem. Biophys. Res. Commun.*, **160**, 881–6.

48. Kilbourn, R. G., Jubran, A., Gross, S. S., Griffith, O. W., and Levi, R. (1990). Reversal of endotoxin-mediated shock by N^G-methyl-L-arginine, an inhibitor of nitric oxide synthase. *Biochem. Biophys. Res. Commun.*, **172**, 1132–8.

49. Petros, A., Lamb, G., Leone, A., Moncada, S., and Bennet, D. (1994). effects of a nitric oxide synthase inhibitor in humans with septic shock. *Cardiovasc. Res.*, **28**, 34–9.

50. Luscher, T. F. and Vanhoutte, P. M. (1986). Endothelium-dependent contractions to acetylcholine in the aorta of the spontaneously hypertensive rat. *Hypertension*, **8**, 344–8.

51. Tesmafariam, B. and Halpern, W. (1988). Endothelium-dependent and endothelium-independent vasodilation in resistance arteries from hypertensive rats. *Hypertension*, **11**, 440–4.

52. Harrison, D. G., Armstrong, M. L., Frieman, P. C., and Heistaad, D. D. (1987). Restoration of endothelium-dependent relaxation by dietary treatment by dietary treatment of atherosclerosis. *J. Clin. Invest.*, **80**, 1808–11.

53. Forstermann, U., Mugge, A., Alheid, U., Haverisch, A., and Frolich, J. C. (1987). Selective attenuation of endothelium-mediated vasodilation in atherosclerotic human coronary arteries. *Circ. Res.*, **62**, 185–90.

54. Davies, P. F. (1995). Flow mediated endothelial mechano-transduction. *Physiol. Rev.*, **75**, 519–60.

55. Felisch, M. and Noack, E. A. (1987). Correlation between nitric oxide formation during degradation of organic nitrates and activation of guanylate cyclase. *Eur. J. Pharmacol.*, **139**, 19–30.

56. Waldman, S. A. and Murad, F. (1987). Cyclic GMP synthesis and function. *Pharmacol. Rev.*, **39**, 163–96.

57. Wolin, M. S., Wood, K. S., and Ignarro, L. J. (1982). Guanylate cyclase from bovine lung: a kinetic analysis of the purified soluble enzyme by protoporphyrin IX, heme and nitrosyl heme. *J. Biol. Chem.*, **257**, 13312–20.

58. Kon, H. and Kataoka, N. (1969). Electron paramegnetin resonance of nitric oxide prohaem complexes with some nitrogenousbases. Model systems of nitrin oxide hemo-proteins. *Biochemistry*, **8**, 4757–62.

59. Marczin, N., Ryan, J., and Catravas, J. (1992). Methylene blue inhibits nitrovasodilator- and endothelium-induced cGMP accumulation in cultured pulmonary arterial smooth muscle cells via generation of superoxide anion. *J. Pharmacol. Exp. Ther.*, **263**, 1–10.

60. Saran, M., Miichel, C., and Bors, W. (1990). Reaction of NO with O_2^-. Implications for the action of endothelium-derived relaxing factor (EDRF). *Free Rad. Res. Commun.*, **10**, 221–6.

61. Waldman, S. A., Rapaport, R. M., and Murad, F. (1987). Desensitization to nitroglycerin in cascular smooth muscle from rat and human. *Biochem. Pharmacol.*, **35**, 3525–31.

62. Schmidt, K., Graier, W. F., Kostner, G. M., Mayer, B., Bohme, E., and Kudovetz, W. R. (1991). Stimulation of soluble guanylate cyclase by endothelium-derived relaxing factor is antagonised by oxidized low-density lipoprotein. *J. Cardiovasc. Pharmacol.*, **17**, S83–8.

63. Andrade, S. P., Hart, I. R., and Piper, P. J. (1992). Inhibitors of nitric oxide synthase selectively reduce flow in tumour-associated neovasculature. *Br. J. Pharmacol.*,

107, 1092–5.

64. Tozer, G. M., Prise, V. E., and Bell, K. M. (1995). The influence of nitric oxide on tumour vasvular tone. *Acta Oncol.*, **34**, 373–7.

65. Dworkin, M. J., Carnochan, P., and Allen-Mersh, T. G. (1995). Nitric oxide inhibition sustains vasopressin-induced vasoconstriction. *Br. J. Cancer*, **71**, 942–4.

66. Freemantle, C. N., Buttery, L. D. K., Springall, D. R., Riveros-Moreno, V., Polak, J. M., and Piper, P. J. (1994). Inhibition of expression of inducible nitric-oxide synthase and reduction of blood flow in murine tumors by dexamethasone. *Br. J. Pharmacol.*, **112**, U38.

67. Meyer, R. E., Shan, S., DeAngelo, J., Dodge, R. K., Bonaventura, J., Ong, E. T., and Dewhirst, M. W. (1995). Nitric oxide synthase inhibition irreversibly decreases per-fusion in the R3230Ac rat mammary adenocarcinoma. *Br. J. Cancer*, **71**, 1169–74.

68. Benninghoff, B., Lehmann, V., Eck, H-P., and Droge, W. (1991). Production of citrulline and ornithine by interferon-γ treated macrophages. *Int. Immunol.*, **3**, 413–7.

69. Albina, J. E. (1990). Temporal expression of different pathways L-arginine metabolism in healing wounds. *J. Immunol.*, **144**, 3877–80.

70. Kennovin, G. D., Flitney, F. W., and Hirst, D. G. (1994). 'Upstream' modification of vasoconstrictor responses in rat epigastric artery supplying an implanted tumour. *Adv. Exp. Med. Biol.*, **277**, 411–6.

71. Kennovin, G. D., Hirst, D. G., Stratford, M. R. L., and Flitney, F. W. (1995). Inducible nitric oxide synthase is ex-pressed in tumour-associated vasculature:inhibition retards tumour growth. In *The biology of nitric oxide* (ed. S. Moncada, M. Feelisch, M. R. Busse, and E. A. Higgs), pp. 259–63. Portland Press, London.

72. Jackson, W. F., Mulsch, A., and Busse, R. (1991). Rhythmic smooth-muscle activity in hamster aortas is mediated by continuous release of no from the endothelium. *Am. J. Physiol.*, **260**, H248–53.

73. Trotter, M. J., Chaplin, D. J., Durand, R. E., and Olive, P. E. (1989). The use of fluorescent probes to identify regions of transient perfusion in murine tumours. *Int. J. Radiat. Oncol. Biol. Phys.*, **16**, 31.

74. Rees, D. D., Cellek, S., Palmer, R. J., and Moncada, S. (1990). Dexamethasone prevents the induction by endo-toxin of nitric oxide *in vitro* and *in vivo. Biochem. Biophys. Res. Commun.*, **173**, 541–7.

75. Amber, I. J., Hibbs, J. B., Taintor, R. R., and Vavrin, Z. (1988). The L-arginine dependent effector mechanism is induced in murine adenocarcinoma cells by culture super-natant from cytotoxic activated macrophages. *J. Leukocyte Biol.*, **43**, 187–92.

76. Radomski, M. W., Jenkins, D. C., Holmes, L., and Moncada, S. (1991). Human colorectal adenocarcinoma cells: differential nitric oxide synthesis determines their ability to aggregate platelets. *Cancer Res.*, **51**, 6073–8.

77. Jenkins, D. C., Charles, I. G., Baylis, S. A., Lelchuk, R., Radomski, M. W., and Moncada, S. (1994). Human colon cancer cell lines show a diverse pattern of nitric oxide syn-thase gene expression and nitric oxide generation. *Br. J. Cancer*, **70**, 847–9.

78. Janssens, S. P., Shimouchi, A., Quertermous, T., Bloch, D. B., and Bloch, K. D. (1992). Cloning and expression of a cDNA encoding human endothelium derived relaxing factor/nitric oxide. *J. Biol. Chem.*, **267**, 14519–22.

79. Geller, D. A., Lowenstein, C. J., and Shapiro, R. A. (1993). Molecular cloning and expression of inducible nitric oxide synthase from human hepatocytes. *Proc. Natl Acad. Sci. USA*, **90**, 3491–5.

80. Nussler, A. K., Di Silvo, M., Billiar, T. R., Hoffman, R. A., Geller, D. A., Selby, R., *et al.* (1992). Stimulation of the nitric oxide synthase pathway in human hepatocytes by cytokines and endotoxin. *J. Exp. Med.*, **176**, 261–4.

81. Wood, P. J., Stratford, I. J., Adams, G. E., Szabo, C., Thiemermann, C., and Vane, J. R. (1993). Modification of energy metabolism and radiation response of a murine tumourby changes in nitric oxide availability. *Biochem. Biophys. Res. Commun.*, **192**, 505–10.

82. Nunokawa, Y., Ishida, N., and Tanaka, S. (1993). Cloning of inducible nitric oxide synthase in rat vascular smooth muscle cells. *Biochem. Biophys. Res. Commun.*, **191**, 89–94.

83. Galea, E., Feinstein, D. L., and Reis, D. J. (1992). Induction of calcium-independent nitric-oxide synthase activity in primary rat glial cultures. *Proc. Natl Acad. Sci. USA*, **22**, 10945–9.

84. Niemann, A., Bjorklund, A., and Eizirik, D. L. (1994). Studies on the molecular regulation of the inducible form of nitric-oxide synthase (inos) in insulin-producing cells. *Diabetologia*, **37**, A52.

85. Eizirik, D. L. Sandler, S. Welsh, N. Hallgren, I. B., Tornelius, E., Bendtzen, K., and Hellerstrom, C. (1993). Exposure of human pancreatic-islets to combinations of cytokines induces nitric-oxide (NO) production and impairment in b-cell function. *Diabetologia*, **36**, A95.

86. Lyons, C. R., Orloff, G. L., and Cunningham, J. M. (1992). Molecular cloning and functional expression of an inducible nitric oxide synthase from a murine macrophage cell line. *J. Biol. Chem.*, **267**, 6370–4.

87. Lorsbach, R. B., Murphy, W. J., Snyder, S. H., and Russell, S. W. (1993). Expression of the nitric oxide synthase gene in mouse macrophages activated by tumour cell killing. *J. Biol. Chem.*, **268**, 1908–13.

88. Cunha, F. Q., Assreuy, J., Moss, D. W., Rees, D., Leal, L. M. C., Moncada, S., and Carrier, M. (1994). Differential induction of nitric oxide synthase in various organs of the mouse during endotoxaemia — role of TNF-alpha and IL-1 beta. *Immunology*, **81**, 211–5.

89. Feldman, P. L., Griffith, O. W., and Stuehr, D. J. (1993). The surprising life of nitric oxide. *Chem. Eng. News*, **71**, 26–38.

90. Thomsen, L., Ching, L-M., Zhuang, L., Gavin, J. B., and Baguley, B. C. (1991). Tumor-dependent increased plasma nitrate concentrations as an indication of the antitumor effect of flavone-8-acetic acid and analogues in mice. *Cancer Res.*, **51**, 77–81.

91. Sherman, P. A., Laubach, V. E., Reep, B. R., and Wood, E. R. (1993). Purification and cDNA sequence of an inducible nitric oxide synthase from a human tumour cell line. *Biochemistry*, **32**, 11600–5.

92. Werner-Felmeyer, G., Werner, E. R., Fuchs, D., Hausen, A., Mayer, B., Reibnegger, G., and Wachter, H. (1993). Ca²⁺/calodulin-dependent nitric oxide synthase activity in the human cervix carcinoma cell line ME-180. *Biochem. J.*, **289**, 357–61.

93. Buttery, L. D. K., Springall, D. R., Andrade, S. P., Riveros-Moreno, V., Hart, I., Piper, P. J., and Polak, J. M. (1993). Induction of nitric oxide synthase in neo-vasculature of experimental tumours in mice. *J. Pathol.*, 311–9.

94. Thomsen, L. L., Lawton, F. G., Knowles, R. G., Beesley, J. E., Riveros-Moreno, V., and Moncada, S. (1994). Nitric oxide synthase activity in human gynecological cancer. *Cancer Res.*, **54**, 1352–4.

95. Erroi, A., Sironi, M., Chiaffarino, F., Chen, Z-G., Mengozzi, M., and Mantovani, A. (1989). IL-1 and IL-6 release by tumour-associated macrophages from human ovarian carcinoma. *Int. J. Cancer*, **44**, 795–801.

96. Vitolo, D., Zerbe, T., Kanbour, A., Dahl, C., Herberman, R. B., and Whiteside, T. L. (1992). Expression of mRNA for cytokines in tumour infiltrating mononuclear cells in ovarian adenocarcinoma and invasive breast cancer. *Int. J. Cancer*, **51**, 573–80.

97. Hibbs, J. B., Traintor, R. R., Vavrin, Z., and Rachlin, E. M. (1988). Nitric oxide: a cytotoxic activated macrophage effector molecule. *Biochem. Biophys. Res. Commun.*, **157**, 87–94.

98. Hibbs, J. B., Traintor, R. R., Vavrin, Z., Granger, D. L., Drapier, J-C., Amber, I. J., and Lancaster, J. R. (1990). Synthesis of nitric oxide from a terminal guanidino nitrogen atom of L-arginine: a molecular mechanism for regulating cellular proliferation that targets intracellular iron. In: *Nitric oxide from L-arginine: a bioregulatory system* (ed. S, Moncada and E. A. Higgs), pp. 189–223. Elsevier, New York.

99. Li, L., Kilbourn, R. G., Adams, J., and Fidler, I. J. (1991). Role of nitric oxide in lysis of tumour cells by cytokine-activated endothelial cells. *Cancer Res.*, **51**, 2531–5.

100. Granger, D. L. and Lehninger, A. L. (1982). Sites of inhibition of mitochondrial electron transport in macrophage-injured neoplastic cells. *J. Cell Biol.*, **95**, 527–35.

101. Draper, J-C. and Hibbs, J. B. (1986). Murine cytotoxic activated macrophages inhibit aconitase in tumour cells. Inhibition involves the iron-sulfur prosthetic group and is reversible. *J. Clin. Invest.*, **78**, 790–7.

102. Lepoivre, M., Fieschi, F., Coves, J., Thelander, L., and Fontecave, M. (1991). Inactivation of ribonucleotide reductase by nitric oxide. *Biochem. Biophys. Res. Commun.*, **179**, 442–8.

103. Lancaster, J. R. and Hibbs, J. B. (1990). EPR demonstration of iron–nitrosyl complex formation by cytotoxic activated macrophages. *Proc. Natl Acad. Sci. USA*, **87**, 1223–7.

104. Xie, K. P., Huang, S. Y., Dong, Z. Y., and Fidler, I. J. (1993). Cytokine-induced apoptosis in transformed murine fibroblasts involves synthesis of endogenous nitric-oxide. *Int. J. Oncol.*, **3**, 1043–8.

105. Cui, S. C., Reichner, J. S., Mateo, R. B., and Albina, J. E. (1994). Activated murine macrophages induce apoptosis in tumour cells through nitric oxide-dependent or independent mechanisms. *Cancer Res.*, **54**, 2462–7.

106. Dong, Z. Y., Staroselsky, A. H., Qi, X. X., Xie, K. P., and Fidler, I. J. (1994). Inverse correlation between expression of inducible nitric-oxide synthase activity and production of metastasis in k-1735 murine melanoma-cells. *Cancer Res.*, **54**, 789–93.

107. Xie, K. P. Huang, S. Y. Dong, Z. Y., Juang, S. H., Gutman, M., Xie, Q. W., *et al.* (1995). Transfection with the inducible nitric-oxide synthase gene suppresses tumorigenicity and abrogates metastasis by m-1735 murine melanoma-cells. *J. Exp. Med.*, **181**, 133–43.

108. Wood, P. J., Sanson, J. M., Stratford, I. J., Adams, G. E., Szabo, C., Thiemermann, C., Vane, J. R. (1994). Modification of metabolism of transplantable and spontaneous murine tumours by the nitric-oxide synthase

inhibitor nitro-L-arginine. *Int. J. Radiat. Oncol. Biol. Phys.*, **29**, 443–7.

109. Wood, P. J., Sanson, J. M., Butler, S. A., Stratford, I. J., Cole, S. M., Szabo, C., *et al.* (1994). Induction of hypoxia in experimental murine tumors by the nitric oxide synthase inhibitor, NG-nitro-L-arginine. *Cancer Res.*, **54**, 6458–63.

110. Stratford, I. J., Adams, G. E., Godden, J., and Howells, N. (1989). Induction of tumour hypoxia post irradiation: a method for increasing the sensitizing efficiency of misonidazole and RSUi1069 *in vivo*. *Int. J. Radiat. Oncol. Biol. Phys.*, **55**, 411–22.

111. Leibmann, J., DeLuca, A. M., Coffin, D., Keeler, L. K., Venzon, D., Wink, D. A., *et al.* (1994). *In vivo* radiation protection by nitric oxide modulation. *Cancer Res.*, **54**, 3365–8.

112. Buttery, L. D. K., Springall, D. R., Andrade, S. P., Riveros-Moreno, V., Hart, I., Piper, P. J., and Polak, J. M. (1994). Induction of nitric-oxide synthase in the neo-vasculature of experimental-tumors in mice. *J. Pathol.*, **171**, 311–9.

113. Jenkins, D. C., Charles, I. G., Thomsen, L. L., Moss, D. W., Holmes, L. S., Baylis, S. A., *et al.* (1995). Roles of nitric oxide in tumor growth. *Proc. Natl Acad. Sci. USA*, **92**, 4392–6.

114. Pipili-Synetos, E., Sakkoula, E., and Maragoudakis, M. E. (1993). Nitric oxide is involved in the regulation of angiogenesis. *Br. J. Pharmacol.*, **108**, 855–7.

115. Folkman, J. (1985). Tumour angiognesis. *Adv. Cancer Res.*, **43**, 175–203.

116. Garg, U. C. and Hassid, A. (1989). Inhibition of rat messangial cell mitogens by nitric oxide-generating vasodilators. *Am. J. Physiol.*, **257**, F60–6.

117. Ziche, M., Morbidelli, L., Masini, E., Amerini, S., Granger, H. J., Maggi, C. A., *et al.* (1994). Nitric-oxide mediates angiogenesis *in-vivo* and endothelial-cell growth and migration *in-vitro* promoted by substance-P. *J. Clin. Invest.*, 2036–44.

118. Leibovich, S. J. (1994). Production of angiogenic activity by human monocytes requires an L-arginine/nitric oxide-dependent effector mechanism. *Proc. Natl Acad. Sci. USA*, **91**, 4190–4.

119. Kubes, P. and Granger, D. N. (1992). Nitric oxide modulates microvascular permeability. *Am. J. Physiol.*, **262**, H611–15.

120. Senger, D. R., Peruzzi, C. A., Feder, J., and Dvorak, H. F., (1986). A highly conserved vascular permeability factor secreted by a variety of human and rodent tumor cell lines. *Cancer Res.*, **46**, 5629–32.

121. Ferrara, N. (1989). Pituitary follicular cells secrete a novel heparin-binding growth factor specific for vascular endothelial cells. *Biochem. Biophys. Res. Commun.*, **161**, 851–8.

122. de Vries, C., Escobedo, J. A., Ueno, H., Houck, K., Ferrara, N., and Williams, L. T. (1992). The fms–like tyrosine kinase, a receptor for vascular endothelial growth factor. *Science*, **255**, 989–91.

123. Terman, B. I., Carrion, M. E., Kovacs, E., Rasmussen, E., Eddy, R. L., and Shows, T. B., (1991). Identification of a new endothelial growth factor receptor tyrosine kinase. *Oncogene*, **6**, 1677–83.

124. Connolly, D. T., Heuvelman, D. M., Nelson, R., Olander, J. V., Eppley, B. L., Delfino, J. J., *et al.* (1989). Tumour vascular permeability factor stimulates endothelial cell growth and angiogenesis. *J. Clin. Invest.*, **84**, 1470–8.

125. Leung, D. W., Cachiancs, G., Kuang, W., Goedell, D. V., and Ferrara, N. (1989). Vascular endothelial growth factor is a sectreted angiogenic mitogen. *Science*, 1306–9.

126. Plate, K. H., Breier, G., Weich, H. A., and Risau, W. (1992). Vascular endothelial growth factor is a potential tumour angiogenesis factor in human gliomas *in vivo*. *Nature*, **259**, 845–8.

127. Tuder, R. M., Flook, B. E., and Voelkel, N. F. (1995). Increased gene expression for VEGF and VEGF receptors kdr/flk and flt in lungs exposed to acute or to chronic hypoxia-modulation of gene expression by nitric oxide. *J. Clin. Invest.*, **95**, 1798–807.

15. Vascular-derived growth factors: potential role in the development of the tumour vasculature

A. Bobik, A. Agrotis, and P. J. Little

Introduction

There are now strong indications that the growth of many solid tumours is dependent on a high level of vascularization via angiogenesis. Angiogenesis, the formation of new capillaries from pre-existing blood vessels appears also necessary (but alone is not sufficient) for subsequent tumour infiltrations and metastases of a tumour (1–3). In many organs such as the bladder (4), cervix (5), and the breast (6–8) the commencement of angiogenic activity marks the end of the prevascular phase of the developing carcinoma, which may have persisted for years with only evidence of hyperplastic growth. However, once a dense pattern of vascularization is formed, neoplastic growth becomes apparent and tumour size increases rapidly; bleeding may occur from the newly formed capillaries and the risk of metastases increases dramatically (2,3,8,9).

The sequence of events which led to the development of a vascularizing tumour phenotype are complex and involve many growth factor-dependent mechanisms, including those dependent on interactions with vascular-derived growth factors. The initial switching of a tumour from a hyperplastic phenotype into an angiogenic phenotype is associated with the loss of control by various cancer suppressor genes; also the genes encoding angiogenesis inhibitor proteins such as thrombospondin are down-regulated (10,11). Changes in the localization of basic fibroblast growth factor (bFGF) from its normal cell-associated state to secretion have also been associated with neovascularization and tumorigenicity (12). Angiogenic tumours may produce a binding protein that promotes secretion of both bFGF and acid fibroblast growth factor (aFGF), neither of which possess hydrophobic signalling sequences normally required for secretion (12–14). However, while a tumour can produce and release a variety of angiogenic factors such as bFGF and vascular endothelial growth factor (VEGF), these alone are unlikely to explain fully the mechanisms involved in tumour angio-genesis. Rather, tumour angiogenesis results from many complex interactions between different cell types, such as fibroblasts, smooth muscle cells, pericytes, endothelial cells, and cells of the immune system, all releasing and responding to or secreting various cytokines/growth factors (15). Here we focus on vascular cells, some of their growth factors, and how they can interact with cytokine networks of a tumour to promote its vascularization.

Vascular cells and angiogenesis

A growing tumour contains a heterogeneous, highly interactive cell population comprised of malignant cells surrounded by a stromal compartment of fibroblasts, endothelial cells, neutrophils, natural killer (NK) cells, lymphocytes, mast cells, and macrophages. The immune cells within the tumour or at its periphery are recruited from the circulation and are often markedly compromised with respect to their immunocompetence; they appear to be reprogrammed to promote the growth and metastasis of the tumour (15–17). Newly formed blood vessels invading the tumour parenchyma provide the additional nutrients and oxygen requirements for the rapidly growing malignant cell population and an exit route for metastasizing cells into the general circulation. The growing tips of capillary buds forming new vessels for the expanding tumour secrete an array of proteolytic enzymes such as collagenases, urokinases, and cathepsin, to degrade the extracellular matrix.

The stimulus for the early components of angiogenesis is likely to involve the same growth factors as those involved in ocular neovascularization (18–20), capillary invasion of arthritic joints, contact dermatitis (21), wound healing (22), and various physiological vascularizations (23,24). Malignant cells and endothelial cells produce monocyte chemotactic protein (MCP-1), and granulocyte/macrophage colony-stimulating factor (GM-CSF) to attract and activate macrophages. Once activated these cells increase vascular permeability by releasing various vasoactive substances such as substance P, platelet-activating factor, and vascular permeability factor (VPF). Macrophages and granulocytes can also affect tissue permeability by secreting a variety of proteases. Other factors (see Table 15.1) secreted by vascular cells have the ability to modulate endothelial cell migration, proliferation, and capillary formation. By secreting such factors, activated macrophages can influence both tumour growth and neovascularization. Indeed, some neoplastic tissues exhibit angiogenic activity *in vivo* and *in vitro* only in the presence of macrophages. Tumour-associated macrophages have been shown to secrete a wide variety of angiogenic factors including interleukin 8 (IL-8), VEGF, tumour necrosis factor α (TNF-α), transforming growth factor α (TGF-α), and transforming growth factor β (TGF-β) (25,26). In addition to being angiogenic, TGF-β inhibits the *in vitro* cytotoxicity of NK cells and lymphokine-activated killer (LAK) cells (27,28). NK and LAK cells also have an ability to produce a variety of interleukins, in particular IL-4 (29) which can stimulate endothelial cells to proliferate (30).

It has now become apparent that the contribution which neovascularization makes to tumour growth lies not only in perfusing the tumour with blood-borne nutrients, but also in the many paracrine effects of vascular endothelial cells on tumour cells. A significant proportion of cells in solid tumours are normal host-derived endothelial cells; occasionally they represent as much as 90% of the cell population. Endothelial cells within or adjacent to a tumour may affect tumour growth and spreading by releasing various cytokines and proteases which act to alter the proliferative and/or invasive behaviour of adjacent tumour cells. Endothelial cells are capable of producing a plethora of cytokines and growth factors which influence angiogenesis and tumour growth (see Table 15.1). Frequently, endothelial cells are located at 'strategic' sites of the tumour–blood vessel interface where tumour cell proliferation is most rapid; such places are also often regions where metastases originate. In these areas in, for example, breast cancer, the release of IL-6 by the endothelial cells can decrease tumour cell association and increase cell mobility, affecting both tumour invasive and metastatic capacity. By adhering to endothelial cells tumour cells are frequently protected from lysis by NK cells. Thus, endothelial cells have unique functions among the different tumour-associated host stromal cells, in addition to forming microvascular networks via angiogenesis.

The angiogenic activity of endothelial cells is very much dependent on the nature of the malignant cells, the cell types that are associated with them, and the growth

Table 15.1. Vascular-derived factors stimulating/promoting endothelial cell migration, proliferation, 'capillary tube' formation, or angiogenesis

Factor	Vascular cell
Basic fibroblast growth factor	Endothelial cells
	Macrophages
Transforming growth factor β	Endothelial cells
	Macrophages
	T lymphocytes
Vascular endothelial growth factor	Macrophages
Tumour necrosis factor α	Macrophages
B61 protein	Endothelial cells
Transforming growth factor α	Macrophages
Interleukin 1	Endothelial cells
	Macrophages
Interleukin 3	Endothelial cells
	T lymphocytes
Interleukin 4	T lymphocytes
Interleukin 8	Endothelial cells
	Macrophages
	Neutrophils
Colony stimulating factors	Endothelial cells
	T lymphocytes
	Monocytes
Platelet-derived endothelial cell growth factor	Macrophages
Platelet-derived growth factor	Endothelial cells
	Macrophages

factors produced, acting either alone or in concert with other factors. Known angiogenic growth factors derived from tumours and vascular cells include VEGF, aFGF and bFGF, TGF-α and TGF-β, epidermal growth factor (EGF), TNF-α, platelet-derived endothelial cell growth factor (PD-ECGF), angiogenin, and various interleukins. The rate at which angiogenesis proceeds in the presence of these cytokines is also influenced by variability in endothelial cell types. Capillary endothelial cells from different organs are not uniform in their responses to growth factors. For example, EGF and TGF-α are potent mitogens for lung-derived endothelial cells (31); skin-derived endothelial cells are also highly responsive to these growth factors and in addition to IL-2 (32). However, endothelial cells of the adrenal glands are not affected by these growth factors (33), but are highly responsive to IL-4 (30). Platelet-derived growth factor (PDGF) and angiogenin are potent mitogens for endothelial cells in the brain (33,34).

Endothelial cells are also capable of influencing the angiogenic process and tumour growth by producing other factors such as IL-6, which is up-regulated during angio-genesis. Angiogenic endothelial cells can attenuate early tumour growth by secreting growth inhibitory agents. A rapid increase in tumour vascularity has been reported to be accompanied by focal histological regression of melanomas at a very early stage of their development; this is most probably due to the sudden exposure of the pro-liferating melanoma cells to multiple growth inhibitors released by endothelial cells. The later stages of tumour growth are resistant to such inhibition. It would appear that through this early inhibitory process, mediated by the vas-cular cells involved in angiogenesis, there is a gradual selection of the most competent subpopulations of human melanoma cells which are capable of replicating and metastasizing rapidly (35).

Endothelial cell phenotypes in angiogenesis

Normally in capillaries there exists a single layer of quies-cent, flattened endothelial cells whose basal surface interacts with the extracellular matrix; the apical non-thrombogenic surface delimits the lumen of the vessel. Endothelial cell quiescence is maintained by the secretory products of pericytes (36). However, once the endothelial cells are stimulated or activated they can alter their pheno-type and take up new functions required for vessel for-mation. The endothelial cells can become spindle-like in shape and then are no longer subject to the negative growth control of pericytes secreting TGF-β-like substances; rather the cells are now capable of dissolving the capillary base-ment membrane and the local extracellular matrix (37–39). They are now also capable of replicating while still in the vessel. Sprouting endothelial cells which form the bud of a developing new vessel secrete serine proteases, tissue-type and urokinase-type plasminogen activator (tPA and uPA) and collagenases, to open a path for their migration through the tissue requiring neovascularization (40). Activated macrophages chemoattracted to the site of angiogenesis can also participate in extracellular matrix degradation by se-creting various metalloproteases, including collagenases (41,42) and serine proteases.

A changing extracellular environment at the tips of capillary sprouts plays an important part in the angiogenic process by further influencing the properties of endothelial cells and their responsiveness to angiogenic factors and cytokines (43,44). Depending on whether the endothelial cells interact with laminin or collagen type IV, their responses to angiogenic substances differ, including their ability to proliferate or form 'capillary tubes' (45–47). As non-proliferating 'leader' endothelial cells of a capillary

bud migrate through the degraded matrix they are followed by proliferating endothelial cells which utilize a variety of growth factors, some of which are derived from the degraded extracellular matrix (Fig. 15.1). Other extra-cellular matrix proteolytic products such as the peptide fragments of hyaluronic acid can also participate in neo-vascularization (48); similarly, peptide fragments resulting from plasmin degradation of fibrin and SPARC (secreted protein, acidic and rich in cysteine) also promote neovas-cularization (49). Endothelial-derived SPARC binds to the endothelial surface membrane with high-affinity, disrupt-ing focal adhesions and regulating cell proliferation and shape *in vitro*. Growth factors which facilitate the angio-genesis are stored in the extracellular matrix to be released during proteolysis, including bFGF, TGF-β, GM-CSF, and IL-3 (50,51).

Vascular-derived growth factors stimulating neovascularization

Vascular cells secrete or produce a variety of growth factors that promote angiogenesis (Table 15.1). Of these, the most extensively studied include bFGF, TGF-βs, VEGFs, TNF-α, TGF-α, and various interleukins. They are general stimulators of angiogenesis, activating many endothelial cell types and capable of acting either alone or in concert with other growth factors to ensure that the affected endothelial cells transit through the different stages of angiogenesis (see Fig. 15.1).

Basic fibroblast growth factors

bFGF can be produced by many cell types including tumour-associated macrophages and endothelial cells (52–55). It is encoded by a single copy gene containing three exons and spans at least 38 kilobases of genomic DNA. Under normal conditions bFGF mRNA transcripts in endothelial cells and macrophages are generally of low abundance, and are relatively unstable (56). Their regula-tion occurs in part through post-transcriptional processes, via A + U-rich sequences in the 3′-untranslated region of the DNA, which consist of the motifs $(TATT)_n$ or $(TAAT)_n$, potential recognition sequences for specific nucleases (57,58). The generation of anti-sense transcripts may also influence bFGF expression post-transcriptionally (59). Anti-sense transcripts are generated from the same genetic locus and result in the presence of two reverse complementary RNA molecules which leads to the for-mation of double-stranded RNA. This dramatically alters bFGF mRNA processing, translation and nuclear/

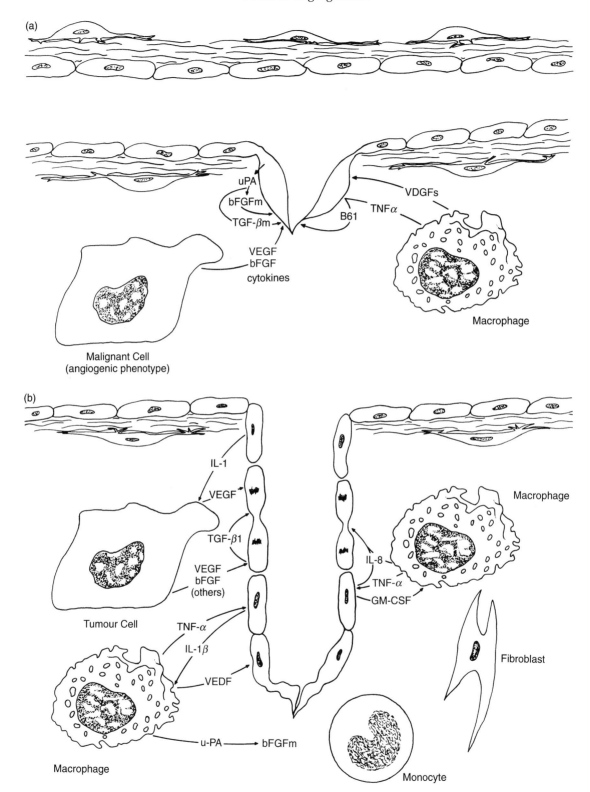

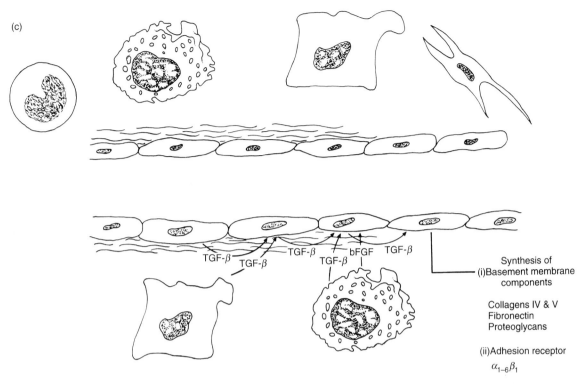

Figure 15.1. Potential roles of some vascular-derived growth factors. (a) Enhancement of an angiogenic stimulus through the release of matrix deposited growth factors (bFGFm and TGF-βm) derived from endothelial cells. Urokinase plasminogen activator (uPA) and other proteolytic enzymes release bFGF and TGF-β during cell endothelial stimulation by vascular-derived growth factors (VDGF) and/or angiogenic factors secreted by tumour cells. (b) Potential cytokine networks between tumour cells and endothelial cells as well as activated macrophages and endothelial cells. All promote angiogenesis either by enhancing endothelial cell proliferation, migration, or invasive capability. (c) Vascular-derived TGF-β participating in the biosynthesis of basement membrane proteins required by a newly formed vessel.

cytoplasmic export. At present, little is known about how this anti-sense transcript is regulated. In activated endothelial cells bFGF mRNA transcripts are usually relatively high in abundance and translated into peptides of multiple size depending on whether translation commences at codons encoding methionine (AUG) or leucine (CUG; GUG). Three forms (18, 24, and 26 kDa) are frequently present in endothelial cells; the lower molecular weight form is normally located in the cytoplasm while the larger peptides are transported into the nucleus (55). A nucleolar localization of bFGF has been correlated with the stimulation of transcription of ribosomal genes during G_0 to G_1 transition, induced by extracellular bFGF (60). Tumour-associated endothelial cells frequently have a different cellular distribution of bFGF compared with quiescent endothelial cells. In phaeochromocytomas endothelial cells contain high levels of bFGF in their cytoplasm and nuclei, but in normal adrenal medulla, endothelial bFGF is predominantly localized in the nucleus (61).

As bFGF is without a hydrophobic signal peptide sequence its secretion by endothelial and other cells is normally compromised (62). As a consequence it is only very slowly deposited into the surrounding extracellular matrix, immobilized, and stabilized by tight binding to proteins such as heparan sulphate proteoglycans and high-affinity soluble FGF receptors (63). Tumours secreting a 17 kDa binding protein for heparin-binding growth factors solubilize matrix-bound FGF associated with adjacent capillaries and microvessels, enabling the growth factor to reach high concentrations, sufficient to activate FGF membrane receptors (13, 64). The secretion by tumour-associated macrophages of heparinases and plasmin also facilitate bFGF release from the matrix. In capillaries this solubilization of endothelial cell-derived bFGF completes the autocrine loop for endothelial cells to stimulate the early stages of angiogenesis (see Fig. 15.1). At present it is not known whether activated macrophages and/or endothelial cells are capable of secreting transport proteins to

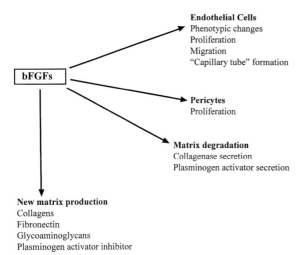

Figure 15.2. Processes in angiogenesis stimulated by basic fibroblast growth factors (bFGFs).

transport bFGF across their cell membranes, in a manner analogous to some tumours (13).

Released bFGF is potentially a multifunctional substance and depending on the receptors expressed by endothelial cells it is capable of altering their phenotype, stimulating uPA production, procollagenase and prostromelysin production, cell migration, proliferation, 'tube' formation *in vitro*, and other cellular events, many of which are critical components of the complex angiogenic process (see Fig. 15.2).

Four closely related receptor types (FGFR-1, -2, -3, and -4) are likely to account for many of the multifunctional effects of bFGF in angiogenesis. They are composed of up to three immunoglobulin (Ig)-like domains, an acidic box of eight amino acids located between the first and second immunoglobulin-like domains, a single transmembrane domain followed by a relatively long juxtamembrane region, and a split tyrosine kinase domain which at its carboxy-terminal tail contains tyrosine which may be phosphorylated upon FGF binding (65). Many variants of this general FGFR structure have been identified, arising from varying pre-mRNA splicing and differential polyadenylation signals within the respective genes. FGFRs-1 and -2 can exist without the first immunoglobulin domain or the acidic box and secreted antagonist forms of FGFR-1 have been reported (66). Endothelial cells can also secrete truncated forms of the FGFR-1 which are deposited into the extracellular matrix (63).

Receptor affinity and selectivity for different FGFs is to a large extent dependent on amino acid sequences within the carboxy-terminus of the third immunoglobulin-like domain and is contingent on whether exons 6 or 7 (the

'IIIb' and 'IIIc' exons), of the respective genes are incorporated into the mRNA (for details see reference 67). Depending on which exons are spliced, the FGFR-1, for example, is capable of binding both bFGF and aFGF. High-affinity receptors for bFGF possess amino acid sequences encoded in exon 7 (IIIc) of the FGFR-1 and FGFR-2 genes. FGFR-3 and -4 possess highest affinities for aFGF and other members of the FGF family, FGF-4 and K-FGF. At present little is known about which receptors are expressed by endothelial cells during the various stages of angiogenesis. However, *in vitro* they can express at least three subtypes, FGFR-1, -3, and -4 (68,69). The high-affinity forms of these receptors are responsible for the many effects of the FGFs; lower-affinity cell surface binding proteins, predominantly heparan sulphate proteoglycans also participate in inducing these cellular events by facilitating the binding of FGF to the high-affinity receptors (62,70–72). The heparin-binding properties of bFGF are important in promoting *in vitro* angiogenesis (71). Both matrix proteins and variations in endothelial cell phenotype are also likely to influence the nature and characteristics of the low-affinity binding FGF binding sites on the endothelial cell surface and the FGF signalling receptors (73,74). Other factors such as IL-1 and interferon γ (IFN-γ) are capable of down-regulating FGFRs on endothelial cells, thereby attenuating angiogenesis (75). It is likely that a combination of such influences regulates the expression of different endothelial cell FGFR genes as they perform their various functions during neovascularization (75,76).

Transforming growth factor β

TGF-β can markedly influence both the phenotype of endothelial cells and their many actions. TGF-β can be produced within an expanding tumour by a number of vascular cells including T lymphocytes, macrophages, and endothelial cells (62,77,78). Depending on the environmental conditions three different isoforms may be produced, TGF-β1, -β2, -β3; these are encoded by different genes and possess between 60 and 80% amino acid sequence homology. Although in two-dimensional (2D) cell culture they appear to exert similar effects, their actions *in vivo* are not necessarily always the same (79).

Because of the close association of tumour cells with endothelial cells in a vascularizing tumour, the effects of tumour-derived TGF-β can be potentially amplified by stimulating endothelial cells to also produce this cytokine (see Fig. 15.1). This autoinduction of the TGF-β1 gene is dependent on elevations in AP-1 and Sp1 transcription factors (80,81). Growth factors which act via receptor tyrosine kinases may also induce TGF-β1 gene activation, at least in part, via such mechanisms. TGF-β1 gene activation can also be influenced by other mechanisms, for example, via the retinoblastoma gene product RB (82) and post-transcriptionally. For the TGF-β2 and TGF-β3 genes the presence of consensus cAMP-responsive elements/activating transcription factor elements (CREs/ATFs) in their promoter regions are thought to regulate their expression (83,84). During stimulation with growth factors which activate receptor tyrosine kinase activity, such as with bFGF, TGF-β1 mRNA expression becomes elevated while mRNA encoding TGF-β2 and TGF-β3 is down-regulated (Agrotis and Bobik, unpublished). Under these conditions TGF-β1 may become the predominant form of TGF-β produced by endothelial cells.

In the normal capillary, shear-stress on endothelial cells can also activate the TGF-β1 gene, via mechanosensitive K^+ channels on their surface membranes (85,86). Under such conditions TGF-β1 is produced in a latent, inactive form and deposited in the extracellular matrix. Latent TGF-β1 is composed of three components, the mature TGF-β1, the propeptide region of its precursor molecule, and a TGF-β-binding protein possessing many matrix-binding sites. Latency is conferred by the electrostatic forces between the propeptide and TGF-β1 (87). Completion of an autocrine cycle for endothelial cell-derived TGF-β1 frequently depends on its release from the extracellular matrix. Acidic microenvironments in areas of necrotic tissues are capable of activating latent TGF-β1. Limited proteolysis by plasmin or related enzymes (88) and the thrombospondin secreted by endothelial cells are also capable of activating latent TGF-β1 (89). As TGF-β1 induces cells to secrete thrombospondin (90), the growth factor can potentially enhance its own effects by regulating thrombospondin production (91).

Vascular-derived TGF-β can influence angiogenesis at many stages (see Figs. 15.1 and 15.3). Phenotypic modulation of endothelial cells by TGF-β is one event early in angiogenesis. When microvascular endothelial cells grown in 3D collagen gels are exposed to TGF-β a rapid and extensive formation of complex, branching, tube-like structures occurs without inhibition of cell proliferation (92,93). In 2D cell culture endothelial cell proliferation is markedly inhibited by TGF-β (92). TGF-β is also capable of modulating cell migration (94), bFGF-induced proteolysis (95), and the ability of VEGF to elicit invasion by endothelial cells (96). It is chemotactic for human monocytes, and induces the expression of TNF-α, bFGF, PDGF, IL-1 mRNAs (97) as well stimulating angiogenic activity (98). Endothelial cell- or monocyte-derived TGF-β can also participate in 'tumour angiogenesis' by altering the composition of the extracellular matrix and influencing the extent of cell adhesion to the pericellular matrix, via various cell surface receptors (see references 62,91,93). Matrix accumulation/modification may occur not only through the ability of TGF-β to induce

extracellular matrix biosynthesis, but also by inhibiting its degradation. Urokinase secretion is reduced by TGF-β and plasminogen activator inhibitor-1 protein secretion is increased (99); a number of collagens, thrombospondin, tenasin, and various heparan sulphate proteoglycans are also induced by this cytokine (62,100,101). These and the many other effects of TGF-β are to a large extent dependent on the nature of cell surface receptors expressed by the different endothelial cell types and their phenotypes (see section on 'Vascular cells and angiogenesis').

Three species of high-affinity receptors for TGF-β have been identified on endothelial cells by their ability to bind and be chemically cross-linked to [^{125}I]TGF-β1 (102). Types I, II, and III receptors have molecular weights of approximately 55, 80, and 280 kDa, respectively (102,103). The type III receptor is a proteoglycan and the most abundant of the receptor classes (104). It is composed of a large extracellular domain, a single transmembrane segment, and a short cytoplasmic region of 41 amino acid with no obvious signalling motif. A major function of this receptor is to modulate the binding of TGF-β to the signalling types I and II receptors, most likely by presenting the ligand to the type II receptor (105). This purported binding function of the type III receptor is indicated by recent observations demonstrating that the expression of soluble type III receptors or the release of type III receptors from the cell's surface can prevent TGF-β-mediated cell signalling by sequestering TGF-β. At present it is uncertain whether the ability of low concentrations of TGF-β1 to enhance endothelial cell

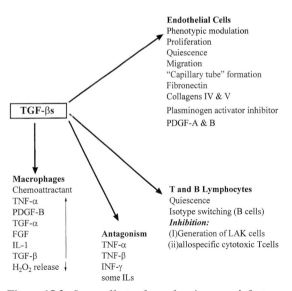

Figure 15.3. Some effects of transforming growth factor (TGF) β potentially important for tumour angiogenesis.

proliferation (102) and *in vitro* angiogenesis (106), and high concentrations to inhibit proliferation/angiogenesis is related to the extent to which the type III receptor alters the presentation of the growth factor to the signalling receptors.

An interaction of TGF-β with the type II receptor is a prerequisite for intracellular signalling in all cells examined so far, including endothelial cells (102). The type II receptor is a member of a family of transmembrane serine/threonine kinases which includes type II activin receptors (for reviews see references 104,105,107). The human type II TGF-β receptor is characterized by a short extracellular region containing a cysteine-rich domain, a hydrophobic transmembrane-spanning region, and an intracellular region containing a serine/threonine kinase domain. It is composed of 565 amino acids whose sequence homology in the extracellular domain is very different from other type II receptors of the family; in the intracellular kinase domain there is up to 40% homology. The type I family of receptors with which TGF-βs interact are also transmembrane serine/threonine kinases. These receptors contain a short motif rich in glycines and serines N-terminal to the kinase domain, which is absent in the type II receptors and serves as a site for phosphorylation (105,108); the type I and II receptors also differ in their intracellular kinase domain.

A stable ternary complex between the type I and type II TGF-β receptors and TGF-β is considered essential for cell signalling (105,108). The complex is thought to initiate a diverse array of signalling events, which are dependent on the precise nature of the type II and type I receptors. In the receptor model proposed by Massagué and co-workers (108), TGF-β exerts its effects by initially binding to the type II receptor, a constitutively active kinase; the type I receptor is then recruited into the complex, transphosphorylated by the type II receptor and signalling initiated. As there are different type I receptors with which the type II TGF-β receptor can complex, different combinations of type I and type II complexes most likely elicit the many gene transcriptional events and cellular responses. For example, the ability of TGF-β to enhance aFGF-induced proliferation in human umbilical vein endothelial cells has been associated with an apparent lack of type I TGF-β receptors (102) and inhibition of proliferation of fetal bovine heart endothelial cell cultures with the presence of all three receptor types (102). Recently other receptor subtypes have been implicated in the effects of TGF-β. The TGF-β/activin binding type I receptor, Tsk7L, accounts for TGF-β-mediated epithelial to mesenchymal cell transition (109,110). Truncated Tsk7L type I receptors lacking most of the cytoplasmic kinase domain and functioning as dominant negative mutants inhibit this transdifferentiation process. At present it is unknown which type I receptor participates in

TGF-β-mediated phenotypic changes in endothelial cells (92,93). The dependence of receptor expression on endothelial cell phenotype is also unclear; endothelial cells exhibiting angiogenesis *in vitro* are known to proliferate in response to TGF-β1 (93). The nature of TGF-β receptors involved in TGF-β actions during angiogenesis require further defining as do those expressed by monocytes/macrophages attracted into tumours. Truncated receptors and alternatively spliced members of the types I and II receptor family are all likely to participate in the neovascularization of a tumour (111).

Vascular endothelial growth factor

VEGF (VPF), a heparin-binding protein is an important multifunctional cytokine that promotes vasculogenesis, physiological/developmental angiogenesis (112,113), and tumour angiogenesis (114–116). It can be produced and secreted by various cell types including many tumour cells (112,114–118) and activated macrophages (117,119,120). Four VEGF isoforms of varying amino acid lengths, $VEGF_{121}$, $VEGF_{165}$, $VEGF_{189}$, and $VEGF_{206}$, have been detected in human tissues (121), arising through alternate splicing of RNA from a single gene (122). $VEGF_{121}$ and $VEGF_{165}$ are the secreted, 'more soluble' forms, whereas the larger isoforms tend to remain mostly cell associated (119). $VEGF_{165}$ and larger isoforms most likely account for the high amounts of VEGF immunoreactivity detected in vessels close to tumours (123). Presumably the cell associated isoforms are bound to 'heparin-containing proteoglycans' and are released by budding/migrating endothelial cells secreting proteolytic enzymes (124). Macrophages are also capable of releasing matrix-bound VEGF by secreting heparinase. Local concentrations may also be increased through gene activation. The VEGF gene contains in its 5′-region consensus sequences for Sp1 binding sites and four potential AP-1 binding sites; a section of the region immediately upstream is also very GC rich, similar to that in the TGF-β1 gene (122). Both phorbol esters, serum and hypoxia are capable of activating the gene. As VEGF activates phospholipase C to elevate inositol trisphosphates and diacyl glycerol, there is also the potential for autoinduction of the VEGF gene in a manner similar to that observed with the TGF-β1 gene (81,125).

VEGF can promote angiogenesis through a variety of mechanisms (118). It stimulates the proliferation of endothelial cells and increases their migratory ability, in part by activating genes participating in proteolysis. In many instances these effects are synergistically enhanced by the presence of other angiogenic factors, such as bFGF (126). VEGF is also a powerful permeabilizer of many small vessels: capillaries, venules, and small veins.

Through this property VEGF influences the production of specific extracellular matrix by promoting the extravasation of plasma fibrinogen leading to fibrin deposition and ultimately to more extensive angiogenesis through the participation of invading activated macrophages (118,127). It can also directly promote macrophage migration into a tumour (128). These and other effects of VEGF on endothelial cells are mediated through cell surface receptors. Two high-affinity VEGF receptors have been identified, *flt*-1 and *flk*-1; both receptors are tyrosine kinases and are somewhat analogous to the PDGF receptors (129,130). The receptor type *flk*-1 is markedly up-regulated in proliferating endothelial cells associated with vascular sprouts, but drastically down-regulated once proliferation has ceased.

Tumour necrosis factor α

Tumour necrosis factor (TNF) α is an important cytokine produced by macrophages (131). It is an anionic polypeptide of 154–157 amino acids initially synthesized as a pro-hormone containing a precursor extension of 76–80 amino acids. Its production in macrophages can be induced by a number of agents that activate these cells and also by hypoxia (132). TNF-α has been proposed as the major cytokine responsible for the angiogenic capability of macrophages (133) and is a potent stimulator of angiogenesis *in vivo* (134). Its actions may, in part, be regulated through the secretion of soluble high-affinity receptors (135).

TNF-α is a multifunctional peptide with respect to its angiogenic capability and can promote the expression, synthesis, and secretion of uPA by endothelial cells (136,137). It can also enhance collagenase synthesis by endothelial cells (138). *In vitro*, TNF-α stimulates endothelial cell migration and tube formation, but inhibits the proliferation of these cells (133,134,138). It can maintain monocyte viability within a tumour by inducing endothelial cells to produce GM-CSF. These and other actions of TNF-α, including the induction of IL-1 synthesis, ICAM-1 expression, and chemotaxis are at least in part due to indirect mechanisms. TNF-α has been reported to enhance the production and secretion of bFGF by endothelial cells (138); also, enhanced collagenase activity has been attributed to the production of this cytokine. It is also possible that bFGF contributes to other aspects of TNF-α's effects on endothelial cells. Under some conditions TNF-α has been reported to inhibit capillary endothelial cell proliferation (139).

Recently, TNF-α has been shown to induce endothelial cells to secrete a 25 kDa protein, known as B61 (140). This inducible endothelial cell gene product binds to and signals through a protein tyrosine kinase receptor, Eck, and contributes to the angiogenic capability of TNF-α (141). *In vivo* B61 is angiogenic and *in vitro* it is a

chemoattractant for endothelial cells. B61 may also exist in a cell associated form, anchored to the cell membrane through a glycosylphosphatidylinositol (GPI) linked protein (142) and can be released through the hydrolytic actions of phosphatidylinositol (PI)-specific phospholipase C. This GPI-linked B61 is also capable of activating the Eck receptor protein–tyrosine kinase without being released from the cell surface (142). Released prostaglandins (143) and platelet-activating factor (144) have also been implicated in TNF-α induced angiogenesis.

Interleukins

Interleukin 1

IL-1 possesses a number of properties which affect both endothelial cell function and angiogenesis. It is composed of two polypeptides with different isoelectric points, IL-1α and IL-1β; they are the products of two separate genes and possess no signal peptide (62). Despite this, endothelial cells and activated macrophages produce and secrete IL-1α (145,146). IL-1 secretion can be elevated by TNF-α or IL-1 itself (145).

IL-1 can influence angiogenesis through a number of mechanisms and affects both endothelial cell morphology and function. In the presence of IL-1 endothelial cells take on a fibroblast-like spindle-shaped appearance (147). Also, by inducing granulocyte colony-stimulating factor (G-CSF) and GM-CSF it may stimulate the endothelial cells to migrate and proliferate (148–150). The production of G-CSF and GM-CSF assists in maintaining viable angiogenic monocytes associated with a tumour. IL-1β release by endothelial cells can also contribute to VEGF release by both tumour- and tumour-associated cells (151). As might be expected from these properties both IL-1α and IL-1β are angiogenic *in vivo* (152); however, IL-1α is the more potent of the two interleukins.

Although IL-1 is an autocrine regulator of endothelial cell growth (153), its effects are not always associated with growth promotion (154) and its ability to either stimulate or inhibit tumour angiogenesis is dependent on the nature of other factors participating in the neovascularization process. For example, simultaneous release of substance P by macrophages will enhance interleukin's angiogenic activity (155). In contrast, bFGF-induced angiogenesis is attenuated by IL-1 through a down-regulation of FGF receptors (75); this effect is specific to FGF-induced angiogenesis as epidermal growth factor receptors are unaffected.

Interleukin 8

IL-8 is a cytokine produced by a number of different cell types including some carcinoma cells (156,157), neutrophils (158,159), mononuclear cells (160), and endothelial cells (149). It is chemotactic for endothelial cells and induces their proliferation (161). It is also a potent stimulator of angiogenesis (162,163) and as IL-8 antisense oligonucleotides inhibit monocyte-induced angiogenic activity (161), it has been proposed as a significant contributor to the overall angiogenic activity of many tumour-associated macrophages. As IL-8 gene expression is increased by TNF-α and IL-1α it is likely to contribute to their angiogenic activity (149).

The effects of IL-8 on endothelial cells appear to be mediated via low-affinity receptors, in particular the IL-8 type I receptor (164). Recently, a prime role for IL-8 in tumour angiogenesis was demonstrated; neutralizing antisera to IL-8 were capable of attenuating angiogenesis in bronchogenic carcinoma (165).

Transforming growth factor α

TGF-α is an angiogenic factor also released by both tumour-associated macrophages (166,167) and many tumour cells. Its release from activated macrophages may occur together with other growth factors and this can potentially modify the endothelial cell's response to TGF-α (167). *In vitro*, it is capable of inducing endothelial cell proliferation, migration (31) and capillary-like tube formation in collagen gels (168). This ability of TGF-α to induce capillary-like structures is dependent on the release by endothelial cells of additional substances such as tPA and probably FGF (168).

Vascular-derived growth factors in tumour angiogenic networks

As many angiogenic growth factors within a tumour have seemingly very similar properties, based on *in vitro* studies, it has been proposed that within any vascularizing tumour there is a large redundancy of factors and cells which ensure adequate neovascularization (26). Tumours may, for example, in addition to secreting bFGF also secrete additional angiogenic members of the FGF family: hst (169,170), int-2 (171), or FGF-5 (172). It is also possible that in addition to ensuring adequate redundancy the many cytokines/growth factors involved in vascularizing a tumour regulate specific cellular events which are not necessarily required for angiogenesis, but rather ensure tumour viability, growth, and metastases. For example, bFGF is not always involved in angiogenesis within a tumour (173). Also, different forms of bFGF are likely to have different functions in angiogenesis (174). TGF-β is likely to be involved in the selection of tumour cells resistant to inhibitory growth factors in addition to promoting endothelial cells through the different stages of angiogenesis (see section on 'Transforming growth factor β', and Fig. 15. 1). It may also participate in other cytokine functions required for tumour survival (see Fig. 15.3). Also, the susceptibility of endothelial cells to the various angiogenic factors will depend on whether they are associated with the appropriate extracellular matrix proteins and expressing appropriate growth factor receptors. At present little is known about the temporal expression of particular receptors during angiogenesis and how they are modulated by the various cytokine networks; only recently IL-1 has been shown to down-regulate FGF receptors and FGF-mediated angiogenesis (75).

Interactions between different angiogenic factors/ growth factors derived from tumour and vascular cells may enhance the formation of capillaries with different physical characteristics. *In vitro* bFGF alone appears to induce capillary-like endothelial tubes of greater dimension than when TGF-β1 is also present (175). Those capillaries formed in the presence of VEGF are likely to be more permeable than those formed in its absence. Their characteristics are also likely to be modified by other cytokines. It is likely that the degree to which particular tumours become vascularized is dependent on precisely when and the extent to which the different angiogenic substances participate in new vessel formation; they may be derived from either tumour cells, vascular cells, or other cell types. For example, early mast cell accumulation, most probably secreting heparin-like substances and activating heparin-binding growth factors, have been associated with very high vascularization of some tumours (176). The extent to which matrix can be degraded by various growth factor-activated cells within a tumour and the nature of the degradation products will also influence the responsiveness of endothelial cells to various growth factors and their ability to participate in the angiogenic process. The production of TNF-resistant triggering proteins induced by vascular or tumour-derived TGF-β1 will, for example, attenuate the angiogenic stimulus of macrophage- or tumour-derived TNF-α on endothelial cells (177).

Summary and conclusions

Although tumour angiogenesis is a very complex process involving many cell types and many cytokine networks, it is very likely that in most angiogenic tumours vascular-derived growth factors will play a significant part in neovascularization. Initially they may either stimulate angiogenesis, if secreted by activated macrophages, or enhance the effects of tumour-derived angiogenic factors by stimulating endothelial cells to release growth factors deposited within their basement membranes. Also, by secreting cytokines such as IL-1 endothelial cells may indirectly promote angiogenesis, stimulating tumour cells and associated macrophages to secrete VEGF. Endothelial cells involved in angiogenesis may also secrete various angiogenic factors such as IL-8 and protein B61. In the latter stages of angiogenesis vascular-derived growth factors may contribute to the synthesis by endothelial cells of basement membrane components. Interference in these cytokine networks at the level of the endothelial cell is one approach to limit angiogenesis. Theoretically, this might be achieved through therapy targeting activated endothelial cells so that they are programmed to express inactive or truncated receptors which interfere with cytokine cell signalling.

References

1. Russell, R. (1989). Successful growth of tumors. *Nature*, **339**, 16–7.
2. Folkman, J. and Klagsbrun, M. (1987). Angiogenic factors. *Science*, **235**, 442–7.
3. Cross, M. and Dexter, T. M. (1991). Growth factors in development, transformation and tumorigenesis. *Cell*, **64**, 271–80.
4. Chodak, G. W., Haudenschild, C., Gittes, R. F., and Folkman, J. (1980). Angiogenic activity as a marker of neoplastic and of preneoplastic lesions of the human bladder. *Ann. Surg.*, **192**, 762–71.
5. Sillman, F., Boyce, J., and Fruchter, R. (1981). The significance of atypical vessels and neovascularization in cervical neoplasia. *Am. J. Obstet. Gynecol.*, **139**, 154–9.
6. Brem, S. S., Gullino, P. M., and Medina, D. (1977). Angiogenesis: a marker to neoplastic transformation of mammary papillary hyperplasia. *Science*, **195**, 880–2.
7. Jensen, H. M. (1987). Angiogenesis induced by normal human breast tissue. In, *Angiogenesis — mechanisms and pathology. Current communications in molecular biology* (e.d. D. B. Rifkin and M. Klagsbrun), pp. 155–7. Cold Spring Harbor Laboratory, Cold Spring Harbor, NY.
8. Liotta, L. A., Steeg, P. S., and Stetler-Stevenson, W. G. (1991). Cancer metastasis and angiogenesis: an imbalance of positive and negative regulation. *Cell*, **64**, 327–36.
9. Weidner, N., Semple, J. P., Welch, W. R., and Folkman, J. (1991). Tumor angiogenesis and metastasis — correlation in invasive breast carcinoma. *T. N. Engl. J. Med.*, **324**, 1–8.
10. Rastinejad, F., Polverini, P. J., and Bouck, N. P. (1989). Regulation of the activity of a new inhibitor of angiogenesis by a cancer suppressor gene. *Cell*, **56**, 345–55.
11. Iruela-Arispe, M. L., Bornstein, P., and Sage, H. (1991). Thrombospondin exerts an antiangiogenic effect on cord formation by endothelial cells *in vitro*. *Proc. Natl Acad. Sci. USA*, **88**, 5026–30.
12. Kandel, J., Bossy-Wetzel, E., Radvanyi, F., Klagsbrun, M., Folkman, J., and Hanahan, D. (1991). Neovascularization is associated with a switch to the export of bFGF in the multistep development of fibrosarcoma. *Cell*, **66**, 1095–104.
13. Czubayko, F., Smith, R. V., Chung, H. C., and Wellstein, A. (1994). Tumor growth and angiogenesis induced by a secreted binding protein for fibroblast growth factors. *J. Biol. Chem.*, **269**, 28243–8.
14. Ensoli, B., Markham, P., Kao, V., Barillari, G., Fiorelli, V., Gendelman, R., *et al.* (1994). Block of AIDS–Kaposi's sarcoma (KS) cell growth, angiogenesis and lesion formation in nude mice by antisense oligonucleotides targeting basic fibroblast growth factor. *J. Clin. Invest.*, **94**, 1736–46.
15. O'Sullivan, C. and Lewis, C. E. (1994). Tumor-associated leukocytes: friends or foes in breast cancer. *J. Pathol.*, **172**, 229–35.
16. Mantovani, A., Bottazzi, B., Colotta, F., Sozzani, S., and Ruco, L. (1992). The origin and function of tumor-associated macrophages. *Immunol. Today*, **13**, 265–70.
17. O'Sullivan, C., Lewis, C. E., Harris, A. L., and McGee, J. O. (1993). Secretion of epidermal growth factor by macrophages associated with breast carcinoma. *Lancet*, **342**, 148–9.
18. Folkman, J., Watson, K., Ingber, D., and Hanahan, D. (1989). Induction of angiogenesis during the transition from hyperplasia to neoplasia. *Nature*, **339**, 58–61.
19. Soubrane, G., Cohen, S. Y., Delayre, T., Tassin, J., Hartmann, M-P., Coscas, G. J., *et al.* (1994). Basic fibroblast growth factor experimentally induced choroidal angiogenesis in the minipig. *Curr. Eye Res.*, **13**, 183–95.
20. Hanneken, A., De Juan, E. Jr., Lutty, G. A., Fox, G. M., Shiffer, S., and Hjelmeland, L. M. (1991). Altered distribution of basic fibroblast growth factor in diabetic retinopathy. *Arch. Ophthalmol.*, **109**, 1005–11.
21. Polverini, P. J., Cotran, R. S., and Sholley, M. M. (1977). Endothelial proliferation in the delayed hypersensitivity reaction: an autoradiographic study. *J. Immunol.*, **118**, 529–32.
22. Di Pietro, L. A. and Polverini, P. J. (1993). Role of the macrophage in the positive and negative regulation of wound neovascularization. *Bohring. Inst. Mitt.*, **92**, 238–47.
23. Ferrara, N. and Henzel, W. J. (1989). Pituitary follicular cells secrete a novel heparin-binding growth factor specific for vascular endothelial cells. *Biochem. Biophys. Res. Commun.*, **161**, 851–8.
24. Phillips, H. S., Hains, J., Leung, D. W., and Ferrara, N. (1990). Vascular endothelial growth factor is expressed in rat corpus luteum. *Endocrinology*, **127**, 965–7.
25. Scannell, G., Waxman, K., Kam, G. J., Ioli, G., Gatanaga, T., Yamamoto, R., and Granger, G. A. (1993). Hypoxia induces a human macrophage cell line to release tumor necrosis factor-α and its soluble receptor *in vitro*. *J. Surg. Res.*, **54**, 281–5.
26. Sunderkötter, C., Steinbrink, K., Goebeler, M., Bhardwaj, R., and Sorg, C. (1994). Macrophages and angiogenesis. *J. Leukocyte Biol.*, **55**, 410–22.
27. Rook, A. H., Kehrl, J. H., Wakefield, L. M., Roberts, A. B., Sporn, M. B., Burlington, D. B., *et al.* (1986). Effects of transforming growth factor-β on the functions of natural killer cells: depressed cytolytic activity and blunting of interferon responsiveness. *J. Immunol.*, **136**, 3916–20.
28. Wahl, S. M., Hunt, M., Wong, H. L., Dougherty, S., McCartney-Francis, N., Wahl, L. M., *et al.* (1988). Transforming growth factor-β is a potent immunosuppressive agent that inhibits IL-1-dependent lymphocyte proliferation. *J. Immunol.*, **140**, 3026–32.
29. Lewis, C. E. and O'Sullivan, C. (1994). Cytokines: mediators of cell to cell communication in solid tumors. *Surgery*, **21**, 22–3.

30. Toi, M., Harris, A. L., and Bicknell, R. (1991). Interleukin-4 is a potent mitogen for capillary endothelium. *Biochem. Biophys Res. Commun.*, **174**, 1287–93.

31. Schreiber, A. B., Winkler, M. E., and Derynck, R. (1986). Transforming growth factor: a more potent angiogenic mediator than epidermal growth factor. *Science*, **232**, 1250–3.

32. Hicks, C., Breit, S. N., and Penny, R. (1989). Response of microvascular endothelial cells to biological response modifiers. *Immunol. Cell Biol.*, **67**, 271–7.

33. Bar, R. S., Boes, M., Booth, B. A., Dake, B. L., Henley, S., and Hartman, M. N. (1989). The effects of platelet-derived growth factor in cultured microvessel endothelial cells. *Endocrinology*, **124**, 1841–8.

34. Chamoux, M., Dehouck, M. P., Fruchart, J. C., Spik, G., Montreuil, J., and Cecchelli, R. (1991). Characterization of angiogenin receptors on bovine brain capillary endothelial cells. *Biochem. Biophys. Res. Commun.*, **176**, 833–9.

35. Rak, J. W., Hegman, E. J., Lu, C., and Kerbel, R. S. (1994). Progressive loss of sensitivity to endothelium-derived growth inhibitors expressed by human melanoma cells during disease progression. *J. Cell. Physiol.*, **159**, 245–55.

36. Sato, Y. and Rifkin, D. B. (1989). Inhibition of endothelial cell movement by pericytes and smooth muscle cells: activation of a latent transforming growth factor-β_1-like molecule by plasmin during co-culture. *J. Cell Biol.*, **109**, 309–15.

37. Ausprunk, D. H. and Folkman, J. (1977). Migration and proliferation of endothelial cells in preformed and newly formed blood vessels during tumor angiogenesis. *Microvasc. Res.*, **14**, 53–65.

38. Ingber, D. E. and Folkman, J. (1989). How does extracellular matrix control capillary morphogenesis? *Cell*, **58**, 803–5.

39. Mignatti, P., Tsuboi, R., Robbins, E., and Rifkin, D. B. (1989). *In vitro* angiogenesis on the human amniotic membrane: requirement for basic fibroblast growth factor-induced proteinases. *J. Cell Biol.*, **108**, 671–82.

40. Van Hinsbergh, V. W., Kooistra, T., Emeis, J. J., and Koolwijk, P. (1991). Regulation of plasminogen activator production by endothelial cells: role in fibrinolysis and local proteolysis. *Int. J. Radiat. Biol.*, **60**, 261–72.

41. Falcone, D. J., McCaffrey, T. A., Haimovilt-Friedman, A., Vergilio, J. A., and Nicholson, A. C. (1993). Macrophage and foam cell release of matrix-bound growth factors. Role of plasminogen activation. *J. Biol. Chem.*, **268**, 11951–8.

42. Adams, D. O. and Hamilton, T. A. (1992). Macrophages as destructive cells in host defence. In *Inflammation: basic principles and clinical correlates*. (ed. J. I. Gallin, I. M. Goldstein, and R. Synderman, pp. 637–62. Raven Press, New York.

43. Gospodarowicz, D. and Ill, C. (1980). Extracellular matrix and control of proliferation of vascular endothelial cells. *J. Clin. Invest.*, **65**, 1351–64.

44. Madri, J. A. and Williams, S. K. (1983). Capillary endothelial cell cultures: phenotypic modulation by matrix components. *J. Cell Biol.* **97**, 153–65.

45. Kubota, Y., Kleinman, H. K., Martin, G. R., and Lawley, T. J. (1988). Role of laminin and basement membrane in the morphological differentiation of human endothelial cells into capillary-like structures. *J. Cell Biol.*, **107**, 1589–98.

46. Montesano, R., Orci, L., and Vassalli, P. (1983). *In vitro* rapid organization of endothelial cells into capillary-like networks is promoted by collagen matrices. *J. Cell Biol.*, **97**, 1648–52.

47. Ingber, D. E. and Folkman, J. (1989). Mechanochemical switching between growth and differentiation during fibroblast growth factor-stimulated angiogenesis *in vitro*: role of extracellular matrix. *J. Cell Biol.*, **109**, 317–30.

48. West, D. C. and Kumar, S. (1989). The effect of hyaluronate and its oligosaccharides on endothelial cell proliferation and monolayer integrity. *Exp. Cell Res.*, **183**, 179–96.

49. Thompson, W. D., Smith, E. B., Strik, C. M., Marshall, F. I., Stout, A. J., and Kocchar, A. (1992). Angiogenic activity of fibrin degradation products is located in fibrin fragment E. *J. Pathol.*, **168**, 47–53.

50. Rogelj, S., Klagsbrun, M., Atzmon, R., Kurokawa, M., Haimovitz, A., Fuks, Z., and Vlodavsky, I. (1989). Basic fibroblast growth factor is an extracellular matrix component required for supporting the proliferation of vascular endothelial cells and the differentiation of PC12 cells. *J. Cell Biol.*, **109**, 823–31.

51. Gordon, M. Y., Riley, G. P., Watt, S. M., and Greaves, M. F. (1987). Compartmentalization of a haematopoietic growth factor (GM-CSF) by glycosaminoglycans in the bone marrow microenvironment. *Nature*, **326**, 403–5.

52. Hori, A., Sasada, R., Matsutani, E., Naito, K., Sakura, Y., Fujita, T., and Kozai, Y. (1991). Suppression of solid tumor growth by immunoneutralizing monoclonal antibody against human basic fibroblast growth factor. *Cancer Res.*, **51**, 6180–4.

53. Schultz-Hector, S. and Haghayegh, S. (1993). Beta-fibroblast growth factor expression in human and murine squamous cell carcinomas and its relationship to regional endothelial cell proliferation. *Cancer Res.*, **53**, 1444–9.

54. Joseph-Silverstein, J., Moscatelli, D., and Rifkin, D. B. (1988). The development of quantitative RIA for basic fibroblast growth factor using polyclonal antibodies against the 157 amino acid form of human bFGF. The identification of bFGF in adherent elicited murine peritoneal macrophages. *J. Immunol. Methods*, **110**, 183–92.

55. Yu, Z-X., Biro, S., Fu, Y-M., Sanchez, J., Smale, G., Sasse, J., *et al.* (1993). Localization of basic fibroblast growth factor in bovine endothelial cells: immuno-histochemical and biochemical studies. *Exp. Cell Res.*, **204**, 247–59.

56. Murphy, P. R., Guo, J. Z., and Friesen, H. G. (1990). Messenger RNA stabilization accounts for elevated basic fibroblast growth factor transcript levels in a human astrocytoma cell line. *Mol. Endocrinol.*, **4**, 196–200.

57. Reeves, R., Elton, T. S., Nissen, M. S., Lehn, D., and Johnson, K. R. (1987). Post-translational gene regulation and specific binding of the non-histone protein HMG-1 by the 3'-untranslated region of bovine interleukin-2 cDNA. *Proc. Natl Acad. Sci. USA*, **84**, 6531–5.

58. Kurokawa, T., Sasada, R., Iwane, M., and Igarashi, K. (1987). Cloning and expression of cDNA encoding human basic fibroblast growth factor. *FEBS Lett.*, **213**, 189–94.

59. Volk, R., Köster, M., Pöting, A., Hartmann, L., and Knöchel, W. (1989). An antisense transcript from the *Xenopus laevis* bFGF gene coding for an evolutionary conserved 24 kd protein. *EMBO J.*, **8**, 2983–8.

60. Bouche, G., Gas, N., Prats, H., Baldwin, V., Tauber, J-P., Teissie, J., and Amalric, F. (1987). Basic fibroblast growth factor enters the nucleolus and stimulates the transcription

of ribosomal genes in ABAE cell undergoing G_0 to G_1 transition. *Proc. Natl Acad. Sci. USA*, **84**, 6770–4.

61. Statuto, M., Ennas, M. G., Zanboni, G., Bonnetti, F., Pea, M., Bernardello, F., *et al.* (1993). Basic fibroblast growth factor in human phaeochromocytoma: a bifunctional and immunohistochemical study. *Int. J. Cancer*, **53**, 5–10.

62. Bobik, A. and Campbell, J. H. (1993). Vascular-derived growth factors: cell biology, pathophysiology and pharmacology. *Pharmacol. Rev.*, **45**, 1–42.

63. Hanneken, A., Maher, P. A., and Baird, A. (1995). High affinity immunoreactive FGF receptors in the extracellular matrix of vascular endothelial cells — implications for the modulation of FGF-2. *J. Cell Biol.*, **128**, 1221–8.

64. Wu, D. Q., Kan, M. K., Sato, G. H., Okamoto, T., and Sato, J. D. (1991). Characterization and molecular cloning of a putative binding protein for heparin-binding growth factors. *J. Biol. Chem.*, **266**, 16778–85.

65. Shi, E., Kan, M., Xu, J., Wang, F., Hou, J., and McKeehan, W. L. (1993). Control of fibroblast growth factor receptor kinase signal transduction by heterodimerization of combinatorial splice variants. *Mol. Cell. Biol.*, **13**, 3907–18.

66. Givol, D. and Yayon, A. (1992). Complexity of FGF receptors: genetic basis for structural diversity and functional specificity. *FASEB J.*, **6**, 3362–9.

67. Cheon, H. G., La Rochelle, W. J., Bottaro, D. P., Burgess, W. H., and Aaronson, S. A. (1994). High affinity binding sites for related fibroblast growth factor ligands reside within different receptor immunoglobulin-like domains. *Proc. Natl Acad. Sci. USA*, **91**, 989–93.

68. Brogi, E., Winkles, J. A., Underwood, R., Clinton, S. K., Alberts, G. F., and Libby, P. (1993). Distinct patterns of expression of fibroblast growth factors and their receptors in human atheroma and nonatherosclerotic arteries. *J. Clin. Invest.*, **92**, 2408–18.

69. Zhao, X-M., First, W. H., Yeoh, T-K., and Miller, G. G. (1994). Modification of alternative messenger RNA splicing of fibroblast growth factor receptors in human cardiac allografts during rejection. *J. Clin. Invest.*, **94**, 992–1003.

70. Klagsbrun, M. (1992). Mediators of angiogenesis: the biological significance of basic fibroblast growth factors (bFGF)-heparin and heparan sulfate interactions. *Cancer Biol.*, **3**, 81–7.

71. Yayon, A., Klagsbrun, M., Esko, J., Leder, P., and Ornitz, D. (1991). Cell surface, heparin-like molecules are required for the binding of basic fibroblast growth factor to its high affinity receptor. *Cell*, **64**, 841–8.

72. Li, L-Y., Safran, M., Aviezer, D., Böhlen, P., Seddon, A. P., and Yayon, A. (1994). Diminished heparin binding of a basic fibroblast growth factor mutant is associated with reduced receptor binding, mitogenesis, plasminogen activator induction and *in vitro* angiogenesis. *Biochemistry*, **33**, 10999–1007.

73. Mummery, C. L., van Rooyen, M., Bracke, M., van den Eijnden-van Raaij, J., van Zoelen, E. J., and Alitalo, K. (1993). Fibroblast growth factor-mediated growth regulation and receptor expression in embryonal carcinoma and embryonic stem cells and human germ cell tumours. *Biochem. Biophys. Res. Commun.*, **191**, 188–95.

74. Saltis, J., Thomas, A., Agrotis, A., Campbell, J. H., Campbell, G. R., and Bobik, A. (1995). Expression of growth factor receptors in arterial smooth muscle cells. Dependency on cell phenotype and serum factors. *Atherosclerosis*, **118**, 77–87.

75. Norioka, K., Mitaka, T., Mochizuki, Y., Hara, M., Kawagoe, M., and Nakamura, H. (1994). Interaction of interleukin-1 and interferon-γ on fibroblast growth factor-induced angiogenesis. *Jpn. J. Cancer Res.*, **85**, 522–9.

76. Bacharach, E., Itin, A., and Keshet, E. (1992). *In vivo* patterns of expression of urokinase and its inhibitor PAI-1 suggest a concerted role in regulating physiological angiogenesis. *Proc. Natl Acad. Sci. USA*, **89**, 10686–90.

77. Leek, R. D., Harris, A. L., and Lewis, C. E. (1994). Cytokine networks in solid human tumours: regulation of angiogenesis. *J. Leukocyte Biol.*, **56**, 423–35.

78. Arrick, B. A., Korc, M., and Derynck, R. (1990). Differential regulation of expression of three transforming growth factor-β species in human breast cancer cell lines by estradiol. *Cancer Res.*, **50**, 299–303.

79. Shah, M., Foreman, D. M., and Ferguson, M. W. J. (1995). Neutralization of TGF-β_1 and TGF-β_2 or exogenous addition of TGF-β_3 to cutaneous rat wounds reduces scarring. *J. Cell Sci.*, **108**, 985–1002.

80. Kim, S-J., Park, K., Rudkin, B. B., Dey, B. R., Sporn, M. B., and Roberts, A. B. (1994). Nerve growth factor induces transcription of transforming growth factor-β_1 through a specific promoter element in PC12 cells. *J. Biol. Chem.*, **269**, 3739–44.

81. Agrotis, A., Saltis, J., and Bobik, A. (1994). Transforming growth factor-β_1 gene activation and growth of smooth muscle cells from hypertensive rats. *Hypertension.*, **23**, 593–9.

82. Kim, S-J., Lee, H-D., Robbins, P. D., Busam, K., Sporn, M. B., and Roberts, A. B. (1991). Regulation of transforming growth factor-β_1 gene expression by the product of the retinoblastoma-susceptibility gene. *Proc. Natl Acad. Sci. USA*, **88**, 3052–6.

83. Lafyatis, R., Lechleider, R., Kim, S-J., Jakowlew, S., Roberts, A. B., and Sporn, M. B. (1990). Structural and functional characterization of the transforming growth factor-β_3 promoter: a cAMP-responsive element regulates basal and induced transcription. *J. Biol. Chem.*, **265**, 19128–36.

84. Bang, Y-J., Kim, S-J., and Danielpour, D. (1992). Cyclic AMP induces transforming growth factor β_2 gene expression and growth arrest in the human androgen-independent prostatic carcinoma cell line PC-3. *Proc. Natl Acad. Sci. USA*, **89**, 3556–60.

85. Malek, A. M., Gibbons, G. H., Dzau, V. J., and Izumo, S. (1993). Fluid shear-stress differentially modulates expression of genes encoding basic fibroblast growth factor and platelet-derived growth factor B-chain in vascular endothelium. *J. Clin. Invest.*, **92**, 2013–21.

86. Ohno, M., Cooke, J. P., and Gibbons, G. H. (1993). Shear-stress-induced TGF-β_1 gene transcription via a flow-activated potassium channel. *Circulation*, **88**, I-183.

87. Gentry, L. E., Webb, N. R., and Lim, G. J. (1987). Type I transforming growth factor beta: amplified expression and secretion of mature and precursor polypeptides in Chinese hamster ovary cells. *Mol. Cell. Biol.*, **7**, 3418–27.

88. Sato, Y. and Rifkin, D. B. (1989). Inhibition of endothelial cell movement by pericytes and smooth muscle cells: activation of a latent transforming growth factor-β1-like molecule by plasmin during co-culture. *J. Cell Biol.*, **109**, 309–15.

89. Schultz-Cherry, S. and Murphy-Ullrich, J. E. (1993). Thrombospondin causes activation of latent transforming

growth factor-β secreted by endothelial cells by a novel mechanism. *J. Cell Biol.*, **122**, 923–32.

90. Penttinen, R. P., Kobayashi, S., and Bornstein, P. (1988). Transforming growth factor-β increases mRNA for matrix proteins both in the presence and in the absence of changes in mRNA stability. *Proc. Natl Acad. Sci. USA*, **85**, 1105–8.

91. Canfield, A. E. and Schor, A. M. (1995). Evidence that tenascin and thrombospondin-1 modulate sprouting of endothelial cells. *J. Cell Sci.*, **108**, 797–809.

92. Madri, J. A., Pratt, B. M., and Tucker, A. M. (1988). Phenotypic modulation of endothelial cells by transforming growth factor-β depends upon the composition and organization of the extracellular matrix. *J. Cell Biol.*, **106**, 1375–84.

93. Iruela-Arispe, M. L. and Sage, E. H. (1993). Endothelial cells exhibiting angiogenesis *in vitro* proliferate in response to TGF-β$_1$. *J. Cell Biochem.*, **52**, 414–30.

94. Yang, E. Y. and Moses, H. L. (1990). Transforming growth factor-β$_1$-induced changes in cell migration, proliferation and angiogenesis in the chicken chorioallantoic membrane. *J. Cell Biol.*, **111**, 731–41.

95. Pepper, M. S., Belin, D., Montesano, R., Orci, L., and Vassalli, J-D. (1990). Transforming growth factor-beta 1 modulates basic fibroblast growth factor-induced proteolytic and angiogenic properties of endothelial cells *in vitro*. *J. Cell Biol.*, **111**, 743–55.

96. Pepper, M. S., Vassalli, J-D., Orci, L., Montesano, R. (1993). Biphasic effect of transforming growth factor-β1 on *in vitro* angiogenesis. *Exp. Cell Res.*, **204**, 356–63.

97. McCartney-Francis, N., Mizel, D., Wong, H., Wahl, L., and Wahl, S. (1990). TGF-β regulates production of growth factors and TGF-β by human peripheral blood monocytes. *Growth Factors*, **4**, 27–35.

98. Wiseman, D. M., Polverini, P. J., Kamp, D. W., and Leibovich, S. J. (1988). Transforming growth factor-beta (TGF-β) is chemotactic for human monocytes and induces their expression of angiogenic activity. *Biochem. Biophys. Res. Commun.*, **157**, 793–800.

99. Slivka, S. R. and Loskutoff, D. (1991). Platelets stimulate endothelial cells to synthesize plasminogen activator inhibitor. Evaluation of the role of transforming growth factor-beta. *Blood*, **77**, 1013–19.

100. Quaglino, D., Nanney, L. B., Kennedy, R., and Davidson, J. M. (1990). Transforming growth factor-β stimulates wound healing and modulates extracellular matrix gene expression in pig skin. *Lab. Invest.*, **63**, 307–19.

101. Nugent, M. A. and Edelman, E. R. (1992). Transforming growth factor-β$_1$ stimulates the production of basic fibroblast growth factor binding proteoglycans in balb/c373 cells. *J. Biol. Chem.*, **267**, 21256–64.

102. Myoken, Y., Kan, M., Sato, G. H., McKeehan, W. L., and Sato, J. D. (1990). Bifunctional effects of transforming growth factor-β (TGF-β) on endothelial cell growth correlate with phenotypes of TGF-β binding sites. *Exp. Cell Res.*, **191**, 299–304.

103. Massagué, J. (1990). The transforming growth factor-β family. *Annu. Rev. Cell Biol.*, **6**, 597–641.

104. Massagué, J., Attisano, L., and Wrana, J. L. (1994). The TGF-β family and its composite receptors. *Trends Cell Biol.*, **4**, 172–8.

105. Kingsley, D. M. (1994). The TGF-β superfamily: new members, new receptors and new genetic tests of function in different organisms. *Genes Dev.*, **8**, 133–46.

106. Pepper, M. S., Vassalli, J-D., Orci, L., and Montesano, R. (1993). Biphasic effect of transforming growth factor-β$_1$ on *in vitro* angiogenesis. *Exp. Cell Res.*, **204**, 356–63.

107. Lin, H. Y. and Moustakas, A. (1994). TGF-β receptors: structure and function. *Cell Mol. Biol.*, **40**, 337–49.

108. Wrana, J. L., Attisano, L., Wieser, R., Ventura, F., and Massagué, J. (1994). Mechanisms of activation of the TGF-β receptor. *Nature*, **370**, 341–7.

109. Ebner, R., Chen, R-H., Shum, L., Lawler, S., Zioncheck, T. F., Lee, A., *et al.* (1993). Cloning of a type I TGF-β receptor and its effects on TGF-β binding to the type II receptor. *Science*, **260**, 1344–8.

110. Miettinen, P. J., Ebner, R., Lopez, A. R., and Derynck, R. (1994). TGF-beta induced transdifferentiation of mammary epithelial cells to mesenchymal cells: involvement of type I receptors. *J. Cell Biol.*, **127**, 2021–36.

111. Xu, J., Matsuzaki, K., McKeehan, K., Wang, F., Kan, M., and McKeehan, W. L. (1994). Genomic structure and cloned cDNAs predict that four variants in the kinase domain of serine/threonine kinase receptors arise by alternative splicing and poly(A) addition. *Proc. Natl Acad. Sci. USA*, **91**, 7957–61.

112. Shweiki, D., Itin, A., Neufeld, G., Gitay-Goren, H., and Keshet, E. (1993). Patterns of expression of vascular endothelial growth factor (VEGF) and VEGF receptors in mice suggest a role in hormonally regulated angiogenesis. *J. Clin. Invest.*, **91**, 2235–43.

113. Millauer, B., Wizigmann-Voos, S., Schnürch, H., Martinez, R., Møller, N. P., Risau, W., and Ullrich, A. (1993). High affinity VEGF binding and developmental expression suggest Flk-1 as a major regulator of vasculogenesis and angiogenesis. *Cell*, **72**, 835–46.

114. Strugar, J., Rothbart, D., Herrington, W., and Criscuolo, G. R. (1994). Vascular permeability factor in brain metastasis: correlation with vasogenic brain edema and tumor angiogenesis. *J. Neurosurg.*, **81**, 560–6.

115. Toi, M., Hoshina, S., Takayanagi, T., and Tominaga, T. (1994). Association of vascular endothelial growth factor expression with tumor angiogenesis and with early relapse in primary breast cancer. *Jpn. J. Cancer. Res.*, **85**, 1045–9.

116. Brown, L. F., Berse, B., Jackman, R. W., Tognazzi, K., Manseau, E. J., Senger, D. R., and Dvorak, H. F. (1993). Expression of vascular permeability factor (vascular endothelial factor) and its receptors in adenocarcinomas of the gastrointestinal final tract. *Cancer Res.*, **53**, 4727–35.

117. Berse, B., Brown, L. F., Van de Water, L., Dvorak, H. F., and Senger, D. R. (1992). Vascular permeability factor (vascular endothelial growth factor) gene is expressed differentially in normal tissues, macrophages and tumors. *Mol. Biol. Cell*, **3**, 211–20.

118. Senger, D. R., Van de Water, L., Brown, L. F., Nagy, J. A., Yeo, K-T., Yeo, T-K., *et al.* (1993). Vascular permeability factor (VPF, VEGF) in tumor biology. *Cancer Metastasis Rev.*, **12**, 303–24.

119. Brown, L. F., Yeo, K-T., Berse, B., Yeo, T-K., Senger, D. R., Dvorak, H. F., and Van de Water, L. (1992). Expression of vascular permeability factor (vascular endothelial growth factor) by epidermal keratinocytes during wound healing. *J. Exp. Med.*, **176**, 1375–9.

120. Yeo, K-T., Wang, H. H., Nagy, J. A., Sioussat, T. M., Ledbetter, S. R., Hoogewerf, A. J., *et al.* (1993). Vascular permeability factor (vascular endothelial growth factor) in

guinea pig and human tumor and inflammatory effusions. *Cancer Res.*, **53**, 2912–8.

121. Ferrara, N., Houck, K., Jakeman, L., and Leung, D. W. (1992). Molecular and biological properties of the vascular endothelial growth factor family of proteins. *Endocr. Rev.*, **13**, 18–32.

122. Tischer, E., Mitchell, R., Hartman, T., Silva, M., Godspodarowicz, D., Fiddes, J. C., and Abraham, J. A. (1991). The human gene for vascular endothelial growth factor. Multiple protein forms are encoded through alternative exon splicing. *J. Biol. Chem.*, **266**, 26031–7.

123. Dvorak, H. F., Sioussat, T. M., Brown, L. F., Berse, B., Nagy, J. A., Sotrel, A., *et al.* (1991). Distribution of vascular permeability factor (vascular endothelial growth factor) in tumors: concentration in tumor blood cells. *J. Exp. Med.*, **174**, 1275–8.

124. Houck, K. A., Leung, D. W., Rowland, A. M., Winer, J., and Ferrara, N. (1992). Dual regulation of vascular endothelial growth factor bioavailability by genetic and proteolytic mechanism. *J. Biol. Chem.*, **267**, 26031–7.

125. Kim, S-J., Angel, P., Lafyatis, R., Hattori, K., Kim, K-Y., Sporn, M. B., *et al.* (1990). Autoinduction of TGF-β_1 is mediated by the AP-1 complex. *Mol. Cell. Biol.*, **10**, 1492–7.

126. Pepper, M. S., Ferrara, N., Orci, L., and Montesano, R. (1992). Potent synergism between vascular endothelial growth factor and basic fibroblast growth factor in the induction of angiogenesis *in vitro*. *Biochem. Biophys. Res. Commun.*, **189**, 824–31.

127. Lanir, N., Ciano, P. S., Van de Water, L., McDonagh, J., Dvorak, A. M., and Dvorak, H. F. (1988). Macrophage migration in fibrin gel matrices. II. Effects of clotting factor XIII, fibronectin and glycosaminoglycan content in cell migration. *J. Immunol.*, **140**, 2340–9.

128. Clauss, M., Gerloch, M., Gerloch, H., Brett, J., Wang, F., Familletti, P. C., *et al.* (1990). Vascular permeability factor: a tumor-derived polypeptide that induces endothelial cell and monocyte procoagulant activity and promotes monocyte migration. *J. Exp. Med.*, **172**, 1535–45.

129. Millauer, B., Wizigmann-Voos, S., Schnürch, H., Martinez, R., Møller, N. P., Risau, W., and Ullrich, A. (1993). High affinity VEGF binding and developmental expression suggest Flk-1 as a major regulatory of vasculogenesis and angiogenesis. *Cell*, **72**, 835–46.

130. Millauer, B., Shawver, L. K., Plate, K. H., Risau, W., and Ullrich, A. (1994). Glioblastoma growth inhibited *in vivo* by a dominant-negative Flk-1 mutant. *Nature*, **367**, 576–9.

131. Sherry, B. and Cerami, A. (1988). Cachectin/tumor necrosis factor exerts endocrine, paracrine, and autocrine control of inflammatory responses. *J. Cell Biol.*, **107**, 1269–77.

132. Scannell, G., Waxman, K., Kaml, G. J., Ioli, G., Gatanaga, T., Yamamoto, R., and Granger, G. A. (1993). Hypoxia induced in human macrophage cell line to release tumor necrosis factor-α and its soluble receptor. *J. Surg. Res.*, **54**, 281–5.

133. Leibovich, S. J., Polverini, P. J., Shepard, H. M., Wiseman, D. M., Shively, V., and Nuseir, N. (1989). Macrophage-induced angiogenesis is mediated by TNF-α. *Nature*, **329**, 630–2.

134. Frater-Schroder, M. F., Risau, W., Hallmann, R., Gautschi, P., and Bohlen, P. (1987). Tumor necrosis factor-α, a potent inhibitor of endothelial cell growth *in vitro*, is angiogenic *in vivo*. *Proc. Natl Acad. Sci. USA*, **84**, 5277–81.

135. Gatanaga, T., Hwang, C., Kohr, W., Cappuccini, F., Lucci, J. A., Jeffes, E. W., *et al.* (1990). Purification and characterization of an inhibitor (soluble tumor necrosis factor receptor) for tumor necrosis factor and lymphotoxin obtained from the serum ultrafiltrates of human cancer patients. *Proc. Natl Acad. Sci. USA*, **87**, 8781–4.

136. van Hinsbergh, V. W., van der Berg, E. A., Fiers, W., and Dooijewaard, G. (1990). Tumor necrosis factor induces the production of urokinase-type plasminogen activator by human endothelial cells. *Blood*, **75**, 1991–8.

137. Niedbala, M. J. and Picarella, M. S. (1992). Tumor necrosis factor induction of endothelial cell urokinase-type plasminogen activator-mediated proteolysis of extracellular matrix and its antagonism by gamma interferon. *Blood*, **79**, 678–87.

138. Okamura, K., Sato, Y., Matsudi, T., Haeanaka, R., Ono, M., Kohno, K., and Kuwano, M. (1991). Endogenous basic fibroblast growth factor-dependent induction of collagenase and interleukin-6 in tumor necrosis factor-treated human microvascular endothelial cells. *J. Biol. Chem.*, **266**, 19162–5.

139. Schweigerer, L., Malerstein, B., and Gospodarowicz, D. (1987). Tumor necrosis factor inhibits the proliferation of cultured capillary endothelial cells. *Biochem. Biophys. Res. Commun.*, **143**, 997–1004.

140. Holzman, L. B., Marks, R. M., and Dixit, V. M. (1990). A novel immediate-early response gene of endothelium is induced by cytokines and encodes a secreted protein. *Mol. Cell. Biol.*, **10**, 5830–8.

141. Pandey, A., Shao, H., Marks, R. M., Polverini, P. J., and Dixit, V. M. (1995). Role of B61, the ligand for the Eck receptor tyrosine kinase in TNF-α-induced angiogenesis. *Science*, **268**, 567–9.

142. Shao, H., Pandy, A., O'Shea, K. S., Seldin, M., and Dixit, V. M. (1995). Characterization of B61, the ligand for the Eck receptor protein-tyrosine kinase. *J. Biol. Chem.*, **270**, 5636–41.

143. Fajardo, L. F., Kwan, H. H., Kowalski, J., Prionas, S. D., and Allison, A. C. (1992). Dual role of tumor necrosis factor-alpha in angiogenesis. *Am. J. Pathol.*, **140**, 539–44.

144. Montrucchio, G., Lupia, E., Battaglia, E., Passerini, G., Bussolino, F., Emanuelli, G., and Camussi, G. (1994). Tumor necrosis factor alpha-induced angiogenesis depends on *in situ* platelet activating factor biosynthesis. *J. Exp. Med.*, **180**, 377–82.

145. Shingu, M., Nobunaga, M., Ezaki, I., and Yoshioka, K. (1991). Recombinant human IL-1 and TNF-α stimulate production of IL-1α and IL-1β by vascular smooth muscle and IL-1α by vascular endothelial cells. *Life Sci.*, **49**, 241–6.

146. Muthukkaruppan, V. R. and Auerbach, R. (1979). Angiogenesis in the mouse cornea. *Science*, **205**, 1416–8.

147. Montesano, R. L., Orci, L., and Vassalli, P. (1995). Human endothelial cell cultures: phenotypic modulation by interleukins. *J. Cell Biol.*, **122**, 424–34.

148. Broudy, V. C., Kaushansky, K., Harlan, J. M., and Adamson, J. W. (1988). Interleukin-1 stimulates human endothelial cells to produce granulocyte–macrophage colony-stimulating factor and granulocyte colony-stimulating factor. *J. Immunol.*, **139**, 464–8.

149. Strieter, R. M., Kunkel, S. L., Showell, H. J., Remick, D. G., Phan, S. H., Ward, P. A., and Marks, R. M. (1989).

Endothelial cell gene expression of a neutrophil chemotactic factor by TNF-α, LPS and IL-1α. *Science*, **243**, 1467–9.

150. Bussolino, F., Ziche, M., Wang, J. M., Alessi, D., Morbidelli, L., Cremona, O., *et al.* (1991). *In vitro* and *in vivo* activation of endothelial cells by colony-stimulating factors. *J. Clin. Invest.*, **87**, 986–95.

151. Li, J., Perrella, M. A., Tsai, J-C., Yet, S-F., Hsieh, C-M., Yoshizum, M., *et al.* (1995). Induction of vascular endothelial growth factor gene expression by interleukin-1β in rat aortic smooth muscle cells. *J. Biol. Chem.*, **270**, 308–12.

152. Benezra, D., Hemo, I., and Maftzir, G. (1990). *In vivo* angiogenic activity of interleukins. *Arch. Ophthalmol.*, **108**, 573–6.

153. Cozzolino, F., Torcia, M., Aldinucci, D., Ziche, M., Almerigogna, F., Bani, D., and Stern, D. M. (1990). Interleukin-1 is an autocrine regulator of human endothelial cell growth. *Proc. Natl Acad. Sci. USA*, **87**, 6487–91.

154. Norioka, K., Hara, M., Kitani, A., Hirose, T., Hirose, W., Harigai, M., *et al.* (1987). Inhibitory effect of human recombinant interleukin-1α and -1β on growth of human vascular endothelial cells. *Biochem. Biophys. Res. Commun.*, **145**, 969–75.

155. Fan, T-P., Hu, D-E., Guard, S., Gresham, A., and Watling, K. J. (1993). Stimulation of angiogenesis by substance P and interleukin-1 in the rat and its inhibition by NK₁ or interleukin-1 receptor antagonist. *Br. J. Pharmacol.*, **110**, 43–9.

156. Hotta, K., Hayashi, K., Ishikawa, J., Tagawa, M., Hashimoto, K., Mizuno, S., and Suzuki, K. (1990). Coding region structure of interleukin-8 gene of human lung giant cell carcinoma LU65C cells that produce LUCT/interleukin-8 homogeneity in interleukin-8 genes. *Immunol. Lett.*, **24**, 165–9.

157. Van Meir, E., Ceska, M., Effenberger, F., Walz, A., Grouzmann, E., Desbaillets, I., *et al.* (1992). Interleukin-8 is produced in neoplastic and infectious diseases of the human control nervous system. *Cancer Res.*, **52**, 4297–305.

158. Matsushima, K., Morishita, K., Yoshimura, T., Lavu, S., Kobayashi, Y., Lew, W., *et al.* (1988). Molecular cloning of a human monocyte-derived neutrophil chemotactic factor (MDNCF) and the induction of MDCNF mRNA by interleukin-1 and tumour necrosis factor. *J. Exp. Med.*, **167**, 1883–93.

159. Bazzoni, F., Cassatella, M. A., Rossi, F., Ceska, M., Dewald, B., and Baggiolini, M. (1991). Phagocytosing neutrophils produce and release high amounts of the neutrophil-activating peptide-1/interleukin-8. *J. Exp. Med.*, **173**, 771–4.

160. Gregory, H., Young, J., Schroder, J. M., Mrowetz, U., and Christophers, E. (1988). Structure determination of a human lymphocyte derived neutrophil activating peptide. *Biochem. Biophys. Res. Commun.*, **151**, 883–90.

161. Koch, A. E., Polverini, P. J., Kunkel, S. L., Harlow, L. A., Di Pietro, L. A., Elner, V. M., *et al.* (1992). Interleukin-8 as a macrophage-derived mediator of angiogenesis. *Science*, **258**, 1799–801.

162. Strieter, R. M., Kunkel, S. L., Elner, V. M., Martonyi, C. L., Koch, A. E., Polverini, P. J., and Elner, S. G. (1992). Interleukin-8. A corneal factor that induces neovascularization. *Am. J. Pathol.*, **141**, 1279–84.

163. Hu, D. E. K., Hori, Y., and Fan, T. P. (1993). Interleukin-8 stimulates angiogenesis in rats. *Inflammation*, **17**, 135–43.

164. Schonbeck, U., Brandt, E., Petersen, F., Flad, H. D., and Loppnow, H. (1995). IL-8 specifically binds to endothelial but not to smooth muscle cells. *J. Immunol.*, **154**, 2375–83.

165. Smith, D. R., Polverini, P. J., Kunkel, S. L. Orringer, M. B., Whyte, R. I., Burdick, M. D., *et al.* (1994). Inhibition of interleukin-8 attenuates angiogenesis in bronchogenic carcinoma. *J. Exp. Med.*, **179**, 1409–15.

166. Madtes, D. K., Raines, E. W., Sakariassen, K. S., Assoian, R. K., Sporn, M. B., Bell, G. I., and Ross, R. (1988). Induction of transforming growth factor-α in activated human alveolar macrophages. *Cell*, **53**, 285–93.

167. Rappolee, D. A., Mark, D., Banda, M. J., and Werb, Z. (1988). Wound macrophages express TGF-α and other growth factors *in vivo*: analysis by mRNA phenotyping. *Science*, **241**, 708–12.

168. Sato, Y., Okamura, K., Morimoto, A., Hamanaka, R., Hamaguchi, K., Shimoda, T., *et al.* (1993). Indispensable role of tissue-type plasminogen activator in growth factor-dependent tube formation of human microvascular endothelial cells *in vitro*. *Exp. Cell Res.*, **204**, 223–9.

169. Delli Bovi, P., Curatola, A. M., Kern, F. G., Greco, A., Ittman, M., and Basililco, C. (1987). An oncogene isolated by transfection of Kaposi's sarcoma DNA encodes a growth factor that is a member of the FGF family. *Cell*, **50**, 729–37.

170. Taira, M., Yoshida, T., Miyagawa, K., Sakamoto, H., Terada, M., and Sugimura, T. (1987). cDNA sequence of human transforming gene hst and identification of the coding sequence required for transforming activity. *Proc. Natl Acad. Sci. USA*, **84**, 2980–4.

171. Yoshida, T., Miyagawa, K., Odagiri, H., Sakamoto, H., Little, P. F., Terada, M., and Sugimura, T. (1987). Transforming gene encoding a protein homologous to fibroblast growth factors and the int-2-encoded protein. *Proc. Natl Acad. Sci. USA*, **84**, 7305–9.

172. Zhan, X., Bates, B., Hu, X., and Goldfarb, M. (1988). The human FGF-5 oncogene encodes a novel protein related to fibroblast growth factors. *Mol. Cell. Biol.*, **8**, 3487–97.

173. Matsuzaki, K., Yoshitake, Y., Matuo, Y., Sasaki, H., and Nishikawa, K. (1989). Monoclonal antibodies against heparin-binding growth factor II/basic fibroblast growth factor that blocks its biological activity: invalidity of the antibodies for tumour angiogenesis. *Proc. Natl Acad. Sci. USA*, **86**, 9911–5.

174. Bikfalvi, A., Klein, S., Pintucci, G., Quatro, N., Mignatti, P., and Rifkin, D. (1995). Differential modulation of cell phenotype by different molecular weight forms of basic fibroblast growth factor: possible intracellular signalling by the high molecular weight forms. *J. Cell Biol.*, **129**, 233–43.

175. Gajdusek, C. M., Luo, Z., and Mayberg, M. R. (1993). Basic fibroblast growth factor and transforming growth factor-beta 1: synergistic mediators of angiogenesis *in vitro*. *J. Cell Biol.*, **157**, 133–44.

176. Blood, C. H. and Zetter, B. R. (1990). Tumor interactions with the vasculature: angiogenesis and tumor metastasis. *Biochim. Biophys. Acta*, **1032**, 89–118.

177. Chang, N-S. (1995). Transforming growth factor-β₁ induction of novel extracellular matrix proteins that trigger resistance to tumor necrosis factor cytotoxicity in murine L929 fibroblasts. *J. Biol. Chem.*, **270**, 7765–72.

16. The role of vascular endothelial growth factor in the regulation of blood vessel growth

Napoleone Ferrara

Introduction

The development of a vascular supply is a fundamental requirement for organ development and differentiation in multicellular organisms (1). Blood vessel formation is also necessary for tissue repair and reproductive functions in the adult (2,3). Substantial experimental evidence also indicates that neovascularization (angiogenesis) plays an important part in the pathogenesis of a variety of disorders. These include: proliferative retinopathies, age-related macular degeneration, tumours, rheumatoid arthritis, psoriasis, etc. (2,4). In the case of proliferative retinopathies and age-related macular degeneration, the new blood vessels are directly responsible for many of the destructive events characteristic of these conditions, as leakage and bleeding, followed by organization of the clot and fibrosis, may ultimately lead to retinal detachment or irreversible damage to the macula (5). Conversely, in neoplasms the role of the neovascularization consists in providing nourishment to the growing tumour, thus allowing the tumour cells to express their critical growth advantage, and permitting the establishment of continuity with the vasculature of the host (4). Therefore, one would anticipate the existence of a correlation between aggressive behaviour and vascularity in tumours. Accordingly, a strong correlation has been noted between density of microvessels in primary breast carcinoma sections and nodal metastases and survival (6–9). Similarly, a correlation has been reported between vascularity and invasive behaviour in bladder (10), prostate (11,12) non-small cell lung (13), and uterine cervix (14) carcinomas and in cutaneous melanomas (15). Furthermore, recent studies have shown a statistically significant increase in microvessel count in severe uterine cervix dysplasia (CIN III) as compared with low-grade lesions (CIN I) (16). Therefore, the number of vessels in tumour sections, which reflects the extent of angiogenesis, may be considered as an important independent predictor of outcome in breast cancer and, possibly, in other malignancies.

Angiogenesis requires at least three steps: (i) degradation of the extracellular matrix (ECM) of a venule, (ii) chemotaxis of endothelial cells toward an angiogenic stimulus; and (iii) proliferation of endothelial cells (2,3). A variety of factors have been previously identified as potential positive regulators of angiogenesis: acid fibroblast growth factor (aFGF), basic fibroblast growth factor (bFGF), endothelial growth factor (EGF), transforming growth factor (TGF) α, TGF-β, monobutyrin, human growth factor (HGF), tumour necrosis factor (TNF) α, PD, endothelial cell growth factor (ECGF, angiogenin, and interleukin 8. Some of these factors are able to stimulate directly endothelial cell growth, while others lack direct stimulatory effects on endothelial cells and thus their angiogenic actions are thought to require the paracrine release of direct-acting factors from macrophages or other cells (2,3).

This chapter will review the molecular properties of vascular endothelial growth factor (VEGF), an endothelial cell mitogen and angiogenesis inducer and will discuss the role of this factor in the regulation of normal and pathological angiogenesis. By alternative splicing of mRNA of a single gene, multiple molecular forms of VEGF are generated (17–19). There are several indications that VEGF and its receptors play a major part in the regulation of physiological angiogenesis, such as embryonic (20–23) and reproductive (24–26) angiogenesis. Also, VEGF is sufficient to achieve a therapeutic end-point in animal models of coronary or limb ischaemia (27). Furthermore, recent studies point to VEGF as a crucial mediator of neovascularization associated with tumours and proliferative retinopathies (28,29).

Biological activities of vascular endothelial growth factor

VEGF is a potent mitogen for vascular endothelial cells but it is apparently devoid of appreciable mitogenic activity for other cell types (30–32). Consequently, VEGF has been regarded as an endothelial cell-specific mitogen. VEGF is also able to induce a marked angiogenic response in a variety of *in vivo* models including the chick chorioallantoic membrane (17,31), the rabbit cornea (33), the primate iris (34), the rabbit bone (35), etc. VEGF has been shown to promote angiogenesis in a tridimensional *in vitro* model, inducing confluent microvascular endothelial cells to invade a collagen gel and form tube-like structures (36). Also, VEGF induces sprouting from rat aortic rings cultured in a tridimensional collagen gel (37). This model emphasizes the specificity of the growth factor for endothelial cells, as the proliferation induced by VEGF consisted almost exclus-ively of vascular endothelial cells. In contrast, insulin growth-like factor (IGF)-1- or platelet-derived growth factor (PDGF)-induced endothelial cell sprouting was accompanied by extensive fibroblastic proliferation (37).

Furthermore, VEGF induces expression of the serine proteases urokinase-type (uPA) and tissue-type (tPA) plasminogen activators (PAs) and also PA inhibitor 1 (PAI-1) in cultured bovine microvascular endothelial cells (38). Furthermore, VEGF induces expression of the metalloproteinase interstitial collagenase in human umbilical vein endothelial cells but not in dermal fibroblasts (39). Interstitial collagenase is able to degrade type I and III collagen (40). The co-induction of PAs and collagenase by VEGF is expected to promote a pro-degradative environment that facilitates migration of endothelial cells. The expression of PAI-1 may serve to regulate and balance the process (41). Very recent studies have shown that VEGF induces expression of urokinase receptor in vascular endothelial cells (42). Given the fact that the PA–plasmin system and in particular the interaction of uPA with uPA receptor is an important element in the chain of cellular processes that mediate cellular invasion and tissue remodelling (43,44), these findings are consistent with the known pro-angiogenic activities of VEGF.

VEGF has been independently purified and cloned as a vascular permeability factor (VPF) based on its ability to induce vascular leakage in the guinea-pig skin (45,46). It has been proposed that an increase in microvascular permeability is a crucial step in angiogenesis associated with tumours and wounds (47,48). According to this hypothesis, a major function of VPF/VEGF in the angiogenic process would be inducing plasma protein leakage. This would result in the formation of an extravascular fibrin gel, a substrate for endothelial and tumour cell growth (49,50).

An additional effect of VEGF on the vascular endothelium is the stimulation of hexose transport (51). Exposure of bovine aortic endothelial cells to VEGF or TNF-α resulted in a significant increase in the rate of hexose transport. The combination of factors had an additive effect. It is tempting to speculate that such an effect is important for an increased glucose metabolism in circumstances of increased demand, such as endothelial cell proliferation or inflammation. Furthermore, it has been shown that VEGF induces tissue factor expression in cultured endothelial cells (52). It has been proposed that the induction of such a procoagulant protein (53) may contribute to the abnormal coagulative properties of tumour vessels in response to TNF-α (54).

VEGF has also been shown to induce vasodilatation *in vitro* in a dose-dependent fashion (55), which translates into a transient hypotension *in vivo* (56). Such effects appear to be mediated primarily by endothelial cell-derived nitric oxide, as assessed by the requirement for an intact endothelium and the blocking by *N*-methyl-arginine (55,56).

Recent studies (57) indicate that the mitogenic and the permeability enhancing activity of VEGF can be potentiated by placenta growth factor (PlGF), a molecule having a significant degree of structural homology with VEGF (58,59). While PlGF has little or no direct mitogenic or permeability enhancing activity, it is able to potentiate significantly the activity of low, marginally efficacious, concentrations of VEGF (57). This effect requires a 10–20-fold molar excess of PlGF over VEGF. Therefore, it may be that PlGF serves to enhance the bioactivity of VEGF in situations where the concentrations of the latter are limiting.

The vascular endothelial growth factor gene

cDNA sequence analysis of a variety of human VEGF clones indicated that VEGF may exist as one of four different molecular species, having 121, 165, 189, and 206 amino acids respectively ($VEGF_{121}$, $VEGF_{165}$, $VEGF_{189}$, $VEGF_{206}$ (17–19). $VEGF_{165}$ is the predominant isoform secreted by a variety of normal and transformed cells. Transcripts encoding $VEGF_{121}$ and $VEGF_{189}$ are detected in the majority of cells and tissues expressing the VEGF gene (18). In contrast, $VEGF_{206}$ is a very rare form, so far identified only in a human fetal liver cDNA library (18). Compared with $VEGF_{165}$, $VEGF_{121}$ lacks 44 amino acids; $VEGF_{189}$ has an insertion of 24 amino acids highly enriched in basic residues and $VEGF_{206}$ has an additional insertion of 17 amino acids. Rodent and bovine VEGF isoforms are shorter by one amino acid (17,32). The organization of the human VEGF gene has been elucidated (18,19). It is known that alternative splicing of RNA, rather than transcription of separate genes, is the basis for the molecular heterogeneity evidenced by cDNA sequence analysis (18,19). The human VEGF gene is organized in eight exons and the size of its coding region has been estimated to be approximately 14 kb (19). $VEGF_{165}$ lacks the residues encoded by exon 6, while $VEGF_{121}$ lacks the residues encoded by exons 6 and 7. Interestingly, there is no intron between the coding sequence of the 24 amino acid insertion in VEGF and the additional 17 amino acid insertion found in $VEGF_{206}$. The 5′ end of the 51 base pair insertion of $VEGF_{206}$ begins with GT, the consensus sequence for the 5′-splice donor necessary for mRNA processing. Therefore, the definition of the 5′-splice donor site for removal of a 1 kb intron sequence is variable (18). Analysis of the VEGF gene promoter region reveals a single major transcription start which lies near a cluster of potential Sp1 factor binding sites. Also, several potential binding sites for the transcription factors AP-1 and AP-2 are present in the promoter region (19).

Analysis of the 3′ untranslated region of the rat VEGF mRNA has revealed the presence of four potential polyadenylation sites (60). A frequently used site is about 1.9 kb further downstream from the previously reported transcription termination codon (32). The sequence within this 3′ untranslated region reveals a number of sequence motifs that are known to be involved in the regulation of mRNA stability (60).

Regulation of vascular endothelial growth factor

Several mechanisms have been shown to be involved in the regulation of VEGF gene expression.

Oxygen tension appears to play a major regulatory part, both *in vitro* and *in vivo*. VEGF mRNA expression is rapidly and reversibly induced by exposure to low Po_2 in a variety of cultured cells including retinal pigmented epithelial cells (61), myoblasts (62), cardiomyocytes (63), and tumour cells (62). In sections of glioblastoma multiforme, VEGF mRNA is highly expressed in ischaemic tumour cells that are juxtaposed to areas of necrosis (62,64). Furthermore, occlusion of the left anterior descending coronary artery results in a dramatic increase in VEGF RNA levels in the pig myocardium, suggesting that VEGF is a mediator of the spontaneous revascularization that occurs in the ischaemic myocardium (63).

It has been shown recently that similarities exist between the mechanisms leading to hypoxic regulation of VEGF and erythropoietin (Epo) (65). The expression of both genes is significantly enhanced by cobalt chloride. Also, the hypoxic induction of both VEGF and Epo genes is inhibited by carbon monoxide, suggesting the involve-

ment of a haem protein in the process of sensing oxygen levels (65). Furthermore, hypoxia-inducibility appears to be conferred to both genes by homologous sequences. By deletion and mutation analysis, a 28-base sequence has been identified in the 5′ promoter of the rat VEGF gene which mediated hypoxia-induced transcription in transient assays (60). Such sequence reveals a high degree of homology and similar protein-binding characteristics as the hypoxia-inducible factor 1 (HIF-1) binding site within the Epo gene, which behaves like a classic 3′ transcriptional enhancer (66). HIF-1 has been purified and cloned as a mediator of transcriptional responses to hypoxia (67,68). Intriguingly, VEGF and Epo may be part of the same homeostatic cascade: Epo increases the oxygen-carrying capacity of the blood by stimulating red cell production, while VEGF-induced angiogenesis permits the delivery of oxygen to ischaemic tissues.

It has been shown that accumulation of adenosine, which occurs under hypoxic conditions, is involved in the hypoxic induction of the VEGF gene (69). According to these studies, adenosine, by activating adenosine A_2 receptors, results in elevated cyclic adenosine monophosphate concentrations which in turn increase VEGF mRNA levels, possibly through a protein kinase A mediated pathway. Very recent studies have provided evidence that activation of c-*src* also participates in the hypoxic up-regulation of VEGF gene (70). Hypoxia increases the kinase activity of pp60 [c-]*src* and its phosphorylation on tyrosine 416. Expression of a negative dominant mutant of c-*src* significantly reduced the hypoxic induction of VEGF.

Consistent with the presence of AP-1 and AP-2 sites in the VEGF gene promoter, phorbol esters and forskolin, a potent activator of adenylate cyclase, induce VEGF mRNA expression (71). Accordingly, luteotrophic hormone, a known activator of adenylate cyclase, has been shown to induce expression of VEGF mRNA in cultured bovine ovarian granulosa cells (71).

Several cytokines or growth factors have been shown to up-regulate VEGF mRNA expression and/or induce release of VEGF protein. For example, exposure of quiescent human keratinocytes to serum, EGF, TGF-β, or keratinocyte growth factor resulted in a marked induction of VEGF mRNA expression (72). In addition, treatment of quiescent cultures of several epithelial and fibroblastic cell lines with TGF-β resulted in induction of VEGF mRNA and release of VEGF protein in the medium (73). Based on these findings, it has been proposed that VEGF may function as a paracrine mediator for indirect-acting angiogenic agents such as TGF-β (73). Furthermore, IL-1 β induces VEGF expression in aortic smooth muscle cells (74). In view of the fact that IL-1 is expressed in atherosclerotic plaques, it is possible that IL-1-induced VEGF release accelerates the progression of atherosclerotic lesions by promoting the development of a neovascular supply.

Differentiation also appears to play a pivotal role in the regulation of VEGF gene expression, at least in some models of cellular differentiation (75). The VEGF mRNA was markedly up-regulated during the conversion of 3T3 pre-adipocytes into adipocytes or during the myogenic differentiation of C2C12 cells. Conversely, VEGF gene expression was dramatically suppressed during the differentiation of the pheochromocytoma cell line PC12 into non-malignant, neuron-like, cells. These studies also indicate that induction of VEGF mRNA expression in pre-adipocytes requires pathways mediated by both protein kinase C and protein kinase A activation (75).

Specific transforming events also result in the induction of VEGF gene expression. For example, a mutated form of the murine p53 tumour suppressor gene (ala135> val) has been shown to induce VEGF mRNA expression and potentiate phorbol ester stimulated VEGF mRNA expression in NIH 3T3 cells in transient transfection assays (76). Likewise, oncogenic mutations or amplification of *ras* lead to VEGF up-regulation in transfected cells (77). This effect is blocked by treatment with inhibitors of *ras* farnesyl transferase. Therefore, it is tempting to speculate that VEGF-induced angiogenesis is a final common pathway for multiple and apparently unrelated alterations in cell growth regulatory pathways, leading to uncontrolled proliferation and tumorigenesis.

The vascular endothelial growth factor isoforms

VEGF purified from a variety of species and sources is a basic, heparin-binding, homodimeric glycoprotein of 45 000 daltons (78). VEGF is inactivated by reducing agents, but it is heat-stable and acid-stable. These properties correspond to those of $VEGF_{165}$, the predominant isoform. $VEGF_{121}$ is a weakly acidic polypeptide that fails to bind to heparin (79). $VEGF_{189}$ and $VEGF_{206}$ are more basic and bind to heparin with greater affinity than $VEGF_{165}$ (79). Such differences in the isoelectric point and in affinity for heparin profoundly affect the bioavailability of the VEGF isoforms (79,80). $VEGF_{121}$ is secreted as a freely soluble protein in the conditioned medium of transfected cells. $VEGF_{165}$ is also secreted but a significant fraction remains bound to the cell surface or the ECM. In contrast, $VEGF_{189}$ and $VEGF_{206}$ are almost completely sequestered in the ECM (80). However, they may be released from the bound state by heparin or heparinase suggesting that their binding site is represented by heparin-

containing proteoglycans. Furthermore, the long forms may be released by plasmin (79,80) following cleavage at the COOH terminus. This action generates a bioactive proteolytic fragment having a molecular weight of ~34 000 daltons (80). Recent studies have shown that the bioactive product of plasmin action is comprised of 110 amino acids (81). Plasminogen activation and generation of plasmin have been shown to play an important part in the angiogenesis cascade (43). However, it is possible that this property is not confined to plasmin. It may be that cleavage of VEGF can be brought about by several inflammation-associated proteases. Thus, the VEGF proteins may become available to endothelial cells by at least two different mechanisms: as freely diffusible proteins ($VEGF_{121}$, $VEGF_{165}$) or following protease activation and cleavage of the longer isoforms. Generation of bioactive VEGF by proteolytic cleavage may be especially important in the microenvironment of a tumour where increased expression of proteases, including PAs, is well documented (44,82). However, loss of heparin binding, whether due to alternative splicing or plasmin cleavage, results in a substantial loss of mitogenic activity for vascular endothelial cells (81).

Interestingly, recent studies have demonstrated the existence of naturally occurring heterodimers between $VEGF_{164}$ and PlGF in the conditioned medium of a rat glioma cell line (83). The VEGF.PlGF heterodimer was approximately sevenfold less potent than the VEGF homodimer in promoting endothelial cell growth.

The vascular endothelial growth factors receptors

Two classes of high-affinity VEGF-binding sites have been identified on the cell surface of cultured bovine endothelial cells. The K_d values are 10 pM and 100 pM, respectively (84,85). Lower-affinity binding sites on mononuclear phagocytes (K_d ~300–500 pM) have been also described (86). It has been suggested that such binding sites are involved in mediating chemotactic effects for monocytes by VEGF. Thieme *et al.* (87) have shown that hypoxia increases VEGF receptor number by 50%, without changing the affinity, in cultured bovine retinal capillary endothelial cells.

Ligand autoradiography studies on fetal and adult rat tissue sections revealed that high-affinity VEGF-binding sites are localized to the vascular endothelium of large or small vessels but not to other cell types (21,88). These findings provide direct evidence for the hypothesis that vascular endothelium is the target of VEGF action. Specific binding co-localizes with factor VIII-like immunoreactivity and is apparent on both proliferating and quiescent endothelial cells (21,88).

Two tyrosine kinases have been identified as VEGF receptors (89–92). The Flt-1 (fms-like-tyrosine kinase) (93) and KDR (kinase domain region) (94) proteins have been shown to bind VEGF with high affinity. Flk-1 (fetal liver kinase-1), the murine homologue of KDR, shares 85% sequence identity with human KDR (95). Both Flt-1 and KDR/Flk-1 have seven immunoglobulin (Ig)-like domains in the extracellular domain, a single transmembrane region and a consensus tyrosine kinase sequence which is interrupted by a kinase-insert domain (93–95). An additional member of the family of tyrosine kinases with seven immunoglobulin-like domains in the extracellular portion is Flt-4, which, however, is not a receptor for VEGF (96). Flt-1 has the highest affinity for rh $VEGF_{165}$, with a K_d of approximately 10–20 pM (89). KDR has a somewhat lower affinity for VEGF: the K_d has been estimated to be approximately 75–125 pM (90). In addition, a soluble form of Flt-1, lacking the seventh immunoglobulin-like domain, transmembrane sequence, and the cytoplasmic domain, has been identified in human umbilical vein endothelial cells (97). This soluble Flt-1 receptor is able to inhibit VEGF-induced mitogenesis and has been proposed to be a physiological negative regulator of VEGF action (97).

In situ hybridization studies have revealed that the Flk-1 mRNA is expressed in the vascular endothelium in the mouse embryo (91,92). There is evidence that the Flk-1 mRNA is down-regulated in adult endothelial cells as compared with fetal endothelial cells (91,92). The Flt-1 mRNA is selectively expressed in vascular endothelial cells, both in fetal and adult mouse tissue (98). Similarly to the high-affinity VEGF binding (21,88), the Flt-1 mRNA is expressed in both proliferating and quiescent endothelial cells (98).

The Flt-1 and KDR proteins have been shown to have different signal transduction properties (99). Porcine aortic endothelial cells lacking endogenous VEGF receptors display chemotaxis and mitogenesis in response to VEGF when transfected with an expression vector coding for KDR. In contrast, transfected cells expressing Flt-1 lack such responses (99,100). While Flk-1/KDR undergoes strong ligand-dependent tyrosine phosphorylation in intact cells (91,92), Flt-1 reveals a very weak or undetectable response (89,99,100). Transfection of Flt-1 cDNA in NIH 3T3 led to a weak VEGF-dependent tyrosine phosphorylation but did not generate any mitogenic signal (100). While a weak induction of c-*fos* was observed in such transfected cells in response to VEGF, c-*myc* was not induced (100). These findings are in agreement with other studies showing that PlGF, which binds with high affinity

to Flt-1 but not to Flk-1/KDR, lacks direct mitogenic or permeability-enhancing properties or the ability to stimulate effectively tyrosine phosphorylation in endothelial cells (57). Therefore, it appears that interaction with Flk-1/KDR is a critical requirement to induce the full spectrum of VEGF biological responses. Whether VEGF induces formation of heterodimers between Flt-1 and Flk-1/KDR, which could confer new properties or ligand specificity upon these receptors, remains to be established. Further studies are required to characterize the molecular events involved in VEGF signal transduction.

Very recent studies have demonstrated that both Flt-1 and Flk-1/KDR are essential for normal development of embryonic vasculature, although their respective roles in endothelial cell proliferation and differentiation appear to be distinct (22,23). Mouse embryos homozygous for a targeted mutation in the flt-1 locus died *in utero* at day 8.5 (22). Endothelial cells developed in both embryonic and extra-embryonic sites but failed to organize in normal vascular channels. Mice where the flk-1 gene had been inactivated revealed a more profound deficit, because they lacked vasculogenesis and also failed to develop blood islands (23). Haematopoietic precursors were severely disrupted and organized blood vessels failed to develop throughout the embryo or the yolk sac resulting in death *in utero* between days 8.5 and 9.5. These findings indicate that the VEGF–Flk-1 system is essential not only for vasculogenesis but also for early haematopoiesis. Flt-1 is also essential but its role appears to be primarily in regulating the assembly of endothelial cells into tubes. Future studies will be required to establish the relative contribution of VEGF and the alternative Flt-1 ligand, PlGF, to such regulatory functions mediated by Flt-1.

The role of vascular endothelial growth factors in the regulation of physiological angiogenesis and maintenance of the vascular endothelium

The proliferation of blood vessels is crucial for a wide variety of physiological processes such as embryonic development, normal growth and differentiation, wound healing and reproductive functions. The VEGF mRNA is expressed within the first few days following implantation in the giant cells of the trophoblast (21,101), suggesting a role for VEGF in the induction of vascular growth in the decidua, placenta, and vascular membranes. At later developmental stages in the mouse or rat embryos, the VEGF mRNA is expressed in several organs, including heart, vertebral column, kidney, and along the surface of the spinal cord and brain (21,101). These studies indicate that a variety of cells express the VEGF mRNA. However, there is no evidence that endothelial cells express the VEGF mRNA, suggesting that VEGF is a purely paracrine mediator. In the developing mouse brain, the highest levels of mRNA expression are associated with the choroid plexus and the ventricular epithelium (101). This argues for a spatial relation between VEGF mRNA expression and angiogenesis, as the vascularization of the cerebral cortex in late prenatal and early postnatal ages proceeds from the pial surface toward the ventricular epithelium (102).

In the human fetus (16–22 weeks), VEGF mRNA expression is detectable in virtually all tissues and is most abundant in lung, kidney, and spleen. VEGF protein, as assessed by immunocytochemistry, is expressed in epithelial cells and myocytes, but not vascular endothelial cells (103). Interestingly, VEGF expression is also detectable, both in fetus and in the adult, around microvessels in areas where endothelial cells are quiescent, such as kidney glomerulus, pituitary, heart, lung, and brain (78,103,104). These findings raise the possibility that VEGF is required not only to induce active vascular proliferation but also for the maintenance of the differentiated state of blood vessels, at least in some circumstances (78).

The first evidence supporting the hypothesis that VEGF may be a physiological regulator of angiogenesis was provided by *in situ* hybridization studies on the rat ovary (24). Angiogenesis is a prominent aspect of the cyclical development of the corpus luteum. Following ovulation, vessels from the theca interna invade the ruptured follicle and a complex microvascular network that nourishes the developing corpus luteum (105). The VEGF mRNA was temporally and spatially related to the proliferation of microvessels. Minimal hybridization was detected in the avascular granulosa cells of pre-ovulatory follicles while a strong hybridization signal was present in the corpus luteum where 50–60% of the total cell population is represented by capillary endothelial cells and pericytes. A similar expression pattern has been recently described in the primate ovary (25).

Cultured human keratinocytes express the VEGF mRNA, suggesting the involvement of VEGF in a major pathophysiological process such as wound healing (72). Interestingly, a decreased expression of VEGF mRNA has been observed in the skin of genetically diabetic db/db mice (72). These findings suggest that an altered regulation of VEGF gene expression contributes to defective angiogenesis and impaired wound healing characteristic of this genetic disorder.

The role of vascular endothelial growth factor in pathological angiogenesis

Tumour angiogenesis

Numerous tumour cell lines express the VEGF mRNA and secrete a VEGF-like protein in the medium (106,107). Furthermore, *in situ* hybridization studies have shown that the VEGF mRNA is markedly up-regulated in virtually all human tumours so far examined. These include: kidney and bladder (108,109), breast (110,111), ovary (112), and gastrointestinal tract (113) carcinomas, and several intracranial tumours including glioblastoma multiforme (62,64,114) and sporadic as well as von Hippel–Lindau syndrome-associated capillary haemangioblastoma (115, 116). Only sections of lobular carcinoma of the breast and papillary carcinoma of the bladder failed to reveal significant VEGF mRNA expression (50). In all of these circumstances, the VEGF mRNA is expressed in tumour cells but not in endothelial cells. This is consistent with the hypothesis that VEGF is a purely paracrine mediator (78). Immunohistochemical studies have localized the VEGF protein not only to the tumour cells but also to the vasculature (64,108,113). This localization indicates that tumour-secreted VEGF accumulates in the target cells. A strong correlation exists between degree of vascularization of the malignancy and VEGF mRNA expression (115). In addition, the mRNA for the VEGF receptors, Flt-1 and KDR, is up-regulated in the tumour-associated endothelial cells in comparison with the vasculature of the surrounding tumour-free tissue (64,108,113,117). Recent studies indicate that the VEGF and PlGF mRNAs are co-expressed in renal cell carcinoma, suggesting that, at least in this tumour, the two factors may play a cooperative role in the induction of angiogenesis (109). Interestingly, a correlation has been observed between VEGF expression, as assessed by immunohistochemistry, and microvessel density in primary breast cancer sections (118). Postoperative survey indicated that the relapse-free survival rate of VEGF-rich tumours was significantly worse than that of VEGF-poor, suggesting that expression of VEGF is associated with stimulation of angiogenesis and with early relapse in primary breast cancer (118). In tumours with a significant component of necrosis such as glioblastoma multiforme, VEGF mRNA expression is not uniform but occurs primarily in clusters of tumour cells at the border between viable tumour and necrotic areas (62,64,114). This localization is consistent with local hypoxia being a major inducer of VEGF gene expression and suggests that a VEGF gradient is responsible for angiogenesis and tumour expansion toward ischaemic areas.

These findings provide strong correlative evidence in support of the hypothesis that VEGF-expressing tumour cells may have a growth advantage *in vivo* due to stimulation of angiogenesis. This is consistent with previous studies showing that expression of $VEGF_{165}$ or $VEGF_{121}$ confers on a non-tumorigenic clone of Chinese hamster ovary cells the ability to form vascularized tumours in nude mice (119). However, VEGF expression did not result in a growth advantage *in vitro* for such cells, indicating that their ability to grow *in vivo* was due to paracrine rather than autocrine mechanisms. Expression of $VEGF_{121}$ has been shown to enhance tumour growth and vascular density also in transfected MCF-7 breast carcinoma cells (120).

More direct evidence for a role of VEGF in tumorigenesis has been made possible by the availability of specific monoclonal antibodies capable of inhibiting VEGF-induced angiogenesis *in vivo* and *in vitro* (121). Such antibodies exert a dramatic inhibitory effect on the growth of a variety of human tumour cell lines injected subcutaneously in nude mice, including glioblastoma multiforme, rhabdomyosarcoma, leiomyosarcoma, colon and epidermoid carcinoma (28,117,122). However, the antibodies (or VEGF) have no effect on the *in vitro* growth of the tumour cells. In agreement with the hypothesis that inhibition of angiogenesis is the mechanism of tumour suppression, the density of microvessels was significantly lower in sections of tumours from antibody-treated animals as compared with controls (28,117). Intravital microscopy techniques have recently provided a direct demonstration that anti-VEGF antibodies indeed block tumour angiogenesis (123). Tumour spheroids of A673 rhabdomyosarcoma cells were implanted in dorsal skinfold chambers inserted in nude mice. Non-invasive visualization of the vasculature, 3, 7, 14 days following tumour spheroid implant, revealed a dramatic suppression of tumour angiogenesis in anti-VEGF treated animals as compared with controls, at all time points.

Warren *et al.* (117) have demonstrated that VEGF is a major mediator of the *in vivo* growth of human colon carcinoma cells in a nude mouse model of liver metastasis where the tumour cells are injected in the spleen. Similarly to human tumours, in this murine model the expression of Flk-1 mRNA was markedly up-regulated in the vasculature associated with liver metastases. Treatment with anti-VEGF monoclonal antibodies resulted in a dramatic decrease in the number and size of metastases. Most of the tumours in the treated group were under 1 mm in diameter and all were under 3 mm. Also, neither blood vessels nor Flk-1 mRNA expression could be demonstrated in such metastases. Administration of anti-VEGF antibodies also results in dramatic suppression of both primary growth and metastasis of A431 cells (122).

An independent verification of the hypothesis that VEGF action is necessary for tumorigenesis has been provided by the finding that retrovirus-mediated expression of a negative dominant Flk-1 mutant suppresses the growth of glioblastoma cells *in vivo* (124).

Angiogenesis associated with other disorders

Diabetes mellitus, occlusion of central retinal vein, or prematurity with subsequent exposure to oxygen can all be associated with intraocular vascular proliferation (125,126). Chronic retinal detachment secondary to tumours or other conditions can also result in neovascularization. The new blood vessels may lead to vitreous haemorrhage, retinal detachment, neovascular glaucoma, and eventual blindness (5). Diabetic retinopathy is the leading cause of blindness in the working population (127). All of these conditions are known to be associated with retinal ischaemia (126). As early as in 1948, Michaelson proposed that the ischaemic retina is able to release into the vitreous diffusible angiogenic factor(s) responsible for retinal and iris neovascularization. Even though IGF-1 and bFGF have been implicated in this process, these factors do not show a consistent increase as it would be expected if they played a significant causative role (128,129). VEGF, by virtue of its diffusible nature and hypoxia inducibility, is an attractive candidate as a retina-derived mediator of intraocular neovascularization. Recently, elevations of VEGF levels in the aqueous and vitreous of eyes with proliferative retinopathy have been reported (29,130,131). In a large series where 164 patients and 210 samples of ocular fluid were examined, a strong correlation was found between levels of immunoreactive VEGF in the aqueous and vitreous humors and active proliferative retinopathy (29). VEGF levels were undetectable or very low (<0.5 ng/ml) in the eyes of individuals affected by non-neovascular disorders or diabetes without proliferative retinopathy. In contrast, the VEGF levels were in the range of 3–10 ng/ml in the presence of active proliferative retinopathy associated with diabetes, occlusion of central retinal vein, or prematurity. Remarkably, the VEGF levels were again very low in the eyes of patients with quiescent proliferative retinopathy, a phase of vascular regression that follows the period of active vascular proliferation in diabetic and other retinopathies (29). Thus, although the involvement of other factors cannot be ruled out, VEGF is the molecule that correlates best with ocular angiogenesis (132).

In agreement with the above findings, *in situ* hybridization studies demonstrated up-regulation of VEGF mRNA in the retina of patients with proliferative retinopathies secondary to diabetes, central retinal vein occlusion, retinal detachment, or intraocular tumours (133). Remarkably, VEGF mRNA expression was confined to the specific retinal layer(s) expected to be ischaemic. For example, in chronic retinal detachment secondary to tumours, VEGF mRNA expression was detected in the outer retinal layer (ORL). Unlike the inner layers, which are supplied by retinal capillaries, the ORL derives oxygen by long-range diffusion from the extraretinal choriocapillaris. When the retina is detached, the continuity between the ORL and the retinal pigmented epithelium and underlying choriocapillaris is interrupted, leading to hypoxia in the ORL but not in inner layers. Conversely, in proliferative diabetic retinopathy without retinal detachment or in retinal vein occlusion, VEGF mRNA expression was not evidenced in the ORL but rather in the inner retinal layer or ganglion cell layer or both (133). These findings provide an anatomical verification of the hypothesis that ischaemia, regardless of its aetiology, is the major factor responsible for VEGF mRNA up-regulation in the retina.

More direct evidence for the hypothesis that VEGF is a mediator of intraocular neovascularization has been recently provided in a primate model of iris neovascularization that closely mimics human disease (134) and in a mouse model of retinopathy of prematurity (135). In the primate model, intraocular administration of anti-VEGF antibodies dramatically inhibits the neovascularization that follows occlusion of central retinal veins (136). Likewise, soluble Flt-1 or Flk-1 fused to an IgG suppresses retinal angiogenesis in the mouse model (137). These findings suggest that treatment with inhibitors of VEGF action may prevent the consequences of neovascularization secondary to ischaemic retinal disorders.

It has been also proposed that VEGF is involved in the pathogenesis of another important disease where angiogenesis plays a significant part, rheumatoid arthritis (RA) (138,139). The RA synovium is characterized by the formation of pannus, an extensively vascularized tissue that invades and destroys the articular cartilage (140). By its vascularity and rapid proliferation rate, the RA synovium has been likened to a tumour (141). Levels of immunoreactive VEGF were high in the synovial fluid of RA patients while they were very low or undetectable in the synovial fluid of patients affected by other forms of arthritis or by degenerative joint disease. Furthermore, anti-VEGF antibodies significantly reduced the endothelial cell chemotactic activity of the RA synovial fluid, indicating that immunoreactive VEGF was bioactive (139).

It has been shown that VEGF expression is increased in psoriatic skin (111). Increased vascularity and permeability are characteristic of psoriasis. Also, VEGF mRNA expression has been recently examined in three bullous dermatological disorders with subepidermal blister formation, bullous pemphigoid, erythema multiforme, and dermatitis herpetiforme (110,111). In all of these conditions, VEGF mRNA was markedly up-regulated not only in the epidermis over blisters but also at a distance from blisters, in areas adjacent to dermal inflammatory infiltrates.

Intriguingly, at least two sequences having a significant homology to VEGF have been identified in the genome of two different strains of *orf* virus, a parapoxvirus that affects goats, sheep, and occasionally humans (142). This suggests that the viral VEGF-like gene has been acquired from a mammalian host and is undergoing genetic drift. Interestingly, the lesions of goats and humans following *orf* virus infection are characterized by extensive microvascular proliferation in the skin, raising the possibility that the product of the viral VEGF-like gene is responsible for such lesions.

Vascular endothelial growth factor as a potential therapeutic agent

The availability of agents able to promote the growth of new collateral vessels would be potentially of major therapeutic value for disorders characterized by inadequate tissue perfusion and might constitute an alternative to surgical reconstruction procedures. For example, chronic limb ischaemia, most frequently caused by obstructive atherosclerosis affecting the superficial femoral artery, is associated with a high rate of morbidity and mortality and treatment is currently limited to surgical revascularization or endovascular interventional therapy (143,144). No pharmacological therapy has been shown to be effective for this condition. Previous studies where bFGF was administered suggest that an angiogenic therapy may be able to restore perfusion following vascular injury (145). It has been recently shown that intra-arterial or intramuscular administration of rhVEGF$_{165}$ may significantly augment perfusion and development of collateral vessels in a rabbit model where 'chronic' hindlimb ischaemia was created by surgical removal of the femoral artery (146,147). These studies provided angiographic evidence of neovascularization in the ischaemic limbs. Arterial gene transfer with a cDNA encoding VEGF$_{165}$ also led to revascularization of rabbit ischaemic limbs to an extent comparable with that achieved with the recombinant protein (148). In addition, the hypothesis that the angiogenesis initiated by the administration of VEGF improved muscle function in ischaemic limbs was recently tested (149). A single intra-arterial injection of rhVEGF$_{165}$ augmented muscle function in this rabbit model of peripheral limb ischaemia. It is also a characteristic of this model that the ischamic limb cannot augment blood flow in response to oxygen demand during exercise. This exercise-induced hyperaemia was significantly improved in ischaemic limbs treated with rh VEGF$_{165}$ (149). Such improvement in perfusion was, however, not seen in other non-ischaemic tissues including the contralateral limb. Similarly, Bauters et al. (150) have shown that both maximal flow velocity and maximal blood flow, as assessed by Doppler, are significantly increased in ischaemic limbs following VEGF administration. Therefore, it appears that the neovascularization seen in response to rhVEGF$_{165}$ result in improvements in physiological parameters, suggesting that this type of therapy may represent a significant advancement in the treatment of peripheral vascular disease. Recent studies have shown that VEGF administration also leads to a recovery of normal endothelial reactivity in dysfunctional endothelium (151). Following obstruction of a large artery and development of collateral vessels, a limiting factor to the restoral of normal flow is the abnormal reactivity of newly formed vessels. For example, the increase in blood flow following acetylcholine infusion is severely blunted; serotonin paradoxically leads to a decrease in blood flow (152). Thirty days after a single intra-arterial bolus of VEGF$_{165}$, restoral of normal increase in blood flow in ischaemic rabbit hindlimb following acetylcholine or serotonin infusion was demonstrated (151). These findings indicate that VEGF action results in the development of blood vessels with a normal and functional endothelium.

Furthermore, it has been shown that VEGF administration may result in increase in coronary blood flow in a dog model of coronary insufficiency (153). Following occlusion of the left circumflex coronary artery, daily injections of rh VEGF distal to the occlusion resulted in a significant enhancement in collateral blood flow over a 4-week period. In addition, Harada et al. (154) have recently demonstrated that extraluminal administration of as little as 2 µg of rhVEGF by an osmotic pump results in a significant increase in coronary blood flow in a pig model of chronic myocardial ischaemia created by ameroid occlusion of proximal circumflex artery. Remarkably, VEGF treatment led to 2.6-fold decrease in the size of left ventricular infarct in this model (154).

Another potential therapeutic application of VEGF is the prevention of restenosis following percutaneous transluminal angioplasty (PTA). Between 15 and 75% of patients undergoing PTA for occlusive coronary or peripheral arterial disease develop restenosis within 6 months. The frequency of clinical stenosis depends on the size and location of the artery and the definition of stenosis (155). It has been proposed that damage to the endothelium is the crucial event triggering fibrocellular intimal proliferation (156). Recent studies have shown that VEGF accelerates re-endotheliazation and attenuates intimal hyperplasia in balloon-injured rat carotid artery or rabbit aorta (157,158). Therefore, it is tempting to speculate that rapid re-endothelialization promoted by VEGF may prove effective at preventing the cascade of events leading to neointima formation and restenosis in patients.

Conclusions

VEGF has been identified and characterized only recently but already appears to play a critical part in the regulation of blood vessel growth as well as having considerable therapeutic potential.

The finding that targeted mutations inactivating the VEGF receptors genes result in a profound deficit in vasculogenesis and blood island formation, leading to early intrauterine death, emphasizes the pivotal role played by the VEGF/VEGF-receptor system in the development of the vascular system.

An attractive possibility is that recombinant VEGF or gene therapy with the VEGF gene may be used in the future to promote endothelial cell growth and collateral vessel formation. This would represent a novel therapeutic modality for conditions that frequently are refractory to conservative measures and unresponsive to pharmacological therapy.

The high expression of VEGF mRNA in the vast majority of human tumours, the presence of the VEGF protein in ocular fluids of individuals with proliferative retinopathies and in the synovial fluid of RA patients strongly supports the hypothesis that VEGF is a key mediator of angiogenesis associated with various pathological conditions. Therefore, anti-VEGF antibodies or VEGF antagonists have the potential to be of therapeutic value for a variety of highly vascularized and aggressive malignancies as well as for other angiogenic disorders. An anti-VEGF therapy may have low toxicity, perhaps limited to inhibition of wound healing and ovarian and endometrial function, as endothelial cells are essentially quiescent in most adult tissues.

In conclusion, recent evidence strongly suggest that, in spite of the plurality of factors potentially involved in pathological angiogenesis, strategies aimed at antagonizing one specific endothelial cell mitogen, VEGF, may form the basis for an effective treatment of a variety of tumours and proliferative retinopathies.

Update: spring 1997

After the completion of this manuscript (summer 1995), significant progress has been made in the VEGF field. The knockout of the VEGF gene has been reported and has provided direct evidence for an irreplaceable role played by this growth factor in the development of the vascular system. Loss of a single VEGF allele results in defective vascularization and early embryonic lethality in mice (159,160). Thus, even a partial loss of VEGF is not compatible with a normal pattern of development and organogenesis. Also, our understanding of the mechanisms of transcriptional and post-transcriptional regulation of VEGF expression has been furthered (161,162). Two additional members of the VEGF family have been described: VEGF-B and VEGF-C (163–5). The latter is a ligand for the Flt-4 tyrosine kinase receptor. Although the biological role of these factors is unclear, their structural homology with VEGF suggests that they may participate in the regulation of blood vessel growth. Progress has been made also in structure/function aspects of VEGF and its receptors. By alanine scanning mutagenesis, the determinants in VEGF required for binding KDR and Flt-1 receptors have been identified (166). The second immunoglobulin-like domain has been shown to contain the major determinants for ligand binding and specificity in Flt-1 and KDR (167). Furthermore, a gene therapy trial using naked plasmid cDNA encoding VEGF165 has been initiated in patients with severe limb ischaemia. A case report of an interim analysis of this trial has been published and reveals histologic and angiographic evidence of angiogenesis in the ischaemic area (168).

References

1. Hamilton, W. J., Boyd, J. D. and Mossman, H. W. (1962). *Human embryology.* Williams & Wilkins, Baltimore.
2. Klagsbrun, M. and D'Amore, P. A. (1991). Regulators of angiogenesis. *Annu. Rev. Physiol.*, **53**, 217–39.
3. Folkman, J and Shing, Y. (1992). Angiogenesis. *J. Biol. Chem.*, **267**, 10931–4.
4. Folkman, J. (1991). What is the evidence that tumors are angiogenesis-dependent? *J. Natl Cancer Inst.*, **82**, 4–6.
5. Garner, A. (1994). Vascular diseases. In *Pathobiology of ocular disease. A dynamic approach* (ed. A. Garner, and G. K. Klintworth), 2nd edn pp. 1625–710 Marcel Dekker, New York.
6. Weidner, N., Semple, P., Welch, W., and Folkman, J. (1991). Tumor angiogenesis and metastasis. Correlation in invasive breast carcinoma. *N. Engl. J. Med.*, **324**, 1–6.
7. Weidner, N., Folkman, J., Pozza, F., Bevilacqua, P., Allred, E. N., Moore, D. H., *et al.* (1992). Tumor angiogenesis: a new significant and independent prognostic indicator in early-stage breast carcinoma. *J. Natl Cancer Inst.*, **84**, 1875–88.
8. Horak, E. R., Leek, R., Klenk, N., Lejeune, S., Smith, K., Stuart, M., *et al.* (1992). Quantitative angiogenesis assessed by anti-PECAM antibodies: correlation with node metastasis and survival in breast cancer. *Lancet*, **340**, 1120–4.
9. Vartanian, R. K. and Weidner, N. (1994). Correlation of intramural endothelial cell proliferation with microvessel density (tumor angiogenesis) and tumor cell proliferation. *Am. J. Pathol.*, **144**, 1188–94.
10. Chodak, G. W., Haudenschild, C., Gittes, R. F. and Folkman, J. (1980). Angiogenic activity as a marker of neoplastic and preneoplastic lesions of the human bladder. *Ann. Surg.*, **192**, 762–71.
11. Wakui, S., Furusato, M., Sasaki, H., Akiyama, A., Kinoshito, I., Asano, K., *et al.* (1992). Tumor angiogenesis in prostatic carcinoma with and without bone metastasis: a morphometric study. *J. Pathol.*, **168**, 257–62.
12. Bigler, S. A., Deering, R. E. and Brawer, M. K. (1993). Comparison of microscopic vascularity in benign and malignant prostatic tissue. *Hum. Pathol.*, **24**, 220–6.
13. Macchiarini, P., Fontanini, G., Hardin, M. J., Squartini, F. and Angeletti, C. A. (1992). Relation of neovascularization to metastasis of non-small cell lung carcinoma. *Lancet*, **340**, 145–6.
14. Sillman, F., Boyce, J. and Fruchter, R. (1981). The significance of atypical vessels and neovascularization in cervical neoplasias. *Am. J. Obstet. Gynecol.*, **139**, 154–7.
15. Srivastava, A., Laidler, P., Davies, R., Horgan, K. and Hughes, L. E. (1988). The prognostic significance of tumor vascularity in intermediate-thickness (0.76–4.0 mm thick) skin melanoma. *Am. J. Pathol.*, **133**, 419–23.
16. Smith-McCune, K. S. and Weidner, N. (1994). Demonstration and characterization of the angiogenic properties of cervical dysplasia. *Cancer Res.*, **54**, 804–8.
17. Leung, D. W., Cachianes, G., Kuang, W-J., Goeddel, D. V. and Ferrara, N. (1989). Vascular endothelial growth factor is a secreted angiogenic mitogen. *Science*, **246**, 1306–9. 1989.
18. Houck, K. A., Ferrara, N., Winer, J., Cachianes, G., Li, B., and Leung, D. W. (1991). The vascular endothelial growth factor family: identification of a fourth molecular species and characterization of alternative splicing of RNA. *Mol. Endocrinol.*, **5**, 1806–14.
19. Tisher, E., Mitchell, R., Hartmann, T., Silva, M., Gospodarowicz, D., Fiddes, J. and Abraham, J. (1991). The human gene for vascular endothelial growth factor. *J. Biol. Chem.*, **266**, 11947–54.
20. Michaelson, I. C. (1948). The mode of development of the vascular system of the retina with some observations on its significance for certainretinal disorders. *Trans. Ophthalmol. Soc. UK*, **68**, 671–821.
21. Jakeman, L. B., Armanini, M., Phillips, H. S., Ferrara, N. (1993). Developmental expression of binding sites and mRNA for vascular endothelial growth factor suggests a role or this protein in vasculogenesis and angiogenesis. *Endocrinology*, **133**, 848–59.
22. Fong, G-H, Rassant, J., Gertenstein, M. and Breitman, M. (1995). Role of Flt-1 receptor tyrosine kinase in regulation of assembly of vascular endothelium. *Nature*, **376**, 6670.
23. Shalabi, F., Rossant, J., Yamaguchi, T. P., Gertenstein, M., Wu, X-F., Breitman, M. L. and Schuh, A. C. (1995). Failure of blood island formation and vasculogenesis in Flk-1 deficient mice. *Nature*, **376**, 62–6.

24. Phillips, H. S., Hains, J., Leung, D. W. and Ferrara, N. (1990). Vascular endothelial growth factor is expressed in rat corpus luteum. *Endocrinology*, **127**, 965–68.

25. Ravindranath, N., Little-Ihrig, L., Phillips, H. S., Ferrara, N. and Zeleznick, A. J. (1992). Vascular endothelial growth factor mRNA expression in the primate ovary. *Endocrinology*, **131**, 254–60.

26. Shweiki, D., Itin, A., Neufeld, G., Gitay-Goren, H. and Keshet, E. (1993). Patterns of expression of vascular endothelial growth factor (VEGF) and VEGF receptors in mice suggest a role in hormonally regulated angiogenesis. *J. Clin. Invest.*, **91**, 2235–43.

27. Ferrara, N. (1993). Vascular endothelial growth factor. *Trends Cardiovasc. Med.*, **3**, 244–50.

28. Kim, K. J., Li, B., Winer, J., Armanini, M., Gillett, N., Phillips, H. S. and Ferrara, N. (1993). Inhibition of vascular endothelial growth factor-induced angiogenesis suppresses tumour growth *in vivo*. *Nature* **362**, 841–4.

29. Aiello, L. P., Avery, R., Arrigg, R., Keyt, B., Jampel, H., Shah, S., *et al.* (1994). Vascular endothelial growth factor in ocular fluid of patients with diabetic retinopathy and other retinal disorders. *N. Engl. J. Med.*, **331**, 1480–7.

30. Ferrara, N. and Henzel, W. J. (1989). Pituitary follicular cells secrete a novel heparin-binding growth factor specific for vascular endothelial cells. *Biochem. Biophys. Res. Commun.*, **161**, 851–9.

31. Plöuet, J., Schilling, J. and Gospodarowicz, D. (1989). Isolation and characterization of a newly identified endothelial cell mitogen produced by AtT20 cells. *EMBO J.*, **8**, 3801–7.

32. Conn, G., Bayne, M., Soderman, L., Kwok, P. W., Sullivan, K. A., Palisi, T. M., *et al.* (1990). Amino acid and cDNA sequence of a vascular endothelial cell mitogen homologous to platelet-derived growth factor. *Proc. Natl Acad. Sci. USA*, **87**, 2628–32.

33. Phillips, G. D., Stone, A. M., Jones, B. D., Schultz, J. C., Whitehead, R. A. and Knighton, D. R. (1995). Vascular endothelial growth factor (rh VEGF165) stimulates direct angiogenesis in the rabbit cornea. *In Vivo*, **8**, 961–5.

34. Tolentino, M. J., Miller, J. W., Gragoudas, E. S., Chatzistefanou, K., Ferrara, N. and Adamis, A. P. (1996). VEGF is sufficient to produce iris neovascularization and neovascular glaucoma in a non-human primate. *Arch. Ophthalmol.*, **114**, 964–70.

35. Connolly, D. T., Heuvelman, D. M., Nelson, R., Olander, J. V., Eppley, B. L., Delfino, J. J., *et al.* (1989). Tumor vascular permeability factor stimulates endothelial cell growth and angiogenesis. *J. Clin. Invest.*, **84**, 1470–8.

36. Pepper, M. S., Ferrara, N., Orci, L. and Montesano, R. (1992). Potent synergism between vascular endothelial growth factor and basic fibroblast growth factor in the induction of angiogenesis. *in vitro. Biochem. Biophys. Res. Commun.*, **189**, 824–31.

37. Nicosia, R. F., Nicosia, S. V., and Smith, M. (1995). Vascular endothelial growth factor, platelet-derived growth factor and insulin-like growth factor-1 promote rat aortic angiogenesis *in vitro. Am. J. Pathol.*, **145**, 1023–9.

38. Pepper M. S., Ferrara, N., Orci, L. and Montesano, R. (1991). Vascular endothelial growth factor (VEGF) induces plasminogen activators and plasminogen activator inhibitor type 1 in microvascular endothelial cells. *Biochem. Biophys. Res. Commun.*, **181**, 902–8.

39. Unemori, E., Ferrara, N., Bauer, E. A. and Amento, E. P. (1992). Vascular endothelial growth factor induces interstitial collagenase expression in human endothelial cells. *J. Cell. Physiol.*, **153**, 557–62.

40. Gross, J. and Nagai, Y. (1965). Specific degradation of the collagen molecule by tadpole collagenolytic enzyme. *Proc. Natl Acad. Sci. USA*, **54**, 1197–204.

41. Pepper, M. S. and Montesano, R. (1990). Proteolytic balance and capillary morphogenesis. *Cell Differ. Dev.*, **32**, 319–31.

42. Mandriota, S., Montesano, R., Orci, L., Seghezzi, G., Vassalli, J-D., Ferrara, N, *et al.* (1995). Vascular endothelial growth factor increases urokinase receptor expression in vascular endothelial cells. *J. Biol. Chem.*, **270**, 9709–16.

43. Mignatti, P., Tsuboi, R., Robbins, E. and Rifkin, D. B. (1989). *In vitro* angiogenesis on the human amniotic membrane: requirement for basic fibroblast growth factor-induced proteinases. *J. Cell Biol.*, **108**, 671–82.

44. Rifkin, D. B., Moscatelli, D., Bizik, J., Quarto, N., Blei, F., Dennis, P., *et al.* (1990). Growth factor control of extracellular proteolysis. *Cell Differ. Dev.* **32**, 313–18.

45. Connolly, D. T., Olander, J. V., Heuvelman, D., Nelson, R., Monsell, R., Siegel, N., *et al.* (1989). Human vascular permeability factor. Isolation from U937 cells. *J. Biol. Chem.*, **254**, 20017–24.

46. Keck, P. J., Hauser, S. D., Krivi, G., Sanzo, K., Warren, T., Feder, J. and Connolly, D. T. (1989). Vascular permeability factor, an endothelial cell mitogen related to platelet derived growth factor. *Science*, **246**, 1309–12.

47. Senger, D. R., Galli, S. J., Dvorak, A. M., Perruzzi, C. A., Harvey, V. S. and Dvorak, H. F. (1983). Tumor cells secrete a vascular permeability factor that promotes accumulation of ascites fluid. *Science*, **219**, 983–85.

48. Dvorak, H. F. (1986). Tumors: wound that do not heal. Similarity between tumor stroma generation and wound healing. *N. Engl. J. Med.*, **315**, 1650–8.

49. Dvorak, H. F., Harvey, V. S., Estrella, P., Brown, L. F., McDonagh, J. and Dvorak, A. M. (1987). Fibrin containing gels induce angiogenesis: implications for tumor stroma generation and wound healing. *Lab. Invest.*, **57**, 673–86.

50. Dvorak, H. F., Brown, L. F., Detmar, M. and Dvorak, A. M. (1995). Vascular permeability factor/ vascular endothelial growth factor, microvascular permeability and angiogenesis. *Am. J. Pathol.*, **146**, 1029–39.

51. Pekala, P., Marlow, M., Heuvelman, D. and Connolly, D. (1990). Regulation of hexose transport in aortic endothelial cells by vascular permeability factor and tumor necrosis factor-alpha, but not by insulin. *J. Biol. Chem.*, **265**, 18051–4.

52. Clauss, M., Gerlach, M., Gerlach, H., Brett, F., Wang, F., Familletti, P. C., *et al.* (1990). Vascular permeability factor: a tumor-derived polypeptide that induces endothelial cell and monocyte procoagulant activity, and promotes monocyte migration. *J. Exp. Med.*, **172**, 1535–45.

53. Nemerson, Y. and Bach, R. (1982). Tissue factor revisited. *Prog. Hemost. Thromb.*, **6**, 237–45.

54. Nawroth, P. and Stern, D. (1988). Modulation of endothelial cell hemostatic properties by tumor necrosis factor. *J. Exp. Med.*, **164**, 470–78.

55. Ku, D. D., Zaleski, J. K., Liu, S. and Brock, T. (1993). Vascular endothelial growth factor induces EDRF-dependent relaxation of coronary arteries. *Am. J. Physiol.*, **265**, H586–92.

56. Yang, R., Thomas, G. R., Bunting, S., Ko, A., Keyt, B., Ferrara, N., *et al.* (1996). Effects of VEGF on hemodynamics and cardiac performance. *J. Cardiovasc. Pharmacol.*, **27**, 838–41.

57. Park, J. E., Chen, H., Winer, J., Houck, K. and Ferrara, N. (1994). Placenta growth factor. Potentiation of vascular endothelial growth factor bioactivity, *in vitro*, and *in vivo*, and high affinity binding to Flt-1 but not to Flk-1/KDR. *J. Biol. Chem.*, **269**, 25646–54.

58. Maglione, D., Guerriero, V., Viglietto, G., Delli-Bovi, P. and Persico, M. G. (1991). Isolation of a human placenta cDNA coding for a protein related to the vascular permeability factor. *Proc. Natl Acad. Sci. USA*, **88**, 9267–71.

59. Hauser, S. and Weich, H. A. (1993). A heparin-binding form of placenta growth factor (PlGF-2) is expressed in human umbilical vein endothelial cells and in placenta. *Growth Factors*, **9**, 259–68.

60. Levy, A. P., Levy, N. S., Wegner, S. and Goldberg, M. A. (1995). Transcriptional regulation of the rat vascular endothelial growth factor gene by hypoxia. *J. Biol. Chem.*, **270**, 13333–40.

61. Shima, D. T., Adamis, A. P., Ferrara, N., Yeo, K-T., Yeo, T-K., Allende, *et al.* (1995). Hypoxic induction of vascular endothelial cell growth factors in the retina: Identification and characterization of vascular endothelial growth factor (VEGF) as the sole mitogen. *Mol. Med.*, **2**, 64–71.

62. Shweiki D., Itin, A., Soffer, D. and Keshet, E. (1992). Vascular endothelial growth factor induced by hypoxia may mediate hypoxia-initiated angiogenesis. *Nature*, **359**, 843–5.

63. Banai, S., Shweiki, D., Pinson, A., Chandra, M., Lazarovici, G. and Keshet, E. (1994). Upregulation of vascular endothelial growth factor expression induced by myocardial ischemia: implications for coronary angiogenesis. *Cardiovasc. Res.* **28**, 1176–9.

64. Plate, K. H., Breier, G., Weich, H. A. and Risau, W. (1992). Vascular endothelial growth is a potential tumour angiogenesis factor *in vivo*. *Nature*, **359**, 845–7.

65. Goldberg, M. A. and Schneider, T. J. (1994). Similarities between the oxygen-sensing mechanisms regulating the expression of vascular endothelial growth factor and erythropoietin. *J. Biol. Chem.*, **269**, 4355–61.

66. Madan, A. and Curtin, P. T. (1993). A 24-base pair sequence 3' to the human erythropoietin contains a hypoxia-responsive transcriptional enhancer. *Proc. Natl Acad. Sci. USA*, **90**, 3928–32.

67. Wang, G. L. and Semenza, G. L. (1995) Purification and characterization of hypoxia-inducible factor-1. *J. Biol. Chem.*, **270**, 1230–7.

68. Wang, G. L., Jiang, B. H., Rue, E. A. and Semenza, G. L. (1995). Hypoxia-inducible factor-1 is a basic helix–loop helix–PAS heterodimer regulated by cellular O_2 tension. *Proc. Natl Acad. Sci. USA*, **92**, 5510–4.

69. Takagi, H., King, G. L., Ferrara, N. and Aiello, L. P. (1996). Hypoxic induction of VEGF is mediated by adenosine through A_2 receptors and elevation of cAMP in retinal microvascular pericytes and endothelial cells *Inv. Oph. Vis. Sci.*, **37**, 2165–76.

70. Mukhopadhyay, D., Tsilokas, L., Zhou, X-M., Foster, D., Brugge, J. S. and Sukhatme, V. P. (1995). Hypoxic induction of human vascular endothelial growth factor expression through c-Src activation, *Nature*, **375**, 577–81.

71. Garrido, C., Saule, S. and Gospodarowicz, D. (1993). Transcriptional regulation of vascular endothelial growth factor gene expression in ovarian bovine granulosa cells. *Growth Factors*, **8**, 109–17.

72. Frank, S., Hubner, G., Breier, G., Longaker, M. T., Greenhalgh, D. G., and Werner, S. (1995). Regulation of

VEGF expression in cultured keratinocytes. Implications for normal and impaired wound healing. *J. Biol. Chem.*, **270**, 12607–13.

73. Pertovaara, L., Kaipainen, A., Mustonen, T., Orpana, A., Ferrara, N., Saksela, O., and Alitalo, K. (1994). Vascular endothelial growth factor is induced in response to transforming growth factor-β in fibroblastic and epithelial cells. *J. Biol. Chem.*, **2**, (69), 6271–4.

74. Li, J., Perrella, M. A., Tsai, J. C., Yet, S. F., Hsieh, C. M., Yoshizumi, M., *et al.* (1995). Induction of vascular endothelial growth factor gene expression by interleukin-1 beta in rat aortic smooth muscle cells. *J. Biol. Chem.*, **270**, 308–12.

75. Claffey, K. P., Wilkinson, W. O., and Spiegelman, B. M. (1992). Vascular endothelial growth factor. Regulation by cell differentiation and activated second messenger pathways. *J. Biol. Chem.*, **267**, 16317–22.

76. Kieser, A., Weich, H., Brandner, G., Marme', D., and Kolch, W. (1994) Mutant p53 potentiates protein kinase C induction of vascular endothelial growth factor expression. *Oncogene*, **9**, 963–9.

77. Rak, J., Mitsuhashi, Y., Bayko, L., Filmns, J., Shirasawa, S., Sasazuki, T., and Kerbel, R. S. (1995). Mutant ras oncogenes upregulate VEGF/VPF expression: implications for induction and inhibition of tumour angiogenesis. *Cancer Res.*, **55**, 4575–80.

78. Ferrara, N., Houck, K., Jakeman, L., and Leung, D. W. (1992). Molecular and biological properties of the vascular endothelial growth factor family of proteins. *Endocr. Rev.*, **13**, 18–32.

79. Houck, K. A., Leung, D. W., Rowland, A. M., Winer, J., and Ferrara, N. (1992). Dual regulation of vascular endothelial growth factor bioavailability by genetic and proteolytic mechanisms. *J. Biol. Chem.*, **267**, 26031–7.

80. Park, J. E., Keller, G-A., and Ferrara, N. (1993). The vascular endothelial growth factor (VEGF) isoforms: differential deposition into the subepithelial extracellular matrix and bioactivity of ECM-bound VEGF. *Mol. Biol. Cell.*, **4**, 1317–26.

81. Keyt, B., Berleau, L., Nguyen, H., Heinshin, H., Chen H., Vandlen, R., and Ferrara, N. (1996). The heparin-binding domain in VEGF: loss of an heparin binding, due to alternative splicing or proteolysis, results in severely decrease mitogenic activity *J. Biol. Chem.*, **271**, 7788–95.

82. Sreenath, T., Matrisian, L. M., Stetler-Stevenson, W., Gattoni-Celli, S., and Pozzatti, R. O. (1992). Expression of matrix metalloproteinases in transformed rat cell lines of high and low metastatic potential. *Cancer Res.*, **52**, 4942–7.

83. DiSalvo, J., Bayne, M. L., Conn, G., Kwok, P. W., Trivedi, P. G., Soderman, D. D., *et al.* (1995). Purification and characterization of a naturally occurring vascular endothelial growth factor placenta growth factor heterodimer. *J. Biol. Chem.*, **270**, 7717–23.

84. Vaisman, N., Gospodarowicz, D., and Neufeld, G. (1990). Characterization of the receptors for vascular endothelial growth factor. *J. Biol. Chem.*, **265**, 19461–9.

85. Plöuet, J. and Moukadiri, H. J. (1990). Characterization of the receptors to vasculotropin on bovine adrenal cortex-derived capillary endothelial cell. *J. Biol. Chem.*, **265**, 22071–5.

86. Shen, H., Clauss, M., Ryan, J., Schmidt, A. M., Tijburg, P., Borden, L., *et al.* (1993). Characterization of vascular permeability factor/vascular endothelial growth factor receptors in mononuclear phagocytes. *Blood*, **81**, 2767–73.

87. Thieme, H., Aiello, L. P., Ferrara, N., and King, G. L. (1995). Comparative analysis of VEGF receptors on retinal and aortic endothelial cells. *Diabetes*, **44**, 98–103.

88. Jakeman, L. B., Winer, J., Bennett, G. L., Altar, C. A., and Ferrara, N. (1992). Binding sites for vascular endothelial growth factor are localized on endothelial cells in adult rat tissues. *J. Clin. Invest.*, **89**, 244–53.

89. deVries, C., Escobedo, J. A., Ueno, H., Houck, K. A., Ferrara, N., and Williams, L. T. (1992). The fms-like tyrosine kinase, a receptor for vascular endothelial growth factor. *Science*, **255**, 989–91.

90. Terman, B. I., Vermazen, M. D., Carrion, M. E., Dimitrov, D., Armellino, D. C., Gospodarowicz, D., and Bohlen, P. (1992). Identification of the KDR tyrosine kinase as a receptor for vascular endothelial growth factor. *Biochem. Biophys. Res. Commun.*, **34**, 1578–86.

91. Millauer, B., Wizigmann-Voos, S., Schnurch, H., Martinez, R., Moller, N. P., Risau, W., and Ullrich A. (1993). High affinity binding and developmental expression suggest Flk-1 as a major regulator of vasculogenesis and angiogenesis. *Cell*, **72**, 835–46.

92. Quinn, T., Peters, K. G., deVries, C., Ferrara, N., and Williams L. T. (1993). Fetal liver kinase 1 is a receptor for vascular endothelial growth factor and is selectively expressed in vascular endothelium. *Proc. Natl Acad. Sci. USA*, **90**, 7533–7.

93. Shibuya, M., Yamaguchi, S., Yamane, A., Ikada, T., Tojo, T., Matsushime, H., and Sato, M. (1990). Nucleotide sequence and expression of a novel human receptor-type tyrosine kinase (*flt*) closely related to the *fms*, family. *Oncogene*, **8**, 519–27.

94. Terman, B. I., Carrion, M. E., Kovacs, E., Rasmussen, B. A., Eddy, R. L., and Shows, T. B. (1991). Identification of a new endothelial cell growth factor receptor tyrosine kinase. *Oncogene*, **6**, 519–24.

95. Matthews, W., Jordan, C. T., Gavin, M., Jenkins, N. A., Copeland, N. G., and Lemischka, I. R. (1991). A receptor tyrosine kinase cDNA isolated from a population of enriched primitive hematopoietic cells and exhibiting close genetic linkage to c-kit. *Proc. Natl Acad. Sci. USA*, **88**, 9026–30.

96. Mustonen, T. and Alitalo, K. (1995). Endothelial receptor tyrosine kinases involved in angiogenesis. *J. Cell Biol.*, **129**, 895–98.

97. Kendell, R. L. and Thomas, K. A. (1993). Inhibition of vascular endothelial growth factor by an endogenously encoded soluble receptor. *Proc. Natl Acad. Sci. USA*, **90**, 10705–9.

98. Peters, K. G., deVries, C., and Williams, L. T. (1993). Vascular endothelial growth factor receptor expression during embryogenesis and tissue repair suggests a role in endothelial differentiation and blood vessel growth. *Proc. Natl Acad. Sci. USA*, **90**, 8915–9.

99. Waltenberger, J., Claesson-Welsh, L., Siegbahn, A., Shibuya, M., and Heldin, C-H. (1994). Different signal transduction properties of KDR and Flt1, two receptors for vascular endothelial growth factor. *J. Biol. Chem.*, **269**, 26988–5.

100. Seetharam, L., Gotoh, N., Maru, Y., Neufeld, G., Yamaguchi, S., and Shibuya, M. (1995). A unique signal transduction pathway for the FLT tyrosine kinase, a receptor for vascular endothelial growth factor. *Oncogene*, **10**, 135–37.

101. Breier, G., Albrecht, U., Sterrer, S., and Risau, W. (1992). Expression of vascular endothelial growth factor during embryonic angiogenesis and endothelial cell differentiation. *Development*, **114**, 521–32.

102. Evans, H. M. (1909). On the development of aortae, cardinal, umbilical veins, and other blood vessels of vertebrate embryos from capillaries. *Anat. Rec.*, **3**, 498–516.

103. Shifren, J. L., Doldi, N., Ferrara, N., Mesiano, S., and Jaffe, R. B. (1994). In the human fetus, vascular endothelial growth factor (VEGF) is expressed in epithelial cells and myocytes, but not vascular endothelium: implications for mode of action. *J. Clin. Endocrinol. Metab.*, **79**, 316–22.

104. Monacci, W., Merrill, M., and Oldfield, E. (1993). Expression of vascular permeability factor/vascular endothelial growth factor in normal rat tissues. *Am. J. Physiol.*, **264**, C995–1002.

105. Bassett, D. L. (1943). The changes in vascular pattern of the ovary of the albino rat during the estrous cycle. *Am. J. Anat.*, **73**, 251–9.

106. Senger, D., Perruzzi, C. A., Feder, J., and Dvorak, H. F. (1986). A highly conserved vascular permeability factor secreted by a variety of human and rodent tumor cell lines. *Cancer Res.*, **46**, 5269–75.

107. Rosenthal, R., Megyesi, J. F., Henzel, W. J., Ferrara, N., and Folkman, J. (1990). Conditioned medium from mouse sarcoma 180 cells contains vascular endothelial growth factor. *Growth Factors*, **4**, 53–9.

108. Brown, L. F., Berse, B., Jackman, R. W., Tognazzi, K., Manseau, E. J., Dvorak, H. F., and Senger, D. R. (1993). Increased expression of vascular permeability factor (vascular endothelial growth factor) and its receptors in kidney and bladder carcinomas. *Am. J. Pathol.*, **143**, 1255–62.

109. Takahashi, A., Sasaki, H., Kim, S. J., Tobisu, K., Kakizoe, T., Tsukamoto, T., *et al.*. (1994). Markedly increased amounts of messenger RNA for VEGF and PlGF in renal cell carcinoma associated with angiogenesis. *Cancer Res.*, **54**, 4233–7.

110. Brown, L. F., Berse, B., Jackman, R. W., Guidi, A. J., Dvorak, H. F., Senger, D. R., *et al.* (1995). Expression of vascular permeability factor (vascular endothelial growth factor) and its receptors in breast cancer. *Hum. Pathol.*, **26**, 86–91.

111. Brown, L. F., Harris, T. J., Yeo, K. T., Stahle-Backdahl, M., Jackman, R. W., Berse, B., *et al.* (1995). Increased expression of vascular permeability factor (vascular endothelial growth factor) in bullous pemphigoid, dermatitis herpetiformis and herythema multiforme. *J. Invest. Dermatol.*, **104**, 744–9.

112. Olson, T. A., Mohanraj, D., Carson, L. F., and Ramakrishnan, S. (1994). Vascular permeability factor gene expression in normal and neoplastic human ovaries. *Cancer Res.*, **54**, 276–80.

113. Brown, L. F., Berse, B., Jackman, R. W., Tognazzi, K., Manseau, E. J., Senger, D. R., and Dvorak, H. F. (1993). Expression of vascular permeability factor (vascular endothelial growth factor) and its receptors in adenocarcinomas of the gastrointestinal tract. *Cancer Res.*, **53**, 4727–35.

114. Phillips, H. S., Armanini, M., Stavrou, D., Ferrara, N., and Westphal, M. (1993). Intense focal expression of vascular endothelial growth factor mRNA in human intracranial neoplasms: association with regions of necrosis. *Int. J. Oncol.*, **2**, 913–9.

115. Berkman, R. A., Merrill, M. J., Reinhold, W. C., Monacci, W. T., Saxena, A., Clark, W. C., *et al.* (1993). Expression of the vascular permeability/vascular endothelial growth

factor gene in central nervous system neoplasms. *J. Clin. Invest.*, **91**, 153–9.

116. Wizigmann-Voss, S., Breier, G., Risau, W., and Plate, K. (1994). Up-regulation of vascular endothelial growth factor and its receptors in von Hippel-Lindau disease-associated and sporadic hemangioblastoma. *Cancer Res.*, **55**, 1358–64.

117. Warren, R. S., Yuan, H, Matli, M. R., Gillett, N. A., and Ferrara, N. (1995). Regulation by vascular endothelial growth factor of human colon cancer tumorigenesis in a mouse model of experimental liver metastasis. *J. Clin. Invest.*, **95**, 1789–97.

118. Toi, M., Hoshima, S., Takayanagi, T., and Tominaga, T. (1994). Association of vascular endothelial growth factor expression with tumor angiogenesis and with early relapse in primary breast cancer. *Jpn. J. Cancer Res.*, **85**, 1045–9.

119. Ferrara, N., Winer, J., Burton, T., Rowland, A., Siegel, M., Phillips, H. S., *et al.* (1993). Expression of vascular endothelial growth factor does not promote transformation but confers a growth advantage *in vivo* to Chinese hamster ovary cells. *J. Clin. Invest.*, **91**, 160–70.

120. Zhang, H. T., Craft, P., Scott, P. A., Ziche, M., Weich, H. A., Harris, A. L., and Bicknell, R. (1995). Enhancement of tumor growth and vascular density by transfection of vascular endothelial growth factor into MCF-7 human breast carcinoma cells. *J. Natl Cancer Inst.*, **87**, 213–9.

121. Kim, K. J., Li, B., Houck, K., Winer, J., and Ferrara, N. (1992). The vascular endothelial growth factor proteins: identification of biologically relevant regions by neutralizing monoclonal antibodies. *Growth Factors*, **7**, 53–64.

122. Melnyk, O., Schuman, M., Kim, K. J. (1996). Vascular endothelial growth factor promotes tumour dissemination by a mechanism distinct from its effect on primary tumour growth. *Cancer Res.*, **56**, 921–4.

123. Borgström, P., Hillan, K. J., Sriramarao, P., and Ferrara, N. (1996). Complete inhibition of angiogenesis and growth of microtumours by anti-vascular endothelial growth factor neutralizing antibody: novel concepts of angiostatic therapy from intravital videomicroscopy. *Cancer Res.*, **56**, 4032–9.

124. Millauer, B., Shawver, L. K., Plate, K. H., Risau, W., and Ullrich A. (1994). Glioblastoma growth is inhibited *in vivo* by a negative dominant Flk-1 mutant. *Nature*, **367**, 576–9.

125. Henkind (1978).

126. Patz, A. (1980). Studies on retinal neovascularization. *Invest. Ophthalmol. Vis. Sci.*, **19**, 1133–8.

127. Olk, R. J. and Lee, C. M. (1993). *Diabetic retinopathy: practical management*. J. B. Lippincott.

128. Hannehan, A., deJuan, E., Lutti, G. A., Fox, G. M., Schiffer, S., and Hjelmeland, L. M. (1991). Altered distribution of basic fibroblast growth factor in diabetic retinopathy. *Arch. Ophthalmol.*, **109**, 1005–11.

129. Meyer-Schwickerath, R., Pfeiffer, A., Blum, W. F., Freyberger, H., Klein, M., Losche, C., *et al.* (1993). Vitreous levels of the insulin-like growth factors I and II, and the insulin-like growth factor binding proteins 2 and 3 increase in neovascular disease. *J. Clin. Invest.*, **92**, 2620–5.

130. Adamis, A. P., Miller, J. W., Bernal, M-T., D'Amico, D., Folkman, J., Yeo, T-K., and Yeo, K-T (1994). Increased vascular endothelial growth factor in the vitreous of eyes with proliferative diabetic retinopathy. *Am. J. Ophthalmol.*, **118**, 445–50.

131. Malecaze, F., Clemens, S., Simorer-Pinotel, V., Mathis, A., Chollet, P., Favard, P., *et al.* (1994). Detection of vascular endothelial growth factor mRNA and vascular endothelial growth factor-like activity in proliferative diabetic retinopathy. *Arch. Ophthalmol.*, **112**, 1476–82.

132. Ferrara, N. (1995). Vascular endothelial growth factor — the trigger for neovascularization in the eye (Editorial). *Lab. Invest.*, **72**, 615–18.

133. Pe'er, J., Shweiki, D., Itin, A., Hemo, I., Gnessin, H., and Keshet, E. (1995). Hypoxia-induced expression of vascular endothelial growth factor (VEGF) by retinal cells is a common factor in neovascularization. *Lab. Invest.*, **72**, 638–45.

134. Miller, J. W., Adamis, A. P., Shima, D. T., d'Amore, P. A., Moulton, R. S., O'Reilly, M. S., *et al.* (1994). Vascular endothelial growth factor/vascular permeability factor is temporally and spatially correlated with ocular neovascularization in a primate model. *Am. J. Pathol.*, **145**, 574–84.

135. Pierce, E. A., Avery, R. L., Foley, E. D., Aiello, L. P., and Smith, L. E. (1995). Vascular endothelial growth factor/vascular permeability factor expression in a mouse model of retinal neovascularization. *Proc. Natl Acad. Sci. USA*, **92**, 905–9.

136. Adamis, A. P., Shima, D. T., Tolentino, M., Gragoudas, E., Ferrara, N., Folkman, J., *et al.* (1996). Inhibition of VEGF prevents ocular neovascularization in a primat. *Arch. Ophthalmol.*, **114**, 66–71.

137. Aiello, L. P., Pierce, E. A., Foley, E. D., Takagi, H., Riddle, L., Chen, H., *et al.* (1995). Suppression of retinal neovascularization *in vivo* by inhibition of vascular endothelial growth factor (VEGF) using VEGF-receptor chimeric proteins. *Proc. Natl Acad. Sci. USA*, **12**, 10453–61.

138. Fava, R. A., Olsen, N. J., Spencer-Green, G., Yeo, T-K., Yeo, K-T., Berse, B., *et al.* (1994). Vascular permeability factor/vascular endothelial growth factor (VPF/VEGF): accumulation and expression in human synovial fluids and rheumatoid arthritis. *J. Exp. Med.*, **180**, 340–6.

139. Koch, E., Harlow, L., Haines, G. K., Amento, E. P., Unemori, E. N., Wong, W-L., *et al.* (1994). Vascular endothelial growth factor: a cytokine modulating endothelial function in rheumatoid arthritis. *J. Immunol.*, **152**, 4149–5.

140. Fassbender, H. J. and Simling-Annefeld, M. (1983). The potential aggressiveness of synovial tissue in rheumatoid arthritis. *J. Pathol.*, **139**, 399–406.

141. Hamilton, J. (1976). Hypothesis: *in vitro* evidence for the invasive and tumor-like properties of the rheumatoid pannus. *J. Rheumatol.*, **10**, 845–51.

142. Lyttle, D. J., Fraser, K. M., Flemings, S. B., Mercer, A. A., and Robinson, A. J. (1994). Homologs of vascular endothelial growth factor are encoded by the poxvirus orf virus. *J. Virol.* **68**, 84–92.

143. Topol, E. J. (1990). *Textbook of interventional cardiology*. W. B. Saunders, Philadelphia, P. A.

144. Thompson, R. W. and D'Amore, P. A. (1990). Recruitment of growth and collateral circulation. In *Clinical ischemic syndromes: mechanisms and consequences of tissue injury*. (ed. G. B., Zelenock, L. G., D'Alecy, J. C., III, Fantone, M., Shlafer, and J. C., Stanley), pp. 117–34. C. V. Mosby, St Louis.

145. Baffour, R., Berman, J., Garb, J. L., Rhee, S. W., Kaufman, J., and Friedmann, P. (1992). Enhanced angiogenesis and growth of collaterals by *in vivo* administration of recombinant basic fibroblast growth factor in a rabbit model of acute lower limb ischemia: dose–response effect of basic fibroblast growth factor. *J. Vasc. Surg.* **16**, 181–91.

146. Takeshita, S., Zhung, L., Brogi, E., Kearney, M., Pu, L-Q., Bunting, S., *et al.* (1994). Therapeutic angiogenesis: a single intra-arterial bolus of vascular endothelial growth

factor augments collateral vessel formation in a rabbit ischemic hindlimb model. *J. Clin. Invest.*, **93**, 662–70.

147. Takeshita, S., Pu, L-Q., Stein, L. A., Sniderman, A. D., Bunting, S., Ferrara, N., *et al.* (1994). Intramuscular administration of vascular endothelial growth factor induces dose-dependent collateral artery augmentation in a rabbit model of chronic limb ischemia. *Circulation*, **90**, II228–34.

148. Takeshita, S., Zheng, L. P., Cheng, D., Riessen, R., Weir, L., Symes, J. F., *et al.* (1996). Therapeutic angiogenesis following arterial gene transfer of vascular endothelial in a rabbit model of hindlimb ischemia. *Biochem. Biophys. Res. Commun.*, **227**, 628–35.

149. Walder, C. E., Errett, C. J., Ogez, J., Heinshon, H., Bunting, S., Lindquist, P., *et al.* Vascular endothelial growth factor (VEGF) improves blood flow and function in a chronic ischemic hind-limb model. *J. Cardiovasc. Res.* (in press).

150. Bauters, C., Asahara, T., Zheng, L. P., Takeshita, S., Bunting, S., Ferrara, N., *et al.* (1994). Physiologic assessment of augmented vascularity induced by VEGF in a rabbit ischemic hindlimb model. *Am. J. Physiol.*, **267**, H1263–71.

151. Bauters, C., Asahara, T., Zheng, L. P., Takeshita, S., Bunting, S., Ferrara, N., *et al.* (1995) Recovery of disturbed endothelium-dependent flow in collateral-perfused rabbit ischemic hindlimb following administration of VEGF. *Circulation*, **91**, 2793–801.

152. Sellke, F. W., Kagaya, Y., Johnson, R. G., Shafique, T., Schoen, F. J., Grossman, W., and Weintraub, R. M. (1992). Endothelial modulation of porcine corinary microcirculation perfused via immature vessels. *Am. J. Physiol.*, **262**, H1669–95.

153. Banai, S., Jaktlish, M. T., Shou, M., Lazarous, D. F., Scheinowitz, M., Biro, S., *et al.* (1994). Angiogenic-induced enhancement of collateral blood flow to ischemic myocardium by vascular endothelial growth factor in dogs. *Circulation*, **89**, 2183–9.

154. Harada, K., Friedman, M., Lopez, J., Prasad, P. V., Hibberd, M., Pearlman, J. D., *et al.* Vascular endothelial growth factor improves coronary flow and myocardial function in chronically ischemic porine hearts. *Am. J. Physiol.* (in press).

155. Graor, R. A. and Gray, B. H. (1991). Interventional treatment of peripheral vascular disease. In *Peripheral vascular diseases* (ed. J. R., Young, R. A., Graor, J. W., Olin, and J. R., Bartholomew), pp. 111–33 Mosby, St Louis, MO.

156. Essed, C. D., Brand, M. V. D., and Becker, A. E. (1983). Transluminal coronary angioplasty and early restenosis. *Br. Heart J.*, **49**, 393–402.

157. Callow, A. D., Choi, E. T., Trachtenberg, J. D., Stevens, S. L., Connolly, D. T., Rodi, C., and Ryan, U. S. (1994). Vascular permeability factor accelerates endothelial

regrowth following balloon angioplasty. *Growth Factors*, **10**, 223–8.

158. Asahara, T., Bauters, C., Pastore, C., Bunting, S., Ferrara, N., Symes, J. F., and Isner. (1995). Local delivery of vascular endothelial growth factor accelerates re-endothelialization and attenuates intimal hyperplasia in balloon-injured rat carotid artery. *Circulation*, **91**, 2802–9.

159. Carmeliet, P., Ferreira, V., Breier, G., Pollefeyt, S., Kieckens, L., Gertenstein, M., *et al.* (1996). Abnormal blood vessel development and lethality in embryos lacking a single VEGF allele. *Nature*, **380**, 435–9.

160. Ferrara, N., Carver-Moore, K., Chen, H., Dowd, M., Lu, L., O'Shea, K. S., *et al.* (1996). Heterozygous embryonic lethality induced by targeted inactivation of the VEGF gene. *Nature*, **380**, 439–42.

161. Levy, A. P., Levy, N. S., and Goldberg, M. A. (1996). Post-transcriptional regulation of vascular endothelial growth factor by hypoxia. *J. Biol. Chem.*, **271**, 2746–53.

162. Iliopulos, O., Levy, A. P., Jiang, C., Kaelin, W. G., and Goldberg, M. A. (1996). Negative regulation of hypoxia-inducible genes by the von Hippel-Lindau protein. *Proc. Natl Acad. Sci. USA*, **93**, 10595–99.

163. Olofsson, B., Pajusola, K., Kaipaineen, A., VonEuler, G., Joukov, V., Saksela, O,. *et al.* (1996). Vascular endothelial growth factor B, a novel growth factor for endothelial cells. *Proc. Natl Acad. Sci. USA*, **93**, 2576–81.

164. Joukov, V., Pajusola, K., Kaipainen, A., Chilov, D., Lahtinen, I., Kukk, E., Saksela, O,. *et al.* (1996). A novel vascular endothelial growth factor, VEGF-C, is a ligand for the FLT4 (VEGFR-3) and KDR (VEGFR-2) receptor tyrosine kinases. *EMBO J.*,**15**, 290–8.

165. Lee, L., Gray, A., Yuan, J., Luoh, S.-M., Avraham, H., and Wood, W. I. (1996). Vascular endothelial growth factor-related protein: A ligand and specific activator of the tyrosine kinase receptor Flt4. *Proc. Natl Acad. Sci. USA*, **93**, 1988–92.

166. Keyt, B., Nguyen, H., Berleau, L., Duarte, C., Park, J., Chen, H., and Ferrara, N. (1996). Identification of VEGF determinants for binding Flt-1 and KDR receptors. Generation of receptor-selective VEGF variants by site-directed mutagenesis. *J. Biol. Chem.*, **271**, 5638–46.

167. Davis-Smyth, T., Chen, H., Park, J., Presta, L. G., and Ferrara, N. (1996). The second immunoglobulin-like domain of the VEGF tyrosine kinase receptor Flt-1 determines ligand binding and may initiate a signal transduction cascade. *EMBO J.*, **15**, 4919–27.

168. Isner, J. M., Pieczek, A., Schainfeld, R., Blair, R., Haley, L., Asahara, T., Rosenfield, K., Razvi, S., Walsh, K., Symes, J. F. (1996). Clinical evidence of angiogenesis following arterial gene transfer of ph VEGF$_{165}$ in patient with ischaemic limb. *Lancet*, **348**, 370–74.

17. The role of fibroblast growth factors in tumour progression and angiogenesis

Gerhard Christofori

Introduction

Already in 1939 and 1945 it had been demonstrated that tumours induce the formation of new capillaries from pre-existing blood vessels, a process termed angiogenesis (1,2). Subsequently, it was shown that soluble angiogenic factors released by tumours were responsible for this process (3,4). The finding that many of these growth factors bound to heparin allowed the purification and classification of a family of heparin-binding growth factors (5). The prototypes of this family are fibroblast growth factor (FGF) 1 and FGF-2, and they have been studied in great detail in many physiological and pathological processes (reviewed in references 6–10). To date the family has expanded to nine distinct, but closely related family members. Based on their pattern of expression and their biological activities they are thought to be involved in many physiological and pathological processes, including embryonic development, differentiation, cell survival, angiogenesis, oncogenic transformation, and tumour cell proliferation.

The vast number of biological activities together with the variety of target cells makes FGFs highly pleiotropic growth factors. This is further complicated by the fact that four distinct FGF receptors exist in many alternative isoforms with varying binding affinities and different signal transduction pathways. The combination of these variables make it difficult to dissect the functions of FGFs *in vivo*. Most knowledge about specific activities of FGFs and their receptors originates from experiments conducted *in vitro*, examining one specific activity and target cell type at a time. Consequently, pleiotropic as well as synergistic effects have not been resolved, and the functional roles of FGFs *in vivo* are not well understood.

The scope of this chapter is to review the current knowledge about the FGF family members and their receptors, and about their specific activities and biological functions. In particular, recent experimental results that address the actual role of FGFs in the autocrine and paracrine stimulation of tumour cell proliferation will be discussed, in physiological and pathological angiogenesis and in tumour angiogenesis and potential pathways that may regulate FGF activity will be described.

Fibroblast growth factor family members

The nine members of the FGF family are structurally related with up to ~55% sequence identity at the amino acid level. They are also highly conserved between species. All FGFs are 18–30 kDa proteins with high-heparin-binding affinity, which has given them their early family name of heparin-binding growth factors (HBGF) (6). The genes for FGFs are all structured in three exons separated by two introns exhibiting dramatically different lengths within the family members; the total length of the introns is 1.1 kb in the FGF-4 gene, 19 kb in the FGF-5 gene, and more than 30 kb in the FGF-2 gene. The coding regions are highly conserved within a central core region, whereas the more N-terminal and C-terminal regions have diverged (Fig. 17.1). FGFs are mitogens for a wide variety of cells of mesodermal and neuroectodermal origin, and the various FGF family members exhibit diverse biological activities by targeting a large number of different cell types. They have been implicated in many physiological and pathological processes, including embryonic development, wound healing, angiogenesis, differentiation, neuronal outgrowth, cell survival, migration, invasion, and transformation. Some of the features of the nine FGF family members are summarized in Table 17.1.

Acidic fibroblast growth factor (FGF-1)

FGF-1 was first identified as mitogenic activity in neural tissue extracts and in bovine brain and was named acidic FGF because of its acidic pI value of 5. FGF-1 is a 18 kDa 154 amino acid protein with truncated forms of 140 and 134 amino acids that possibly originate from a combination of proteolytic cleavage and disulphide rearrangement. Truncation probably has no physiological relevance (6,11). The N-terminus of the 154 amino acid form is

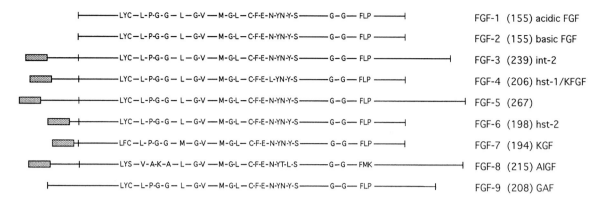

Figure 17.1. Schematic representation of the members of the fibroblast growth factor (FGF) family of proteins. Amino acid residues that are highly conserved among human members of the FGF family, with the exception of murine FGF-8, are shown. Stipled boxes at the N-terminus represent signal peptides. The length of the proteins (in amino acids) is given in parentheses.

Table 17.1. Properties of human FGF family members

Growth factor	Primary translation product[a]	Subcellular localization	Heparin affinity[b]	Gene mapping (human)
FGF-1 (aFGF)	155	no signal peptide cytosol (endo)[d] nuclear (exo)[d]	1.0 M	5q31–33
FGF-2 (bFGF)	155	no signal peptide cytosol (endo)[d] nuclear (exo)[d]	1.5 M	4q25
	196[c] 201[c] 210[c]	no signal peptide nuclear and cytosol		
FGF-3 (int-2)	239	secreted nuclear and cytosol	ND	11q13
	271[c]	nuclear and cytosol		
FGF-4 (hst-1; KGF)	206	secreted	1.0–1.2 M	11q13
FGF-5	267	secreted	1.0–1.5 M	4q21
FGF-6 (hst-2)	198	secreted	ND	12p13
FGF-7 (KGF)	194	secreted	0.6 M	ND
FGF-8 (AIGF)	215 (mouse)	secreted	ND	ND
FGF-9 (GAF)	208	no signal peptide, but secreted	ND	ND

[a] Number of amino acids.
[b] NaCl concentration required for the elution from heparin affinity columns.
[c] Products of initiation at upstream CUG codons.
[d] exo, exogenously added FGF is bound to FGF receptors, internalized and targeted to the nucleus; endo; endogenously synthesized FGF is predominantly present in the cytoplasm, but also found at low levels in the nucleus (see text).
ND: binds to heparin, but the exact affinity has not been determined.

acetylated; however, non-acetylated FGF-1 produced in bacteria or mammalian cells has equivalent activity (12). The primary translation product is 155 amino acids based on the cDNA sequence indicating that some form of protein processing may occur. There is no evidence for a N-terminal extended form of FGF-1, as a termination codon is found at −1 of the AUG initiation codon. Most curiously, FGF-1 does not have a signal peptide for secretion.

Heparin enhances the mitogenic activity of FGF-1 on target cells, by stabilizing the relatively labile FGF-1 in an active conformation and protecting it against denaturation by heat, extreme pH, and proteolysis (13). The resolution of the crystal structure of FGF-1 together with peptide competition experiments has revealed that the heparin and receptor binding domains differ (14–17). FGF-1 has three cysteine residues, two of which are conserved in the other FGF family members. Substitution of any of the three cysteines by serine results in stabilization of FGF-1 independent of heparin and does not affect its biological activities (18,19). FGF-1 binds copper, and it has been shown that copper induced the formation of biologically inactive homodimers (20). Such dimer formation may be involved in the export of FGF-1 from producer cells (see section on 'Export of FGF-1 and FGF-2', p. 222).

FGF-1 is found in the nucleus of many cells, and a putative nuclear localization signal has been located at amino acids 21–27. Deletion of this nuclear localization sequence resulted in loss of mitogenic activity of FGF-1, which could be restored by addition of the yeast histone 2B nuclear localization site (21). Notably, FGF-1 was targeted to the nucleus when added exogenously to endothelial cells, whereas internal synthesized FGF-1 was only inefficiently localized to the nucleus, implicating a novel signal transduction/import pathway (22,23; also see section on 'Internalization and subcellular localization of FGFs', p. 211).

FGF-1 is predominantly expressed in neural and neuroendocrine tissues, and it is found in distinct regions of kidney, cardiac muscle, prostate, islets of Langerhans, cerebrum, and cerebellum. It is also expressed by a variety of cultured cell lines including vascular smooth muscle cells and a number of tumour cell lines. FGF-1 is a potent inducer of DNA synthesis, proliferation, cell survival, differentiation, and cell migration in a large number of normal diploid cell types and established cell lines of mesodermal origin, including fibroblasts, endothelial cells, myoblasts, chondrocytes, osteoblasts, and of neuroectodermal origin, including neuroblasts and astroglial cells (for other examples see references 6,9).

Attempts to dissect the biological role of FGF-1 in specific bioassays revealed many different functions. Among them, FGF-1 may play an important part in the autocrine and paracrine growth regulation of tumour cells and in angiogenesis.

Basic fibroblast growth factor (FGF-2)

FGF-2 was initially purified from bovine pituitary and based on the pI of 9.6 it was named basic FGF. Subsequently, it was also purified from many other tissues. FGF-2 is a 18 kDa, 155 amino acid protein. Nine amino acids at the N-terminus are sometimes proteolytically removed during the experimental extraction procedure. FGF-2, like FGF-1, does not have a signal sequence for secretion (reviewed in references 6,7,9,10). However, N-terminal extended isoforms of approximately 22, 23, and 25 kDa have been described. They originate from unusual translational initiation at CUG codons upstream of the original AUG initiation codon (22–24). While the 18 kDa form of FGF-2 is localized to the cytosol, these high-molecular weight forms are predominantly associated with the nucleus due to a nuclear localization signal in the alternatively expressed N-terminal region (22). Similar to FGF-1, the 18 kDa form of FGF-2 is translocated to the nucleus and nucleolus when added exogenously. A potential nuclear localization site has been described at amino acids 26–31. Mutation in this region did not affect mitogenic activity; however, stimulation of plasminogen activator production was reduced (25). Further investigation is warranted to elucidate the functional role of the nuclear localization of FGF-1 and FGF-2 (see also section on 'Internalization and subcellular localization of FGFs', p. 211).

FGF-2 has a higher affinity for heparin than FGF-1; it elutes at a salt concentration of 1.4–1.6 mol/l from heparin columns (Table 17.1). However, unlike FGF-1, heparin does not exhibit a stimulatory effect on the activity of FGF-2. FGF-2 contains four cysteines including the two that are conserved in the other family members. Mutation of the cysteine residues in FGF-2 resulted in stabilization and resistance against acidic pH, but did not affect its mitogenic activity (26). This feature of mutated FGF-2 is currently being exploited therapeutically in the treatment of duodenal ulcers (27).

Resolution of the crystal structure of FGF-2, peptide competition experiments and specific neutralizing antibodies have localized the receptor binding site to two regions distinct from the heparin-binding sites (15,28–30). FGF is a substrate for phosphorylation by protein kinase C at Ser-72 and protein kinase A at Thr-120 resulting in an increased receptor binding affinity of the protein. Indeed, phosphorylated FGF-2 has been found in extracts of cultured endothelial cells (31).

FGF-2 is expressed in almost all organs and tissues examined. It is found in many cultured cell types, including fibroblasts, endothelial cells, glial cells, and smooth muscle cells. Many tumours and tumour cell lines express FGF-2 as an autocrine growth regulatory factor (see section on 'Oncogenic activity of FGF family members', p. 000). FGF-2 has essentially the same target cell types as FGF-1 (6,7). The only exception may be melanocytes which respond to FGF-2, but not to FGF-1 (32).

The biological activities of FGF-2 have been extensively studied and documented *in vivo* and *in vitro*. For example, the direct involvement of FGF-2 in *Xenopus* embryonic development has been demonstrated (reviewed in reference 33). FGF-2 stimulates DNA synthesis, cell proliferation, and migration in a variety of cell types. It also stimulates cell differentiation. For example, exposure to FGF-2 induces the differentiation of sheep pre-adipocyte fibroblasts into adipocytes. Moreover, FGF-2 as a competence factor stimulates haematopoiesis (34) and it may function as a mitogen in megakaryocytopoiesis (35). FGF-2 is also a survival factor for a number of neuronal cell types, such as injured cholinergic neurons (36). Finally, FGF-2 is angiogenic *in vitro* and *in vivo*. Based on its pleiotropic activities, FGF-2 has been proposed to be involved in many different physiological and pathological processes, including embryonic development, cell differentiation, cell survival, angiogenesis, and tumorigenesis.

int-2 (FGF-3)

FGF-3 was originally identified due to the insertion of mouse mammary tumour virus next to the FGF-3 gene causing transcriptional activation of FGF-3 (37). Inspired by the insertion event, the gene was named int-2. It was later discovered that int-2 had 44% identity to FGF-2, and it was renamed as FGF-3 (38). Alternative use of three distinct promoters and two poly(A) sites result in different mRNA species (39,40). FGF-3 usually is a protein of 239 amino acids in human and of 245 amino acids in mice. However, FGF-3 that has been transcribed from its P2 promoter initiates translation from a CUG initiation codon upstream of the conventional AUG initiation codon resulting in a 271 and 274 amino acid protein, respectively. The CUG initiated forms of FGF-3 were found in both the secretory pathway and in the nucleus due to a competition between a rather atypical signal peptide and a bipartite nuclear localization signal. The differential subcellular localization also resulted in diverse biological effects. Once imported to the nucleus, FGF-3 was localized to the nucleolus, and the exclusive expression of a mutant form that localizes to the nucleolus resulted in inhibition of cell proliferation (40,41). Secretion of FGF-3 is rather inefficient, and it has been shown that immature forms of FGF-3 accumulate in the Golgi from where they were only slowly released into the extracellular matrix. N-terminal modification and glycosylation were suspected to be involved in the retention of the protein (42).

FGF-3 is mainly expressed during embryonic development, during early gestation to mid-somite stage in mesodermal cells of the primitive streak and of parietal endoderm. It is also found in migrating mesoderm, neuroepithelial cells of the hindbrain and pharyngeal pouches. Based on its expression pattern and secretion it has been proposed to induce migration of cells during development, and to be involved in spatial patterning (43). FGF-3 is not expressed in adult tissues and is usually not found in cultured cell lines. However, the gene for FGF-3 was found to be amplified in a number of different tumour types, including breast cancer and squamous cell carcinoma of head and neck (44,45). The biological activities of FGF-3 are not well understood. FGF-3 is able to transform NIH 3T3 cells, however, only when expressed at high levels (46). FGF-3 is not angiogenic in a variety of bioassays. Disruption of the genes for FGF-3 by homologous recombination in mice led to tail and inner ear abnormalities among other deficiencies (47).

hst-1, KFGF (FGF-4)

FGF-4 was discovered by its transforming activity in DNA derived from human stomach cancer (named hst-1) and as KFGF in DNA extracted from Kaposi sarcoma lesions (48,49). FGF-4 is a 206 amino acid protein in humans and 202 amino acids in mice. The N-terminal region (30–31 amino acids) contains the signal peptide that is cleaved to give a secreted protein of 175 or 176 amino acids. Together with N-linked glycosylation, the molecular weight is approximately 22–23 kDa. FGF-4 is efficiently secreted by cells that produce it. Mutation of the glycosylation site does not affect secretion, but gives rise to cleavage products (13 and 15 kDa) that exhibit stronger biological activity than wild-type FGF-4 (50).

FGF-4 is expressed early during embryonic development, but not in adult tissues or normal cell lines in culture. Mice that carry a disruption of both alleles of the FGF-4 gene die shortly after implantation of the blastocyst. Apparently, the inner cell mass is impaired, and growth and differentiation of the FGF-4-deficient inner cell mass can be rescued by addition of recombinant FGF-4 (51). Later in development FGF-4 is expressed in the primitive streak and myotomes, spatially restricted within many sites. The expression pattern partially overlaps, but is distinct from FGF-5 (52). FGF-4 has been demonstrated to play a pivotal part in limb development, myogenesis, and tooth development (reviewed in references 53–55). During the development of the limb in chicken and mouse, FGF-4 is expressed in the apical–ectodermal ridge directing the outgrowth and patterning of the limb. It provides all signals necessary for outgrowth of the limb and for maintaining the polarizing activity of limb bud cells *in vivo* and *in vitro*. Indeed, polymeric beads releasing the factor can induce ectopic limb formation, further emphasizing the central part FGF-4 plays in this developmental process (56).

Transfection and high expression of FGF-4 leads to autocrine transformation of cells via FGF receptors on the cell surface. Furthermore, gene amplification and/or up-regulated expression of FGF-4 has been found to correlate with the malignant phenotype in many types of cancer cells suggesting that FGF-4 plays a major part in oncogenic transformation and tumour progression (see section on 'Oncogenic activity of FGF family members'). FGF-4 is a mitogen for fibroblasts and vascular endothelial cells, and is angiogenic *in vitro* and *in vivo* (57).

FGF-5

FGF-5 was identified by transformation of NIH 3T3 cells with DNA extracted from human bladder tumours (58). The core region of FGF-5 exhibits 50% identity to FGF-2. FGF-5 is a protein of 267 amino acids, and N-linked and possibly O-linked glycosylation result in a secreted protein of 32.5–38.5 kDa (59). FGF-5 is expressed at spatially and temporally restricted sites in the developing mouse embryo (60), and a role in gastrulation has been suggested (61). FGF-5 mRNA is detectable in adult brain with distinct spatial expression, at least in part, in neurons (62,63). However, no protein could be found in tissue extracts. Targeted mutation of the FGF-5 gene by homologous recombination or spontaneous mutation of the FGF-5 gene in the angora (go) mouse result in abnormally long hair due to a defect of hair growth cycle regulation (64). Although FGF-5 and FGF-4 have partially overlapping patterns of expression during embryonic development, inactivation of FGF-4 gene function causes early embryonic lethality, whereas the loss of FGF-5 only results in this mild hair growth defect, suggesting that the FGF family members exert dramatically different functions in embryonic development. FGF-5 is expressed in some tumour cell lines, and in normal fibroblasts it can be induced by serum growth factors (65,66). FGF-5 is mitogenic for BALB/c 3T3 cells and fetal bovine heart endothelial cells in culture (58). Furthermore, it exerts neurotrophic activity on motoneurons, rat septal cholinergic and raphe serotonergic neurons and, thus, may play an important part in neural development (67,68).

FGF-6

FGF-6 was cloned by its homology to FGF-4 and by its transforming activity (69,70). It is structurally very similar to FGF-4 with 70% identity at the amino acid level. FGF-6 is secreted as a glycosylated protein of 25 kDa (71). Little is known about the expression of FGF-6 or its biological role. In mouse embryos, expression of FGF-6 is detected first at embryonic day 9.5. It is expressed exclusively in the myotomal compartment of the somite. In later stages of development expression of FGF-6 is restricted to the skeletal muscle lineage, and it is postulated that FGF-6 is involved in body wall and skeletal muscle development (72). In the adult, expression of FGF-6 has been detected in skeletal muscle, heart, and testis (71). While FGF-6 is mitogenic for BALB/c 3T3 fibroblasts, only a limited heparin-dependent response has been described in bovine aortic endothelial cells (73).

Keratinocyte growth factor (KGF) (FGF-7)

FGF-7 was isolated as a mitogen for cultured keratinocytes from fibroblasts (74). It consists of 194 amino acids, the 64 amino acids at the N-terminus are unique, and the remainder exhibits 30% identity to FGF-3 (75). It has a hydrophobic signal sequence and is efficiently secreted as a 28 kDa, N-glycosylated protein.

FGF-7 is produced by fibroblasts *in vivo*, and its mRNA is expressed in adult kidney, colon, and ileum, but not in brain or lung (75). FGF-7 is mitogenic for many epithelial and stromal cells, but exhibits only little activity on mesenchyme-derived cell lines. The highest mitogenic activity is found with keratinocytes. During embryonic development FGF-7 is transiently expressed in the developing myocardium, myotomes, cleaved muscles, and in the ventricular zone of the developing forebrain. Later in development it is expressed in mesenchymal cells, suggesting that it might play an important part in mesenchymal–epithelial interactions (76). FGF-7 is highly up-regulated upon wounding of the skin, suggesting that it has a part in the wound healing process (77).

Androgen-induced growth factor (AIGF) (FGF-8)

FGF-8 was purified and cloned from the androgen-dependent mouse mammary carcinoma cell line SC3 (78,79). It is a polypeptide chain of 215 amino acids in length and is 30–40% identical to the other FGF family members. FGF-8 carries a signal peptide and is efficiently secreted as 28 and 32 kDa proteins. A potential alternative splice pattern would result in molecular weights of 22 and 28 kDa, thus the two isoforms are probably glycosylated. Its expression is induced by testosterone in SC3 cells; it is the first growth factor to show such an inducibility. Only one of the two conserved cysteine residues is present in FGF-8, corresponding to Cys-100 in FGF-2. Also, the domain which supposedly binds to the receptor exhibits only 44% identity to the other family members, indicating that FGF-8 might have diverged from the other members of the family. FGF-8 is an autocrine growth factor for androgen dependent mammary carcinoma cells.

Glia-activating factor (GAF) (FGF-9)

FGF-9 is the most recent member of the FGF family. It has been purified and cloned from human glioma cell lines and rat brain (80,81). Its amino acid sequence in the conserved core region is approximately 30% identical to the other family members and is conserved to 94% between human and rat. The cDNA sequence predicts an amino acid sequence of 208 amino acids in length. Curiously, FGF-9 does not have a signal peptide for secretion, yet it is found as a glycoprotein in the conditioned medium of transfected COS or Chinese hamster ovary (CHO) cells. Proteins with molecular weights of 30, 29, and 25 kDa have been purified from the culture medium. These isoforms probably arise due to N-terminal truncation during the purification procedure. FGF-9 is known to be expressed in brain and kidney of adult rats. It is a mitogen for O-2A progenitor cells, PC12 cells, BALB/c rat glial cells but not for human umbilical cord endothelial cells, even in the presence of heparin. FGF-9 may further have transforming activity on BALB/c 3T3 cells.

Fibroblast growth factor receptors

Two types of FGF-binding sites have been identified on a large number of different tissues and cell types, first indirectly by binding of radiolabelled ligands to cells and tissues, and subsequently by detailed biochemical characterization and isolation of cDNAs (reviewed in references 82–84). High-affinity receptors for FGF represent low number (10^4–10^5 receptors per cell), but high-affinity binding sites (K_d of ~20–600 pM) for FGF. They are typical members of the transmembrane tyrosine kinase family of receptors. Thus far, at least four members have been identified and cDNAs isolated; however, an enormous diversity of alternative mRNA processing possibilities results in different extracellular domains with variable ligand specificity and affinity (Table 17.2). Alternative splicing also produces soluble forms of some of the high-affinity FGF receptors.

Low-affinity binding sites have been characterized that exhibit high capacity ($1–2 \times 10^6$ sites per cell), but low affinity for ligand binding (K_d of ~2–20 nM). Low-affinity receptors for FGF are predominantly proteoglycans carrying heparan sulphate side chains that bind FGFs. They sequester and present FGFs to their high-affinity receptors, but are unable to activate a signal transduction cascade on their own (13,85–87).

High-affinity fibroblast growth factor receptors

The first receptor for FGF was purified and the cDNA isolated as a high-affinity receptor for FGF-2 from chicken (88). This receptor was highly homologous to the flg tyro-

Table 17.2. Properties of high affinity FGF receptors

Receptor	Other names	Apparent molecular weight[a]	mRNA length	Gene mapping (human)	FGF binding[b]
FGFR-1	flg, cek 1	150 kDa	4.2 kb 4.3 kb	8pl2	IIIa: 1, 2 IIIb: 1 IIIc: 1, 2, 4, 5, 6
FGFR-2	KGF receptor bek, cek 3	135 kDa	4.4 kb	10q26	IIIb: 7, 1 IIIc: 1, 2, 4
FGFR-3	cek 2	135 kDa	4.5 kb	4p16.3	IIIb: 1 IIIc: 1, 2, 4
FGFR-4		110 kDa	3.0 kb	5q35	1, 4, 6

[a] Apparent molecular weight of transmembrane isoforms.
[b] FGFs that bind with high affinity to the different Ig loop III splice variants are presented (see text). Note that not all members of the FGF family have been tested for their binding to the alternative isoforms of the FGF receptors.

sine kinase cDNA previously cloned from human endothelial cells, and it was named FGF receptor 1 (FGFR-1). Subsequently, FGFR-1 was shown to bind FGF-1, FGF-2, and FGF-4 (89–92).

FGFR-2 was first identified by screening of a mouse liver expression library with anti-phosphotyrosine antibodies and called bek (93). Subsequent molecular cloning of human, murine, and chicken homologues to bek revealed that it is a receptor for FGF-1 and FGF-2 (89,94,95). It was also identified and cloned as an amplified gene in stomach cancer (K-sam; 96). FGFR-2 binds FGF-1, FGF-2, and FGF-4 with high affinity, but not FGF-5 or FGF-7 (KGF). A variant of FGFR-2 was identified by expression cloning as KGF receptor and was shown to be a splice variant of the bek gene (see below; (97,98).

FGFR-3 was cloned from human leukaemia cell lines by low stringency hybridization and degenerate polymerase chain reaction methods (99,100). FGFR-3 turned out to be highly homologous to the previously cloned orphan tyrosine kinase receptor cek-2 (94).

FGFR-4 was also cloned by degenerate PCR methods targeting the conserved tyrosine kinase domain of receptor tyrosine kinases from human leukaemia cell lines (100). FGFR-4 binds FGF-1 and FGF-6 with high affinity, FGF-4 with lower affinity, and FGF-2 with an even lower affinity (101,102).

The overall structure of the four members of the FGF receptor family is identical and can be summarized from N- to C-terminus as follows (Fig. 17.2A): signal peptide, two or three extracellular immunoglobulin like loops

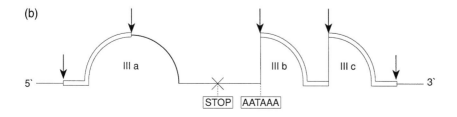

Figure 17.2. (a) Schematic representation of the structural domains of the fibroblast growth factor (FGF) receptor family. The different functional domains are indicated to the right. Location of the domains in FGFR-1 are given in amino acid number from N- to C-terminus on the left. (b) Schematic representation of the genomic structure for the region encoding the third immunoglobulin domain of FGFR-1. The two alternative exons IIIb and IIIc are used for transmembrane forms of the receptor. Alternative usage of the exon IIIa results in the use of the polyadenylation site (indicated as AATAAA) and translational termination at an stop codon (STOP) resulting into a soluble receptor. Arrows indicate the different alternative splice sites.

(immunoglobulin domains), characteristic acidic region between first and second immunoglobulin domain, trans-membrane domain, cytoplasmic domain with the catalytic tyrosine kinase domain split by a 14 amino acid kinase insert similar to platelet-derived growth factor (PDGF) receptor, and a carboxy-terminal tail (reviewed in reference 103). All four receptors are highly homologous to each other with 70–80% amino acid identity in the ligand binding domains (immunoglobulin loops II and III) and in the tyrosine kinase domain. Other less conserved regions still exhibit 50–60% homology (100).

Complex alternative splicing combined with alternative polyadenylation creates a high diversity in receptor iso-forms for FGFR-1 to -3, but not for FGFR-4, resulting both in receptors with distinct and others with redundant functions, ligand specificities, and signal transduction pathways (82,83,104 and references therein). Some of these receptor variants are described below.

One of the more general splicing variations found in FGFR-1, FGFR-2, and FGFR-3 affects the FGF binding domain and, thus, the ligand specificity of the receptors (Fig. 17.2). Alternative usage of exons IIIb and IIIc encoding the alternative second halves of the third immunoglobulin domain, creates different membrane spanning forms (Fig. 17.2B). In comparison with FGFR-1 containing the immunoglobulin loop IIIc, use of immuno-globulin loop IIIb reduces the affinity for FGF-2 about 50-fold, whereas the affinity for FGF-1 is not affected (92,105). Use of a polyadenylation site preceding these alternative exons produces a receptor variant that lacks transmembrane and cytoplasmic domains and is soluble (IIIa; 106,107). This soluble form of FGFR-1 is functional in that it can bind FGF-1 and FGF-2 (105).

With FGFR-2 this alternative splicing event results in a dramatic difference in ligand-binding specificity: use of immunoglobulin loop IIIc gives a receptor which binds FGF-1 and FGF-2 with high affinity, but not FGF-7 (KGF). FGFR-2 containing immunoglobulin loop IIIb binds FGF-7 (KGF) with very high and FGF-1 and FGF-2 with 50-fold lower affinity. Thus, two growth factor receptors with different ligand specificities are encoded by alternate transcripts from the same gene (98,108).

The alternative immunoglobulin loop III isoforms of FGFR-3 also exhibit different ligand specificities. FGF-1, FGF-4, and to a lesser extent FGF-2 bind and activate the immunoglobulin loop IIIc isoform of FGFR-3. In contrast, the immunoglobulin loop IIIb isoform exclusively binds FGF-1 (92). A soluble IIIa isoform of FGFR-3 has also been detected; however, the function of these soluble receptors remains unknown.

That the binding specificity is predominantly defined by the immunoglobulin loop III domain was demonstrated by

experiments where the immunoglobulin loop III of FGFR-3 was replaced by the immunoglobulin loop IIIc of FGFR-1. Similar to FGFR-1 the resulting chimeric receptor bound FGF1, FGF-2, FGF-4, FGF-5, and FGF-6, but not FGF-7. Replacement of the immunoglobulin loop III of FGFR-3 by the FGFR-2 immunoglobulin loop IIIb resulted in binding of FGF-7. In contrast, fusion of the FGFR-2 IIIb domain on to FGFR-1 did not result in FGF-7 binding indicating that FGFR-1 might also depend on other domains in defining ligand-binding specificity (109,110).

In addition to the splice variants described above, many other alternative products have been described. For example, another splicing event leads to FGFR-1 isoforms that contain only two of the three immunoglobulin loops and that exhibit qualitatively similar ligand-binding activities for FGF-1 and FGF-2 (90,107,111). A po-tentially secreted form of FGFR-1 containing only the first immunoglobulin loop I and the acidic motif has also been described (112). Furthermore, three truncated extracellular domain forms of FGFR-1 have been identified as soluble FGF-binding proteins in blood and in the extracellular matrix and basement membrane of vascular endothelial cells. Their biological function, however, remains unclear (112,113). The structure–function relationship of the splice variant receptors and their biological role has just started to be addressed and mutational analysis has revealed many details of ligand–receptor interaction and of receptor signal transduction (reviewed in reference 82).

FGF receptors that lack an active tyrosine kinase domain can be employed as dominant negative FGF receptors. Such a tyrosine kinase deficient form of FGFR-2 IIIb has been expressed in transgenic mice in lung epi-thelia resulting in dramatic inhibition of branching and development of lung airway epithelia (114), and in the skin of transgenic mice resulting in the perturbation of the organization and differentiation of keratinocytes (115). Such dominant-negative forms of the FGF receptors will be useful tools to investigate the biological functions of FGF ligands and receptors.

FGF receptors, like their ligands, are heparin-binding proteins. It has been shown that heparin binds to immunoglobulin loop II, and that receptor binding and FGF-mediated mitogenicity are dependent on the presence of heparin or heparin-like molecules (92,116–118). Data from many experiments suggest that the high-affinity receptor complex is an intimate ternary complex of the transmembrane tyrosine kinase receptor, heparan sulphate glycosaminoglycans, and FGF ligands. Each of these com-ponents has binding domains, and together these com-ponents define ligand specificity and binding affinity (82; see later).

FGF receptors are expressed in many tissues and cell lines, showing overlapping, but distinct expression patterns during embryonic development (83,119–121). FGFR-1 is predominantly expressed in the central nervous system and skin. The soluble isoform IIIa is expressed in brain, skeletal muscle, and skin, isoform IIIb is predominantly expressed in skin, and isoform IIIc is found in almost all tissues except liver (105,122). FGFR-2 is expressed in adult mouse liver, lung, brain, kidney, but not in heart and spleen (93). During embryonic development it is expressed in embryonic lung epithelia (121,123). A correlation of alternative usage of the immunoglobulin III loop of FGFR-2 has been reported during epithelial–mesenchymal transition and in the malignant progression of the prostate during epithelial to stromal/mesenchymal conversion of the tumour cells. Epithelial cells express exclusively the IIIb isoform of the FGFR-2, the KGF receptor, whereas mesenchymal cells synthesize the IIIc isoform, the FGF-1 and FGF-2 receptor (124,125). FGFR-4 is expressed at particularly high levels in fetal adrenals, but not in brain, bone, skin, and other sites where the others FGFRs are expressed (100). FGFR-4 is also present in definitive endoderm and skeletal muscle lineage in the developing mouse embryo (126).

Inactivation of FGFR-1 gene function by homologous recombination in mice resulted in embryonic lethality during early post-implantation development. From these results it has been concluded that FGFR-1 is required for proper embryo cell proliferation, for correct axial formation and for mesodermal patterning (127,128). Although the four members of the FGF receptor family are very similar to each other in activity and are expressed in partially overlapping patterns during embryonic development, inactivation of one receptor results in a very severe phenotype, indicating that FGF receptors function in a non-redundant manner and exert very specific activities. Recently, unique mutations in FGF receptors have been shown to be associated with human skeletal disorders (reviewed in reference 129). Mutation of FGFR-1 correlated with the Pfeiffer syndrome, and mutation of FGFR-2 were found to be associated with several syndromes including Crouzon, Pfeiffer, Apert, and Jackson–Weis syndromes. Furthermore, dominant mutations in different domains of FGFR-3 correlated with several different skeletal dysplasias. These results suggest an important role for FGF receptors in bone development.

FGFR-1 is also utilized as a specific entry site for herpes simplex virus type I during viral infection. Association of FGF-2 with virus particles has been suggested to allow virus entry (130,131). Furthermore, FGF receptors are frequently up-regulated in many cancers, suggesting that autocrine or paracrine growth stimulation by FGF ligands and FGF receptors plays an important part in tumour progression (see later).

Low-affinity fibroblast growth factor receptors

FGF-2 has been localized to the extracelluar matrix and the basement membrane of endothelial cells and other cell types (reviewed in references (13,85,86)). Using competition experiments, low-affinity binding sites for FGF have been biochemically characterized. Some of these receptors for FGF have been isolated and cloned. Examples of these transmembrane proteoglycan cores are syndecan and perlecan (132,133). In general, low-affinity receptors contain heparan sulphate side chains, and by binding to the heparan sulphate moiety FGFs are sequestered on the cell surface. Heparan sulphate side chains are specific for this binding; other glycosaminoglycans, such as dermatan sulphate, keratan sulphate, or chondroitin sulphate do not bind FGFs (132). These low-affinity receptors for FGF are found in the extracellular matrix, the basement membrane, and the cell surface. It has been suggested that binding of FGFs to the heparan sulphate proteoglycans (HSPGs) will result in protection and storage of FGF in the extracellular matrix and in basement membrane (134). Heparin, heparan sulphates, and heparitinase are able to release stored FGF *in vitro* and *in vivo* from extracellular matrix, basement membrane and from the cell surface (reviewed in references (13,85–87); see also section on 'Export of FGF-1 and FGF-2', p. 222 and Chapter 18).

High-and low-affinity fibroblast growth factor receptor cooperativity

Both FGF ligands and FGF receptors bind heparin and heparin-like molecules, and it has been demonstrated that heparin or heparan sulphate are also required for the binding of FGF to its receptor. The interaction of heparin, heparan sulphate, or HSPGs (low-affinity receptors) with high-affinity FGF receptors and FGF ligands has been examined by several experimental approaches. In mutant CHO cells that lacked any heparan sulphate low-affinity receptors, binding of FGF to its high-affinity receptor was very inefficient, indicating that binding of FGF to HSPG facilitated its binding to the high-affinity FGF receptors (135). Transfection of FGFR-1 or FGFR-2 into 32D cells, a murine haematopoietic cell line that did not express significant levels of HSPG, also resulted in cells that are growth responsive to FGF-1 and FGF-4, but only in the presence of heparin (116). A similar conclusion was reached in studies where HSPG have been removed by digestion with heparitinase or by prevention of sulphation. Under these conditions FGF-2 did not bind to its high-affinity receptors and the biological activity of FGF-2 was impaired. The failure to bind to its receptors could be rescued by the addition of exogenous soluble heparin (117). These experiments were reproduced in cell-free systems using soluble extracellular domains of the FGF receptor, heparan sulphates and FGF ligand (118,136–138). Collectively, these results have been interpreted in a dual receptor model (135,139). According to this model, FGF is sequestered in the extracellular matrix, basement membrane, or on the cell surface upon binding to the heparan sulphate side chains of low-affinity, but high-capacity receptors. The large number of binding sites leads to an accumulation of FGF ligands on the cell surface, resulting in the delivery of FGFs to the high-affinity, but low-capacity FGF receptors.

Both FGF ligands and FGF receptors bind heparin, and two potential mechanisms have been proposed that may mediate the cooperativity between heparan sulphates, FGF ligands, and FGF receptors. First, heparin could induce a conformational change in the ligand and/or in the receptor to bring about ligand–receptor binding (induced-fit model). In a second model, heparin would induce oligomerization of FGF which might be important for receptor dimerization and activation (140). The latter model is supported by several lines of evidence. FGF-1 binds at high density (one molecule every four to five polysaccharide units) and with high affinity to heparin. Resolution of the crystal structures of FGF-1 and FGF-2 complexed with heparin or synthetic heparan-derived oligosaccharides also indicates that several heparin binding sites on FGF-2 mediate dimerization of FGF molecules (14,141). The resulting oligomerized FGF-1 complexes bind to several receptor molecules leading to receptor dimerization, transphosphorylation, and signal transduction (142,143). This conclusion is consistent with data showing that FGF receptors have multiple FGF-binding sites in immuroglobulin loops II and III, and that hetero- or homodimers of FGF can bind to FGF receptors (110).

Recently, it has been reported that heparin by itself in the absence of FGF ligands is able to stimulate autophosphorylation of FGFR-4 (144). FGFR-4 differs from the other FGF receptors in that it has higher affinity to heparin due to two heparin-binding sites in immuroglobulin loops I and II which are not present in the other receptors. Mutation of the ligand-binding domain of FGFR-4 does not affect the activation by heparin suggesting that in FGFR-4 two different ligands may independently activate signal transduction.

Much more remains to be learned about the functional role of HSPG in FGF signalling and the regulatory roles

that might be associated with these interactions. For example, changes in the heparan sulphate side chains of HSPG might modulate the binding of FGF ligands to their receptors resulting in changed bioactivities. Consistent with this proposition is the report that changes in heparan sulphate side chains result in different binding specificity of cells to FGF-1 and FGF-2 during neural development (145).

Signal transduction pathways

Binding of FGFs to their high-affinity receptors causes the activation of the intrinsic tyrosine kinase activity and a cascade of events, leading eventually to the induction of immediate early gene transcription and to cell proliferation. Like all transmembrane tyrosine kinase receptors, FGF receptors dimerize upon ligand binding and transphosphorylate at tyrosine residues (103). Heterodimerization between different FGF receptors and heterologous transphosphorylation between FGFR-1 and FGFR-2 has been demonstrated indicating that hetero- and homodimers of the types 1–1, 2–2, and 1–2 exist (146,147). Similar heterodimerization events between different splice variants of FGFR-1 have also been demonstrated (82). Thus, the question of ligand specificity and affinity is further complicated.

A major target of tyrosine kinase phosphorylation induced by FGF receptor activation is phospholipase C gamma-1 (PLC gamma-1; 150 kDa). PLC gamma-1 binds via its src-homology 2 (SH2) domain to the major autophosphorylation site of FGFR-1, tyrosine 766 (148–150). The presence of tyrosine residue 766 is not only crucial for PLC gamma-1 activation, but also for receptor internalization and down-regulation (151). A residue corresponding tyrosine 766 is also found in the other members of the FGF receptor family.

Binding of FGF and subsequent activation of FGF receptors results in phosphorylation and activation of a number of substrates including raf kinase, Map-2 kinase, erk ser/thr-protein kinase, cortactin, and two additional unknown proteins, p60 and p130 (reviewed in references 82,83,152). Cortactin is a major substrate for c-*src* tyrosine kinase, and it has been shown that c-*src* associates with cortactin in a FGF-dependent manner. It binds to the FGFR-1 via its SH2 domain and can be immunoprecipitated by antibodies specific for FGFR-1. These data indicate that the FGF-dependent association of c-*src* with FGFR-1 induces the phosphorylation of cortactin (153). Subsequent to the phosphorylation of these substrates transcription of immediate early genes and tissue-type plasminogen activator is up-regulated by mechanisms that remain to be elucidated (21,148,154). Notably, FGF-1 must be exposed to BALB/c 3T3 fibroblast for a minimum of 12 h to cause proliferation. Throughout this time period proteins are phosphorylated at tyrosine residues; however, the pattern of tyrosine phosphorylation at earlier time points differs from that at later time points, indicating that continous tyrosine phosphorylation of various proteins is required to carry the cells through the G_0 to G_1 transition of the cell cycle (155).

Binding of FGFs to FGFR-4 causes a pattern of protein phosphorylation that is slightly different from that of FGFR-1. For example, PLC gamma-1 is phosphorylated by the FGFR-4 to a much higher extent (156). Also, FGFR-4 does not have the two conserved tyrosine residues in the kinase split domain, a region where phospho-inositol-3-kinase is thought to bind to the PDGF receptor. In conclusion, the signalling pathway of activated FGF receptors has just begun to be studied. As with many other receptor tyrosine kinases many little pieces are in hand, but they have not been brought together to complete the puzzle.

Internalization and subcellular localization of fibroblast growth factors

Upon binding to their receptors, FGF-1 and FGF-2 are rapidly internalized with concomitant down-regulation of the surface receptors. However, they are not degraded through the lysosomal pathway like other growth factors, instead fragments of various sizes are stabilized and accumulate within the cell (134,157–159). FGF-2 is internalized by using both pathways, i.e. via binding to low-affinity receptors in the absence of high-affinity receptors, or vice versa by binding to high-affinity receptors in the absence of low-affinity receptors (160,161).

Some of the *exogenously* added FGF-2 that is internalized upon binding to its receptors is taken up into the nucleus where it resides within the nucleolus, the nucleo-plasmic network, and the nuclear chromatin (162–164). This nuclear uptake appears to be dependent on the cell's state of proliferation. A putative nuclear translocation signal has been identified in FGF-2 at amino acids 26–31. However, detailed mutational analysis of the nuclear localization sequence revealed that it was not required for nuclear localization, rather it was important for protein stability, thereby modulating the biological activity of FGF-2 (165). This nuclear translocation should not be confused with the nuclear targeting of *endogenous* FGF-2 isoforms that originate from CUG initiation codons upstream of the original AUG start site. The additional N-terminal codon region of these higher molecular weight forms of FGF-2 contains a nuclear localization site which

translocates the endogenously synthesized isoforms of FGF-2 into the nucleus (22).

FGF-1 was also found in considerable amounts in the nucleus (21,166). As with FGF-2, *exogenously* added FGF-1 was imported to the nucleus by binding to its receptors. A putative nuclear localization signal NYKKPKL has been identified that is required for this exogenous pathway (159,167). Mutant FGF-1 that carried a deletion of this sequence still bound to its receptors and was internalized, but failed to stimulate DNA synthesis in target cells, although tyrosine phosphorylation and the induction of c-*fos* expression appeared to be unaffected. However, as with FGF-2, the mutant proteins were less stable, making a straightforward conclusion impossible (21,159,168,169). FGF-1 added to 3T3 fibroblasts was also imported to the nucleus upon binding to its receptors and progression of the cells through the G_1 phase of the cell cycle (155). Upon maximum stimulation of tyrosine kinase activity, during G_1 phase of the cell cycle, FGFR-1 is translocated into the nucleus where it still exhibits tyrosine kinase activity (170).

How FGF-1 or FGF-2 enter the nucleus and how their nuclear translocation affects signal transduction remains to be elucidated. The requirement for long-lasting exposure of endothelial cells or fibroblasts to FGF-1 or FGF-2 for induction of proliferation suggests that receptor binding must be saturated and/or that internalization of the ligand/receptor complex is a rate-limiting step (171,172). The data discussed above can be summarized in a biphasic model of FGF signal transduction. In an early phase, FGF binds to its receptors which are internalized and down-regulated. This phase most probably commits the cells to entering the cell cycle (G_0/G_1 commitment). In a second, late phase of exposure to FGF ligand, low levels of the surface receptors bind ligand, internalize, and trans-locate together with the ligand to the nucleus. As a result, hyperphosphorylation of 'late' tyrosine kinase substrates induces DNA synthesis and G_1 progression (155).

An interesting approach towards the dissection of FGF signalling, receptor internalization, and nuclear import has been reported recently (173). FGF-1 fused to diphtheria toxin was exposed to cells lacking functional FGF receptors, but bearing a high number of diphteria toxin receptors, resulting in stimulation of DNA synthesis. In cells carrying FGF receptors, but lacking diphtheria toxin receptors, only wild-type FGF-1, but not the chimeric protein, were imported into the nucleus and stimulated DNA synthesis. However, both FGF-1 and the FGF–diphtheria toxin fusion protein were able to initiate phosphorylation of tyrosine substrates. This experiment also suggests that FGF receptors utilize several different signal transduction mechanisms.

Fibroblast growth factors in tumorigenesis, angiogenesis, and tumour angiogenesis

Based on their wide spectrum of target cells, FGF family members have been suspected to play important parts in many biological events, and many studies have substantiated this proposition. Some of the members of the FGF family are potent mitogens for a large number of cell types of the mesodermal and neuroectodermal lineage, and thus could be responsible for the proliferative stimulus in tumours derived from these cells. However, at the same time some of the FGFs are mitogenic for endothelial cells, thereby hampering attempts to separate the functional role of FGFs in tumorigenesis from their role in tumour angiogenesis. For this reason, the biological role of FGFs in tumour cell proliferation is discussed separately from their role in physiological and pathological angiogenesis. Finally, we evaluate the evidence for a direct involvement of FGF family members in the induction and regulation of tumour angiogenesis.

Fibroblast growth factors and tumour cell proliferation

Oncogenic activity of fibroblast growth factor family members

FGF-3 (int-2) was identified after insertion of mouse mammary tumour virus (MMTV) in the mouse genome causing the up-regulation of FGF-3 gene expression and tumour induction (37,38). Subsequently, FGF-3 was shown in transgenic mouse models to induce the development of mammary hyperplasia and neoplasia and prostate hyperplasia (174–176). However, in most cases FGF-3 by itself caused only the development of hyperplastic lesions which spontaneously regressed, indicating that additional events are required for complete tumour progression. Such a synergistic cooperation in the progression to full malignancy has been demonstrated between FGF-3 and FGF-4 in transgenic mice (177,178). Consistent with its function in transgenic mice, amplification of the gene for FGF-3 was found in a proportion of human breast cancer biopsies (44) and squamous cell carcinoma of head and neck (45). In addition, FGF-3 was expressed at elevated levels in a significant number of Kaposi sarcomas (179). FGF-3 is able to transform NIH 3T3 cells, however, only at high levels of expression (46).

FGF-4 was identified in NIH 3T3 transformation assays as hst-1 in the DNA from human stomach cancer, colon carcinoma, and hepatoma (48,180,181), and as KFGF from Kaposi sarcoma (49). However, isolation of FGF-4 as a transforming gene might have been coincidental and does not reflect expression in these tumours. For example, FGF-4 is not generally overexpressed in Kaposi sarcoma (182). Expression of FGF-4 in NIH 3T3 fibroblasts completely transforms the cells, as assayed by increased motility, invasiveness, and malignancy in vitro and in vivo (183). Similarly, up-regulated expression of FGF-4 induced spontaneous metastasis in MCF-7 breast carcinoma cell lines (184–186) and transformation of human adrenal cortex carcinoma cell lines (187). Retroviral transfer of FGF-4 into mice induced the development of soft tissue sarcomas and meningeal tumours (188). In cancer patients FGF-4 is expressed in a number of tumours including teratocarcinomas and germ cell tumours (189,190). Amplification of both the genes for FGF-3 and FGF-4 was found in mammary tumours and squamous cell carcinomas at a frequency of 20% (reviewed in reference 7). As both genes are localized in close vicinity of each other on human chromosome 11q13, co-amplification of the two genes is not surprising. The synergistic effect of FGF-4 with FGF-3 has also been demonstrated in transgenic mice and in MMTV tumorigenesis studies, where FGF-4 has also been identified as an insertion site of MMTV (177,178,191). FGF-4 is mitogenic for endothelial cells and it is angiogenic in vitro and in vivo and, thus, might also be involved in the induction of tumour angiogenesis (57).

The cDNA for FGF-5 was cloned by its ability to transform NIH 3T3 fibroblasts. It is expressed by a number of tumour cell lines (58). FGF-5 is a secreted protein, and an autocrine growth regulatory pathway has been suggested (59). However, many details of target cell specificity and tumour cell proliferation remain to be investigated. High levels of FGF-5 expression have been found in patients with bladder carcinoma, hepatoma, and endometrial carcinoma, FGF-5 was also expressed in Kaposi sarcoma lesions, and it has been demonstrated that epidermal growth factor induces expression of FGF-5 in Kaposi sarcoma-derived cell lines, suggesting that FGF-5 might play a part in the development of Kaposi sarcoma (192,193).

FGF-6 was cloned by screening a mouse cosmid library with an FGF-4-specific probe. The human gene for FGF-6 was also cloned by virtue of its transformation activity as hst-2 (70). FGF-6 has the ability to transform NIH 3T3 fibroblasts in focus forming assays in vitro and confers the ability to form tumours in athymic mice in vivo (69). FGF-6 is expressed in some Kaposi sarcoma lesions (193).

FGF-7 is a stromal mediator of epithelial cell proliferation (75; also see above). Under pathological conditions it may play a part in wound healing (77). Its oncogenic potential is not known. FGF-8 was purified and cloned from an androgen-dependent mouse mammary carcinoma cell line. Its expression is induced by androgen and it stimulates the tumour cells in an autocrine fashion (79,194). Recently, FGF-8 was also identified as frequently activated gene in MMTV-infected mice. Owing to alternative splicing, several different isoforms with varying transforming activities on NIH 3T3 fibroblasts have been identified (195). FGF-9 was purified and cloned from a human glioma cell line. It is mitogenic for glial cells, and an autocrine growth regulatory pathway has been suggested (80,81). Its transforming potential on other cell types or a role in human cancers have not yet been reported.

The transforming potential of FGF-1 and FGF-2

By virtue of their secretion the FGF family members described above are able to establish an autocrine pathway of transformation and proliferation. In contrast, FGF-1 and FGF-2 do not contain a signal sequence for secretion and are usually found cell-associated. Thus, in order to explain their growth stimulatory function during tumour development, it is also necessary to explain how these FGFs are exposed to their receptors on the cell surface (see section on 'Inhibition of FGF activity', p. 221).

Many experiments investigating the transforming potential of FGF-1 and FGF-2 have been performed; however, a clear correlation between export of FGF-1 and FGF-2 and transformation was not apparent (reviewed in references 7, 196). For example, expression of the original FGF-2 coding sequence lacking a signal peptide in BALB/c 3T3 fibroblasts or BHK cells resulted in transformation of the cells and the detection of FGF-2 in the culture supernatant. However, transformation was not affected by neutralizing antibodies to FGF-2, indicating that the FGF-2 activation occurred within the cells (197,198). High levels of expression of signalless FGF-2 seemed to be required to induce the transformed phenotype, and in some cases expression of signalless FGF-2 did not result in transformation (157,199–201). Furthermore, none of the cell lines transformed by signalless FGF-2 were tumorigenic in athymic mice. Similarly, melanocytes transfected with FGF-2 acquired similar properties to those of metastatic melanoma cells *in vitro*, but they were not tumorigenic *in vivo* (202).

'Forced secretion' of FGF-2 by fusing a signal peptide onto the N-terminus of FGF-2 resulted in complete autocrine transformation of NIH 3T3 fibroblasts. Cells expressing the signal peptide fusion were highly transformed as assessed by growth in soft agar, focus formation assays, and tumorigenicity and metastasis assays in athymic mice

(196,200,201,203). Despite the attached signal peptide, in two reports, FGF-2 was not detectable in the culture medium, whereas Blam and co-workers reported secretion of FGF-2 as modified high-molecular-weight forms. The observed difference between the reports might be due to the different signal sequences used or to the different levels of expression obtained. Transformation could not be inhibited by neutralizing antibodies, but was reversed by suramin, a polyanionic drug known to inhibit growth factor–receptor interaction (201). This result suggests that FGF binds within the cell to its receptor, thereby establishing an internal autocrine loop of FGF-induced transformation. In similar experiments, BALB/c 3T3 fibroblasts expressing a signal peptide/FGF-2 chimeric protein were able to induce the formation of tumours when injected into athymic mice. However, in these experiments tumour formation could be prevented by intravenous injection of neutralizing antibodies (204).

Similar results were obtained with FGF-1. NIH 3T3 cells tranfected with wild-type FGF-1 synthesized but did not secrete FGF-1 and did not show any sign of transformation (205). In contrast, FGF-1 (amino acids 1–154) fused to a signal peptide was readily secreted by the transfected NIH 3T3 cells resulting in transformation of the cells and the formation of highly vascularized tumours when injected into athymic mice. FGF-1 (amino acids 21–154) fused to a signal peptide was not secreted, but mediated the transition to the transformed phenotype (206).

In conclusion, wild-type FGF-1 and FGF-2 by themselves seems to transform only when expressed at high levels. In contrast, acquisition of a signal peptide converts FGF-1 and FGF-2 into highly transforming proteins analogous to other family members, such as FGF-3, FGF-4, FGF-5, and FGF-6. Consistent with these findings, the deletion of the signal sequence from FGF-4 significantly diminished transformation (207). Despite the attached signal peptide FGF-1 or FGF-2 were not detected in the culture medium and transformation could not be inhibited by specific antibodies to FGF-1 or FGF-2, suggesting that the autocrine transformation by 'forced secretion' of FGF-1 and FGF-2 occurred within the cells.

FGF-1 and FGF-2 in tumour development

Extensive studies on the expression of FGF-1 and FGF-2 in tumour biopsies *in vivo* together with functional studies on tumour cell proliferation *in vitro* provided a plethora of evidence for the involvement of FGF-1 and FGF-2 in tumour development. In some cases expression of FGF-1 or FGF-2 correlated with malignancy, and interference with the activities of FGF-1 or FGF-2 diminished tumour growth and cell transformation.

For example, many research groups have reported increased expression of FGF-1 and FGF-2 in glioblastomas as compared with normal brain (for example references 208–211). FGF-1 and FGF-2 were significantly up-regulated in human gliomas in proportion to the extent of malignancy (212,213). Furthermore, the malignant phenotype of glioblastoma cell lines could be inhibited by FGF-2-specific antibodies indicating that FGF-2 utilized an autocrine pathway to promote tumour progression (214,215). FGF-1 and FGF-2 did not appear to be up-regulated in metastatic brain tumours, and only FGF-2 was expressed in meningiomas (213). FGF-2 and sometimes FGF-1 are constitutively expressed at high levels in melanomas, but not in normal melanocytes (32,216). Proliferation and growth in soft agar was inhibited by anti-sense oligonucleotides to FGF-2 or FGFR-1 in a melanoma cell line, indicating that FGF-2 might be an autocrine growth factor for melanoma cells (217,218). In Kaposi sarcoma, FGF-2 and sometimes FGF-1 were detectable in tissue specimens and Kaposi sarcoma-derived cell lines. In fact, proliferation, angiogenesis, and lesion formation by Kaposi sarcoma-derived cell lines in athymic mice could be prevented by treatment with antisense oligonucleotides to FGF-2 (219).

Elevated expression of either FGF-1 or FGF-2 has also been demonstrated in a variety of other tumour types *in vivo* and in tumour cell lines *in vitro*. In some cases FGF expression correlated significantly with advanced stages of tumour development and malignancy (reviewed in references 6,7,220). Examples are the expression of FGF-2 and FGF-1 in squamous cell carcinoma, human leukaemic cells, human bladder carcinoma, human pancreatic carcinoma, human ovarian cancer, and gastric carcinoma; the expression of FGF-2 in pituitary tumours, renal tumours, mammary carcinoma cell lines, prostate carcinoma cell lines, colon carcinoma cell lines, hepatoma cell lines, chondrosarcoma cell lines, osteosarcoma cell lines, and the expression of FGF-1 in rat Morris hepatoma cell lines. In some tumour cell lines functional experiments towards the role of FGF in tumour cell transformation and proliferation have been performed. For example, FGF-2 was shown to promote proliferation (221) and differentiation (222) of neuroblastoma cells. Similarly, the anchorage independent growth of a human adrenal carcinoma cell line was enhanced by FGF-2 (223). Finally, autocrine growth of human nasopharyngeal carcinoma cell lines was dependent on the expression of FGF-2 and FGF receptors (224).

Fibroblast growth factor receptors and tumorigenesis

Similar to the FGF ligands, expression of FGF receptors is significantly up-regulated in a variety of cancer types. For example, the genes for FGFR-1 and -2 were found to be amplified and overexpressed in a subset of breast cancers. In these cases amplification of FGFR-2 significantly correlated with amplification of the gene for c-*myc*, whereas amplification of FGFR-1 correlated with the amplification of the genes for FGF-3 and FGF-4 (225,226). The gene for FGFR-2 was found to be amplified in stomach cancer where it was isolated as K-sam (96). FGFR-1 expression was found to be up-regulated in glioblastoma, whereas FGFR-2 was present in white matter and low-grade astrocytomas, but absent in glioblastoma (227). Indeed, during progression to the most malignant phenotype of glioblastoma, a gradual shift from FGFR-2 to FGFR-1 with two or three immunoglobulin domains was observed (228). In another report, expression of both FGFR-1 and FGFR-2 was found to be up-regulated in gliomas and meningiomas (229). Inhibition of FGFR-1 expression by anti-sense oligonucleotides resulted in the inhibition of melanoma proliferation (218).

Elevated expression of FGFR-2 IIIb and IIIc were reported in endometrial adenocarcinoma (230) and FGFR-1 and FGFR-2 in Kaposi sarcoma (193). The gene for FGFR-4 appeared to be amplified in human breast and gynaecological cancers (231). FGFR-4 has also been reported to be expressed by melanoma cells (232). All four members of the FGF receptor family are expressed in a variety of tumour cell lines *in vitro*. For example, many breast cancer cell lines have up-regulated FGF receptors; MDA MB 134 breast carcinoma carries an amplified gene for FGFR-1 with high expression of FGFR-1, but also FGFR-4 which is not amplified (233,234). All four members of the FGF receptor family are expressed by the MCF 7 breast carcinoma cell line and in a number of leukaemia cell lines (235,236). However, stimulation of the receptor with FGF-1 or FGF-2 resulted in growth inhibition rather than stimulation of proliferation. In conclusion, up-regulated expression of FGF receptors is frequently found in tumour cells concomitant with the expression of FGF ligands, suggesting that many tumour cells utilize FGF ligands and FGF receptors in an autocrine pathway of transformation and proliferation.

Fibroblast growth factors in angiogenesis

Formation of new blood vessels from pre-existing blood vessels (angiogenesis) is a multistep process. Stages in these process include the activation of quiescent endothelial cells in a pre-existing vessel, degradation of the basement membrane, migration of endothelial cells into the interstitial space and sprouting (not necessarily accompanied by proliferation), endothelial cell proliferation at the migrating tip, lumen formation, generation of new basement membrane with the recruitment of pericytes, formation of anastomoses, and finally initiation of blood flow (see Chapter 1).

With the ability to culture endothelial cells, quantifiable assays could be devised that specifically measure the diverse activities involved in angiogenesis, including proliferation, migration, and tube formation. These *in vitro* assays are complemented by a range of *in vivo* bioassays in which the complete process of angiogenesis is recapitulated and can be studied including the chick chorioallantoic membrane, the cornea pocket, the hamster cheek pouch, and the rabbit ear chamber (see Chapter 6). The utilization of these bioassays allows the identification and characterization of factors that either promote or inhibit angiogenesis. Many of the angiogenesis-promoting (angiogenic) factors have been identified in cell lysates, tissue extracts or culture supernatants of a variety of cell types. Although numerous angiogenic factors have been identified, FGF-1 and FGF-2 served for a long time as prototype polypeptide angiogenic factors.

Angiogenic properties of fibroblast growth factor family members

FGF-1 and FGF-2 are mitogenic for endothelial cells and stimulate endothelial cell migration (reviewed in references 237–240). They induce endothelial cell production of proteases that are capable of degrading basement membranes, such as collagenase and plasminogen activator (241–243). FGF-1 and FGF-2 also cause endothelial cells to migrate and form capillary-like tubes in three dimensional culture systems *in vitro* (243). Both FGF-1 and FGF-2 exhibit potent angiogenic activity in all *in vivo* assays tested. In fact, they are usually employed in these bioassays as positive references. Although there is no doubt about the angiogenic capabilities of FGF-1 and FGF-2, their detailed functional role in defined physiological or pathological angiogenesis is not understood.

Endothelial cells derived from large or small vessels are not only a target for FGF-2, they also synthesize high amounts of FGF-2 *in vitro* (244–246). Most of the FGF-2 produced by the cells is found associated with the extracellular matrix and the basement membrane (reviewed in reference 85). Measureable amounts were also detectable in the culture medium (246). Moreover, addition of neutralizing antibodies to capillary endothelial cell cultures resulted in a moderate, but reproduceable reduction of endothelial cell proliferation (247). Spontaneous migration of endothelial cells has been shown to depend on FGF-2 that has been synthesized and released by the bovine aortic endothelial cells themselves. Neutralizing antibodies to FGF-2 inhibited migration of these cells suggesting an autocrine role of FGF stimulation (248). A similar autocrine role of

endothelial cell-produced FGF-2 has been shown to promote tube formation in collagen gels (249).

Many other FGF-mediated activities on endothelial cells have been reported. These include the prevention of irradiation-induced apoptosis of endothelial cells (250, 251). FGF-2 also induced the down-regulation of lymphocyte adhesion molecules in endothelial cells *in vitro* resulting in a reduced basal adhesion of lymphocytes to endothelial cells (252). FGF-2-mediated prevention of lymphocyte adhesion to tumour endothelium may explain how cancer cells that express FGF-2 may escape the host immune surveillance during the angiogenic phase of tumour growth. Collectively, these data indicate that FGF-2 is an important regulatory factor for endothelial cells, the cell type that is central for angiogenesis.

One approach to study the functional role of FGFs during angiogenesis is the induction of angiogenesis in an experimental system *in vitro* or *in vivo* with the concomitant modulation of FGF activity. In such an *in vitro* experiment, rat aorta specimen were cultured in collagen which resulted in endothelial cell sprouting from the aortic piece (253). Angiogenic sprouting was stimulated by addition of exogenous FGF-2 and inhibited by neutralizing antibodies to FGF-2. Apparently, FGF-2 was released by experimental wounding and the released FGF-2 mediated autocrine stimulation of angiogenesis after injury.

Polyvinyl sponges saturated with FGF-2 and implanted into rats induce neovascularization (254,255), and antibodies to FGF-2 prevent this process (256). Implantation of slow release pellets loaded with FGF-2 under the kidney capsule also resulted in the induction of neovascularization, in the absence of any inflammatory response suggesting that FGF-2 directly induced angiogenesis (257). Similarly, FGF-2 packaged into polymer-based devices and implanted in the periadventitial space of rat carotid artery, or in the rat mesenteric window caused a dose-dependent stimulation of angiogenesis (258,259). These results are in contrast to experiments where the implantation of FGF-2 in Hydron or Elvax pellets into the rabbit cornea elicited an angiogenic response only when it was accompanied by inflammation, suggesting that in this setting FGF-2 was not directly angiogenic (260).

FGF-1 complexed to gelatin caused site-specific angiogenesis when implanted into the neck or peritoneal cavity of the rat (261). Based on these observation, FGF-induced vascularization and formation of organoid structures was proposed as a means for gene therapy. For example, after restoration of their genetic defect autologous cells could be reimplanted into the body. However, in order to stay metabolically active, these cells need to be in a vascularized organoid structure. In the course of these experiments, it has been possible to enhance and stabilize the formation of vascular organoid structures by implantation of collagen I- and IV-coated Goretex to which FGF-1 has been attached (262). In another series of experiments in dogs and rats, implantation of FGF-1 or FGF-2 at the site of islet transplantation resulted in a dramatically accelerated establishment of blood flow in the transplant (263). One of the most direct approaches to utilize the angiogenic capabilities of FGF-1 has been the direct gene transfer of FGF-1 carrying an artifical signal peptide into porcine arteries. Expression of the secreted form of FGF-1 induced intimal thickening, paralleled by increased neovascularization within the expanded intima. Taken together, these experiments demonstrate the capability of FGF-1 to induce neovascularization *in vivo* (264).

Not much is known about the angiogenic properties of the other members of the FGF family. FGF-3 by itself is not mitogenic for endothelial cells. In contrast, recombinant FGF-4 has been shown to be a potent mitogen for vascular endothelial cells (265). It also exhibited strong angiogenic activity in the chick chorioallantoic membrane and the rat corneal assay. Furthermore, NIH 3T3 fibroblasts transfected with FGF-4 appeared to develop highly vascularized tumours in immunodeficient mice (57). FGF-5 has been shown to be a mitogen for fetal bovine heart endothelial cells *in vitro* (58), and FGF-6 exhibited a limited response on bovine aortic endothelial cells (73). The angiogenic activity of FGF-5 and FGF-6 *in vivo* still need to be examined.

Fibroblast growth factors in physiological and pathological angiogenesis

The results summarized above clearly demonstrate that FGF-1 and FGF-2 are able to induce directly angiogenesis *in vitro* and *in vivo*. However, it is not known how FGFs interact with the target endothelial cells *in vivo*, and which of their pleiotropic activities is actually required for the induction of angiogenesis *in vivo*. For instance, it has not been demonstrated that FGF-1 or FGF-2 are directly involved in physiological or pathological angiogenesis, such as ovulation, implantation, wound healing, or vascular disease. Most of the accumulated data have been based predominantly on expression studies that have attempted to correlate expression of FGFs with angiogenic processes. Cause–effect studies have mainly been hampered by the lack of specific tools for the molecular dissection of the functional role of FGFs during angiogenesis *in vivo*. In addition, due to the lack of a signal sequence for secretion, it becomes difficult to explain the molecular mechanisms by which FGF-1 and FGF-2 are exposed to the FGF receptors on the surface of target endothelial cells.

In early embryonic development the *de novo* formation of blood vessels from precursor endothelial cells (vasculogenesis) is distinguished from the formation of blood vessels from the pre-existing blood vessel plexus (angiogenesis). The role of FGFs in vasculogenesis is not known. The involvement of members of the FGF family in embryonic development is undisputed and has been discussed above. However, a functional role of FGFs in developmental angiogenesis has not been unequivocally demonstrated. Conclusions are based mainly on the spatial and temporal correlation of FGF expression and neovascularization. For example, the neovascularization of the renal Anlage might be controlled by a paracrine process mediated in part by FGF-2 (266). Recently, it has been reported that the sedative drug thalidomide inhibited FGF-induced angiogenesis. As FGF-4 has been shown to play a major part in limb development, and thalidomide caused limb defects in babies whose mothers took thalidomide during pregnancy, it is conceivable that the angiogenic activity of FGF-4 was also functionally required for limb development (267). During physiological angiogenesis, such as the menstrual cycle and pregnancy, expression of FGF-1 or FGF-2 has been found in tissues and cells. However, it has not been demonstrated that FGFs are actually required for angiogenesis in these processes (reviewed in reference 9).

Different roles have been shown for FGF family members in wound healing. Whereas FGF-7 has been shown to be responsible for the proliferation of keratinocytes, FGF-2 has been proposed to act in a biphasic fashion to promote angiogenesis and also stromal cell proliferation. Early during wound healing, damaged cells release FGF-2, whereas later wound healing macrophages are a major source of angiogenic activity. After migrating into the wound site macrophages are activated to release FGF-2 and tumour necrosis factor (TNF) α in the depth of the wound where oxygen is low and lactate high (260,268). Application of FGF-2 to injured tympanic membranes of guinea-pigs brings about rapid healing by induction of rapid proliferation of the subepithelial connective tissue layer (269). In a similar tissue repair process, FGF-1 was shown to be dramatically up-regulated in regenerating kidney proximal tubule epithelial cells that had been damaged with nephrotoxic agents (270).

In atherosclerosis, FGF-1 and FGF-2 are expressed in early, simple, and advanced atherosclerotic plaques. FGF-2 is expressed in macrophages and smooth muscle cells, the principal cells involved in the formation of atherosclerotic lesions, and increased expression of FGF-2 and FGFR-1 was associated with neovascularization of atheromatous lesions (271). Intravenous infusion of FGF-2 stimulated endothelial cell regeneration and smooth muscle cell proliferation only after endothelial injury or denudation. These experiments demonstrate that FGF-2 targets both endothelial cells and smooth muscle cells in a vessel, and that the endothelium serves as a barrier preventing the contact of smooth muscle cells with FGFs (272–274). Endothelial cells appear to respond to FGFs in the blood only after injury or another 'activation step'. As mentioned above, expression of a secreted form of FGF-1 in porcine arteries induced intimal thickening and increased neovascularization within the expanded intima. These experiments indicate that FGF-1 has the capability to induce intimal hyperplasia in the arterial wall *in vivo*, and might also be responsible for neovascularization of the atherosclerotic plaques (264). Thus, FGF-1 and FGF-2 may drive angiogenic events that may be central to atheroma development.

Another example of the role of FGF-2 in pathophysiological neovascularization has been reported recently. Experimental duodenal ulcers in rats are relatively deficient in microvessels. FGF-2 is highly expressed in normal gastric mucosa; however, it is most likely degraded by the acidic pH of an ulcerated stomach resulting in dramatically decreased levels of FGF-2. Oral administration of FGF-2 that has been mutated into an acid-resistant form by removing the cysteine residues in the molecule (bFGF-CS23), induced angiogenesis in the ulcer bed and accelerated ulcer healing (27,275,276). Consistent with the involvement of FGF-2 in gastric mucosa vascularization, the anti-ulcer drug sucralfate, a synthetic heparin analogue, has been shown to bind and stabilize FGF-1 and FGF-2 (27,277).

In rheumatoid arthritis the ingrowth of a vascular pannus may be produced by excessive release of angiogenic factors from infiltrating macrophages, immune cells, or inflammatory cells (278,279). FGFs are potent mitogens for synovial fibroblasts, and exhibit synergistic effects with other growth factors thought to be involved in rheumatoid arthritis (280). For example, both FGF-1 and PDGF-B were expressed at elevated levels in rheumatoid synovium and induced specific tyrosine phosphorylation suggesting that locally expressed FGF-1 and PDGF-B were involved in stimulating hyperplasia of rheumatoid synovial fibroblast-like cells. The levels of FGF-1 also correlated with the extent and intensity of synovial mononuclear cell infiltration, suggesting that FGFs may exhibit pleiotropic activities in the development of rheumatoid arthritis (166,281,282).

A final example of angiogenesis occurring during pathological conditions is the formation of collaterals after myocardial infarct. Coronary collateral vessels reduce damage to ischaemic myocardium after coronary obstruction, and the formation of collateral blood vessels is thought to be induced by angiogenic growth factors. FGF-

1 and FGF-2 in combination with heparin are mitogenic for coronary venular endothelial cells, targets for coronary angiogenesis and collateral formation (283). FGF-2 injected intracoronarily in a canine myocardial infarct model stimulated angiogenesis and resulted in improved cardiac systolic function and reduced infarct size (284). Similarly, FGF-2 induced an increase in vessel density and increased collateral blood flow in dogs whose coronary flow was experimentally compromised, when administered as daily bolus injection directly into the collateral dependent zone (285). In contrast, FGF-2 either implanted via an epicardial sponge or applied by arterial infusion, could not induce an angiogenic response in the affected myocardium, but rather caused smooth muscle cell hyperplasia in the ischaemic areas, indicating that the mode of FGFs' delivery to target tissues may be of major relevance (286–288). FGF-1 and FGF-2 also exhibit hypotensive activity that can be separated from their mitogenic activity by protein engineering (289). Systemic administration of FGF decreased arterial blood pressure, probably by raising the concentration of intracellular calcium ions that may induce endothelium-derived relaxing factor (EDRF).

Most of the data described above are based on a correlation between FGF expression and angiogenesis, and it cannot be excluded that FGFs are targeting cell types other than endothelial cells, and that other angiogenic factors are the actual inducers of angiogenesis. Again, the variable activities and the diversity of target cells of FGFs make it difficult to characterize their angiogenic activity *in vivo*. It should be noted that another angiogenic factor, vascular endothelial growth factor (VEGF), has been shown to be expressed at high levels during many physiological and pathological angiogenic processes (see Chapter 10). For example, VEGF is expressed in the granulosa cells during follicle maturation, in lutein cells during corpus luteum formation and in the maternal decidua during placenta development. In pathological events VEGF expression is induced by hypoxia, wound healing, chronic inflammation, and vascular repair. Moreover, VEGF seems to be involved in the collateral blood flow of ischaemic myocardium, in ocular angiogenesis, in psoriasis, and in rheumatoid arthritis. Interestingly, FGF-1 and FGF-2 exhibit a dramatic synergistic effect with VEGF in the induction of endothelial cell migration, proliferation, and capillary-like tube formation in three-dimensional culture systems (290,291). Although this synergistic effect has not been demonstrated *in vivo*, it is conceivable that both angiogenic factors cooperate in the regulation of neovascularization under many physiological or pathological circumstances.

Many inhibitors of angiogenesis and tumour angiogenesis have been described. One of the main criteria for

their activity is the ability to inhibit FGF-induced proliferation of endothelial cells *in vitro* or FGF-induced
angiogenesis *in vivo*. However, most of these compounds
inhibit endothelial cell proliferation as such, regardless of
the angiogenic stimulus.

In a few cases inhibition of FGF-mediated endothelial
cell proliferation *in vitro* might have an important function
in vivo. For example, transforming growth factor β (TGF-
β) is an inhibitor of endothelial cell proliferation *in vitro*
by directly counteracting FGF-2 activity (reviewed in
reference 292). *In vivo*, pericytes inhibit endothelial cell
proliferation thereby regulating the completion of neovascularization. It has been shown that upon close contact
to endothelial cells pericytes or smooth muscle cells
release TGF-β resulting in the inhibition of endothelial
cell proliferation (293,294). FGF and TGF-β also regulate
angiogenesis by modulating proteolysis in the extracellular matrix. Although both FGF-2 and TGF-β
induce the expression of plasminogen activators and
plasminogen activator inhibitors, FGF seems to tilt the
balance towards proteolysis, whereas TGF-β seems to
induce inhibition of proteolysis required for endothelial
cell proliferation (295,296). The detailed role of TGF-β in
angiogenesis and tumour angiogenesis is described in
Chapter 13.

Interleukin (IL) 1α and IL-1β are structurally very
similar to FGF-1 and FGF-2 and also do not carry a signal
sequence for secretion (15,28,29). In addition, IL-1α also
carries a nuclear localization signal and is localized to the
nucleus. As with the FGFs, the biological significance of
this nuclear localization is not understood (297). IL-1α
counteracts the activities of FGF-1 and FGF-2 and inhibits
endothelial cell proliferation and survival. Senescent
human endothelial cells express high levels of IL-1α, as
compared with low levels in young or immortalized
endothelial cells (298–300). Treatment of senescent
endothelial cells with anti-sense oligonucleotides to IL-1α
resulted in decreased expression of IL-1α and subsequently in the prevention of senenescence and the
extension of the proliferative lifespan (298). Endothelial
cell adhesion, proliferation, and angiogenesis in the
skin of mice induced by FGF-2 was also inhibited
by IL-1, thereby exhibiting a synergistic effect with
interferon gamma (301). IL-1, TGF-β, interferon gamma,
TNFα, and the tumour promoter 12-*O*-tetradecanoyl
phorbol-13-acetate (TPA) inhibit FGF-mediated endothelial cell proliferation. It has been suggested that
these factors promote differentiation of endothelial
cells by inducing cellular quiescence (298). The
role of these factors in modulating the activities of
FGFs on endothelial cells *in vivo* warrants further
examination.

Fibroblast growth factor in tumour angiogenesis

As FGF-2 and to a lesser extent FGF-1 are expressed by
many tumours *in vivo* and tumour cell lines *in vitro*, it has
been tacitly assumed that they were responsible for the
induction of angiogenesis during tumour progression.
However, closer inspection of the molecular mechanisms
of tumour angiogenesis on one hand and of the actual role
of FGFs in tumour angiogenesis on the other suggested
that the assumption of a general involvement of FGF-1 or
FGF-2 in tumour angiogenesis was oversimplified. Other
angiogenic factors, such as VEGF, have been shown to
play a lead part during the induction of tumour angiogenesis in some cases and, therefore, additional work is
required to reveal the actual contribution of FGFs to
tumour angiogenesis. In some instances expression of
FGF-1 or FGF-2 *in vivo* correlates with the degree of vascularity of the tumours. However, at the same time FGFs
have other target cell specificities. In most cases the targets
are the tumour cells themselves leading to an autocrine or
paracrine stimulation of tumour cell proliferation (see
section on 'FGF-1 and FGF-2 in tumour development',
p. 213). Other targets could also be the cells within the
remodelling stroma of the growing tumour. Therefore, it
has been very difficult to dissect the pleiotropic activities
of FGFs in functional terms and to assess their actual role
in tumour angiogenesis *in vivo*.

In order to induce tumour angiogenesis, FGFs produced
by the tumour cells need to be released to bind FGF
receptors on the surface of endothelial cells. However,
both FGF-1 and FGF-2 lack a signal sequence for secretion, and although several mechanisms for their release
from cells have been proposed, their export pathway has
not been elucidated (see section on 'Export of FGF-1 and
FGF-2'). Experiments using chimeric FGF-2 carrying a
signal peptide revealed that when cells producing this
secreted form of FGF-2 were injected into athymic mice
they developed vascularized tumours and had no apparent
effect on smooth muscle or fibroblast proliferation (204).
It is also possible that FGFs are produced by cells other
than tumour cells. For example, an increase in FGF-2
synthesis in tumour vasculature has been observed indicating that endothelial cells themselves could be a source of
FGF-2 (302). Tumours also recruit macrophages and
activate them to secrete FGF-2 (303). Furthermore, mast
cells may also be recruited by tumours. They are loaded
with heparin which they might release in the tumour and
amplify the effects of FGF-1 or FGF-2 (304).

In many naturally growing as well as in experimentally
induced tumours the extent of vascularization correlates
with the expression of angiogenic FGF family members.

For example, neural transplants that have been retrovirally transfected with the FGF-4 gene and express high levels of FGF-4 exhibit abundant capillary proliferation and induce the formation of capillary angiosarcomas suggesting that FGF-4 may have a direct role in angiogenesis and endothelial cell transformation (305). Moreover, in glioblastoma and meningioma, the levels of expression of FGF-2 and FGFR-1 correlate significantly not only with tumour cell proliferation, but also with the vascularity of tumours (210–212). In a co-culture assay it has been shown that glioblastoma cell lines that exhibited high levels of FGF-2 expression were able to induce tube formation of bovine aortic endothelial cells. This process was inhibited by neutralizing antibodies to FGF-2, suggesting that FGF-2 plays a paracrine role in tumour angiogenesis (306). However, up-regulated FGFR1 expression appeared to be confined to the tumour cells and not to endothelial cells, suggesting that FGF function was associated with autocrine growth stimulation of the tumour cells (228).

Xenografted DLD-2 human colon tumours exhibited increased growth rates and reduced hypoxic fractions when FGF-2 was systemically applied to the mice suggesting that the extent of vascularization was regulated by FGF-2 (307). In another experiment DLD-2 human colon carcinoma and C6 glioma cells that lacked high-affinity receptors for FGF-2 and that could not be stimulated by FGF-2 were used to form tumours in athymic mice. Systemic injections of FGF-2 resulted in higher vascular density in the tumours and in increased tumour size. In contrast, specific antibodies to FGF-2 significantly retarded tumour growth. The tumour vessels expressed receptors for FGF-2 suggesting that in this case FGF-2 modulated tumour angiogenesis (308).

FGF-1 and FGF-2 have been found to be highly expressed in Kaposi sarcoma lesions of AIDS patients (see section on 'FGF-1 and FGF-2 in tumour development', p. 213). Indeed, FGF-2 injected into the nude mouse elicited the formation of Kaposi sarcoma-like lesions in regard to the extent of vascularization, the morphology of proliferating cells and general pathology. In these experiments, FGF-2 synergized with the *Tat* gene product of human immunodeficiency virus in causing Kaposi sarcoma-like lesions. Fibronectin could replace *Tat* suggesting that FGF-2 induced the lesions and that *Tat* enhanced its activity by mimicking the effect of extracellular matrix molecules (309). Interestingly, a recent report demonstrated that *Tat* by itself was angiogenic as determined in several angiogenesis assays *in vitro* and *in vivo* (310).

Elevated levels of FGF-2, but not FGF-1 were found by highly sensitive immunoassay methods in the serum and urine of bladder cancer patients with highest levels in patients with active metastatic disease (311,312). Similar

elevated levels of FGF-2 were found in the urine of patients with a wide variety of other neoplasms (313). FGF-2 was also detected in the cerebrospinal fluid of children with brain tumours, but not in normal controls. The levels of FGF-2 correlated significantly with the extent of vascularization in the tumours (314). In infantile haemangioma, levels of FGF-2 were abnormally elevated in the urine of patients during the proliferative phase of haemangioma development, but returned to normal levels during involution or therapeutic treatment (315). In an experimental setting, BALB/c 3T3 cells that expressed a mutant, but active form of FGF-2 were transplanted into athymic mice, resulting in elevated levels of the mutated form of FGF-2 in the urine of tumour-bearing mice (316). Taken together, these experiments suggest that the source of circulating FGF in the serum and urine originated, at least in part, from the tumour itself. The presence of FGF-2 in body fluids of cancer patients and experimental animals correlated significantly with the extent of vascularization and metastasis suggesting that expression and release of FGFs might be involved in tumour angiogenesis. Based on these results the detection of FGF in the urine of cancer patients might be a useful diagnostic and prognostic tool. The results also indicate that FGF-2 is released by producer cells despite the lack of a signal peptide (see section on 'Export of FGF-1 and FGF-2', p. 222.)

The association of FGF-2 export with the angiogenic phenotype has also been observed in a transgenic mouse model of tumour development. Transgenic mice harbouring the bovine papilloma virus 1 (BPV-1) genome develop abnormalities in the dermal layer of the skin (317). Initially, two forms of hyperplasia arise: mild and aggressive fibromatosis. Increased overall thickness of the skin, increased density of fibroblasts and neovascularization correlate with the aggressive form of fibromatosis. Subsequently, protuberant tumours (fibrosarcomas) arise out of those regions. Histological examination of the different stages of fibrosarcoma development in the BPV 1 transgenic mice indicates that the transition from mild fibromatosis to aggressive fibromatosis is accompanied by a dramatic increase of capillary blood vessels (318). Cell lines that have been derived from the different stages of tumour development recapitulate this phenotypic difference (319). Aggressive fibromatosis as well as fibrosarcoma cell lines secrete factors including FGF-2 into their culture medium that are mitogenic for capillary endothelial cells. FGF-2 is cell-associated in normal fibroblasts and in mild fibromatosis cell lines. In contrast, FGF-2 is found in the conditioned medium of the aggressive fibromatosis and fibrosarcoma cell lines. Cell death or lysis does not appear to be involved in the release of FGF-2 from the tumour cells (318). Rather, it appears that a switch in the subcellular localization of FGF-2 in the cell lines correlates with the induction of tumour angiogenesis.

The experimental data on the role of FGFs in tumour angiogenesis are still circumstantial and indirect. It remains to be demonstrated that FGFs are actually required for neovascularization during tumour progression. In addition to their angiogenic activity, FGFs as autocrine growth factors are frequently responsible for tumour cell proliferation. Based on these diverse functions, three alternate pathways of FGF activity can be envisioned. First, FGF could be an autocrine or paracrine growth factor for tumour cells only (Fig. 17.3a). Second, FGF might exclusively stimulate endothelial cell migration and proliferation,

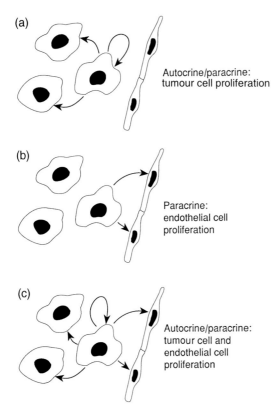

Figure 17.3. The potential mitogenic pathways of fibroblast growth factors (FGFs) during tumorigenesis. (a) Tumour cells that produce FGF may mitogenically stimulate themselves in an autocrine or paracrine manner. (b) FGF that is released by tumour cells exclusively stimulates proliferation of endothelial cells in a paracrine fashion. (c) FGF released by tumour cells induces proliferation of both tumour cells and endothelial cells. Note that upon release of FGF, additional cell types, such as stromal fibroblasts, may respond to FGF.

thus inducing tumour angiogenesis (Fig. 17.3b). Finally, FGF in a paracrine/autocrine fashion might exert mitogenic activity on both tumour cells and endothelial cells (Fig. 17.3). It is also conceivable that other cell types, such as stromal fibroblasts, may be targets of FGF activity or that FGF produced by tumour cells stimulates an additional cell type to secrete an angiogenic factor. Functional experiments involving highly specific inhibitors of FGF activity during tumour angiogenesis *in vivo* or genetic experiments in which the activity of FGF ligands or FGF receptors can be modulated, for example by conditional disruption of gene function in transgenic mice, will be required to fully characterize the diverse roles of FGFs in tumour angiogenesis.

Again, the angiogenic factor VEGF and its receptors have been shown to play an important functional part in tumour angiogenesis (see Chapter 10). Recently, it has been demonstrated that FGF-1 and FGF-2 together with VEGF synergistically induce the formation of capillary-like structures in three-dimensional endothelial cell culture systems (290,291). These results raise the possibility that both of these potent angiogenic factors, FGF and VEGF, might be involved in tumour angiogenesis. Further experimentation is warranted to determine whether a single angiogenic factor is sufficient or whether a combination of factors are necessary for the induction of tumour angiogenesis. However, the balance between angiogenic factors and angiogenic inhibitors seems to be *the* important parameter for the regulation of physiological and pathological angiogenesis and, thus, these experiments will have to assess the interplay of many factors *in vivo* (315).

Regulation of fibroblast growth factor activity

The potent mitogenic activity of FGFs on a variety of target cells requires a strict temporal and spatial regulation of FGF and FGF receptor expression and/or activity. Inhibition of FGF or FGF receptor activities as well as the specific ablation of cells bearing FGF receptors may provide therapeutic tools for the treatment of the pathological conditions in which FGFs may play a part.

Studies on the transcriptional regulation of FGF-1 and FGF-2 are still limited, yet some of them might be of relevance to the role of FGFs in angiogenesis and tumour development. For example, it has been shown that FGF-2 is able to stimulate its own transcription in endothelial cells indicating that FGF-2 can amplify its own activities (320). Similarly, IL-1 is able to up-regulate FGF-2 transcription and protein synthesis in smooth muscle cells suggesting that vascular injury or inflammation could be a trigger for increased FGF-2 synthesis (321). Most interestingly for tumorigenesis, it has been shown that the gene product of the tumour suppressor gene p53 bound to the promoter region of FGF-2 and repressed transcription of FGF-2 in glioma and hepatocellular carcinoma cell lines. In contrast, mutated p53 was able to up-regulate FGF-2 transcription (322).

Another potential level for the regulation of FGF activity is the variable subcellular localization of the different isoforms of FGF-2 and FGF-3, and the nuclear targeting of FGF-1 and FGF-2 (see earlier on pp. 211). Although some mechanistic aspects of these processes have been addressed, their functional implications remain to be elucidated. Post-transcriptional modifications of FGF-1 and FGF-2 including protein phosphorylation by protein kinase A or protein kinase C have been reported and might also play an important part in the modulation FGF activity (31).

FGF-1 and FGF-2 lack a signal sequence for the entrance of proteins into the rough endoplasmatic reticulum and subsequent secretion through the conventional secretory pathway, and the molecular pathway by which these growth factors are secreted from the cytoplasm to the extracellular space is not known. Two steps for the release of FGF-1 or FGF-2 from cells have to be considered: first, the actual translocation through the plasma membrane into the extracellular space, and second, the release of FGF-1 and FGF-2 from their sequestration sites in the extracellular matrix and basement membranes. Export and release of FGFs are presumably tightly regulated. For example, despite its potent mitogenic activity on endothelial cells, FGF-2 has been found in the walls of quiescent blood vessels (323).

Inhibition of fibroblast growth factor activity

Experimental approaches towards the functional role of FGF ligands and FGF receptors during tumorigenesis and angiogenesis are still hampered by the lack of specific tools to interfere with their activities. As described above, specific neutralizing antibodies to FGF and their receptors inhibited proliferation of various cell lines *in vitro*; however, when injected into athymic mice they did not affect tumour size, tumour cell proliferation, or tumour vascularization (324). Suramin, a polyanion, disrupts binding of FGFs to their receptors (201,325). It has been used in clinical trials on cancer patients with some promising effects (326,327). However, suramin is not specific for FGFs and also interferes with binding of several other growth factors to their receptors. Also, treatment of Kaposi sarcoma-derived cells with suramin or protamine had no inhibitory effect. Instead it resulted in the up-regulation of FGF-2, FGF-5, and FGF receptors, consistent with clinical

observations that suramin caused stimulation of Kaposi sarcoma growth in patients (328).

Pentosan polysulphate, another polyanionic heparin analogue, has been reported to inhibit proliferation of tumour cell lines derived from breast cracinoma, prostate carcinoma, lung carcinoma, epidermoid tumors, and rhabdomyosarcomas in culture and in athymic mice (329). Human adrenal cancer cell lines that have been transfected with FGF-4 were dramatically inhibited in their proliferation and tumour formation by pentosan polysulphate, whereas suramin or dextran sulphate exhibited only a slight inhibitory effect (325). However, treatment of HIV-associated Kaposi sarcoma in patients with pentosan polysulphate did not reveal a significant tumour response (330).

One approach to inhibit the biological activities mediated by FGF ligands and FGF receptors is the utilization of dominant-negative receptor constructs which, when co-expressed with FGF receptors, can block activation and signal transduction. Some of these tools have already been employed to study the functional role of FGFs and their receptors in airways epithelia development and in wound healing (section on 'High-affinity FGF receptors', p. 206; 114,115). In a similar manner, NIH 3T3 cells transformed by FGF-4 were supressed by expression of tyrosine kinase-deficient dominant-negative FGF receptors. In these experiments a truncated version of FGFR-2 was significantly more efficient than a truncated version of FGFR-1, and the inhibition could be overcome by the addition of excess growth factor (331).

Another approach to interfere with tumour growth is the ligand-specific targeting of toxins to tumour cells expressing FGF receptors. For example, a fusion protein consisting of FGF-2 and saporin, a cell toxin isolated from the plant *saponaria*, was specifically targeted to FGF receptors and exhibited anti-tumour activity *in vitro* and *in vivo* (332,333). Recombinant versions of these fusion proteins expressed in *Escherichia* coli inhibited growth of B16F10 melanoma cell lines *in vitro* and retarded tumour growth and metastasis *in vivo* (334,335).

Alternatively, fusion of FGF-1 to *Pseudomonas* exotoxin A resulted in specific cytotoxicity to a variety of tumour cell lines expressing FGF receptors including those of prostate, colon, or breast carcinoma (336). This approach has also specifically affected glioblastoma cells *in vitro* and *in vivo*, but was less efficient than TGF-α/*Pseudomonas* exotoxin A fusion that was targeted to the EGF receptor on the surface of the tumour cells (337). Systemic application in athymic mice grafted with several different tumour cell lines slowed tumour growth, but did not induce complete regression. Most likely, the exotoxin attacked tumour mass rather than the tumour endothelium

(336). *Pseudomonas* exotoxin FGF-1 fusion proteins also inhibited endothelial cells proliferation and tube formation *in vitro* by inducing dose-dependent cell death (338).

Other inhibitory compounds have been developed that bind and inactivate FGF ligands. However, their specificity towards FGFs and/or other growth factors is not yet established. For example, using systemic evolution of ligands by exponential enrichment (SELEX) high-affinity RNA ligands to FGF-2 have been isolated that inhibit binding of FGF-2 to its receptor (339). Recently, it has also been reported that phosphorothioate oligodeoxynucleotides bind to FGF-1, -2, and -4, thereby preventing their binding to FGF receptors and removing FGF ligands from low-affinity binding sites on the cell surface (340).

In conclusion, based on a multitude of expression studies in tumour biopsies and in tumour cell lines, FGFs and their receptor are likely to play a part in the growth regulation of many cancers. Experiments utilizing tools that interfere with FGF ligand and receptor activity demonstrated such a functional role. However, better and more specific reagents need to be developed in order to interfere efficiently with either tumour cell proliferation or tumour angiogenesis.

Export of FGF-1 and FGF-2

Low levels of FGF-2 have been detected in the conditioned medium of endothelial cells (246,248) and some tumour cell lines (341–343). Using a sensitive immunoassay, elevated levels of FGF-2 were detected in the conditioned medium of endothelial cells after mitogenic stimulation, suggesting that proliferating endothelial cells might release FGF-2 as well (344). However, the exported forms of FGF-2 and the export pathway has not been further investigated. Neutralizing antibodies could interfere with an autocrine loop of FGF-2 and FGF receptors in endothelial cells (247). Furthermore, cell migration was caused by FGF release from cells that have been transformed with signalless FGFs (345–347). However, in all these cases the mechanism of FGF export, namely the actual translocation of FGF-1 or FGF-2 through the plasma membrane, remains unknown. Other examples of cytokines that are secreted in the absence of an apparent signal peptide include IL-1α and IL-1β, patelet-derived endothelial cell growth factor (PD-ECGF), ciliary neurotrophic factor (CNTF), adult T-cell leukaemia-derived factor (ADF), thymosin, and parathymosin. In all these cases, the mechanism of export remains undefined; however, possible novel pathways for these secretory proteins have been proposed (348).

Cell wounding and cell lysis

It has been suggested that FGF-1, FGF-2, and IL-1 could be released through cell lysis induced by wounding, necrosis or cell death (8,196,247,349,350). Multiple reports argue for such a passive pathway of cytokine export. Lethal injury of aortic endothelial cells by endotoxin resulted in release of FGF-2 and secondary sequestration in the extracellular matrix (351). Furthermore, irradiation of cultured endothelial cells resulted in a dose-dependent release of mitogenic activities, most probably FGF-2 together with PDGF (352). Endothelial, BHK-21, and NIH 3T3 cells injured *in vitro* by scraping, stimulated cell migration that could be inhibited by protamine, suramin, and neutralizing antibodies to FGF-2, indicating that FGF-2 has been released into the extracellular space (248). Export of FGF-2 from viable cells was stimulated by transient, sublethal injury of endothelial cells by scrape-wounding *in vitro*. In these experiments, the release of FGF-2 did not correlate with cell death or a functional secretory pathway, suggesting that mechanical transient disruption of plasma membranes might be involved in the release of cytosolic FGF-2. However, such a release was not observed in all cell lines tested (353,354). Moreover, FGF release appeared to depend on the cell density of the cultures used, suggesting that cell lysis might not be the only pathway for the release of FGF (343).

Rat aorta injured during resection induced capillary sprouting of endothelial cells from the explant. Inhibition by specific antibodies indicated that FGF-2 was released from the tissue (253). Similarly, infarcted myocardial tissue released FGF activity at levels that correlated with the levels of creatine phosphokinase, a marker for cell injury. Subsequently, it has been shown that these FGF activities consisted of FGF-1 and FGF-2 which were already expressed in normal myocardium (355). High amounts of FGF-2 are contained in platelets and macrophages. As these cells are known to release their entire cell constituents upon activation, it is conceivable that FGFs are released by these cells during inflammation, hypoxia, or ischaemia (356–358). However, in some angiogenic processes, such as ovulation, wounding does not occur. This suggests that if signalless FGFs play a part in angiogenesis, they may be exported by an active secretory pathway other than conventional secretion.

Active export of FGF-1 and FGF-2

Several reports during the last 5 years provide evidence that export of FGF-1 and FGF-2 may involve a novel secretory pathway. Stably transfected NIH 3T3 cells that expressed high levels of signalless FGF-1, released FGF-1 upon heat shock in a process that required the *de novo* synthesis of protein (359). The transfected 3T3 cells exported FGF-1 as a functionally inactive homodimer. This export was not prevented by Brefeldin A and methylamine, inhibitors of endoplasmic reticulum–Golgi transport and exocytosis, respectively (360). Three cysteine residues (Cys 30,97 and 131) in FGF-1 were required for export, as mutants that lack them were synthesized, but not exported. These cysteine residues were not required for bioactivity, and intramolecular disulphide bridges were not formed in active molecules (19). Copper-induced homodimer formation, on the other hand, has been shown to inactivate FGF-1 (20). Dimer formation could therefore be an important step in the release of FGF-1 from cells. In HeLa cells, UV irradiation induced the concomitant export of FGF-2 and IL-1α (361). Similar results were reported using Cos cells and NIH 3T3 cells transfected with FGF-2 (346,362). In these cases, high levels of FGF-2 expression resulted in the constitutive export of FGF-2 in a process that was independent from the conventional secretion pathway.

Export of endogenous FGF-2 has also been reported. T lymphocytes isolated from peripheral blood constitutively released FGF-2 into the culture medium (363). It has also been reported that T lymphocytes upon co-culturing with irradiated B lymphoma line were stimulated to secrete FGF-1 in unusual high molecular weight forms (320–600 kDa) (364). A similar active export of FGF-2 has recently been reported in cell lines derived from different stages of fibrosarcoma development in transgenic mice carrying the bovine papilloma virus genome (see also section on 'FGF in tumour angiogenesis'; 318). In the normal dermal fibroblasts and in the mild fibromatosis stage, FGF-2 is exclusively cell associated. However, in cell lines derived from the aggressive fibromatosis stage and from fibrosarcomas, FGF-2 is released by a mechanism that does not involve cell death or cell lysis. However, the nature of the released FGF-2 and the pathway of export have not been further investigated.

In another transgenic mouse model of tumour development the simian virus 40 large T oncogene (SV40 Tag) is expressed under the control of the rat insulin-II promoter (Rip 1Tag2). These mice develop tumours in the β cells of the islets of Langerhans (insulinomas) in a predictable manner (365). Different stages of tumour development are distinguishable. Although all the β cells express T antigen, only 70% of the islets develop 'hyperplasia', as determined by an increased proliferation index (366). Two populations of hyperplastic islets can be identified; most of the hyperplastic islets exhibit normal vascularization, whereas a small proportion (3–10% of the total islets) are hypervascularized and secrete soluble angiogenic factors that are chemotactic and mitogenic for endothelial cells in a three-dimensional culture system (367). The latter class of hyperplastic islets have acquired an additional step towards the development of highly vascularized insulinomas (angiogenic switch). We have recently demonstrated that cell lines established from the β-cell tumours of Rip1 Tag2 transgenic mice (βTC) constitutively secreted FGF-1 into the culture medium (Christofori et al., manuscript submitted). FGF-1 was found to be sequestered in conditioned medium, as assessed by mitogenic activity and heparin affinity. Treatment of conditioned medium with high salt recovered FGF-1 as high molecular weight (HMW) forms with reduced heparin affinity and a molecular mass of approximately 40 kDa. Reducing agents partially converted monomeric FGF-1 from the complexed forms indicating that disulphide bonds were involved in the modification of FGF-1, possibly in forming homodimers. The HMW forms of FGF-1 were found in cell lysates as well as in the culture medium, suggesting that the HMW forms represented intermediates in the export pathway. Brefeldin A, an inhibitor of conventional secretion, did not interfere with FGF-1 export by β tumour cells.

In other established tumour cell lines, including human breast carcinoma and murine fibrosarcoma, a similar export of FGF-2 as HMW forms with reduced heparin affinity was detected. This did not hold true for normal or pre-malignant cell lines that expressed high levels of FGF-2 (Christofori et al., manuscript submitted). Among the different tumour cell lines analysed, the pattern that FGF-1 or FGF-2 were exported as HMW forms, presumably as dimers, with reduced heparin affinity is remarkably similar. Moreover, none of the cell lines analysed were affected in their FGF export by treatment with Brefeldin A or verapamil, inhibitors of the conventional secretion pathway and the multidrug resistance transporters, respectively (346,360,362). Collectively, these data strongly suggest that a similar, non-conventional pathway is utilized by the different cell lines for the export of FGF-1 and FGF-2. Alternatively, FGF-1 could be bound as a heterodimer to another unknown partner to produce the observed HMW forms. One candidate for a partner protein that could associate with FGF-1/2 to produce the ~40 kDa HMW forms is a recently discovered FGF binding protein (FGF-BP) (368).

Elevated levels of FGF-2 were found in the body fluids of cancer patients and experimental animals bearing tumours, indicating that FGF-2 was released during tumour progression (see section on 'FGF in tumour angiogenesis'). Circulating FGF-like activity was also found at elevated levels and with unusual molecular weight forms in the plasma of familial multiple endocrine neoplasia type 1 patients (369). FGF-2 was also found in the uterine luminal fluid concomitant with the expression of FGF-2 at the apical surface of epithelial cells at days 4 and 5 of pregnancy in rat (370) and in uterine luminal fluid in pregnant pigs (371).

In combination these data suggest that FGF-1 and FGF-2 are selectively exported by many tumour cell types and also by normal cell types under stress conditions or during physiological angiogenesis via a non-conventional secretory pathway. A switch in the subcellular localization of FGF may be a general mechanism of tumour promoted angiogenesis. The ability of cells to regulate FGF export may also impact on non-disease roles of FGF-1 and FGF-2.

Extracellular sequestration and release

Another major issue associated with the release pathway of FGF-1 and FGF-2 is the nature of their sequestration to (HSPGs) in the extracellular matrix and basement membrane of cells (see also Chapter 18). When endothelial cells from different sources were analysed, the majority of FGF-2 was cell associated (245,247,372–374). Although the majority of FGF-2 was in the cytosol, reasonably high levels of FGF-2 were detected in the extracellular matrix (85,244,245,374–376) and in the basement membrane (377). FGF-2 has also been found in the basement membrane of cardiac myocytes in culture (378), in the basement membrane of bovine cornea (377), and FGF-1 has been detected in the extracellular matrix of mouse skeletal muscle (377). The sequestered forms of FGF-2 could be released by heparin, heparan sulphate, heparitinase, or by plasminogen activator-mediated proteolytic activity (376,380). Furthermore, infusion of rabbits with heparin released FGF-2, indicating that FGF-2 was sequestered by the luminal surface of vascular endothelium (381).

Matrix-bound FGF-1 or FGF-2 appeared to be active and induced endothelial cell proliferation and plasminogen activator production (382,383). Basement membranes from corneal endothelial cells support the growth of vascular endothelial cells in the absence of exogenous growth factors (384) and induce the differentiation of PC12 cells as visualized by neurite outgrowth (385). Upon binding to heparin and heparan sulphates the FGFs might be stabilized against denaturation and proteolytic degradation (386–389). However, FGF-2 was detected in vivo in the extracellular matrix and basement membranes of tissues, where no cell proliferation or motility could be detected, suggesting that FGF-2 may also be stored in a latent, inactive form.

By binding to the extracellular matrix the activity of soluble stimulators or inhibitors can be locally stored and regulated. HSPGs, such as syndecan or perlecan, function as low-affinity FGF receptors and sequester FGFs. This association is necessary for the efficient binding of FGFs to their high-affinity receptors. In addition, upon cell to cell contact the exposure of sequestered FGFs on one cell's surface to another cell bearing high-affinity receptors could activate FGF receptor signalling. The model that FGFs might be stored in a latent form that can be locally activated by heparin or heparitinases, or by exposure to their high-affinity receptors offers an attractive possibility for the regulation of FGF activities either in cell–cell contact situations or when present as soluble cytokines. However, further investigation is warranted to confirm such mechanisms.

Summary and conclusions

In this review we have focused on the potential functional role of members of the FGF family and their receptors in tumour cell proliferation, in physiological and pathological angiogenesis, and in tumour angiogenesis. Most, if not all, members of the FGF family seem to play an important part in tumour cell proliferation in cancer patients or in experimental systems. FGF-1, FGF-2, and FGF-4 are clearly angiogenic in vitro and in vivo. However, despite a vast and extreme experimental effort, their detailed functional role in physiological angiogenesis and in tumour angiogenesis remains to be elucidated.

Members of the FGF family exhibit a confusing multitude of biological activities and, for this reason, their distinct functions on particular target cells cannot be easily identified in vivo. The picture becomes even more complicated by other growth factors that share some of the activities and target cells of FGFs. Novel experimental strategies need to be utilized, including genetic manipulation in transgenic mice or the development of highly specific inhibitors for growth factor and growth factor receptor activities, in order to clarify the detailed biological role of FGFs. Some of these tools are now available and are being used to unravel the functional role of FGF family members in tumour development and, particularly, in tumour angiogenesis.

Acknowledgements

I am grateful to Drs Douglas Hanahan and Judah Folkman for encouraging me to work on tumour angiogenesis, for many fruitful discussions and for their support. I wish to thank Drs Matt Cotten and Gabor Lamm for their critical comments on the manuscript. The research in the laboratory of the author was supported in part by the Austrian Industrial Research Promotion Fund.

References

1. Algire, G. H., Chalkley, W. H., Legallais, F. Y., and Park, H. D. (1945). Vascular reactions of normal and malignant tumors *in vivo*. I. Vascular reactions of mice to wounds and to normal and neoplastic transplants. *J. Natl Cancer Inst.*, **6**, 73–85.

2. Ide, A. G., Baker, N. H., and Warrem, S. L. (1939). Vascularization of the Brown-Pearce rabbit epithelioma transplant as seen in the transparent ear chamber. *Am. J. Roentgenol.*, **42**, 881–89.

3. Greenblatt, M. and Shubik, P. (1968). Tumor angiogenesis: transfilter diffusion studies in the hamster by transparent chamber technique. *J. Natl Cancer Inst.*, **41**, 111–14.

4. Ehrmann, R. L. and Knoth, M. (1968). Choriocarcinoma: transfilter stimulation of vasoproliferation in the hamster cheek pouch — studied by light and electron microscopy. *J. Natl Cancer Inst.*, **41**, 1329–32.

5. Shing, Y., Folkman, J., Sullivan, R., Butterfield, C., Murray, J., and Klagsbrun, M. (1984). Heparin-affinity: purification of a tumor-derived capillary endothelial cell growth factor. *Science*, **223**, 1296–9.

6. Burgess, W. H. and Maciag, T. (1989). The heparin-binding (fibroblast) growth factor family of proteins. *Annu. Rev. Biochem.*, **58**, 575–606.

7. Basilico, C. and Moscatelli, D. (1992). The FGF family of growth factors and oncogenes. *Adv. Cancer Res.* **59**, 115–65.

8. Thomas, K. A. (1988). Transforming potential of fibroblast growth factor genes. *Trends Biochem. Sci.*, **13**, 327–8.

9. Gospodarowicz, D. (1990). Fibroblast growth factor and the control of vascular endothelial cell proliferation and differentiation. In *Genetic mechanisms in carcinogenesis and tumor progression* (ed. C. L. Harris and L. A. Liotta), pp. 15–30. Wiley-Liss, New York.

10. Gospodarowicz, D. (1990). Fibroblast growth factor and its role in development. In *Growth regulation of cancer II* (ed. M. E. Lippman and R. B. Dickson), pp. 49–63. Alan R. Liss, New York.

11. McKeehan, W. L. and Crabb, J. W. (1987). Isolation and characterization of different molecular and chromatographic forms of heparin binding growth factor 1 from bovine brain. *Anal. Biochem.* **164**, 563–9.

12. Forough, R., Engleka, K., Thompson, J. A., Jackson, A., Imamura, T., and Maciag, T. (1991). Differential expression in *Escherichia coli* of the alpha and beta forms of heparin-binding acidic fibroblast growth factor-1: potential role of RNA secondary structure. *Biochim. Biophys. Acta*, **1090**, 293–8.

13. Klagsbrun, M. (1990). The affinity of fibroblast growth factors (FGFs) for heparin; FGF–heparan sulfate interactions in cells and extracellular matrix. *Curr. Opin. Cell Biol.*, **2**, 857–63.

14. Zhu, X., Hsu, B. T., and Rees, D. C. (1993). Structural studies of the binding of the anti-ulcer drug sucrose octasulfate to acidic fibroblast growth factor. *Structure*, **1**, 27–34.

15. Zhu, X., Komiya, H., Chirino, A., Faham, S., Fox, G. M., Arakawa, T., *et al.* (1991). Three-dimensional structures of acidic and basic fibroblast growth factors. *Science*, **251**, 90–3.

16. Burgess, W. H., Friesel, R., and Winkles, J. A. (1994). Structure-function studies of FGF-1: dissociation and partial reconstitution of certain of its biological activities. *Mol. Reprod. Dev.*, **39**, 56–60.

17. Burgess, W. H., Shaheen, A. M., Ravera, M., Jaye, M., Donohue, P. J., and Winkles, J. A. (1990). Possible dissociation of the heparin-binding and mitogenic activities of heparin-binding (acidic fibroblast) growth factor-1 from its receptor-binding activities by site-directed mutagenesis of a single lysine residue. *J. Cell Biol.*, **111**, 2129–38.

18. Ortega, S., Schaeffer, M. T., Soderman, D., DiSalvo, J., Linemeyer, D. L., Gimenez, G. G., and Thomas, K. A. (1991). Conversion of cysteine to serine residues alters the activity, stability, and heparin dependence of acidic fibroblast growth factor. *J. Biol. Chem.*, **266**, 5842–6.

19. Linemeyer, D. L., Menke, J. G., Kelly, L. J., DiSalvo, J., Soderman, D., Schaeffer, M. T., *et al.* (1990). Disulfide bonds are neither required, present, nor compatible with full activity of human recombinant acidic fibroblast growth factor. *Growth Factors*, **3**, 287–98.

20. Engleka, K. A., and Maciag, T. (1992). Inactivation of human fibroblast growth factor-1 (FGF-1) activity by interaction with copper ions involves FGF-1 dimer formation induced by copper-catalyzed oxidation. *J. Biol. Chem.*, **267**, 11307–15.

21. Imamura, T., Engleka, K., Zhan, X., Tokita, Y., Forough, R., Roeder, D., *et al.* (1990). Recovery of mitogenic activity of a growth factor mutant with a nuclear translocation sequence. *Science*, **249**, 1567–70.

22. Florkiewicz, R. Z., Baird, A., and Gonzalez, A. M. (1991). Multiple forms of bFGF: differential nuclear and cell surface localization. *Growth Factors*, **4**, 265–75.

23. Renko, M., Quarto, N., Morimoto, T., and Rifkin, D. B. (1990). Nuclear and cytoplasmic localization of different basic fibroblast growth factor species. *J. Cell. Physiol.*, **144**, 108–14.

24. Powell, P. P. and Klagsbrun, M. (1991). Three forms of rat basic fibroblast growth factor are made from a single mRNA and localize to the nucleus. *J. Cell. Physiol.*, **148**, 202–10.

25. Isacchi, A., Statuto, M., Chiesa, R., Bergonzoni, L., Rusnati, M., Sarmientos, P., *et al.* (1991). A six-amino acid deletion in basic fibroblast growth factor dissociates its mitogenic activity from its plasminogen activator-inducing capacity. *Proc. Natl Acad. Sci. USA*, **88**, 2628–32.

26. Seno, M., Sasada, R., Iwane, M., Sudo, K., Kurokawa, T., Ito, K., and Igarashi, K. (1988). Stabilizing basic fibroblast growth factor using protein engineering. *Biochem. Biophys. Res. Commun.*, **151**, 701–8.

27. Folkman, J., Szabo, S., Stovroff, M., McNeil, P., Li, W., and Shing, Y. (1991). Duodenal ulcer. Discovery of a new mechanism and development of angiogenic therapy that accelerates healing. *Ann. Surg.*, **214**, 414–25.

28. Zhang, J. D., Cousens, L. S., Barr, P. J., and Sprang, S. R. (1991). Three-dimensional structure of human basic fibroblast growth factor, a structural homolog of interleukin 1 beta [published erratum appears in *Proc. Natl Acad. Sci. USA*, 1991; **88** (12): 5477]. *Proc. Natl Acad. Sci. USA*, **88**, 3446–50.

29. Eriksson, A. E., Cousens, L. S., Weaver, L. H., and Matthews, B. W. (1991). Three-dimensional structure of

human basic fibroblast growth factor. *Proc. Natl Acad. Sci. USA*, **88**, 3441–5.

30. Kurokawa, M., Doctrow, S. R., and Klagsbrun, M. (1989). Neutralizing antibodies inhibit the binding of basic fibroblast growth factor to its receptor but not to heparin. *J. Biol. Chem.*, **264**, 7686–91.

31. Feige, J. J., Ling, N., and Baird, A. (1991). Phosphorylation of basic fibroblast growth factor by purified protein kinase C and the identification of a cryptic site of phosphorylation. *Biochem. Biophys. Res. Commun.*, **175**, 31–6.

32. Halaban, R., Ghosh, S., and Baird, A. (1987). bFGF is the putative natural growth factor for human melanocytes. *In Vitro Cell Dev. Biol.*, **23**, 47–52.

33. Slack, J. M. (1994). Inducing factors in *Xenopus* early embryos. *Curr. Biol.*, **4**, 116–26.

34. Bikfalvi, A. and Han, Z. C. (1994). Angiogenic factors are hematopoietic growth factors and vice versa. *Leukemia*, **8**, 523–9.

35. Bikfalvi, A., Han, Z. C., and Fuhrmann, G. (1992). Interaction of fibroblast growth factor (FGF) with megakaryocytopoiesis and demonstration of FGF receptor expression in megakaryocytes and megakaryocytic-like cells. *Blood*, **80**, 1905–13.

36. Anderson, K. J., Dam, D., Lee, S., and Cotman, C. W. (1988). Basic fibroblast growth factor prevents death of lesioned cholinergic neurons *in vivo*. *Nature*, **332**, 360–1.

37. Dickson, C., Smith, R., Brookes, S., and Peters, G. (1984). Tumorigenesis by mouse mammary tumor virus: proviral activation of a cellular gene in the common integration region int-2. *Cell*, **37**, 529–36.

38. Smith, R., Peters, G., and Dickson, C. (1988). Multiple RNAs expressed from the int-2 gene in mouse embryonal carcinoma cell lines encode a protein with homology to fibroblast growth factors. *EMBO J.*, **7**, 1013–22.

39. Acland, P., Dixon, M., Peters, G., and Dickson, C. (1990). Subcellular fate of the int-2 oncoprotein is determined by choice of initiation codon. *Nature*, **343**, 662–5.

40. Kiefer, P., Acland, P., Pappin, D., Peters, G., and Dickson, C. (1994). Competition between nuclear localization and secretory signals determines the subcellular fate of a single CUG-initiated form of FGF3. *EMBO J.*, **13**, 4126–36.

41. Kiefer, P. and Dickson, C. (1995). Nucleolar association of fibroblast growth factor 3 via specific sequence motifs has inhibitory effects on cell growth. *Mol. Cell. Biol.*, **15**, 4364–74.

42. Kiefer, P., Peters, G., and Dickson, C. (1993). Retention of fibroblast growth factor 3 in the Golgi complex may regulate its export from cells. *Mol. Cell. Biol.*, **13**, 5781–93.

43. Wilkinson, D. G., Bhatt, S., and McMahon, A. P. (1989). Expression pattern of the FGF-related proto-oncogene int-2 suggests multiple roles in fetal development. *Development*, **105**, 131–6.

44. Meyers, S. L. and Dudley, J. P. (1992). Sequence analysis of the int-2/fgf-3 gene in aggressive human breast carcinomas. *Mol. Carcinog.*, **6**, 243–51.

45. Zhou, D. J., Casey, G., and Cline, M. J. (1988). Amplification of human int-2 in breast cancer and squamous carcinomas. *Oncogene*, **2**, 279–82.

46. Goldfarb, M., Deed, R., MacAllan, D., Walther, W., Dickson, C., and Peters, G. (1991). Cell transformation by Int-2 — a member of the fibroblast growth factor family. *Oncogene*, **6**, 65–71.

47. Mansour, S. L. (1994). Targeted disruption of int-2 (fgf-3) causes developmental defects in the tail and inner ear. *Mol. Reprod. Dev.*, **39**, 62–7.

48. Sakamoto, H., Mori, M., Taira, M., Yoshida, T., Matsukawa, S., Shimizu, K., *et al.* (1986). Transforming gene from human stomach cancers and a noncancerous portion of stomach mucosa. *Proc. Natl Acad. Sci. USA*, **83**, 3997–4001.

49. Delli, B. P., Curatola, A. M., Kern, F. G., Greco, A., Ittmann, M., and Basilico, C. (1987). An oncogene isolated by transfection of Kaposi's sarcoma DNA encodes a growth factor that is a member of the FGF family. *Cell*, **50**, 729–37.

50. Bellosta, P., Talarico, D., Rogers, D., and Basilico, C. (1993). Cleavage of K-FGF produces a truncated molecule with increased biological activity and receptor binding affinity. *J. Cell. Biol.*, **121**, 705–13.

51. Feldman, B., Poueymirou, W., Papaioannou, V. E., DeChiara, T. M., and Goldfarb, M. (1995). Requirement of FGF-4 for postimplantation mouse development. *Science*, **267**, 246–9.

52. Drucker, B. J. and Goldfarb, M. (1993). Murine FGF-4 gene expression is spatially restricted within embryonic skeletal muscle and other tissues. *Mech. Dev.*, **40**, 155–63.

53. Tickle, C. and Eichele, G. (1994). Vertebrate limb development. *Annu. Rev. Cell Biol.* **10**, 121–52.

54. Niswander, L., Tickle, C., Vogel, A., and Martin, G. (1994). Function of FGF-4 in limb development. *Mol. Reprod. Dev.*, **39**, 83–8.

55. Johnson, R. L., Riddle, R. D., and Tabin, C. J. (1994). Mechanisms of limb patterning. *Curr. Opin. Genet. Dev.*, **4**, 535–42.

56. Cohn, M. J., Izpisua, B. J., Abud, H., Heath, J. K., and Tickle, C. (1995). Fibroblast growth factors induce additional limb development from the flank of chick embryos. *Cell*, **80**, 739–46.

57. Yoshida, T., Ishimaru, K., Sakamoto, H., Yokota, J., Hirohashi, S., Igarashi, K., *et al.* (1994). Angiogenic activity of the recombinant hst-1 protein. *Cancer Lett.*, **83**, 261–8.

58. Zhan, X., Bates, B., Hu, X. G., and Goldfarb, M. (1988). The human FGF-5 oncogene encodes a novel protein related to fibroblast growth factors. *Mol. Cell. Biol.*, **8**, 3487–95.

59. Bates, B., Hardin, J., Zhan, X., Drickamer, K., and Goldfarb, M. (1991). Biosynthesis of human fibroblast growth factor-5. *Mol. Cell. Biol.*, **11**, 1840–5.

60. Haub, O. and Goldfarb, M. (1991). Expression of the fibroblast growth factor-5 gene in the mouse embryo. *Development*, **112**, 397–406.

61. Hebert, J. M., Boyle, M., and Martin, G. R. (1991). mRNA localization studies suggest that murine FGF-5 plays a role in gastrulation. *Development*, **112**, 407–15.

62. Haub, O., Drucker, B., and Goldfarb, M. (1990). Expression of the murine fibroblast growth factor 5 gene in the adult central nervous system. *Proc. Natl Acad. Sci. USA*, **87**, 8022–6.

63. Gomez, P. F. and Cotman, C. W. (1993). Distribution of fibroblast growth factor 5 mRNA in the rat brain: an *in situ* hybridization study. *Brain Res.*, **606**, 79–86.

64. Hebert, J. M., Rosenquist, T., Götz, J., and Martin, G. R. (1994). FGF5 as a regulator of the hair growth cycle:

evidence from targeted and spontaneous mutations. *Cell*, **78**, 1017–25.

65. Werner, S., Roth, W. K., Bates, B., Goldfarb, M., and Hofschneider, P. H. (1991). Fibroblast growth factor 5 proto-oncogene is expressed in normal human fibroblasts and induced by serum growth factors. *Oncogene*, **6**, 2137–44.

66. Goldfarb, M., Bates, B., Drucker, B., Hardin, J., and Haub, O. (1991). Expression and possible functions of the FGF-5 gene. *Ann. N. Y. Acad. Sci.*, **638**, 38–52.

67. Lindholm, D., Harikka, J., da Penha-Berzaghi, M., Castren, E., Tzimagiorgis, G., Hughes, R. A., and Thoenen, H. (1994). Fibroblast growth factor-5 promotes differentiation of cultured rat septal cholinergic and raphe serotonergic neurons: comparison with the effects of neurotrophins. *Eur. J. Neurosci.*, **6**, 244–52.

68. Hughes, R. A., Sendtner, M., Goldfarb, M., Lindholm, D., and Thoenen, H. (1993). Evidence that fibroblast growth factor 5 is a major muscle-derived survival factor for cultured spinal motoneurons. *Neuron*, **10**, 369–77.

69. Marics, I., Adelaide, J., Raybaud, F., Mattei, M. G., Coulier, F., Planche, J., de Lepeyriere, O., and Birnbaum, D. (1989). Characterization of the HST-related FGF.6 gene, a new member of the fibroblast growth factor gene family. *Oncogene*, **4**, 335–40.

70. Iida, S., Yoshida, T., Naito, K., Sakamoto, H., Katoh, O., Hirohashi, S., *et al.* (1992). Human hst-2 (FGF-6) oncogene: cDNA cloning and characterization. *Oncogene*, **7**, 303–9.

71. de, L. O., Rosnet, O., Benharroch, D., Raybaud, F., Marchetto, S., Planche, J., Galland, F., *et al.* (1990). Structure, chromosome mapping and expression of the murine Fgf-6 gene. *Oncogene*, **5**, 823–31.

72. Han, J. K. and Martin, G. R. (1993). Embryonic expression of Fgf-6 is restricted to the skeletal muscle lineage. *Dev. Biol.*, **158**, 549–54.

73. Pizette, S., Batoz, M., Prats, H., Birnbaum, D., and Coulier, F. (1991). Production and functional characterization of human recombinant FGF-6 protein. *Cell. Growth Differ.*, **2**, 561–6.

74. Rubin, J. S., Osada, H., Finch, P. W., Taylor, W. G., Rudikoff, S., and Aaronson, S. A. (1989). Purification and characterization of a newly identified growth factor specific for epithelial cells. *Proc. Natl Acad. Sci. USA*, **86**, 802–6.

75. Finch, P. W., Rubin, J. S., Miki, T., Ron, D., and Aaronson, S. A. (1989). Human KGF is FGF-related with properties of a paracrine effector of epithelial cell growth. *Science*, **245**, 752–5.

76. Mason, I. J., Fuller, P. F., Smith, R., and Dickson, C. (1994). FGF-7 (keratinocyte growth factor) expression during mouse development suggests roles in myogenesis, forebrain regionalisation and epithelial–mesenchymal interactions. *Mech. Dev.*, **45**, 15–30.

77. Werner, S., Peters, K. G., Longaker, M. T., Fuller, P. F., Banda, M. J., and Williams, L. T. (1992). Large induction of keratinocyte growth factor expression in the dermis during wound healing. *Proc. Natl Acad. Sci. USA*, **89**, 6896–900.

78. Tanaka, A., Lu, J., Yamanishi, H., Nonomura, N., Yasui, T., Maeyama, M., *et al.* (1990). Effects of androgen, fibroblast growth factors or other various growth factors on growth of Shionogi carcinoma cells in a protein-free medium. *Anticancer Res.*, **10**, 1637–41.

79. Tanaka, A., Miyamoto, K., Minamino, N., Takeda, M., Sato, B., Matsuo, H., and Matsumoto, K. (1992). Cloning and characterization of an androgen-induced growth factor essential for the androgen-dependent growth of mouse mammary carcinoma cells. *Proc. Natl Acad. Sci. USA*, **89**, 8928–32.

80. Miyamoto, M., Naruo, K., Seko, C., Matsumoto, S., Kondo, T., and Kurokawa, T. (1993). Molecular cloning of a novel cytokine cDNA encoding the ninth member of the fibroblast growth factor family, which has a unique secretion property. *Mol. Cell. Biol.*, **13**, 4251–9.

81. Naruo, K., Seko, C., Kuroshima, K., Matsutani, E., Sasada, R., Kondo, T., and Kurokawa, T. (1993). Novel secretory heparin-binding factors from human glioma cells (glia-activating factors) involved in glial cell growth. Purification and biological properties. *J. Biol. Chem.*, **268**, 2857–64.

82. McKeehan, W. L. and Kan, M. (1994). Heparan sulfate fibroblast growth factor receptor complex: structure-function relationships. *Mol. Reprod. Dev.*, **39**, 69–81.

83. Partanen, J., Vainikka, S., Korhonen, J., Armstrong, E., and Alitalo, K. (1992). Diverse receptors for fibroblast growth factors. *Prog. Growth Factor Res.*, **4**, 69–83.

84. Ledoux, D., Gannoun, Z. L., and Barritault, D. (1992). Interactions of FGFs with target cells. *Prog. Growth Factor Res.*, **4**, 107–20.

85. Vlodavsky, I., Korner, G., Ishai, M. R., Bashkin, P., Bar, S. R., and Fuks, Z. (1990). Extracellular matrix–resident growth factors and enzymes: possible involvement in tumor metastasis and angiogenesis. *Cancer Metastasis Rev.*, **9**, 203–26.

86. D'Amore, P. A. (1990). Heparin–endothelial cell interactions. *Haemostasis*, **1**, 159–65.

87. Baird, A. (1994). Potential mechanisms regulating the extracellular activities of basic fibroblast growth factor (FGF-2). *Mol. Reprod. Dev.*, **39**, 43–8.

88. Lee, P. L., Johnson, D. E., Cousens, L. S., Fried, V. A., and Williams, L. T. (1989). Purification and complementary DNA cloning of a receptor for basic fibroblast growth factor. *Science*, **245**, 57–60.

89. Dionne, C. A., Crumley, G., Bellot, F., Kaplow, J. M., Searfoss, G., Ruta, M., *et al.* (1990). Cloning and expression of two distinct high-affinity receptors cross-reacting with acidic and basic fibroblast growth factors. *EMBO J.*, **9**, 2685–92.

90. Mansukhani, A., Moscatelli, D., Talarico, D., Levytska, V., and Basilico, C. (1990). A murine fibroblast growth factor (FGF) receptor expressed in CHO cells is activated by basic FGF and Kaposi FGF. *Proc. Natl Acad. Sci. USA*, **87**, 4378–82.

91. Safran, A., Avivi, A., Orr, U. A., Neufeld, G., Lonai, P., Givol, D., and Yarden, Y. (1990). The murine flg gene encodes a receptor for fibroblast growth factor. *Oncogene*, **5**, 635–43.

92. Ornitz, D. M. and Leder, P. (1992). Ligand specificity and heparin dependence of fibroblast growth factor receptors 1 and 3. *J. Biol. Chem.*, **267**, 16305–11.

93. Kornbluth, S., Paulson, K. E., and Hanafusa, H. (1988). Novel tyrosine kinase identified by phosphotyrosine antibody screening of cDNA libraries. *Mol. Cell. Biol.*, **8**, 5541–4.

94. Pasquale, E. B. (1990). A distinctive family of embryonic protein-tyrosine kinase receptors. *Proc. Natl Acad. Sci. USA*, **87**, 5812–6.

95. Houssaint, E., Blanquet, P. R., Champion, A. P., Gesnel, M. C., Torriglia, A., Courtois, Y., and Breathnach, R. (1990). Related fibroblast growth factor receptor genes exist in the human genome. *Proc. Natl Acad. Sci. USA*, **87**, 8180–4.

96. Hattori, Y., Odagiri, H., Nakatani, H., Miyagawa, K., Naito, K., Sakamoto, H., *et al.* (1990). K-sam, an amplified gene in stomach cancer, is a member of the heparin-binding growth factor receptor genes. *Proc. Natl Acad. Sci. USA*, **87**, 5983–7.

97. Miki, T., Fleming, T. P., Bottaro, D. P., Rubin, J. S., Ron, D., and Aaronson, S. A. (1991). Expression cDNA cloning of the KGF receptor by creation of a transforming autocrine loop. *Science*, **251**, 72–5.

98. Miki, T., Bottaro, D. P., Fleming, T. P., Smith, C. L., Burgess, W. H., Chan, A. M., and Aaronson, S. A. (1992). Determination of ligand-binding specificity by alternative splicing: two distinct growth factor receptors encoded by a single gene. *Proc. Natl Acad. Sci. USA*, **89**, 246–50.

99. Keegan, K., Johnson, D. E., Williams, L. T., and Hayman, M. J. (1991). Isolation of an additional member of the fibroblast growth factor receptor family, FGFR-3. *Proc. Natl Acad. Sci. USA*, **88**, 1095–9.

100. Partanen, J., Makela, T. P., Eerola, E., Korhonen, J., Hirvonen, H., Claesson, W. L., and Alitalo, K. (1991). FGFR-4, a novel acidic fibroblast growth factor receptor with a distinct expression pattern. *EMBO J.*, **10**, 1347–54.

101. Ron, D., Reich, R., Chedid, M., Lengel, C., Cohen, O. E., Chan, A. M., *et al.* (1993). Fibroblast growth factor receptor 4 is a high affinity receptor for both acidic and basic fibroblast growth factor but not for keratinocyte growth factor. *J. Biol. Chem.*, **268**, 5388–94.

102. Vainikka, S., Partanen, J., Bellosta, P., Coulier, F., Birnbaum, D., Basilico, C., *et al.* (1992). Fibroblast growth factor receptor-4 shows novel features in genomic structure, ligand binding and signal transduction [published erratum appears in *EMBO J.* 1993; **12**(2): 810]. *EMBO J.*, **11**, 4273–80.

103. Ullrich, A., and Schlessinger, J. (1990). Signal transduction by receptors with tyrosine kinase activity. *Cell*, **61**, 203–12.

104. Johnson, D. E., and Williams, L. T. (1993). Structural and functional diversity in the FGF receptor multigene family. *Adv. Cancer Res.*, **60**, 1–41.

105. Werner, S., Duan, D. S., de, V. C., Peters, K. G., Johnson, D. E., and Williams, L. T. (1992). Differential splicing in the extracellular region of fibroblast growth factor receptor 1 generates receptor variants with different ligand-binding specificities. *Mol. Cell. Biol.*, **12**, 82–8.

106. Johnson, D. E., Lee, P. L., Lu, J., and Williams, L. T. (1990). Diverse forms of a receptor for acidic and basic fibroblast growth factors. *Mol. Cell. Biol.*, **10**, 4728–36.

107. Johnson, D. E., Lu, J., Chen, H., Werner, S., and Williams, L. T. (1991). The human fibroblast growth factor receptor genes: a common structural arrangement underlies the mechanisms for generating receptor forms that differ in their third immunoglobulin domain. *Mol. Cell. Biol.*, **11**, 4627–34.

108. Cheon, H. G., LaRochelle, W. J., Battaro, D. P., Burgess, W. H., and Aaronson, S. A. (1994). High-affinity binding sites for related fibroblast growth factor ligands reside within different receptor immunoglobulin-like domains. *Proc. Natl Acad. Sci. USA*, **91**, 989–93.

109. Zimmer, Y., Givol, D., and Yayon, A. (1993). Multiple structural elements determine ligand binding of fibroblast growth factor receptors. Evidence that both Ig domain 2 and 3 define receptor specificity. *J. Biol. Chem.*, **268**, 7899–903.

110. Chellaiah, A. T., McEwen, D. G., Werner, S., Xu, J., and Ornitz, D. M. (1994). Fibroblast growth factor receptor (FGFR) 3. Alternative splicing in immunoglobulin-like domain III creates a receptor highly specific for acidic FGF/FGF-1. *J. Biol. Chem.*, **269**, 11620–7.

111. Crumley, G., Bellot, F., Kaplow, J. M., Schlessinger, J., Jaye, M., and Dionne, C. A. (1991). High-affinity binding and activation of a truncated FGF receptor by both aFGF and bFGF. *Oncogene*, **6**, 2255–62.

112. Hanneken, A., Ying, W., Ling, N., and Baird, A. (1994). Identification of soluble forms of the fibroblast growth factor receptor in blood. *Proc. Natl Acad. Sci. USA*, **91**, 9170–4.

113. Hanneken, A., Maher, P. A., and Baird, A. (1985). High affinity immunoreactive FGF receptors in the extracellular matrix of vascular endothelial cells — implications for the modulation of FGF-2. *J. Cell Biol.*, **128**, 1221–8.

114. Peters, K., Werner, S., Liao, X., Wert, S., Whitsett, J., and Williams, L. (1994). Targeted expression of a dominant negative FGF receptor blocks branching morphogenesis and epithelial differentiation of the mouse lung. *EMBO J.*, **13**, 3296–301.

115. Werner, S., Weinberg, W., Liao, X., Peters, K. G., Blessing, M., Yuspa, S. H., *et al.* (1993). Targeted expression of a dominant-negative FGF receptor mutant in the epidermis of transgenic mice reveals a role of FGF in keratinocyte organization and differentiation. *EMBO J.*, **12**, 2635–43.

116. Mansukhani, A., Dell'Era, P., Moscatelli, D., Kornbluth, S., Hanafusa, H., and Basilico, C. (1992). Characterization of the murine BEK fibroblast growth factor (FGF) receptor: activation by three members of the FGF family and requirement for heparin. *Proc. Natl Acad. Sci. USA*, **89**, 3305–9.

117. Rapraeger, A. C., Krufka, A., and Olwin, B. B. (1991). Requirement of heparan sulfate for bFGF-mediated fibroblast growth and myoblast differentiation. *Science*, **252**, 1705–8.

118. Kan, M., Wang, F., Xu, J., Crabb, J. W., Hou, J., and McKeehan, W. L. (1993). An essential heparin-binding domain in the fibroblast growth factor receptor kinase. *Science*, **259**, 1918–21.

119. Korhonen, J., Partanen, J., Eerola, E., Vainikka, S., Ilvesmaki, V., Voutilainen, R., *et al.* (1991). Novel human FGF receptors with distinct expression patterns. *Ann. N. Y. Acad. Sci.*, **638**, 403–5.

120. Peters, K., Ornitz, D., Werner, S., and Williams, L. (1993). Unique expression pattern of the FGF receptor 3 gene during mouse organogenesis. *Dev. Biol.*, **155**, 423–30.

121. Peters, K. G., Werner, S., Chen, G., and Williams, L. T. (1992). Two FGF receptor genes are differentially expressed in epithelial and mesenchymal tissues during limb formation and organogenesis in the mouse. *Development*, **114**, 233–43.

122. Wanaka, A., Milbrandt, J., and Johnson, E. J. (1991). Expression of FGF receptor gene in rat development. *Development*, **111**, 455–68.

123. Orr, U. A., Bedford, M. T., Burakova, T., Arman, E., Zimmer, Y., Yayon, A., *et al.* (1993). Developmental localization of the splicing alternatives of fibroblast growth factor receptor-2 (FGFR2). *Dev. Biol.*, **158**, 475–86.

124. Savagner, P., Valles, A. M., Jouanneau, J., Yamada, K. M., and Thiery, J. P. (1994). Alternative splicing in fibroblast

growth factor receptor 2 is associated with induced epithelial-mesenchymal transition in rat bladder carcinoma cells. *Mol. Biol. Cell.*, **5**, 851–62.

125. Yan, G., Fukabori, Y., McBride, G., Nikolaropolous, S., and McKeehan, W. L. (1993). Exon switching and activation of stromal and embryonic fibroblast growth factor (FGF)-FGF receptor genes in prostate epithelial cells accompany stromal independence and malignancy. *Mol. Cell. Biol.*, **13**, 4513–22.

126. Stark, K. L., McMahon, J. A., and McMahon, A. P. (1991). FGFR-4, a new member of the fibroblast growth factor receptor family, expressed in the definitive endoderm and skeletal muscle lineages of the mouse. *Development*, **113**, 641–51.

127. Deng, C. X., Wynshaw, B. A., Shen, M. M., Daugherty, C., Ornitz, D. M., and Leder, P. (1994). Murine FGFR-1 is required for early postimplantation growth and axial organization. *Genes Dev.*, **8**, 3045–57.

128. Yamaguchi, T. P., Harpa, K., Henkemeyer, M., and Rossant, J. (1994). fgfr-1 is required for embryonic growth and mesodermal patterning during mouse gastrulation. *Genes Dev.*, **8**, 3032–44.

129. Muenke, M. and Schell, U. (1995). Fibroblast-growth-factor receptor mutations in human skeletal disorders. *Trends Genet.*, **11**, 308–13.

130. Kaner, R. J., Baird, A., Mansukhani, A., Basilico, C., Summers, B. D., Florkiewicz, R. Z., and Hajjar, D. P. (1990). Fibroblast growth factor receptor is a portal of cellular entry for herpes simplex virus type 1 [see comments]. *Science*, **248**, 1410–3.

131. Baird, A., Florkiewicz, R. Z., Maher, P. A., Kaner, R. J., and Hajjar, D. P. (1990). Mediation of virion penetration into vascular cells by association of basic fibroblast growth factor with herpes simplex virus type 1. *Nature*, **348**, 344–6.

132. Kiefer, M. C., Stephans, J. C., Crawford, K., Okino, K., and Barr, P. J. (1990). Ligand-affinity cloning and structure of a cell surface heparan sulfate proteoglycan that binds basic fibroblast growth factor. *Proc. Natl Acad. Sci. USA*, **87**, 6985–9.

133. Saunders, S., Jalkanen, M., O'Farrell, S., and Bernfield, M. (1989). Molecular cloning of syndecan, an integral membrane proteoglycan. *J. Cell Biol.*, **108**, 1547–56.

134. Moscatelli, D. (1988). Metabolism of receptor-bound and matrix-bound basic fibroblast growth factor by bovine capillary endothelial cells. *J. Cell Biol.*, **107**, 753–9.

135. Yayon, A., Klagsbrun, M., Esko, J. D., Leder, P., and Ornitz, D. M. (1991). Cell surface, heparin-like molecules are required for binding of basic fibroblast growth factor to its high affinity receptor. *Cell*, **64**, 841–8.

136. Guimond, S., Maccarana, M., Olwin, B. B., Lindahl, U., and Rapraeger, A. C. (1993). Activating and inhibitory heparin sequences for FGF-2 (basic FGF). Distinct requirements for FGF-1, FGF-2, and FGF-4. *J. Biol. Chem.*, **268**, 23906–14.

137. Ishihara, M., Tyrrell, D. J., Stauber, G. B., Brown, S., Cousens, L. S., and Stack, R. J. (1993). Preparation of affinity-fractionated, heparin-derived oligosaccharides and their effects on selected biological activities mediated by basic fibroblast growth factor. *J. Biol. Chem.*, **268**, 4675–83.

138. Aviezer, D., Levy, E., Safran, M., Svahn, C., Buddecke, E., Schmidt, A., *et al.* (1994). Differential structural require-

ments of heparin and heparan sulfate proteoglycans that promote binding of basic fibroblast growth factor to its receptor. *J. Biol. Chem.*, **269**, 114–21.

139. Klagsbrun, M. and Baird, A. (1991). A dual receptor system is required for basic fibroblast growth factor activity. *Cell*, **67**, 229–31.

140. Ornitz, D. M., Yayon, A., Flanagan, J. G., Svahn, C. M., Levi, E., and Leder, P. (1992). Heparin is required for cell-free binding of basic fibroblast growth factor to a soluble receptor and for mitogenesis in whole cells. *Mol. Cell. Biol.*, **12**, 240–7.

141. Ornitz, D. M., Herr, A. B., Nilsson, M., Westman, J., Svahn, C.-M., and Waksman, G. (1995). FGF binding and FGF receptor activation by synthetic heparan-derived di- and trisaccharides. *Science*, **268**, 432–36.

142. Mach, H., Volkin, D. B., Burke, C. J., Middaugh, C. R., Linhardt, R. J., Fromm, J. R., *et al.* (1993). Nature of the interaction of heparin with acidic fibroblast growth factor. *Biochemistry*, **32**, 5480–9.

143. Spivak, K. T., Lemmon, M. A., Dikic, I., Ladbury, J. E., Pinchasi, D., Huang, J., *et al.* (1994). Heparin-induced oligomerization of FGF molecules is responsible for FGF receptor dimerization, activation, and cell proliferation. *Cell*, **79**, 1015–24.

144. Gao, G. and Goldfarb, M. (1995). Heparin can activate a receptor tyrosine kinase. *EMBO J.*, **14**, 2183–90.

145. Nurcombe, V., Ford, M. D., Wildschut, J. A., and Bartlett, P. F. (1993). Developmental regulation of neural response to FGF-1 and FGF-2 by heparan sulfate proteoglycan. *Science*, **260**, 103–6.

146. Bellot, F., Crumley, G., Kaplow, J. M., Schlessinger, J., Jaye, M., and Dionne, C. A. (1991). Ligand-induced transphosphorylation between different FGF receptors. *EMBO J.*, **10**, 2849–54.

147. Ueno, H., Gunn, M., Dell, K., Tseng, A. J., and Williams, L. (1992). A truncated form of fibroblast growth factor receptor 1 inhibits signal transduction by multiple types of fibroblast growth factor receptor. *J. Biol. Chem.*, **267**, 1470–6.

148. Burgess, W. H., Dionne, C. A., Kaplow, J., Mudd, R., Friesel, R., Zilberstein, A., *et al.* (1990). Characterization and cDNA cloning of phospholipase C-gamma, a major substrate for heparin-binding growth factor 1 (acidic fibroblast growth factor)-activated tyrosine kinase. *Mol. Cell. Biol.*, **10**, 4770–7.

149. Mohammadi, M., Honegger, A. M., Rotin, D., Fischer, R., Bellot, F., Li, W., *et al.* (1991). A tyrosine-phosphorylated carboxy-terminal peptide of the fibroblast growth factor receptor (Flg) is a binding site for the SH2 domain of phospholipase C-gamma 1. *Mol. Cell. Biol.*, **11**, 5068–78.

150. Mohammadi, M., Dionne, C. A., Li, W., Li, N., Spivak, T., Honegger, A. M., *et al.* (1992). Point mutation in FGF receptor eliminates phosphatidylinositol hydrolysis without affecting mitogenesis. *Nature*, **358**, 681–4.

151. Sorokin, A., Mohammadi, M., Huang, J., and Schlessinger, J. (1994). Internalization of fibroblast growth factor receptor is inhibited by a point mutation at tyrosine 766. *J. Biol. Chem.*, **269**, 17056–61.

152. Maciag, T., Zhan, X., Garfinkel, S., Friedman, S., Prudovsky, I., Jackson, A., *et al.* (1994). Novel mechanisms of fibroblast growth factor 1 function. *Recent Prog. Horm. Res.*, **49**, 105–23.

153. Zhan, X., Plourde, C., Hu, X., Friesel, R., and Maciag, T. (1994). Association of fibroblast growth factor receptor-1 with c-Src correlates with association between c-Src and cortactin. *J. Biol. Chem.*, **269**, 20221–4.

154. Gay, C. G. and Winkles, J. A. (1990). Heparin-binding growth factor-1 stimulation of human endothelial cells induces platelet-derived growth factor A-chain gene expression. *J. Biol. Chem.*, **265**, 3284–92.

155. Zhan, X., Hu, X., Friesel, R., and Maciag, T. (1993). Long term growth factor exposure and differential tyrosine phosphorylation are required for DNA synthesis in BALB/c 3T3 cells. *J. Biol. Chem.*, **268**, 9611–20.

156. Vainikka, S., Joukov, V., Wennstrom, S., Bergman, M., Pelicci, P. G., and Alitalo, K. (1994). Signal transduction by fibroblast growth factor receptor-4 (FGFR-4). Comparison with FGFR-1. *J. Biol. Chem.*, **269**, 18320–6.

157. Moscatelli, D. and Quarto, N. (1989). Transformation of NIH 3T3 cells with basic fibroblast growth factor or the hst/K-fgf oncogene causes downregulation of the fibroblast growth factor receptor: reversal of morphological trans-formation and restoration of receptor number by suramin. *J. Cell Biol.*, **109**, 2519–27.

158. Friesel, R. and Maciag, T. (1988). Internalization and degradation of heparin binding growth factor-I by endo-thelial cells. *Biochem. Biophys. Res. Commun.*, **151**, 957–64.

159. Zhan, X., Hu, X., Friedman, S., and Maciag, T. (1992). Analysis of endogenous and exogenous nuclear trans-location of fibroblast growth factor-1 in NIH 3T3 cells. *Biochem. Biophys. Res. Commun.*, **188**, 982–91.

160. Gannoun, Z. L., Pieri, I., Badet, J., Moenner, M., and Barritault, D. (1991). Internalization of basic fibroblast growth factor by Chinese hamster lung fibroblast cells: involvement of several pathways. *Exp. Cell. Res.*, **197**, 272–9.

161. Roghani, M. and Moscatelli, D. (1992). Basic fibroblast growth factor is internalized through both receptor-mediated and heparan sulfate-mediated mechanisms. *J. Biol. Chem.*, **267**, 22156–62.

162. Walicke, P. A. and Baird, A. (1991). Internalization and processing of basic fibroblast growth factor by neurons and astrocytes. *J. Neurosci.*, **11**, 2249–58.

163. Baldin, V., Roman, A. M., Bosc, B. I., Amalric, F., and Bouche, G. (1990). Translocation of bFGF to the nucleus is G1 phase cell cycle specific in bovine aortic endothelial cells. *EMBO J.*, **9**, 1511–7.

164. Amalric, F., Baldin, V., Bosc, B. I., Bugler, B., Couderc, B., Guyader, M., *et al.* (1991). Nuclear translocation of basic fibroblast growth factor. *Ann. N. Y. Acad. Sci.*, **638**, 127–38.

165. Presta, M., Gualandris, A., Urbinati, C., Rusnati, M., Coltrini, D., Isacchi, A., *et al.* (1993). Subcellular localiza-tion and biological activity of M(r) 18 000 basic fibroblast growth factor: site-directed mutagenesis of a putative nuclear translocation sequence. *Growth Factors*, **9**, 269–78.

166. Sano, H., Forough, R., Maier, J. A., Case, J. P., Jackson, A., Engleka, K., *et al.* (1990). Detection of high levels of heparin binding growth factor-1 (acidic fibroblast growth factor) in inflammatory arthritic joints. *J. Cell Biol.*, **110**, 1417–26.

167. Cao, Y., Ekstrom, M., and Pettersson, R. F. (1993). Characterization of the nuclear translocation of acidic fibroblast growth factor. *J. Cell Sci.*, **104**, 77–87.

168. Imamura, T., Tokita, Y., and Mitsui, Y. (1992). Identification of a heparin-binding growth factor-1 nuclear translocation sequence by deletion mutation analysis. *J. Biol. Chem.*, **267**, 5676–9.

169. Friedman, S., Zhan, X., and Maciag, T. (1994). Mutagenesis of the nuclear localization sequence in EGF-1 alters protein stability but not mitogenic activity. *Biochem. Biophys. Res. Commun.*, **198**, 1203–8.

170. Prudovsky, I., Savion, N., Zhan, X., Friesel, R., Xu, J., Hou, J., *et al.* (1994). Intact and functional fibroblast growth factor (FGF) receptor-1 trafficks near the nucleus in response to FGF-1. *J. Biol. Chem.*, **269**, 31720–4.

171. Presta, M., Rusnati, M., Urbinati, C., Sommer, A., and Ragnotti, G. (1991). Biologically active synthetic fragments of human basic fibroblast growth factor (bFGF): identification of two Asp-Gly-Arg-containing domains involved in the mitogenic activity of bFGF in endothelial cells. *J. Cell. Physiol.*, **149**, 512–24.

172. Zhan, X., Hu, X., Hampton, B., Burgess, W. H., Friesel, R., and Maciag, T. (1993). Murine cortactin is phosphorylated in response to fibroblast growth factor-1 on tyrosine residues late in the G1 phase of the BALB/c 3T3 cell cycle. *J. Biol. Chem.*, **268**, 24427–31.

173. Wiedlocha, A., Falnes, P. O., Madshus, I. H., Sandvig, K., and Olsnes, S. (1994). Dual mode of signal transduction by externally added acidic fibroblast growth factor. *Cell*, **76**, 1039–51.

174. Muller, W. J., Lee, F. S., Dickson, C., Peters, G., Pattengale, P., and Leder, P. (1990). The int-2 gene product acts as an epithelial growth factor in transgenic mice. *EMBO J.*, **9**, 907–13.

175. Stamp, G., Fantl, V., Poulsom, R., Jamieson, S., Smith, R., Peters, G., and Dickson, C. (1992). Nonuniform expression of a mouse mammary tumor virus-driven int-2/Fgf-3 trans-gene in pregnancy-responsive breast tumors. *Cell. Growth Differ.*, **3**, 929–38.

176. Tutrone, R. J., Ball, R. A., Ornitz, D. M., Leder, P., and Richie, J. P. (1993). Benign prostatic hyperplasia in a trans-genic mouse: a new hormonally sensitive investigatory model. *J. Urol.*, **149**, 633–9.

177. Shackleford, G. M., MacArthur, C. A., Kwan, H. C., and Varmus, H. E. (1993). Mouse mammary tumor virus infec-tion accelerates mammary carcinogenesis in Wnt-1 trans-genic mice by insertional activation of int-2/Fgf-3 and hst/Fgf-4. *Proc. Natl Acad. Sci. USA*, **90**, 740–4.

178. Murakami, A., Tanaka, H., and Matsuzawa, A. (1990). Association of hst gene expression with metastatic pheno-type in mouse mammary tumors. *Cell. Growth Differ.*, **1**, 225–31.

179. Huang, Y. Q., Li, J. J., Moscatelli, D., Basilico, C., Nicolaides, A., Zhang, W. G., *et al.* (1993). Expression of int-2 oncogene in Kaposi's sarcoma lesions. *J. Clin. Invest.*, **91**, 1191–7.

180. Taira, M., Yoshida, T., Miyagawa, K., Sakamoto, H., Terada, M., and Sugimura, T. (1987). cDNA sequence of human transforming gene hst and identification of the coding sequence required for transforming activity. *Proc. Natl Acad. Sci. USA*, **84**, 2980–4.

181. Yoshida, T., Miyagawa, K., Odagiri, H., Sakamoto, H., Little, P. F., Terada, M., and Sugimura, T. (1987). Genomic sequence of hst, a transforming gene encoding a protein homologous to fibroblast growth factors and the int-2-encoded protein [published erratum appears in *Proc. Natl*

Acad. Sci. USA, 1988; **85**(6): 1967]. *Proc. Natl Acad. Sci. USA*, **84**, 7305–9.

182. Sinkovics, J. G. (1991). Kaposi's sarcoma: its 'oncogenes' and growth factors. *Crit. Rev. Oncol. Hematol.*, **11**, 87–107.

183. Taylor, W. R., Greenberg, A. H., Turley, E. A., and Wright, J. A. (1993). Cell motility, invasion, and malignancy induced by overexpression of K-FGF or bFGF. *Exp. Cell Res.*, **204**, 295–301.

184. McLeskey, S. W., Kurebayashi, J., Honig, S. F., Zwiebel, J., Lippman, M. E., Dickson, R. B., and Kern, F. G. (1993). Fibroblast growth factor 4 transfection of MCF-7 cells produces cell lines that are tumorigenic and metastatic in ovariectomized or tamoxifen-treated athymic nude mice. *Cancer Res.*, **53**, 2168–77.

185. Kurebayashi, J., McLeskey, S. W., Johnson, M. D., Lippman, M. E., Dickson, R. B., and Kern, F. G. (1993). Quantitative demonstration of spontaneous metastasis by MCF-7 human breast cancer cells cotransfected with fibroblast growth factor 4 and LacZ. *Cancer Res.*, **53**, 2178–87.

186. Kern, F. G., McLeskey, S. W., Zhang, L., Kurebayashi, J., Liu, Y., Ding, I. Y., *et al.* (1994). Transfected MCF-7 cells as a model for breast-cancer progression. *Breast Cancer Res. Treatment*, **31**, 153–65.

187. Wellstein, A., Lupu, R., Zugmaier, G., Flamm, S. L., Cheville, A. L., Delli, B. P., *et al.* (1990). Autocrine growth stimulation by secreted Kaposi fibroblast growth factor but not by endogenous basic fibroblast growth factor. *Cell. Growth Differ.*, **1**, 63–71.

188. Talarico, D., Ittmann, M. M., Bronson, R., and Basilico, C. (1993). A retrovirus carrying the K-fgf oncogene induces diffuse meningeal tumors and soft-tissue fibrosarcomas. *Mol. Cell. Biol.*, **13**, 1998–2010.

189. Yoshida, M. C., Wada, M., Satoh, H., Yoshida, T., Sakamoto, H., Miyagawa, K., *et al.* (1988). Human HST1 (HSTF1) gene maps to chromosome band 11q13 and coamplifies with the INT2 gene in human cancer. *Proc. Natl Acad. Sci. USA*, **85**, 4861–4.

190. Schofield, P. N., Ekstrom, T. J., Granerus, M., and Engstrom, W. (1991). Differentiation associated modulation of K-FGF expression in a human teratocarcinoma cell line and in primary germ cell tumours. *FEBS Lett.*, **280**, 8–10.

191. Peters, G. (1991). Inappropriate expression of growth factor genes in tumors induced by mouse mammary tumor virus. *Semin. Virol.*, **2**, 319–28.

192. Werner, S., Viehweger, P., Hofschneider, P. H., and Roth, W. K. (1991). Low mitogenic response to EGF and TGF alpha: a characteristic feature of cultured Kaposi's sarcoma derived cells. *Oncogene*, **6**, 59–64.

193. Li, J. J., Huang, Y. Q., Moscatelli, D., Nicolaides, A., Zhang, W. C., and Friedman, K. A. (1993). Expression of fibroblast growth factors and their receptors in acquired immunodeficiency syndrome-associated Kaposi sarcoma tissue and derived cells. *Cancer*, **72**, 2253–9.

194. Sato, B., Kouhara, H., Koga, M., Kasayama, S., Saito, H., Sumitani, S., *et al.* (1993). Androgen-induced growth factor and its receptor: demonstration of the androgen-induced autocrine loop in mouse mammary carcinoma cells. *J. Steroid Biochem. Mol. Biol.*, **47**, 91–8.

195. MacArthur, C. A., Lawshe, A., Shankar, D. B., Heikinheimo, M., and Shackleford, G. M. (1995). FGF-8 isoforms differ in NIH3T3 cell transforming potential. *Cell. Growth Differ.*, **6**, 817–25.

196. Yayon, A. and Klagsbrun, M. (1990). Autocrine regulation of cell growth and transformation by basic fibroblast growth factor. *Cancer Metastasis Rev.*, **9**, 191–202.

197. Sasada, R., Kurokawa, T., Iwane, M., and Igarashi, K. (1988). Transformation of mouse BALB/c 3T3 cells with human basic fibroblast growth factor cDNA. *Mol. Cell. Biol.*, **8**, 588–94.

198. Neufeld, G., Mitchell, R., Ponte, P., and Gospodarowicz, D. (1988). Expression of human basic fibroblast growth factor cDNA in baby hamster kidney-derived cells results in autonomous cell growth. *J. Cell Biol.*, **106**, 1385–94.

199. Quarto, N., Talarico, D., Sommer, A., Florkiewicz, R., Basilico, C., and Rifkin, D. B. (1989). Transformation by basic fibroblast growth factor requires high levels of expression: comparison with transformation by hst/K-fgf. *Oncogene Res.*, **5**, 101–10.

200. Rogelj, S., Weinberg, R. A., Fanning, P., and Klagsbrun, M. (1988). Basic fibroblast growth factor fused to a signal peptide transforms cells. *Nature*, **331**, 173–5.

201. Yayon, A. and Klagsbrun, M. (1990). Autocrine transformation by chimeric signal peptide-basic fibroblast growth factor: reversal by suramin. *Proc. Natl Acad. Sci. USA*, **87**, 5346–50.

202. Dotto, G. P., Moellmann, G., Ghosh, S., Edwards, M., and Halaban, R. (1989). Transformation of murine melanocytes by basic fibroblast growth factor cDNA and oncogenes and selective suppression of the transformed phenotype in a reconstituted cutaneous environment. *J. Cell Biol.*, **109**, 3115–28.

203. Blam, S. B., Mitchell, R., Tischer, E., Rubin, J. S., Silva, M., Silver, S., *et al.* (1988). Addition of growth hormone secretion signal to basic fibroblast growth factor results in cell transformation and secretion of aberrant forms of the protein. *Oncogene*, **3**, 129–36.

204. Hori, A., Sasada, R., Matsutani, E., Naito, K., Sakura, Y., Fujita, T., and Kozai, Y. (1991). Suppression of solid tumor growth by immunoneutralizing monoclonal antibody against human basic fibroblast growth factor. *Cancer Res.*, **51**, 6180–4.

205. Jaye, M., Lyall, R. M., Mudd, R., Schlessinger, J., and Sarver, N. (1988). Expression of acidic fibroblast growth factor cDNA confers growth advantage and tumorigenesis to Swiss 3T3 cells. *EMBO J.*, **7**, 963–9.

206. Forough, R., Xi, Z., MacPhee, M., Friedman, S., Engleka, K. A., Sayers, T., *et al.* (1993). Differential transforming abilities of non-secreted and secreted forms of human fibroblast growth factor-1. *J. Biol. Chem.*, **268**, 2960–8.

207. Talarico, D. and Basilico, C. (1991). The K-fgf/hst oncogene induces transformation through an autocrine mechanism that requires extracellular stimulation of the mitogenic pathway. *Mol. Cell. Biol.*, **11**, 1138–45.

208. Stefanik, D. F., Rizkalla, L. R., Soi, A., Goldblatt, S. A., and Rizkalla, W. M. (1991). Acidic and basic fibroblast growth factors are present in glioblastoma multiforme. *Cancer Res.*, **51**, 5760–5.

209. Zagzag, D., Miller, D. C., Sato, Y., Rifkin, D. B., and Burstein, D. E. (1990). Immunohistochemical localization of basic fibroblast growth factor in astrocytomas. *Cancer Res.*, **50**, 7393–8.

210. Ueba, T., Takahashi, J. A., Fukumoto, M., Ohta, M., Ito, N., Oda, Y., *et al.* (1994). Expression of fibroblast growth factor receptor-1 in human glioma and meningioma tissues. *Neurosurgery*, **34**, 221–5.

211. Maxwell, M., Naber, S. P., Wolfe, H. J., Hedley, W. E., Galanopoulos, T., Neville, G. J., and Antoniades, H. N. (1991). Expression of angiogenic growth factor genes in primary human astrocytomas may contribute to their growth and progression. *Cancer Res.*, **51**, 1345–51.

212. Takahashi, J. A., Fukumoto, M., Igarashi, K., Oda, Y., Kikuchi, H., and Hatanaka, M. (1992). Correlation of basic fibroblast growth factor expression levels with the degree of malignancy and vascularity in human gliomas. *J. Neurosurg.*, **76**, 792–8.

213. Takahashi, J. A., Mori, H., Fukumoto, M., Igarashi, K., Jaye, M., Oda, Y., *et al.* (1990). Gene expression of fibroblast growth factors in human gliomas and meningiomas: demonstration of cellular source of basic fibroblast growth factor mRNA and peptide in tumor tissues. *Proc. Natl Acad. Sci. USA*, **87**, 5710–4.

214. Morrison, R. S., Giordano, S., Yamaguchi, F., Hendrickson, S., Berger, M. S., and Palczewski, K. (1993). Basic fibroblast growth factor expression is required for clonogenic growth of human glioma cells. *J. Neurosci. Res.*, **34**, 502–9.

215. Takahashi, J. A., Fukumoto, M., Kozai, Y., Ito, N., Oda, Y., Kikuchi, H., and Hatanaka, M. (1991). Inhibition of cell growth and tumorigenesis of human glioblastoma cells by a neutralizing antibody against human basic fibroblast growth factor. *FEBS Lett.*, **288**, 65–71.

216. Albino, A. P., Davis, B. M., and Nanus, D. M. (1991). Induction of growth factor RNA expression in human malignant melanoma: markers of transformation. *Cancer Res.*, **51**, 4815–20.

217. Becker, D., Meier, C. B., and Herlyn, M. (1989). Proliferation of human malignant melanomas is inhibited by antisense oligonucleotides targeted against basic fibroblast growth factor. *EMBO J.*, **8**, 3685–91.

218. Becker, D., Lee, P. L., Rodeck, U., and Herlyn, M. (1992). Inhibition of the fibroblast growth factor receptor 1 (FGFR-1) gene in human melanocytes and malignant melanomas leads to inhibition of proliferation and signs indicative of differentiation. *Oncogene*, **7**, 2303–13.

219. Ensoli, B., Markham, P., Kao, V., Barillari, G., Fiorelli, V., Gendelman, R., *et al.* (1994). Block of AIDS–Kaposi's sarcoma (KS) cell growth, angiogenesis, and lesion formation in nude mice by antisense oligonucleotide targeting basic fibroblast growth factor. A novel strategy for the therapy of KS. *J. Clin. Invest.*, **94**, 1736–46.

220. Ortega, S. and Thomas, K. A. (1990). The oncogenic potential of fibroblast growth factor genes. In *Molecular biology of cancer genes*. (ed. M. Sluyser) Ellis Horwood, New York.

221. Ludecke, G. and Unsicker, K. (1990). Mitogenic effect of neurotrophic factors on human IMR 32 neuroblastoma cells. *Cancer*, **65**, 2270–8.

222. Lavenius, E., Parrow, V., Nanberg, E., and Pahlman, S. (1994). Basic FGF and IGF-I promote differentiation of human SH-SY5Y neuroblastoma cells in culture. *Growth Factors*, **10**, 29–39.

223. Corin, S. J., Chen, L. C., and Hamburger, A. W. (1990). Enhancement of anchorage-independent growth of a human adrenal carcinoma cell line by endogenously produced basic fibroblast growth factor. *Int. J. Cancer*, **46**, 516–21.

224. Chao, H. H., Yang, V. C., and Chen, J. K. (1993). Acidic FGF and EGF are involved in the autocrine growth stimulation of a human nasopharyngeal carcinoma cell line and sub-line cells. *Int. J. Cancer*, **54**, 807–12.

225. Adnane, J., Gaudray, P., Dionne, C. A., Crumley, G., Jaye, M., Schlessinger, J., *et al.* (1991). BEK and FLG, two receptors to members of the FGF family, are amplified in subsets of human breast cancers. *Oncogene*, **6**, 659–63.

226. Jacquemier, J., Adelaide, J., Parc, P., Penault, L. F., Planche, J., DeLapeyriere, O., and Birnbaum, D. (1994). Expression of the FGFR1 gene in human breast-carcinoma cells. *Int. J. Cancer*, **59**, 373–8.

227. Yamaguchi, F., Saya, H., Bruner, J. M., and Morrison, R. S. (1994). Differential expression of two fibroblast growth factor-receptor genes is associated with malignant progression in human astrocytomas. *Proc. Natl Acad. Sci. USA*, **91**, 484–8.

228. Morrison, R. S., Yamaguchi, F., Saya, H., Bruner, J. M., Yahanda, A. M., Donehower, L. A., and Berger, M. (1994). Basic fibroblast growth factor and fibroblast growth factor receptor I are implicated in the growth of human astrocytomas. *J. Neurooncol.*, **18**, 207–16.

229. Takahashi, J. A., Suzui, H., Yasuda, Y., Ito, N., Ohta, M., Jaye, M., *et al.* (1991). Gene expression of fibroblast growth factor receptors in the tissues of human gliomas and meningiomas. *Biochem. Biophys. Res. Commun.*, **177**, 1–7.

230. Pekonen, F., Nyman, T., and Rutanen, E. M. (1993). Differential expression of keratinocyte growth factor and its receptor in the human uterus. *Mol. Cell. Endocrinol.*, **95**, 43–9.

231. Jaakkola, S., Salmikangas, P., Nylund, S., Partanen, J., Armstrong, E., Pyrhonen, S., *et al.* (1993). Amplification of fgfr4 gene in human breast and gynecological cancers. *Int. J. Cancer*, **54**, 378–82.

232. Easty, D. J., Herlyn, M., and Bennett, D. C. (1995). Abnormal protein tyrosine kinase gene expression during melanoma progression and metastasis. *Int. J. Cancer*, **60**, 129–36.

233. Lafage, M., Pedeutour, F., Marchetto, S., Simonetti, J., Prosperi, M. T., Gaudray, P., and Birnbaum, D. (1992). Fusion and amplification of two originally non-syntenic chromosomal regions in a mammary carcinoma cell line. *Genes Chromosom. Cancer*, **5**, 40–9.

234. McLeskey, S. W., Ding, I. Y., Lippman, M. E., and Kern, F. G. (1994). MDA-MB-134 breast carcinoma cells over-express fibroblast growth factor (FGF) receptors and are growth-inhibited by FGF ligands. *Cancer Res.*, **54**, 523–30.

235. Lehtola, L., Partanen, J., Sistonen, L., Korhonen, J., Warri, A., Harkonen, P., *et al.* (1992). Analysis of tyrosine kinase mRNAs including four FGF receptor mRNAs expressed in MCF-7 breast-cancer cells. *Int. J. Cancer*, **50**, 598–603.

236. Armstrong, E., Vainikka, S., Partanen, J., Korhonen, J., and Alitalo, R. (1992). Expression of fibroblast growth factor receptors in human leukemia cells. *Cancer Res.*, **52**, 2004–7.

237. Gospodarowicz, D., Neufeld, G., and Schweigerer, L. (1987). Fibroblast growth factor: structural and biological properties. *J. Cell. Physiol. Suppl.*, **5**, 15–26.

238. Folkman, J. and Klagsbrun, M. (1987). Angiogenic factors. *Science*, **235**, 442–47.

239. Thomas, K. A. (1987). Purification and characterization of acidic fibroblast growth factor. *Methods Enzymol.*, **147**, 120–35.

240. Klagsbrun, M. and D'Amore, P. A. (1991). Regulators of angiogenesis. *Annu. Rev. Physiol.*, **53**, 217–39.

241. Moscatelli, D., Presta, M., and Rifkin, D. B. (1986). Purification of a factor from human placenta that stimulates

capillary endothelial cell protease production, DNA synthesis, and migration. *Proc. Natl Acad. Sci. USA*, **83**, 2091–5.

242. Mignatti, P., Tsuboi, R., Robbins, E., and Rifkin, D. B. (1989). *In vitro* angiogenesis on the human amniotic membrane: requirement for basic fibroblast growth factor-induced proteinases. *J. Cell Biol.*, **108**, 671–82.

243. Montesano, R., Vassalli, J. D., Baird, A., Guillemin, R., and Orci, L. (1986). Basic fibroblast growth factor induces angiogenesis *in vitro*. *Proc. Natl Acad. Sci. USA*, **83**, 7297–301.

244. Vlodavsky, I., Fridman, R., Sullivan, R., Sasse, J., and Klagsbrun, M. (1987). Aortic endothelial cells synthesize basic fibroblast growth factor which remains cell associated and platelet-derived growth factor like protein which is secreted. *J. Cell. Physiol.*, **131**, 402–8.

245. Vlodavsky, I., Folkman, J., Sullivan, R., Friedman, R., Ishai-Michaeli, R., Sasse, J., and Klagsbrun, M. (1987). Endothelial cell-derived basic fibroblast growth factor: synthesis and deposition into subendothelial extracellular matrix. *Proc. Natl Acad. Sci. USA*, **84**, 2292–6.

246. Schweigerer, L., Neufeld, G., Friedman, J., Abraham, J. A., Fiddes, J. C., and Gospodarowicz, D. (1987). Capillary endothelial cells express basic fibroblast growth factor, a mitogen that promotes their own growth. *Nature*, **325**, 257–9.

247. D'Amore, P. A. (1990). Modes of FGF release *in vivo* and *in vitro*. *Cancer Metastasis Rev.*, **9**, 227–38.

248. Sato, Y. and Rifkin, D. B. (1988). Autocrine activities of basic fibroblast growth factor: regulation of endothelial cell movement, plasminogen activator synthesis, and DNA synthesis. *J. Cell Biol.*, **107**, 1199–205.

249. Sato, Y., Shimada, T., and Takaki, R. (1991). Autocrinological role of basic fibroblast growth factor on tube formation of vascular endothelial cells *in vitro*. *Biochem. Biophys. Res. Commun.*, **180**, 1098–102.

250. Haimovitz, F. A., Balaban, N., McLoughlin, M., Ehleiter, D., Michaeli, J., Vlodavsky, I., and Fuks, Z. (1994). Protein kinase C mediates basic fibroblast growth factor protection of endothelial cells against radiation-induced apoptosis. *Cancer Res.*, **54**, 2591–7.

251. Fuks, Z., Persaud, R. S., Alfieri, A., McLoughlin, M., Ehleiter, D., Schwartz, J. L., *et al.* (1994). Basic fibroblast growth factor protects endothelial cells against radiation-induced programmed cell death *in vitro* and *in vivo*. *Cancer Res.*, **54**, 2582–90.

252. Kitayama, J., Nagawa, H., Yasuhara, H., Tsuno, N., Kimura, W., Shibata, Y., and Muto, T. (1994). Suppressive effect of basic fibroblast growth factor on transendothelial emigration of CD4(+) T-lymphocyte. *Cancer Res.*, **54**, 4729–33.

253. Villaschi, S. and Nicosia, R. F. (1993). Angiogenic role of endogenous basic fibroblast growth factor released by rat aorta after injury. *Am. J. Pathol.*, **143**, 181–90.

254. Davidson, J. M., Klagsbrun, M., Hill, K. E., Buckley, A., Sullivan, R., Brewer, P. S., and Woodward, S. C. (1985). Accelerated wound repair, cell proliferation, and collagen accumulation are produced by a cartilage-derived growth factor. *J. Cell Biol.*, **100**, 1219–27.

255. Hu, D. E., Hori, Y., Presta, M., Gresham, G. A., and Fan, T. P. (1994). Inhibition of angiogenesis in rats by IL-1 receptor antagonist and selected cytokine antibodies. *Inflammation*, **18**, 45–58.

256. Broadley, K. N., Aquino, A. M., Woodward, S. C., Buckley, S. A., Sato, Y., Rifkin, D. B., and Davidson, J. M. (1989). Monospecific antibodies implicate basic fibroblast growth factor in normal wound repair. *Lab. Invest.*, **61**, 571–5.

257. Hayek, A., Culler, F. L., Beattie, G. M., Lopez, A. D., Cuevas, P., and Baird, A. (1987). An *in vivo* model for study of the angiogenic effects of basic fibroblast growth factor. *Biochem. Biophys. Res. Commun.*, **147**, 876–80.

258. Edelman, E. R., Nugent, M. A., Smith, L. T., and Karnovsky, M. J. (1992). Basic fibroblast growth factor enhances the coupling of intimal hyperplasia and proliferation of vasa vasorum in injured rat arteries. *J. Clin. Invest.*, **89**, 465–73.

259. Norrby, K. (1994). Basic fibroblast growth factor and *de novo* mammalian angiogenesis. *Microvasc. Res.*, **48**, 96–113.

260. Knighton, D. R., Phillips, G. D., and Fiegel, V. D. (1990). Wound healing angiogenesis: indirect stimulation by basic fibroblast growth factor. *J. Trauma*, **30**, S134–44.

261. Thompson, J. A., Anderson, K. D., DiPietro, J. M., Zwiebel, J. A., Zametta, M., Anderson, W. F., and Maciag, T. (1988). Site-directed neovessel formation *in vivo*. *Science*, **241**, 1349–52.

262. Thompson, J. A., Haudenschild, C. C., Anderson, K. D., DiPietro, J. M., Anderson, W. F., and Maciag, T. (1989). Heparin-binding growth factor 1 induces the formation of organoid neovascular structures *in vivo* [published erratum appears in *Proc. Natl Acad. Sci. USA*, 1990; **87**(4): 1625] [retracted by Thompson, J. A., Haudenschild, C. C., Anderson, K. D., DiPietro, J. M., Anderson, W. F., and Maciag, T. In *Proc. Natl Acad. Sci. USA*, 1992; **89**(16): 7849]. *Proc. Natl Acad. Sci. USA*, **86**, 7928–32.

263. Stagner, J. I. and Samols, E. (1992). Induction of angiogenesis by growth factors: relevance to pancreatic islet transplantation. *Exs*, **61**, 381–5.

264. Nabel, E. G., Yang, Z. Y., Plautz, G., Forough, R., Zhan, X., Haudenschild, C. C., *et al.* (1993). Recombinant fibroblast growth factor-1 promotes intimal hyperplasia and angiogenesis in arteries *in vivo*. *Nature*, **362**, 844–6.

265. Miyagawa, K., Sakamoto, H., Yoshida, T., Yamashita, Y., Mitsui, Y., Furusawa, M., *et al.* (1988). hst-1 transforming protein: expression in silkworm cells and characterization as a novel heparin-binding growth factor. *Oncogene*, **3**, 383–9.

266. Risau, W. and Ekblom, P. (1986). Production of a heparin-binding angiogenesis factor by the embryonic kidney. *J. Cell Biol.*, **103**, 1101–7.

267. D'Amato, R. J., Loughnan, M. S., Flynn, E., and Folkman, J. (1994). Thalidomide is an inhibitor of angiogenesis. *Proc. Natl Acad. Sci. USA*, **91**, 4082–5.

268. Knighton, D. R., Hunt, T. K., Scheuenstuhl, H., Halliday, B. J., Werb, Z., and Banda, M. J. (1983). Oxygen tension regulates the expression of angiogenesis factor by macrophages. *Science*, **221**, 1283–5.

269. Fina, M., Bresnick, S., Baird, A., and Ryan, A. (1991). Improved healing of tympanic membrane perforations with basic fibroblast growth factor. *Growth Factors*, **5**, 265–72.

270. Zhang, G., Ichimura, T., Maier, J. A., Maciag, T., and Stevens, J. L. (1993). A role for fibroblast growth factor type-1 in nephrogenic repair. Autocrine expression in rat kidney proximal tubule epithelial cells *in vitro* and in the regenerating epithelium following nephrotoxic damage by

S-(1,1,2,2-tetrafluoroethyl)-L-cysteine *in vivo*. *J. Biol. Chem.*, **268**, 11542–7.

271. Hughes, S. E., Crossman, D., and Hall, P. A. (1993). Expression of basic and acidic fibroblast growth factors and their receptor in normal and atherosclerotic human arteries. *Cardiovasc. Res.*, **27**, 1214–9.

272. Lindner, V. and Reidy, M. A. (1991). Proliferation of smooth muscle cells after vascular injury is inhibited by an antibody against basic fibroblast growth factor. *Proc. Natl Acad. Sci. USA*, **88**, 3739–43.

273. Lindner, V., Lappi, D. A., Baird, A., Majack, R. A., and Reidy, M. A. (1991). Role of basic fibroblast growth factor in vascular lesion formation. *Circ. Res.*, **68**, 106–13.

274. Edelman, E. R., Nugent, M. A., and Karnovsky, M. J. (1993). Perivascular and intravenous administration of basic fibroblast growth factor: vascular and solid organ deposition. *Proc. Natl Acad. Sci. USA*, **90**, 1513–17.

275. Szabo, S and Hollander, D. (1989). Pathways of gastrointestinal protection and repair: mechanisms of action of sucralfate. *Am. J. Med.*, **86**, 23–31.

276. Szabo, S., Folkman, J., Vattay, P., Morales, R. E., Pinkus, G. S., and Kato, K. (1994). Accelerated healing of duodenal ulcers by oral administration of a mutein of basic fibroblast growth factor in rats. *Gastroenterology*, **106**, 1106–11.

277. Volkin, D. B., Verticelli, A. M., Marfia, K. E., Burke, C. J., Mach, H., and Middaugh, C. R. (1993). Sucralfate and soluble sucrose octasulfate bind and stabilize acidic fibroblast growth factor. *Biochim. Biophys. Acta*, **1203**, 18–26.

278. Peacock, D. J., Banquerigo, M. L., and Brahn, E. (1992). Angiogenesis inhibition suppresses collagen arthritis. *J. Exp. Med.*, **175**, 1135–8.

279. Wilder, R. L., Case, J. P., Crofford, L. J., Kumkumian, G. K., Lafyatis, R., Remmers, E. F., *et al.* (1991). Endothelial cells and the pathogenesis of rheumatoid arthritis in humans and streptococcal cell wall arthritis in Lewis rats. *J. Cell. Biochem.*, **45**, 162–6.

280. Hamilton, J. A., Butler, D. M., and Stanton, H. (1994). Cytokine interactions promoting DNA synthesis in human synovial fibroblasts. *J. Rheumatol.*, **21**, 797–803.

281. Sano, H., Engleka, K., Mathern, P., Hla, T., Crofford, L. J., Remmers, E. F., *et al.* (1993). Coexpression of phosphotyrosine-containing proteins, platelet-derived growth factor-B, and fibroblast growth factor-1 *in situ* in synovial tissues of patients with rheumatoid arthritis and Lewis rats with adjuvant or streptoccal cell wall arthritis. *J. Clin. Invest.*, **91**, 553–65.

282. Remmers, E. F., Sano, H., Lafyatis, R., Case, J. P., Kumkumian, G. K., Hla, T., *et al.* (1991). Production of platelet derived growth factor B chain (PDGF-B/c-sis) mRNA and immunoreactive PDGF B-like polypeptide by rheumatoid synovium: coexpression with heparin binding acidic fibroblast growth factor-1. *J. Rheumatol.*, **18**, 7–13.

283. Schelling, M. E. (1991). FGF mediation of coronary angiogenesis. *Ann N. Y. Acad. Sci.*, **638**, 467–9.

284. Yanagisawa, M. A., Uchida, Y., Nakamura, F., Tomaru, T., Kido, H., Kamijo, T., *et al.* (1992). Salvage of infarcted myocardium by angiogenic action of basic fibroblast growth factor. *Science*, **257**, 1401–3.

285. Unger, E. F., Banai, S., Shou, M., Lazarous, D. F., Jaklitsch, M. T., Scheinowitz, M., *et al.* (1994). Basic fibroblast growth factor enhances myocardial collateral flow in a canine model. *Am. J. Physiol.*, **266**, 1588–95.

286. Banai, S., Jaklitsch, M. T., Casscells, W., Shou, M., Shrivastav, S., Correa, R., *et al.* (1991). Effects of acidic fibroblast growth factor on normal and ischemic myocardium. *Circ. Res.*, **69**, 76–85.

287. Unger, E. F., Banai, S., Shou, M., Jaklitsch, M., Hodge, E., Correa, R., *et al.* (1993). A model to assess interventions to improve collateral blood flow: continuous administration of agents into the left coronary artery in dogs. *Cardiovasc. Res.*, **27**, 785–91.

288. Unger, E. F., Shou, M., Sheffield, C. D., Hodge, E., Jaye, M., and Epstein, S. E. (1993). Extracardiac to coronary anastomoses support regional left ventricular function in dogs. *Am. J. Physiol.*, **264**, 1567–74.

289. Cuevas, P., Carceller, F., Ortega, S., Zazo, M., Nieto, I., and Gimenez, G. G. (1991). Hypotensive activity of fibroblast growth factor. *Science*, **254**, 1208–10.

290. Goto, F., Goto, K., Weindel, K., and Folkman, J. (1993). Synergistic effects of vascular endothelial growth factor and basic fibroblast growth factor on the proliferation and cord formation of bovine capillary endothelial cells within collagen gels [see comments]. *Lab. Invest.*, **69**, 508–17.

291. Pepper, M. S., Ferrara, N., Orci, L., and Montesano, R. (1992). Potent synergism between vascular endothelial growth factor and basic fibroblast growth factor in the induction of angiogenesis *in vitro*. *Biochem. Biophys. Res. Commun.*, **189**, 824–31.

292. Saunders, K. B. and D'Amore, P. A. (1991). FGF and TGF-beta: actions and interactions in biological systems. *Crit. Rev. Eukaryot. Gene Expr.*, **1**, 157–72.

293. Orlidge, A. and D'Amore, P. A. (1987). Inhibition of capillary endothelial cell growth by pericytes and smooth muscle cells. *J. Cell Biol.*, **105**, 1455–62.

294. Antonelli, O. A., Saunders, K. B., Smith, S. R., and D'Amore, P. A. (1989). An activated form of transforming growth factor beta is produced by cocultures of endothelial cells and pericytes. *Proc. Natl Acad. Sci. USA*, **86**, 4544–8.

295. Flaumenhaft, R., Abe, M., Mignatti, P., and Rifkin, D. B. (1992). Basic fibroblast growth factor-induced activation of latent transforming growth factor beta in endothelial cells: regulation of plasminogen activator activity. *J. Cell Biol.*, **118**, 901–9.

296. Pepper, M. S. and Montesano, R. (1990). Proteolytic balance and capillary morphogenesis. *Cell Differ. Dev.*, **32**, 319–27.

297. Wessendorf, J. H., Garfinkel, S., Zhan, X., Brown, S., and Maciag, T. (1993). Identification of a nuclear localization sequence within the structure of the human interleukin-1 alpha precursor. *J. Biol. Chem.*, **268**, 22100–4.

298. Maier, J. A., Voulalas, P., Roeder, D., and Maciag, T. (1990). Extension of the life-span of human endothelial cells by an interleukin-1 alpha antisense oligomer. *Science*, **249**, 1570–4.

299. Garfinkel, S., Haines, D. S., Brown, S., Wessendorf, J., Gillespie, D. H., and Maciag, T. (1992). Interleukin-1 alpha mediates an alternative pathway for the antiproliferative action of poly(I.C) on human endothelial cells. *J. Biol. Chem.*, **267**, 24375–8.

300. Garfinkel, S., Brown, S., Wessendorf, J. H., and Maciag, T. (1994). Post-transcriptional regulation of interleukin 1 alpha in various strains of young and senescent human umbilical vein endothelial cells. *Proc. Natl Acad. Sci. USA*, **91**, 1559–63.

301. Norioka, K., Mitaka, T., Mochizuki, Y., Hara, M., Kawagoe, M., and Nakamura, H. (1994). Interaction of interleukin-1 and interferon-gamma on fibroblast growth factor-induced angiogenesis. *Jpn. J. Cancer Res.*, **85**, 522–9.

302. Schulze, O. K., Risau, W., Vollmer, E., and Sorg, C. (1990). *In situ* detection of basic fibroblast growth factor by highly specific antibodies. *Am. J. Pathol.*, **137**, 85–92.

303. Polverini, P. J. and Leibovich, S. J. (1984). Induction of neovascularization *in vivo* and endothelial proliferation *in vitro* by tumor-associated macrophages. *Lab. Invest.*, **51**, 635–42.

304. Folkman, J. (1992). The role of angiogenesis in tumor growth. *Semin. Cancer Biol.*, **3**, 65–71.

305. Brustle, O., Aguzzi, A., Talarico, D., Basilico, C., Kleihues, P., and Wiestler, O. D. (1992). Angiogenic activity of the K-fgf/hst oncogene in neural transplants. *Oncogene*, **7**, 1177–83.

306. Abe, T., Okamura, K., Ono, M., Kohno, K., Mori, T., Hori, S., and Kuwano, M. (1993). Induction of vascular endothelial tubular morphogenesis by human glioma cells. A model system for tumor angiogenesis. *J. Clin. Invest.*, **92**, 54–61.

307. Leith, J. T. and Michelson, S. (1993). Effects of administration of basic fibroblast growth factor on hypoxic fractions in xenografted DLD-2 human tumours: time dependence. *Br. J. Cancer*, **68**, 727–31.

308. Gross, J. L., Herblin, W. F., Dusak, B. A., Czerniak, P., Diamond, M. D., Sun, T., *et al.* (1993). Effects of modulation of basic fibroblast growth factor on tumor growth *in vivo*. *J. Natl Cancer Inst.*, **85**, 121–31.

309. Ensoli, B., Gendelman, R., Markham, P., Fiorelli, V., Colombini, S., Raffeld, M., *et al.* (1994). Synergy between basic fibroblast growth factor and HIV-1 Tat protein in induction of Kaposi's sarcoma. *Nature*, **371**, 674–80.

310. Albini, A., Barillari, G., Benelli, R., Gallo, R., and Ensoli, B. (1995). Angiogenic properties of human immunodeficiency virus type 1 Tat protein. *Proc. Natl Acad. Sci. USA*, **92**, 4838–42.

311. Nguyen, M., Watanabe, H., Budson, A. E., Richie, J. P., and Folkman, J. (1993). Elevated levels of the angiogenic peptide basic fibroblast growth factor in urine of bladder cancer patients. *J. Natl Cancer Inst.*, **85**, 241–2.

312. Fujimoto, K., Ichimori, Y., Kakizoe, T., Okajima, E., Sakamoto, H., Sugimura, T., and Terada, M. (1991). Increased serum levels of basic fibroblast growth factor in patients with renal cell carcinoma. *Biochem. Biophys. Res. Commun.*, **180**, 386–92.

313. Nguyen, M., Watanabe, H., Budson, A. E., Richie, J. P., Hayes, D. F., and Folkman, J. (1994). Elevated levels of an angiogenic peptide, basic fibroblast growth factor, in the urine of patients with a wide spectrum of cancers [see comments]. *J. Natl Cancer Inst.*, **86**, 356–61.

314. Li, V. W., Folkerth, R. D., Watanabe, H., Yu, C., Rupnick, M., Barnes, P., *et al.* (1994). Microvessel count and cerebrospinal fluid basic fibroblast growth factor in children with brain tumours. *Lancet*, **344**, 82–6.

315. Folkman, J. (1995). Angiogenesis in cancer, vascular, rheumatoid and other disease. *Nature Med.*, **1**, 27–31.

316. Soutter, A. D., Nguyen, M., Watanabe, H., and Folkman, J. (1993). Basic fibroblast growth factor secreted by an animal tumor is detectable in urine. *Cancer Res.*, **53**, 5297–9.

317. Lacey, M., Alpert, S., and Hanahan, D. (1986). Bovine papillomavirus genome elicits skin tumours in transgenic mice. *Nature*, **322**, 609–12.

318. Kandel, J., Bossy, W. E., Radvanyi, F., Klagsbrun, M., Folkman, J., and Hanahan, D. (1991). Neovascularization is associated with a switch to the export of bFGF in the multistep development of fibrosarcoma. *Cell*, **66**, 1095–104.

319. Sippola, T. M., Hanahan, D., and Howley, P. M. (1989). Cell-heritable stages of tumor progression in transgenic mice harboring the bovine papillomavirus type 1 genome. *Mol. Cell. Biol.*, **9**, 925–34.

320. Weich, H. A., Iberg, N., Klagsbrun, M., and Folkman, J. (1991). Transcriptional regulation of basic fibroblast growth factor gene expression in capillary endothelial cells. *J. Cell Biochem.*, **47**, 158–64.

321. Gay, C. G. and Winkles, J. A. (1991). Interleukin 1 regulates heparin-binding growth factor 2 gene expression in vascular smooth muscle cells. *Proc. Natl Acad. Sci. USA*, **88**, 296–300.

322. Ueba, T., Nosaka, T., Takahashi, J. A., Shibata, F., Florkiewicz, R. Z., Vogelstein, B., *et al.* (1994). Transcriptional regulation of basic fibroblast growth factor gene by p53 in human glioblastoma and hepatocellular carcinoma cells. *Proc. Natl Acad. Sci. USA*, **91**, 9009–13.

323. Cordon, C. C., Vlodavsky, I., Haimovitz, F. A., Hicklin, D., and Fuks, Z. (1990). Expression of basic fibroblast growth factor in normal human tissues. *Lab. Invest.* **63**, 832–40.

324. Dennis, P. A. and Rifkin, D. B. (1990). Studies on the role of basic fibroblast growth factor *in vivo*: inability of neutralizing antibodies to block tumor growth. *J. Cell. Physiol.*, **144**, 84–98.

325. Wellstein, A., Zugmaier, G., Califano, J. 3., Kern, F., Paik, S., and Lippman, M. E. (1991). Tumor growth dependent on Kaposi's sarcoma-derived fibroblast growth factor inhibited by pentosan polysulfate. *J. Natl Cancer Inst.*, **83**, 716–20.

326. LaRocca, R. V., Cooper, M. R., Uhrich, M., Danesi, R., Walther, M. M., Linehan, W. M., and Myers, C. E. (1991). Use of suramin in treatment of prostatic carcinoma refractory to conventional hormonal manipulation. *Urol. Clin. North Am.*, **18**, 123–9.

327. Walz, T. M., Abdiu, A., Wingren, S., Smeds, S., Larsson, S. E., and Wasteson, A. (1991). Suramin inhibits growth of human osteosarcoma xenografts in nude mice. *Cancer Res.*, **51**, 3585–9.

328. Huang, Y. Q., Li, J. J., Nicolaides, A., Zhang, W. G., and Friedman, K. A. (1993). Increased expression of fibroblast growth factors (FGFs) and their receptor by protamine and suramin on Kaposi's sarcoma-derived cells. *Anticancer Res.*, **13**, 887–90.

329. Zugmaier, G., Lippman, M. E., and Wellstein, A. (1992). Inhibition by pentosan polysulfate (PPS) of heparin-binding growth factors released from tumor cells and blockage by PPS of tumor growth in animals. *J. Natl Cancer Inst.*, **84**, 1716–24.

330. Pluda, J. M., Shay, L. E., Foli, A., Tannenbaum, S., Cohen, P. J., Goldspiel, B. R., *et al.* (1993). Administration of pentosan polysulfate to patients with human immunodeficiency virus-associated Kaposi's sarcoma. *J. Natl Cancer Inst.*, **85**, 1585–92.

331. Li, Y., Basilico, C., and Mansukhani, A. (1994). Cell transformation by fibroblast growth factors can be suppressed by truncated fibroblast growth factor receptors. *Mol. Cell. Biol.*, **14**, 7660–9.

332. Lappi, D. A., Maher, P. A., Martineau, D., and Baird, A. (1991). The basic fibroblast growth factor–saporin mitotoxin acts through the basic fibroblast growth factor receptor. *J. Cell. Physiol.*, **147**, 17–26.

333. Beitz, J. G., Davol, P., Clark, J. W., Kato, J., Medina, M., Frackelton, A. J., *et al.* (1992). Antitumor activity of basic fibroblast growth factor–saporin mitotoxin *in vitro* and *in vivo*. *Cancer Res.*, **52**, 227–30.

334. Ying, W., Martineau, D., Beitz, J., Lappi, D. A., and Baird, A. (1994). Anti-B16-F10 melanoma activity of a basic fibroblast growth factor-saporin mitotoxin. *Cancer*, **74**, 848–53.

335. Lappi, D. A., Ying, W., Barthelemy, I., Martineau, D., Prieto, I., Benatti, L., *et al.* (1994). Expression and activities of a recombinant basic fibroblast growth factor–saporin fusion protein. *J. Biol. Chem.*, **269**, 12552–8.

336. Siegall, C. B., Gawlak, S. L., Chace, D. F., Merwin, J. R., and Pastan, I. (1994). *In vivo* activities of acidic fibroblast growth factor–*Pseudomonas* exotoxin fusion proteins. *Bioconjug. Chem.*, **5**, 77–83.

337. Kunwar, S., Pai, L. H., and Pastan, I. (1993). Cytotoxicity and antitumor effects of growth factor–toxin fusion proteins on human glioblastoma multiforme cells. *J. Neurosurg.*, **79**, 569–76.

338. Merwin, J. R., Lynch, M. J., Madri, J. A., Pastan, I., and Siegall, C. B. (1992). Acidic fibroblast growth factor–*Pseudomonas* exotoxin chimeric protein elicits antiangiogenic effects on endothelial cells. *Cancer Res.*, **52**, 4995–5001.

339. Jellinek, D., Lynott, C. K., Rifkin, D. B., and Janjic, N. (1993). High-affinity RNA ligands to basic fibroblast growth factor inhibit receptor binding. *Proc. Natl Acad. Sci. USA*, **90**, 11227–31.

340. Guvakova, M. A., Yakubov, L. A., Vlodavsky, I., Tonkinson, J. L., and Stein, C. A. (1995). Phosphorothioate oligodeoxynucleotides bind to basic fibroblast growth factor, inhibit its binding to cell surface receptors, and remove it from low affinity binding sites on extracellular matrix. *J. Biol. Chem.*, **270**, 2620–7.

341. New, B. A. and Yeoman, L. C. (1992). Identification of basic fibroblast growth factor sensitivity and receptor and ligand expression in human colon tumor cell lines. *J. Cell. Physiol.*, **150**, 320–6.

342. Yamada, K., Yoshitake, Y., Norimatsu, H., and Nishikawa, K. (1992). Roles of various growth factors in growth of human osteosarcoma cells which can grow in protein-free medium. *Cell Struct. Funct.*, **17**, 9–17.

343. Sato, Y., Murphy, P. R., Sato, R., and Friesen, H. G. (1989). Fibroblast growth factor release by bovine endothelial cells and human astrocytoma cells in culture is density dependent. *Mol. Endocrinol.*, **3**, 744–8.

344. Gabra, N., Khiat, A., and Calabresi, P. (1994). Detection of elevated basic fibroblast growth factor during early hours of *in vitro* angiogenesis using a fast ELISA immunoassay. *Biochem. Biophys. Res. Commun.*, **205**, 1423–30.

345. Mignatti, P., Morimoto, T., and Rifkin, D. B. (1992). Basic fibroblast growth factor, a protein devoid of secretory signal sequence, is released by cells via a pathway independent of the endoplasmic reticulum–Golgi complex. *J. Cell. Physiol.*, **151**, 81–93.

346. Mignatti, P. and Rifkin, D. B. (1991). Release of basic fibroblast growth factor, an angiogenic factor devoid of secretory signal sequence: a trivial phenomenon or a novel secretion mechanism? *J. Cell Biochem.*, **47**, 201–7.

347. Mignatti, P., Morimoto, T., and Rifkin, D. B. (1991). Basic fibroblast growth factor released by single, isolated cells stimulates their migration in an autocrine manner. *Proc. Natl Acad. Sci. USA*, **88**, 11007–11.

348. Muesch, A., Hartmann, E., Rohde, K., Rubartelli, A., Sitia, R., and Rapoport, T. A. (1990). A novel pathway for secretory proteins? *Trends Biochem. Sci.*, **15**, 86–8.

349. Young, P. R., Hazuda, D. J., and Simon, P. L. (1988). Human interleukin 1 beta is not secreted from hamster fibroblasts when expressed constitutively from a transfected cDNA. *J. Cell Biol.*, **107**, 447–56.

350. Klagsbrun, M. and Vlodavsky, I. (1988). Biosynthesis and storage of basic fibroblast growth factor (bFGF) by endothelial cells: implication for the mechanism of action of angiogenesis. *Prog. Clin. Biol. Res.*, **266**, 55–61.

351. Gajdusek, C. M. and Carbon, S. (1989). Injury-induced release of basic fibroblast growth factor from bovine aortic endothelium. *J. Cell. Physiol.*, **139**, 570–9.

352. Witte, L., Fuks, Z., Haimovitz, F. A., Vlodavsky, I., Goodman, D. S., and Eldor, A. (1989). Effects of irradiation on the release of growth factors from cultured bovine, porcine, and human endothelial cells. *Cancer Res.*, **49**, 5066–72.

353. McNeil, P. L., Muthukrishnan, L., Warder, E., and D'Amore, P. A. (1989). Growth factors are released by mechanically wounded endothelial cells. *J. Cell Biol.*, **109**, 811–22.

354. Muthukrishnan, L., Warder, E., and McNeil, P. L. (1991). Basic fibroblast growth factor is efficiently released from a cytolsolic storage site through plasma membrane disruptions of endothelial cells. *J. Cell. Physiol.*, **148**, 1–16.

355. Thompson, R. J., Jackson, A. P., and Langlois, N. (1986). Circulating antibodies to mouse monoclonal immunoglobulins in normal subjects — incidence, species specificity, and effects on a two-site assay for creatine kinase–MB isoenzyme. *Clin. Chem.*, **32**, 476–81.

356. Joseph, S. J., Moscatelli, D., and Rifkin, D. B. (1988). The development of a quantitative RIA for basic fibroblast growth factor using polyclonal antibodies against the 157 amino acid form of human bFGF. The identification of bFGF in adherent elicited murine peritoneal macrophages. *J. Immunol. Methods*, **110**, 183–92.

357. Rennard, S. I., Bitterman, P. B., Ozaki, T., Rom, W. N., and Crystal, R. G. (1988). Colchicine suppresses the release of fibroblast growth factors from alveolar macrophages *in vitro*. The basis of a possible therapeutic approach of the fibrotic disorders. *Am. Rev. Respir. Dis.*, **137**, 181–5.

358. Baird, A., Mormede, P., and Bohlen, P. (1985). Immunoreactive fibroblast growth factor in cells of peritoneal exudate suggests its identity with macrophage-derived growth factor. *Biochem. Biophys. Res. Commun.*, **126**, 358–64.

359. Jackson, A., Friedman, S., Zhan, X., Engleka, K. A., Forough, R., and Maciag, T. (1992). Heat shock induces release of fibroblast growth factor 1 from NIH 3T3 cells. *Proc. Natl Acad. Sci. USA*, **89**, 10691–5.

360. Jackson, A., Tarantini, F., Gamble, S., Friedman, S., and Maciag, T. (1995). The release of fibroblast growth factor-1 from NIH 3T3 cells in response to temperature involves the function of cysteine residues. *J. Biol. Chem.*, **270**, 33–6.

361. Krämer, M., Sachsenmaier, C., Herrlich, P., and Rahmsdorf, H. J. (1993). UV irradiation-induced inter-leukin-1 and basic fibroblast growth factor synthesis and release mediate part of the UV response. *J. Biol. Chem.*, **268**, 6734–41.

362. Florkiewicz, R. Z., Majack, R. A., Buechler, R. D., and Florkiewicz, E. (1995). Quantitative export of FGF-2 occurs through an alternative, energy-dependent, non-ER/Golgi pathway. *J. Cell. Physiol.*, **162**, 388–99.

363. Blotnick, S., Peoples, G. E., Freeman, M. R., Eberlein, T. J., and Klagsbrun, M. (1994). T lymphocytes synthesize and export heparin-binding epidermal growth factor-like growth factor and basic fibroblast growth factor, mitogens for vascular cells and fibroblasts: differential production and release by CD4+ and CD8+ T cells [see comments]. *Proc. Natl Acad. Sci. USA*, **91**, 2890–94.

364. Saita, N., Sakata, K. M., Matsumoto, M., Iyonaga, K., Ando, M., Adachi, M., and Hirashima, M. (1994). Production of fibroblast proliferative cytokines from T lym-phocytes stimulated by a B cell lymphoma line and their functional heterogeneity. *Immunol. Lett.*, **41**, 279–86.

365. Hanahan, D. (1985). Heritable formation of pancreatic β-cell tumors in transgenic mice expressing recombinant insulin/simian virus 40 oncogenes. *Nature*, **315**, 115–22.

366. Teitelmann, G., Alpert, S., and Hanahan, D. (1988). Proliferation, senescence, and neoplastic progression of β cells in hyperplastic pancreatic islets. *Cell*, **52**, 97–105.

367. Folkman, J., Watson, K., Ingber, D., and Hanahan, D. (1989). Induction of angiogenesis during the transition from hyperplasia to neoplasia. *Nature*, **339**, 58–61.

368. Czubayko, F., Smith, R. V., Chung, H. C., and Wellstein, A. (1994). Tumor growth and angiogenesis induced by a secreted binding protein for fibroblast growth factors. *J. Biol. Chem.*, **269**, 28243–8.

369. Zimering, M. B., Brandi, M. L., deGrange, D. A., Marx, S. J., Streeten, E., Katsumata, N., *et al.* (1990). Circulating fibroblast growth factor-like substance in familial multiple endocrine neoplasia type 1. *J. Clin. Endocrinol. Metab.*, **70**, 149–54.

370. Carlone, D. L. and Rider, V. (1993). Embryonic modula-tion of basic fibroblast growth factor in the rat uterus. *Biol. Reprod.*, **49**, 653–65.

371. Brigstock, D. R., Heap, R. B., and Brown, K. D. (1989). Polypeptide growth factors in uterine tissues and secretions. *J. Reprod. Fertil.*, **85**, 747–58.

372. Schweigerer, L., Neufeld, G., Mergia, A., Abraham, J. A., Fiddes, J. C., and Gospodarowicz, D. (1987). Basic fibro-blast growth factor in human rhabdomyosarcoma cells: implications for the proliferation and neovascularization of myoblast-derived tumors. *Proc. Natl Acad. Sci. USA*, **84**, 842–6.

373. Vlodavsky, I., Folkman, J., Sullivan, R., Fridman, R., Ishai, M. R., Sasse, J., and Klagsbrun, M. (1987). Endothelial cell-derived basic fibroblast growth factor: synthesis and deposition into subendothelial extracellular matrix. *Proc. Natl Acad. Sci. USA*, **84**, 2292–6.

374. Baird, A. and Ling, N. (1987). Fibroblast growth factors are present in the extracellular matrix produced by endothelial cells *in vitro*: implications for a role of heparinase-like enzymes in the neovascular response. *Biochem. Biophys. Res. Commun.*, **142**, 428–35.

375. Globus, R. K., Plouet, J., and Gospodarowicz, D. (1989). Cultured bovine bone cells synthesize basic fibroblast

376. Bashkin, P., Doctrow, S., Klagsbrun, M., Svahn, C. M., Folkman, J., and Vlodavsky, I. (1989). Basic fibroblast growth factor binds to subendothelial extracellular matrix and is released by heparitinase and heparin-like molecules. *Biochemistry*, **28**, 1737–43.

377. Folkman, J., Klagsbrun, M., Sasse, J., Wadzinski, M., Ingber, D., and Vlodavski, I. (1988). Heparin-binding angiogenic protein — basic fibroblast growth factor — is stored within basement membrane. *Am. J. Pathol.*, **130**, 393–9.

378. Weiner, H. L. and Swain, J. L. (1989). Acidic fibroblast growth factor mRNA is expressed by cardiac myocytes in culture and the protein is localized to the extracellular matrix. *Proc. Natl Acad. Sci. USA*, **86**, 2683–7.

379. DiMario, J., Buffinger, N., Yamada, S., and Strohman, R. C. (1989). Fibroblast growth factor in the extracellular matrix of dystrophic (mdx) mouse muscle. *Science*, **244**, 688–90.

380. Saksela, O. and Rifkin, D. B. (1990). Release of basic fibroblast growth factor–heparan sulfate complexes from endothelial cells by plasminogen activator-mediated proteolytic activity. *J. Cell Biol.*, **110**, 767–75.

381. Thompson, R. W., Whalen, G. F., Saunders, K. B., Hores, T., and D'Amore, P. A. (1990). Heparin-mediated release of fibroblast growth factor-like activity into the circulation of rabbits. *Growth Factors*, **3**, 221–9.

382. Presta, M., Maier, J. A., Rusnati, M., and Ragnotti, G. (1989). Basic fibroblast growth factor is released from endothelial extracellular matrix in a biologically active form. *J. Cell. Physiol.*, **140**, 68–74.

383. Flaumenhaft, R., Moscatelli, D., Saksela, O., and Rifkin, D. B. (1989). Role of extracellular matrix in the action of basic fibroblast growth factor: matrix as a source of growth factor for long-term stimulation of plasminogen activator production and DNA synthesis. *J. Cell. Physiol.*, **140**, 75–81.

384. Gospodarowicz, D., Delgado, D., and Vlodavsky, I. (1980). Permissive effect of the extracellular matrix on cell proliferation *in vitro*. *Proc. Natl Acad. Sci. USA*, **77**, 4094–98.

385. Lander, A. D., Fujii, D. K., Gospodarowicz, D., and Reichardt, L. F. (1982). Characterization of a factor that promotes neurite outgrowth: evidence linking activity to a heparan sulfate proteoglycan. *J. Cell Biol.*, **94**, 574–85.

386. Rosengart, T. K., Johnson, W. V., Friesel, R., Clark, R., and Maciag, T. (1988). Heparin protects heparin-binding growth factor-I from proteolytic inactivation *in vitro*. *Biochem. Biophys. Res. Commun.*, **152**, 432–40.

387. Damon, D. H., Lobb, R. R., D'Amore, P. A., and Wagner, J. A. (1989). Heparin potentiates the action of acidic fibro-blast growth factor by prolonging its biological half-life. *J. Cell. Physiol.*, **138**, 221–6.

388. Saksela, O., Moscatelli, D., Sommer, A., and Rifkin, D. B. (1988). Endothelial cell-derived heparan sulfate binds basic fibroblast growth factor and protects it from proteolytic degradation. *J. Cell Biol.*, **107**, 743–51.

389. Gospodarowicz, D. and Cheng, J. (1986). Heparin protects basic and acidic FGF from inactivation. *J. Cell. Physiol.*, **128**, 475–84.

18. The biphasic effects of transforming growth factors β in angiogenesis

Joseph A. Madri and Sabita Sankar

Introduction

Angiogenesis is a dynamic process which can be defined as the formation of new vessels. Angiogenesis is known to occur during development, in response to injury and tumour angiogenic factors and is thought to be controlled by many diverse, complex factors acting in concert in local environments over finite time periods. The principal cells involved in the process of angiogenesis are microvascular endothelial cells, which are distinct from endothelial cells lining the larger vessels of the circulatory system in their physiological functions as well as in their responses to injury, although both large vessel and microvascular endothelial cells are derived from the same stem cells (1–5). The differences between large vessel and microvascular endothelial cells are clearly noted when one compares their responses with injury. Large vessel endothelia respond to denudation injury caused by angioplasty, endarterectomy, and synthetic and autologous bypass grafting by undergoing sheet migration which is modulated, in part, by soluble factors and the existing and newly synthesized extracellular matrix components. In many instances re-endothelization is incomplete and the affected endothelial cells exhibit altered metabolic and adhesive behaviours which contribute to the development of stenotic lesions and ultimately compromise blood flow (2–4). In contrast, following injury microvascular endothelial cells initiate an angiogenic process also modulated by both existing and newly synthesized extracellular matrix components and soluble factors (6–9). This process consists of local disruption of the basement membrane investing the affected endothelial cells, migration of the endothelial cells into the local interstitial stroma, cell proliferation, new vessel formation, and stabilization. Selective involution of newly formed vascular beds occurs during development and during wound healing as a normal aspect of these complex processes (10). The distinct behavioural patterns exhibited by these two endothelial cell types have given rise to the hypotheses that large vessel endothelial cells sometimes exhibit 'dysfunctional' behaviour in response to injury-induced changes in the extracellular matrix and soluble factor environments, favouring the development of arteriosclerosis (11); while microvascular endothelial cells exhibit a 'plastic' phenotype in response to injury-induced changes in the local extracellular matrix and soluble factor environments, displaying the variety of phenotypes normally observed in the microvasculature during angiogenesis (5,10).

In this chapter we will discuss the effects of modulation of growth factor receptor surface expression and responsiveness during the process of angiogenesis and the roles of extracellular matrix composition and organization in mediating these changes. In particular, extracellular matrix mediated effects on platelet-derived growth factor (PDGF) receptor and transforming growth factor beta (TGF-β) receptor expression and responsiveness will be discussed.

Transforming growth factors beta modulate endothelial cell behaviour in a complex manner

Over the past several years many reports have been published illustrating a wide variety of TGF-β-mediated effects on endothelial cells including changes in proliferative and migration rates, expression of integrin heterodimeric pairs, proteinases and proteinase inhibitors, a variety of extracellular matrix components, and cytoskeletal components (7,9,12–15). On initial review, many of these reports appear contradictory, documenting increases or decreases in the above-mentioned aspects of cell behaviour. Additionally, endothelial cells derived from different vascular beds exhibit distinct behavioural patterns to TGF-β treatment, depending upon the isoform of TGF-β used and its concentration (16–20). For example, bovine aortic endothelial cells (BAEC) (which can be considered a typical large vessel endothelial cell population) respond to TGF-β1 and TGF-β3 but are refractory to TGF-β2; while rat epididymal fat pad microvascular endothelial cells (which typify a microvascular endothelial cell population) are responsive to all three TGF-β isoforms (16–18). Our understanding of these differences is incomplete but the discrepancy may be due, in part, to differences in the surface expression of particular TGF-β receptors and/or their ratios on endothelial cells derived from different vascular beds or to differences in the engagement and activation of selected signalling pathways distal to the receptors (9).

Aortic endothelial cell responsiveness to TGF-β isoforms is dependent upon the surface expression of particular TGF-β receptor proteins

The observation that BAEC proliferation and migration are inhibited, fibronectin and plasminogen activator inhibitor 1 (PAI-1) synthesis are increased and urokinase plasminogen activator (uPA) activity is decreased following TGF-β1 and TGF-β3, but not TGF-β2 treatment correlates with the presence of TGF-β type I and II receptors and the absence of type III receptors on the BAEC surfaces (16,18). BAEC stably transfected with the TFG-β type III receptor (betaglycan) cDNA displayed surface expression of the type III receptor protein and were noted to be responsive to TGF-β2 in proliferation, migration, and PAI-1 synthesis assays to the same levels as TGF-β1 and TGF-β3 (21). These data are consistent with the concept that TGF-β type III receptor does not perform a signalling function. Instead, it serves to present the TGF-β2 ligand to the type II and I receptors, thus modulating the TGF-β isoform response in these cells (21–24). These findings are in agreement with the findings of several investigators who found that introduction of the TGF-β type III receptor into myoblast cell lines lacking this receptor rendered the cells responsive to TGF-β2 (23–25).

In contrast to the above-mentioned studies, BAEC stably transfected with the TGF-β type III receptor (betaglycan) cDNA in the reverse orientation displayed profoundly reduced surface expression of both the type I and type II receptors. Furthermore, BAEC transfected with this construct were noted to be refractory to TGF-β1 and TGF-β2 isoforms in proliferation, migration, and PAI-1 synthesis assays, consistent with the notion that complete down-regulation of the TGF-β type III receptor could alter the surface expression of the TGF-β type II and type I receptors in a fashion that is not currently understood (21).

In recent studies we have shown that BAEC TGF-β receptor expression can be modulated by treatment with soluble factors. Similar to findings observed in osteoblasts (26), BAEC were noted to exhibit changes in their TGF-β

receptor expression profile in response to PGE$_2$, a prostaglandin known to elicit changes in TGF-β receptor expression in osteoblast cultures (27). Specifically, pretreatment with PGE$_2$ rendered BAEC refractory to TGF-β1-mediated inhibition of proliferation. This effect appears to be specific as PGE$_2$-treated cells retain their ability to increase their expression of PAI-1 in response to TGF-β1 treatment. When TGF-β receptor surface expression was analysed, we found that type II receptor expression was significantly reduced, consistent with the notion that the type II receptor is involved in engaging and activating the signalling pathway that modulates proliferation while the type I receptor is involved in mediating the signalling pathway(s) that affect extracellular matrix, proteinase, and proteinase inhibitor synthesis. These findings are consistent with the findings of Chen *et al.* who utilized dominant negative type II receptor constructs in transfection studies (28). In these studies transfection of dominant negative type II receptor constructs resulted in loss of TGF-β's anti-proliferative effect. Additionally, the development of mutant cell lines expressing only the type I receptor revealed the selective loss of TGF-β's antiproliferative effect with retention of TGF-β's ability to upregulate PAI-1 and fibronectin expression (29–31). In addition, in complementation analyses using different cell hybrids, increased type II receptor expression was associated with growth suppression but not the induction of several extracellular matrix proteins (32).

These studies, taken together, support the concept that the absence or presence of particular TGF-β receptors on a cell surface determine, in part, the cell's response to the particular TGF-β isoform. These studies also suggest the possibility that the growth factor receptor profile of an endothelial cell might be dynamic, being responsive to the local extracellular matrix composition and organization and the local soluble factor milieu.

Microvascular endothelial cell responsiveness to growth factors is dependent upon the surface expression of particular receptor proteins

While the effects of TGF-β1 on large vessel endothelial proliferation, migration, extracellular matrix, and proteinase/proteinase inhibitor synthesis are generally accepted (11,33), TGF-β1 mediated effects on microvascular endothelial cell behaviour are somewhat controversial (5,7,9). This is most likely due to the 'plasticity' of the microvascular endothelial cell phenotype and the particular culture conditions used in the various studies (5). The term 'plasticity' is used to describe the great range of phenotypes that the microvascular endothelial cell expresses during the complex process of angiogenesis. Over the past several years many studies examining various effects of TGF-β isoforms on microvascular endothelial cell behaviour have been performed resulting in a somewhat confusing assessment of TGF-β's role in the process of angiogenesis. The observation that TGF-β1 elicited an angiogenic response when injected sub-cutaneously in mice suggested that TGF-β1 might be an angiogenic factor (34). However, several studies utilizing standard two-dimensional culture techniques found microvascular endothelial cell proliferation to be inhibited by TGF-β1, TGF-β2, and TGF-β3 (16,18), casting doubt as to whether TGF-β could function as an angiogenic factor. This apparent discrepancy between *in vivo* and *in vitro* generated data can be resolved by taking into account the complex multifunctional process of angiogenesis that occurs *in vivo* in a growth factor-rich, three-dimensional environment and comparing this with the relatively simple limited processes examined *in vitro* in the context of simple extracellular matrix coatings or in mixtures of matrix components or isolated intact matrices in the presence of defined soluble factors (35–38) (Fig. 18.1). It is not surprising that the endothelial cells cultured under these conditions behave in ways dissimilar to their *in vivo*

counterparts. However, utilizing tissue culture models does offer some benefit, as they allow the analyses of particular cell functions in a defined environment and can mimic certain aspects of the angiogenic process (5,9).

Platelet-derived growth factor receptor modulation

The use of tissue culture models to study the process of angiogenesis has been extensive and fruitful. For example, Battegay *et al.* demonstrated that the 'sprouting' cells observed in some BAEC cultures are cells which invade the space beneath the BAEC monolayer in organized aggregates, mimicking angiogenic sprouts. These investigators have demonstrated that these cells, in contrast to the cells comprising the monolayer, exhibit proliferative responses to PDGF isoforms (38). Nicosia *et al.*, have noted similar behaviour patterns in their rat aortic ring model of angiogenesis. In this model the investigators noted that the angiogenic sprouts growing out radially from the aortic ring were responsive to PDGF isoforms while the endothelial cells associated with the aortic ring were refractory (39). In our studies similar findings were also documented. Namely, Rat epididymal Fat pad derived microvascular endothelial Cells (RFC) cultured in standard two-dimensional culture on a collagen substratum (culture

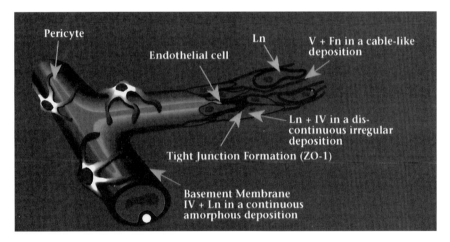

Figure 18.1. Schematic representation of the matrix modulation of microvascular endothelial cell (EC) phenotype during angiogenesis. Cells at the distal tip of the angiogenic sprout deposit and interact with a different matrix composition and organization compared with cells nearer the parent vessel. Cells at the distal tip express features of undifferentiated EC, having high-migratory, proteolytic and proliferative rates, platelet-derived growth factor (PDGF) receptors, α smooth muscle actin and a high transforming growth factor (TGF) β receptor type II–I ratio. In contrast, cells nearer the parent vessel deposit and interact with a mature basement membrane and express features of differentiated EC, having low-migratory, proteolytic and proliferative rates, tight junction formation, loss of both PDGF receptors and α smooth muscle actin and a low TGF-β receptor type II–I ratio. Abbreviations: V = type V collagen; Fn = fibronectin; Ln = laminin; IV = type IV collagen. Based on data from references 6 and 8.

conditions that may mimic the actively proliferating, migratory cells at the tip of an angiogenic sprout) exhibited surface expression of PDGF receptor α and β chains and a proliferative response to PDGF BB and AB. When these cells were cultured in a three-dimensional type I collagen gel (culture conditions that may mimic the differentiated, mitotically quiescent cells at the base of an angiogenic sprout) they were noted to lose expression of both PDGF receptor chains as well as responsiveness to PDGF iso-forms. Switching the cells back and forth from the two-dimensional to the three-dimensional environment caused a reversible transient expression of the PDGF receptor chains, illustrating the 'plastic' phenotype of this cell type (5,40). These three examples illustrate the 'plasticity' of selected endothelial populations and the role of the microenvironment in regulating the expression of growth factor receptors and the cell's responsiveness to growth factors. These studies are supported by several *in vivo* studies in which PDGF receptors were localized to endothelial cells comprising angiogenic sprouts (41–44).

Transforming growth factor beta receptor modulation

Several recent reports have illustrated a mechanism of signal transduction which may be initiated following TGF-β binding (45,46). Based on the data from several reports, investigators have proposed that the TGF-β type II and type I receptors exist as homodimers in the plasma membrane (47). Evidence has been accrued demonstrating that the presence of both receptor types is necessary, namely, that type II receptor is necessary for TGF-β binding to the type I receptor and the type II receptor is necessary for sig-nalling to the type I receptor (45). Investigators have also demonstrated that the type II receptor is constitutively phosphorylated but does not initiate a signal unless it binds its ligand (TGF-β1), after which it phosphorylates the type I receptor and signals downstream events (45). Thus, accordingly, both type I and type II receptors are needed for signal transduction and the specificity of the signalling pathways (differential effects on proliferative rate, extra-cellular matrix, protease, and protease inhibitor synthesis as observed in several cell types) are thought to occur as downstream events (Fig. 18.2).

The phenomenon of growth factor modulation observed in vascular endothelial cells can be evoked to explain dif-ferential TGF-β responsiveness during the process of angiogenesis. Arispe and Sage noted that 'sprouting' BAEC, in addition to being responsive to PDGF, exhibit increases in their proliferative rates in response to TGF-β1 treatment, in contrast to subconfluent monolayer cul-tures of BAEC which are inhibited by TGF-β1 (37).

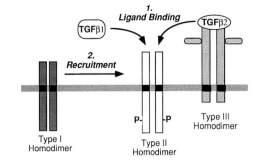

Binding of TGFβ1 to the type II receptor directly or TGFβ2 via the type III receptor elicits binding and phosphorylation and activation of the type I receptor and signal transduction

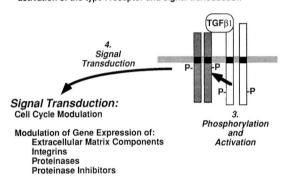

Figure 18.2. General transforming growth factor (TGF) β type I, type II and type III receptor signaling scheme. According to this scheme: 1. TGF-β1 ligand binds to constitutively phosphorylated type II receptor homodimers [TGF-β2 will bind to the type II receptor only in the presence of the type III receptor (betaglycan)]. 2. TGF-β binding to the type II receptors elicits recruitment of type I receptor homodimers. 3. The complexed type I receptors are then phosphorylated by the adjacent type II receptor. 4. The type I receptor kinase then initiates signalling cascades that modulate proliferation and selected gene expression. This scheme is based on data and concepts from references 25 and 45–47.

Although not determined, one could speculate that the 'sprouting' BAEC express a different TGF-β receptor profile on their surfaces than the subconfluent BAEC monolayers or that TGF-β1 activates distinct signalling pathways in the 'sprouting' BAEC compared with the subconfluent BAEC monolayers. In recent studies we have documented such a phenomenon (48). Specifically, when grown in two-dimensional culture, RFC proliferation is known to be inhibited by TGF-β1 treatment (7,16,18). The TGF-β type II to type I receptor ratio is 5:1 in these culture conditions as determined by receptor cross-linking experiments. In contrast, when grown in three-dimensional

(a)

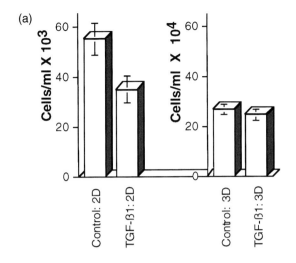

(b)

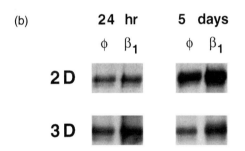

Figure 18.3. (a) Transforming growth factor (TGF) β1 inhibits proliferation of microvessel endothelial cells plated on type I collagen [two-dimensional (2D) cultures] but not in cells plated with gels comprised of type I collagen [three-dimensional (3D) cultures]. Left panel: proliferation assays were performed on RFC grown in 2D culture on a coating of collagen type I for 5 days in the absence and presence of 0.5 ng/ml TGF-β1. 1×10^4 cells were initially plated into the 60 mm dishes. Each point represents quadruplicate samples. The vertical lines represent standard deviations. Right panel: proliferation assay performed on RFC grown in 3D culture in a collagen type I gel for 1 and 5 days in the absence and presence of 0.5 ng/ml TGF-β1. 1×10^6 cells/ml of gel were initially plated into the 60 mm dishes in 200 ml droplets. Each point represents quadruplicate samples. Vertical lines represent standard deviations. (b) TGF-β1 modulates fibronectin protein levels in 2D and 3D cultures differently. Upper panel: autoradiograph of affinity-purified [^{35}S]-methionine labelled fibronectin (Fn) from RFC grown in 2D culture on coatings of collagen type I for and 5 days in the absence (Φ) and presence of 0.5 ng/ml TGF-β1. Lower panel: Autoradiograph of affinity-purified [^{35}S]-methionine labelled Fn from RFC grown in 3D culture in collagen type I GELS for 1 and 5 days in the absence (Φ) and presence of 0.5 ng/ml TGF-β1.

culture, RFC proliferation is not inhibited by TGF-β1 treatment and the TGF-β type II to type I receptor ratio is 1:1 in these culture conditions (48). Thus, lowering the type II to type I receptor ratio appears to modulate the TGF-β1 effect on proliferation (48). Interestingly, under both culture conditions (two- and three-dimensional culture) the effects of TGF-β1 on collagen and fibronectin synthesis is preserved (Fig. 18.3) (48). In additional studies, in order to mimic the effects of three-dimensional culture on TGF-β receptor expression, stable transfection of a cDNA coding for a truncated TGF-β type II receptor missing the cytoplasmic domain and functioning as a dominant negative mutant was used (48). Such RFC grown in two-dimensional culture were noted to be refractory to TGF-β1 treatment when proliferation was examined but they retained their TGF-β1-mediated fibronectin induction. Conversely, stable transfection of cDNA coding for a truncated TGF-β type I receptor missing the cytoplasmic domain and functioning as a dominant negative mutant resulted in these RFC exhibiting inhibition of proliferation in

response to TGF-β1 but lacking any fibronectin synthesis induction (48). These findings illustrate the complexity of TGF-β receptor signalling and the potential of distinct signalling pathways operational for the type I and type II receptors. The recent studies of Centrella *et al.*, in which distinct populations of osteoblasts exhibit distinct type II to type I receptor ratios and differential proliferative and extracellular matrix synthetic responsiveness to TGF-β1, support this concept (26). Further support comes from the studies of Chen *et al.*, in which the investigators utilized stable transfection of cDNA coding for a truncated TGF-β type II receptor missing the cytoplasmic domain and functioning as a dominant-negative mutant as a method of altering TGF-β receptor ratios (28).

Additional support for this hypothesis can be taken from the work of Atfi *et al.* in which a relationship between TGF-β1 mediated inhibition of proliferation, c-*src* activity and protein level, shc phosphorylation and shc-GRB-2 association was noted (49) and recent work performed in our laboratory in which BAEC over-expressing c-*src* were

Microvascular Endothelial Cells

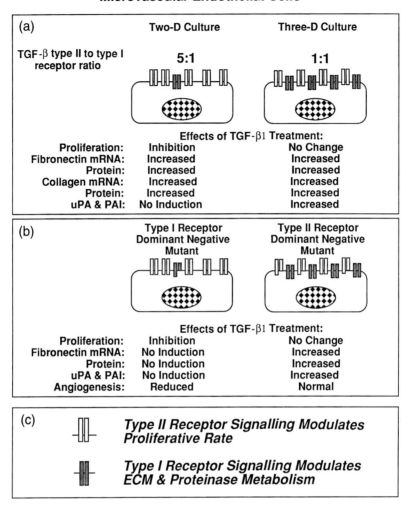

Figure 18.4. Transforming growth factor (TGF) β type I and type II receptor modulation and signalling in microvascular endothelial cells. (a) In two-dimensional culture the cells exhibit a 5:1 type II to type I receptor ratio and respond to TGF-β1 by decreasing their proliferative rate and increasing their extracellular matrix (ECM) synthesis. In contrast, in three-dimensional culture these cells exhibit a 1:1 type II to type I receptor ratio and response to TGF-β1 with no change in their proliferative rate, but increases in their ECM, proteinase, and proteinase inhibitor synthesis. (b) The modulation of receptor ratios and changes in cell behaviour evoked by changes in culture conditions can be mimicked using expression of dominant negative mutants of the type I and type II receptor. Cells expressing the type I receptor dominant negative mutant exhibit decreases in proliferative rate in response to TGF-β1, but do not exhibit changes in ECM, proteinase, and proteinase inhibitor synthesis and exhibit reduced *in vitro* angiogenesis patterns. In contrast, cells expressing the type II receptor dominant negative mutant exhibit no changes in proliferative rate in response to TGF-β1, but do exhibit increases in ECM, proteinase, and proteinase inhibitor synthesis and normal *in vitro* angiogenesis patterns. (c) The findings summarized in (a) and (b) support the concepts of modulation of TGF-β1 receptor surface expression and distinct type I and type II receptor signalling pathways in endothelial cells, with the type I TGF-β receptor signalling modulation of ECM and proteinase and proteinase inhibitor metabolism and the type II TGF-β receptor signalling modulation of proliferative rates. uPA, urokinase plasminogen activator; PAI, plasminogen activator inhibitor.

noted to be resistant to proliferation inhibition by TGF-β1 but were observed to retain their fibronectin and PAI-1 inducibility (50). These data are consistent with at least two signalling pathways following TGF-β engagement, one modulating proliferation and another modulating extracellular matrix, proteinase and proteinase inhibitor synthesis, regulated by the relative ratios of type II to type I receptor surface expression (Fig. 18.4). Much more investigation is needed in this area to develop a clearer, more complete understanding of TGF-β-mediated signalling pathways. It is likely that different cell types may utilize distinct signalling pathways having different specificities and selectivities in response to TGF-β isoforms.

During the process of angiogenesis it is likely that endothelial cells at the tip of the angiogenic sprout express very different surface receptor profiles than the cells nearer the parent vessel, responding to the multitude of factors present differently, depending upon their receptor repertoire and factor interactions (Fig. 18.6).

The role(s) of factor interactions and TGF β receptor surface expression in modulating proteolysis during angiogenesis

In addition to the complexity of the TGF-β receptor signalling system, there is the added complexity of endothelial cell responses to other soluble factors during the process of angiogenesis. Several groups have been investigating the coordinate roles of combinations of soluble factors present during the process of angiogenesis (14,35,36,51). Pepper *et al.* examined the interactions of basic fibroblast growth factor (bFGF) and TGF-β1 during *in vitro* angiogenesis (14,36,52). These investigators showed that proteolysis is tightly regulated during angiogenesis and necessary for new vessels to develop and mature. Specifically, they demonstrated that bFGF induces microvascular endothelial cell invasion and tube formation in fibrin gels (36,52). This behaviour was correlated with

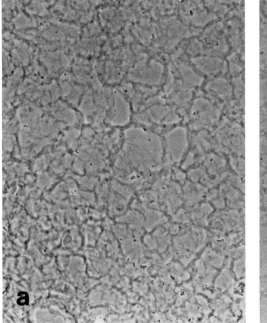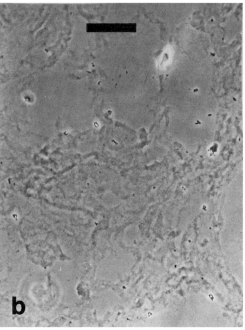

Figure 18.5. Trasylol inhibits transforming growth factor (TGF) β1 mediated tube formation in microvascular endothelial cells (RFC) cultured three-dimensional (3D) collagen gels. Photomicrographs of phase microscopic analyses of sections of 1 day 3D cultures of RFCs grown in the absence and presence of 0.5 ng/ml TGF-β1. (a) Typical phase microscopy field of a section of a 1 day 3D culture of RFC treated with 0.5 ng/ml TGF-β1. Note the extensive organization of the cells into multicellular aggregates forming a network of tubes. (b) Typical phase microscopy field of a section of a 1 day 3D culture of RFC treated with 0.5 ng/ml TGF-β1 and 1 mmol/l Trasylol. Note the relative lack of organization of the cells into multicellular aggregates compared with (a). Original magnification = 200×. Black bar = 500 mm.

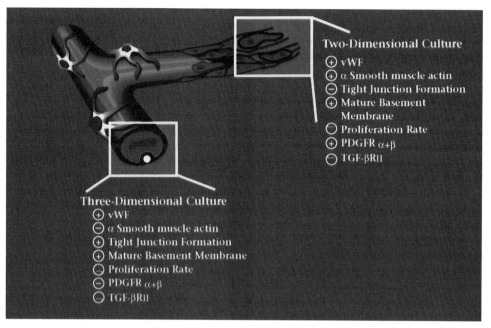

Figure 18.6. Schematic representation of the specific culture conditions which mimic the modulation of microvascular endothelial cell (EC) phenotypes during angiogenesis. Specific culture conditions mimic either EC at the distal tip of an angiogenic sprout (two-dimensional culture) or differentiated EC nearer the parent vessel (three-dimensional culture). Data used in generating this figure were taken from references 1, 2, 4–7, 9, 10, 16–18, and 40. vWF, von Willebrand's factor; TGF, transforming growth factor; PDGFR, platelet-derived growth factor receptor.

increased uPA activity and mRNA levels. These investigators showed that levels of PAI-1 protein and mRNA are also elevated in response to bFGF, suggesting that a tight local control of proteolysis is necessary for normal angiogenesis to occur. The relative inductions of uPA and PAI-1 would be expected to vary depending upon the factors present and the state of the endothelial cells. Investigations have demonstrated differences in the induction of uPA and PAI-1 by bFGF and TGF-β1 (52). It was noted that bFGF induced an increase in proteolysis while TGF-β1 elicited a net anti-proteolysis. Cultures treated with bFGF were found to have widely patent lumina while cultures treated with bFGF and TGF-β1 displayed only superficial invasion of the gel in the form of solid cords. The importance of this tight dynamic control of proteolysis in the process of angiogenesis was also illustrated using transduced endothelial cells. In these studies endothelial cells transduced with the middle T (mT) oncogene from polyoma virus (which induces haemangiomas in mice) formed large, ectatic sac-like structures resembling haemangiomas when cultured in fibrin gels. These cells were found to express increased uPA activity and decreased PAI-1 activity compared with normal endothelial cells. When these cells were

cultured in fibrin gels in the presence of the plasmin inhibitors TRASYLOL or ε-amino caproic acid (ε-ACA) the cells formed branching networks of tube-like structures with patent lumina similar to normal endothelial cells (53). These studies illustrate the importance of tight regulation of factor-driven control of proteolysis during angiogenesis.

The importance of TGF-β receptor surface expression has also been shown in the regulation of uPA and PAI-1. In recent studies we have demonstrated that when RFC are grown in two-dimensional culture (exhibiting a 5:1 TGF-β type II to type I receptor ratio) they do not exhibit either a uPA or PAI-1 response to TGF-β1 treatment. In contrast, when RFC are grown in three-dimensional culture (exhibiting a 1:1 TGF-β type II to type I receptor ratio) they respond to TGF-β1 treatment by undergoing tube formation in the collagen gel and exhibiting a transient increase in both uPA and PAI-1 activities (48). Perturbation of this tightly regulated activity by treatment of these cultures with TRASYLOL inhibited tube formation (Fig. 18.5). These data are consistent with and support the concept that tight regulation of proteolysis is necessary during the angiogenic response and that the TGF-β1-mediated responses will depend upon the relative cell surface expression of the type

I and type II TGF-β receptors as well as the presence of other growth factors and their receptors.

Summary and conclusions

In spite of intense investigations, the complex behaviour of vascular endothelial cells during the process of angiogenesis is still incompletely understood. The observations of independent modulation of selected growth factor receptors by these cells undergoing *in vitro* angiogenesis correlates well with the complex proliferative and extracellular matrix synthetic behaviour of the microvascular endothelial cell at different stages during this process (Fig. 18.6). An example of the importance of TGF-β receptor surface expression modulation in the vasculature can be found in the recent work of McAllister *et al.* (54). Data presented in this paper suggest that mutations in a TGF-β-binding protein, endoglin, which like betaglycan does not have a direct signalling activity, is the cause of hereditary haemorrhagic telangiectasia type I, an autosomal dominant disorder characterized by multisystemic vascular dysplasia and recurrent haemorrhages (54). The data summarized in this chapter support the concept of an as yet still undefined extracellular matrix organization/composition-modulated events, possibly integrin mediated, driving the observed changes in receptor expression (40). The recent work of several laboratories (55–57) illustrate the profound effects of modulating integrin-mediated adhesive processes on both *in vitro* and *in vivo* angiogenesis. While the specific signal transduction pathways which are responsible for the modulation of PDGF receptor and TGF-β receptor expression in microvascular endothelial cells and their effects during angiogenesis are unknown, the continuing advances in receptor and signalling biology should allow for a more complete understanding of this phenomenon in the near future.

References

1. Madri, J. A. and Pratt, B. M. (1988). Angiogenesis. In *The molecular and cellular biology of wound healing* (ed. R. F. Clark, and P. Henson), pp. 337–58. Plenum Press, New York.
2. Madri, J. A., Kocher, O., Merwin, J. R., Bell, L., and Yannariello-Brown, J. (1989). The interactions of vascular cells with solid phase (matrix) and soluble factors. *J. Cardiovasc. Pharmacol.*, **14**, S70–5.
3. Madri, J. A., Bell, L., Marx, M., Merwin, J. R., Basson, C. T., and Prinz, C. (1991). The effects of soluble factors and extracellular matrix components on vascular cell behavior *in vitro* and *in vivo*: models of de-endothelialization and repair. *J. Cell. Biochem.*, **45**, 1–8.
4. Madri, J. A., Merwin, J. R., Bell, L., Basson, C. T., Kocher, O., Perlmutter, R., and Prinz, C. (1992). Interactions of

matrix components and soluble factors in vascular cell responses to injury: modulation of cell phenotype. In *Endothelial cell dysfunction* (ed. N. Simionescu, and M. Simionescu), pp. 11–30. Plenum Press, New York.
5. Madri, J. A. and Marx, M. (1992). Matrix composition, organization and soluble factors: modulators of microvascular cell differentiation *in vitro*. *Kidney Int.*, **41**, 560–5.
6. Form, D. M., Pratt, B. M., and Madri, J. A. (1986). Endothelial cell proliferation during angiogenesis: *in vitro* modulation by basement membrane components. *Lab. Invest.*, **55**, 521–30.
7. Madri, J. A., Pratt, B. M., and Tucker, A. M. (1988). Phenotypic modulation of endothelial cells by transforming growth factor-β depends upon the composition and organization of the extracellular matrix. *J. Cell Biol.*, **106**, 1375–84.
8. Nicosia, R. F. and Madri, J. A. (1987). The microvascular extracellular matrix: developmental changes during angiogenesis in the aortic ring–plasma clot model. *Am. J. Pathol.*, **128**, 78–90.
9. Madri, J. A., Bell, L., and Merwin, J. R. (1992). Modulation of vascular cell behavior by transforming growth factors beta. *Mol. Reprod. Dev.*, **32**, 121–6.
10. Madri, J. A., Sankar, S., and Romanic, A. M. (1995). Angiogenesis. In *The molecular and cellular biology of wound healing* (ed. R. A. F. Clark, 2nd edn), pp. 335–71. Plenum Press, New York.
11. Madri, J. A. and Bell, L. (1992). Vascular cell responses to injury: modulation by extracellular matrix and soluble factors. In *Ultrastructure, membranes and cell interactions in atherosclerosis* (ed. H. Robenek and N. Severs), pp. 165–79. CRC Press, Boca Raton, FL.
12. Kocher, O. and Madri, J. A. (1989). Modulation of actin mRNAs in vascular cells by matrix components and TGF-β1. *In Vitro*, **25**, 424–34.
13. Muller, G., Behrens, J., Nussbaumer, U., Bohlen, P., and Birchmeier, W. (1987). Inhibitory effect of transforming growth factor β on endothelial cells. *Proc. Natl Acad. Sci. USA*, **84**, 5600–4.
14. Pepper, M. S., Belin, D., Montesano, R., Orci, L., and Vassali, J-D. (1990). Transforming growth factor β-1 modulates basic fibroblast growth factor-induced proteolytic and angiogenic properties of endothelial cells *in vitro*. *J. Cell Biol.*, **111**, 743–55.
15. Basson, C. T., Kocher, O., Basson, M. D., Asis, A., and Madri, J. A. (1992). Differential modulation of vascular cell integrin and extracellular matrix expression *in vitro* by TGF-β1 correlates with reciprocal effects on cell migration. *J. Cell. Physiol.*, **153**, 118–28.
16. Merwin, J. R., Newman, W., Beall, D., Tucker, A., and Madri, J. A. (1991). Vascular cells respond differentially to transforming growth factors-beta₁ and beta₂ *in vitro*. *Am. J. Pathol.*, **138**, 37–51.
17. Merwin, J. R., Anderson, J., Kocher, O., van Itallie, C., and Madri, J. A. (1990). Transforming growth factor β1 modulates extracellular matrix organization and cell–cell junctional complex formation during *in vitro* angiogenesis. *J. Cell. Physiol.*, **142**, 117–28.
18. Merwin, J. R., Tucker, A., Roberts, A., Kondaiah, P., and Madri, J. A. (1991). Vascular cell responses to transforming growth factor beta₃ mimic those of transforming growth factor beta₁ *in vitro*. *Growth Factors*, **5**, 149–58.
19. Qian, S. W., Burmester, J. K., Merwin, J. R., Madri, J. A., Sporn, M. B., and Roberts, A. B. (1992). Identification of a

structural domain that distinguishes the actions of the type 1 and 2 isoforms of TGF-β on endothelial cells. *Proc. Natl Acad. Sci. USA*, **89**, 6290–4.

20. Burmester, J. K., Qian, S. W., Roberts, A. B., Huang, A. Amatayakul-Chantler, S., Suardet, L., *et al.* (1993). Characterization of distinct functional domains of transforming growth factor-β. *Proc. Natl Acad. Sci. USA*, **90**, 8628–32.

21. Sankar, S., Mahooti-Brooks, N., Centrella, M., McCarthy, T. L., and Madri, J. A. (1995). Expression of transforming growth factor beta type III receptor in vascular endothelial cells increases their responsiveness to transforming growth factor β2. *J. Biol. Chem.*, **270**, 13567–71.

22. Cheifetz, S., Bellon, T., Cales, C., Vera, S., Bernabeu, C., Massague, J., and Letarte, M. (1992). Endoglin is a component of the TGF-β receptor system in human endothelial cells. *J. Biol. Chem.*, **267**, 19027–30.

23. Lopez-Casillas, F., Payne, H. M., Andres, J. L., and Massague, J. (1994). Betaglycan can act as a dual modulator of TGFβ access to signaling receptors: mapping of ligand binding and GAG attachment sites. *J. Cell Biol.*, **124**, 557–68.

24. Lopez-Casillas, F., Wrana, J. L., and Masssague, J. (1993). Betaglycan presents ligand to the TGF-β signaling receptor. *Cell*, **73**, 1435–44.

25. Moustakas, A., Lin, H. Y., Henis, Y. I., Plamondon, J., O'Connor-McCourt, M. D., and Lodish, H. F. (1993). The transforming growth factor β receptors types I, II, III form hetero-oligomeric complexes in the presence of ligand. *J. Biol. Chem.*, **266**, 22215–18.

26. Centrella, M., Casinghino, S., Kim, J., Pham, T., Rosen, V., Wozney, J., and McCarthy, T. L. (1995). Independent changes in type I and type II receptors for transforming growth factor β induced by bone morphogenetic protein 2 parallel expression of the osteoblast phenotype. *Mol. Cell. Biol.*, **15**, 3273–81.

27. Sankar, S., Mahooti-Brooks, N., Centrella, M., McCarthy, T. L., and Madri, J. A. (1995). Modulation of transforming growth factor beta receptor profiles differentially regulate TGF-β mediated responsiveness in vascular endothelial cells (submitted).

28. Chen, R-H, Ebner, R., and Derynck, R. (1994). Inactivation of the type II receptor reveals two receptor pathways for the diverse TGF-β activities. *Science*, **260**, 1335–8.

29. Arrick, B. A., Lopez, A. R., Elfman, F., Ebner, R., Damsky, C. H., and Derynck, R. (1992). Altered metabolic and adhesive properties and increased tumorigenesis associated with increased expression of transforming growth factor beta 1. *J. Cell Biol.*, **118**, 715–26.

30. Fafeur, V. B., Terman, I., Blum, J., and Bohlen, P. (1990). Basic FGF treatment of endothelial cells downregulates the 85 kDa TGF beta receptor subtype and decreases the growth inhibitory response to TGF-beta 1. *Growth Factors*, **3**, 237–45.

31. Franzen, P., Ichijo, H., and Miyazono, K. (1993). Different signals mediate transforming growth factor-β1 induced growth inhibition and extracellular matrix production in prostate carcinoma cells. *Exp. Cell Res.*, **207**, 1–7.

32. Geiser, A. G., Burmester, J. K., Webbink, R., Roberts, A. B., and Sporn, M. B. (1992). Inhibition of growth by transforming growth factor β following fusion of two non-responsive human carcinoma cell lines: implications of the type II receptor in growth inhibitory responses. *J. Biol. Chem.*, **267**, 2588–93.

33. Madri, J. A., Reidy, M., Kocher, O., and Bell, L. (1989). Endothelial cell behaviour after denudation injury is modulated by TGF-β and fibronectin. *Lab. Invest.*, **60**, 755–65.

34. Roberts, A. B., Sporn, M. B., Assoian, R. K., Smith, J. M., Roche, W. S., Wakefield, L. A., *et al.* (1986). Transforming growth factor β: rapid induction of fibrosis and angiogenesis *in vivo* and stimulation of collagen formation *in vitro*. *Proc. Natl Acad. Sci. USA*, **83**, 4167–71.

35. Gajdusek, C. M., Luo, Z., and Mayberg, M. R. (1993). Basic fibroblast growth factor and transforming growth factor beta-1: synergistic mediators of angiogenesis *in vitro*. *J. Cell. Physiol.*, **157**, 133–44.

36. Pepper, M. S., Vassalli, J-D., Orci, L., and Montesano, R. (1993). Biphasic effect of transforming growth factor-β1 on *in vitro* angiogenesis. *Exp. Cell Res.*, **204**, 356–63.

37. Iruela-Arispe, M. L. and Sage, H. (1993). Endothelial cells exhibiting angiogenesis *in vitro* proliferate in response to TGF-β1. *J. Cell. Biochem.*, **52**, 414–30.

38. Battegay, E. J., Rupp, J., Iruela-Arispe, L., Sage, H., and Pech, M. (1994). PDGF-BB modulates endothelial proliferation and angiogenesis *in vitro* via PDGFβ-receptors. *J. Cell Biol.*, **125**, 917–28.

39. Nicosia, R. F., Nicosia, S. V., and Smith, M. (1994). Vascular endothelial growth factor, platelet-derived growth factor, and insulin-like growth factor-1 promote rat aortic angiogenesis *in vitro*. *Am. J. Pathol.*, **145**, 1023–9.

40. Marx, M., Perlmutter, R., and Madri, J. A. (1994). Modulation of PDGF-receptor expression in microvascular endothelial cells during *in vitro* angiogenesis. *J. Clin. Invest.*, **93**, 131–9.

41. Smits, A., Hermansson, M., Nister, M., Karnushina, I., Heldin, C-H., Westermark, B., and Funa, K. (1989). Rat brain capillary endothelial cells express functional PDGF B-type receptors. *Growth Factors*, **2**, 1–8.

42. Bar, R. S., Boes, M., Booth, B. A., Dake, B. L., Henley, S., and Hart, M. N. (1989). The effects of platelet-derived growth factor in cultured microvessel endothelial cells. *Endocrinology*, **124**, 1841–8.

43. Beitz, J. G., Kim, I-S., Calabresi, P., and Frackelton, A. F. (1991). Human microvascular endothelial cells express receptors for platelet-derived growth factor. *Proc. Natl Acad. Sci. USA*, **88**, 2021–5.

44. Heldin, P., Pertoft, H., Norlinder, H., Heldin, C-H., and Laurent, T. C. (1991). Differential expression of platelet-derived growth factor α- and β-receptors on fat-storing cells and endothelial cells of rat liver. *Exp. Cell Res.*, **193**, 364–9.

45. Wrana, J. L., Attisano, L., Wiener, R., Ventura, F., and Massague, J. (1994). Mechanism of activation of the TGFβ receptor. *Nature*, **370**, 341–6.

46. Derynck, R. (1994). TGFβ-receptor-mediated signaling. *Trends Biochem. Sci.*, **19**, 548–53.

47. Heldin, C-H. (1995). Dimerization of cell surface receptors in signal transduction. *Cell*, **80**, 213–23.

48. Sankar, S., Mahooti-Brooks, N., Centrella, M., McCarthy, T. L., and Madri, J. A. (1995). Modulation of transforming growth factor beta receptor expression in microvascular endothelial cells during *in vitro* angiogenesis. *J. Clin. Invest.*, **97**, 1436–46.

49. Atfi, A., Drobetsky, E., Boissonneault, M., Chapdelaine, A., and Chevalier, S. (1994). Transforming growth factor β down-regulates src family protein tyrosine kinase signaling pathways. *J. Biol. Chem.*, **269**, 30688–93.

50. Sankar, S., Mahooti-Brooks, N., Centrella, M., McCarthy, T. L., and Madri, J. A. (1995). Over-expression of c-src selectively abrogates TGF-β1 mediated inhibition of proliferation in bovine aortic endothelial cells (in preparation).

51. Saksela, O., Moscatelli, D., and Rifkin, D. B. (1987). The opposing effects of basic fibroblast growth factor and TGF-β1 on the regulation of plasminogen activator activity in capillary endothelial cells. *J. Cell Biol.*, **105**, 957–63.

52. Pepper, M. S. and Montesano, R. (1990). Proteolytic balance and capillary morphogenesis. *Cell Differ. Dev.*, **32**, 319–28.

53. Montesano, R., Pepper, M. S., Mohle-Steinlein, U., Risau, W., Wagner, E. F., and Orci, L. (1990). Increased proteolytic activity is responsible for the aberrant morphogenetic behavior of endothelial cells expressing middle T oncogene *Cell*, **62**, 435–45.

54. McAllister, K. A., Grogg, K. M., Johnson, D. W., Gallione, C. J., Baldwin, M. A., Jackson, C. E., *et al.* (1994). Endoglin, a TGF-β binding protein of endothelial cells, is the gene for hereditary haemorrhagic telangiectasia type 1. *Nature Genet.*, **8**, 345–51.

55. Gamble, J. R., Matthias, L. J., Meyer, G., Kain, P., Russ, G., Faull, R., *et al.* (1993). Regulation of *in vitro* capillary tube formation by anti-integrin antibodies. *J. Cell Biol.*, **121**, 931–943.

56. Brooks, P. C., Montgomery, A. M. P., Rosenfeld, M., Reisfeld, R. A., Hu, T., Klier, G., and Cheresh, D. A. (1994). Integrin αvβ3 antagonists promote tumor regression by inducing apoptosis of angiogenic blood vessels. *Cell*, **78**, 1157–64.

57. Meredith, J. E., Fazeli, B., and Schwartz, M. A. (1993). The extracellular matrix as a cell survival factor. *Mol. Biol. Cell*, **4**, 953–61.

19. Thymidine phosphorylase/platelet-derived endothelial cell growth factor: an angiogenic enzyme

Amir Moghaddam, Rangana Choudhuri, and Roy Bicknell

Introduction

Thymidine phosphorylase is an angiogenic enzyme which is overexpressed in many solid tumours. In contrast to other well characterized angiogenic molecules such as vascular endothelial growth factor (VEGF) and basic fibroblast growth factor (bFGF) it is not a mitogen for endothelial cells nor is it heparin binding. The fact that thymidine phosphorylase is an angiogenic molecule, an enzyme involved in nucleotide homeostasis and not a classic growth factor makes it a particularly intriguing molecule to study. It is now known that the product of thymidine/phosphorylase action on thymidine, 2-deoxy-D-ribose, is angiogenic and it is release of this that mediates the angiogenic activity of the enzyme. This chapter reviews the studies that have led to the identification of thymidine phosphorylase as a potential regulator of both physiological (*e.g.* endometrial) as well as tumour angiogenesis.

Thymidine phosphorylase, the enzyme

Platelet-derived endothelial cell growth factor is thymidine phosphorylase

In 1987 Miyazono *et al.* identified an angiogenic activity in platelet lysates which was not due to known angiogenic peptides (1). This peptide was named platelet-derived endothelial cell growth factor (PD-ECGF) in the light of its putative growth stimulatory properties. PD-ECGF was shown to stimulate the uptake of [methyl-^{3}H]thymidine by endothelial cells *in vitro* when the cultured endothelial cells were incubated with PD-ECGF in the presence of low serum for 24–48 h and subsequently pulsed with [methyl-^{3}H]thymidine for 4 h (2). Later this activity was shown to result from depletion of serum-derived thymidine by the thymidine phosphorylase activity of PD-ECGF, resulting in rapid uptake when the cells were subsequently pulsed with [methyl-^{3}H]thymidine. PD-ECGF did not stimulate the growth or DNA synthesis of endothelial cells (3). Thus the name PD-ECGF is inappropriate for this molecule.

When a partial clone of the gene for human thymidine phosphorylase was sequenced, it matched that of PD-ECGF (4). In addition, there is 40% amino acid sequence homology between PD-ECGF and the *Escherichia coli* thymidine phosphorylase (5). This led to the realization that PD-ECGF is thymidine phosphorylase.

Metabolic activity of thymidine phosphorylase

Thymidine phosphorylase has been purified from a variety of mammalian tissues, as well as several bacterial sources. It consists of two identical subunits, the molecular weight of each subunit being 45 kDa in bacteria and 55 kDa in mammals. Thymidine phosphorylase catalyses the reversible phosphorolysis of thymidine and other pyrimidine 2-deoxyribosides (with the exception of 4-amino substituted compounds) to 2-deoxyribose 1-phosphate and their respective bases, (see below) (6,7). 2-deoxyribose 1-phosphate is rapidly dephosphorylated to 2-deoxyribose and believed to be transported out of the cell (8).

$$\text{Pyrimidine deoxyribonucleoside} + P_i \Longleftrightarrow \text{pyrimidine base} + \text{deoxyribose} - 1\text{-phosphate}$$

The biochemical reactions catalysed by thymidine phosphorylase are involved in the base and nucleotide salvage pathway and hence thymidine phosphorylase may be considered to play a part in the modulation of DNA precursor pools. An imbalance of nucleotide pools and their precursors will affect DNA replication, integrity, and repair leading to genetic lesions (9). Although the enzyme reaction is reversible, the role of thymidine phosphorylase is thought to be catabolic, maintaining nucleoside pool balance. For further details of the role of thymidine phosphorylase nucleotide balance, the reader is referred to other articles (9–11).

Angiogenic activity of thymidine phosphorylase

The angiogenic activity of thymidine phosphorylase has been confirmed in a number of *in vivo* assays. These include the chick chorioallantoic membrane (CAM) assay, the rabbit corneal assay, the rat subcutaneous sponge model, a cryo-injured skin graft assay, the gelatin implant assay, and in xenografted thymidine phophorylase transfected cell lines.

The first demonstration of the angiogenic activity of thymidine phosphorylase was in the chick CAM assay where a polymer disc containing thymidine phosphorylase was placed on the CAM and slowly released the protein over time. Ishikawa *et al.* showed that thymidine phosphorylase partially purified from platelets induced a 'spoke wheel' vascularization response on the chick CAM (12). This activity was neutralized by polyclonal anti-thymidine phosphorylase. These results were later confirmed by Haraguchi *et al.* who along with Miyadera *et al.* also reported that in the mouse gelatin sponge implant assay, 10 µg of thymidine phosphorylase enhanced neovascularization, as determined by the haemoglobin content of the gelatin sponges (13,14).

In the rabbit corneal assay the test material is placed at a distance from the corneal limbus (see Chapter 2). Endothelial cells then migrate from the limbal vasculature into the subepithelial space between the corneal epithelium and the stromal cells (15). M. Ziche and R. Bicknell (personal communication) found that the MCF-7 adenocarcinoma cell line stably expressing thymidine phosphorylase induced a strong angiogenic response when injected into the limbus when compared with negative control cells. As the cornea is avascular a positive response is easier to score than the chick CAM assay. However, this property of the corneal assay has also led to major criticisms, one of which is that as the cornea is kept avascular by an active process (16); thus many of the triggers for vascularization must exist in the tissue but be suppressed by an active inhibitory process.

Detailed analysis of the angiogenic activity of thymidine phosphorylase has been carried out using the rat sponge model (3). Unlike the chick CAM assay and the rabbit corneal assay it allows continuous and reproducible analysis of blood flow in vessels by measuring the rate of clearance of radioactive xenon from the sponge. Injection of 10 pmol of recombinant thymidine phosphorylase daily into a subcutaneously implanted sponge resulted in increased vascularity of the sponge compared with controls. Polyclonal antisera inhibited the thymidine phosphorylase enhanced vascularization. Histological examination of the implanted sponges revealed the presence of capillaries in the thymidine phosphorylase treated sponges along with enhanced invasion of fibrotic cells compared with the control sponge (Fig. 19.1).

A novel freeze-injured skin graft model (17) has also been used to examine the angiogenic activity of thymidine phosphorylase (3). This assay involves freeze-injuring full

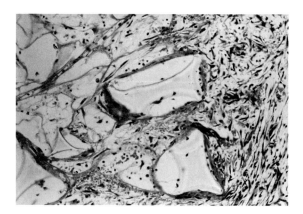

(a)

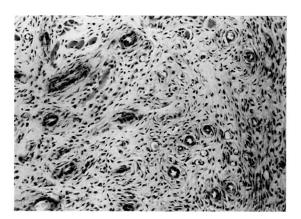

(b)

Figure 19.1. Histological study of thymidine phosphorylase induced neovascularization in the rat sponge model. Subcutaneously implanted sponges were removed from the rat then sectioned and stained with eosin/haematoxylin. The fibres and infiltration of fibrotic tissue is evident in the control sponges (a), while infiltration of host cells in thymidine phosphorylase treated sponges (b) is more prominent. Well-differentiated vessels with smooth muscle cell walls are apparent in the thymidine phosphorylase treated sponges.

thickness rat skin grafts by incubation for a short time in liquid nitrogen. After autografting, slow release polymer pellets containing thymidine phosphorylase were sutured around the periphery of the graft. Vascularization was assessed quantitatively by laser Doppler flowmetry and by measuring the rate at which injected radioactive xenon was cleared from the graft. Freeze injury delayed revascularization of the graft compared with grafts that had not been freeze injured. Moghaddam et al. found that 500 ng of thymidine phosphorylase placed in the periphery of the graft significantly accelerated healing of the grafts (3).

Even though each of the angiogenic assays described have inherent limitations, the fact that activity was seen in a varied range of established assays suggests that it is reasonable to conclude that the enzyme thymidine phosphorylase is clearly angiogenic.

Thymidine phosphorylase is chemotactic for endothelial cells *in vitro*

The *in vivo* angiogenesis models described above are time consuming and expensive. Hence it is useful to have an *in vitro* assay for angiogenesis. Endothelial cell migration in response to a stimulus is one such assay which has been shown to correlate well with angiogenesis. The Boyden chamber is commonly used to analyse chemotactic activity of molecules. In this chamber Ishikawa et al. demonstrated that thymidine phosphorylase is chemotactic for bovine aortic endothelial cells (12). The optimum concentration was 2 ng/ml and this activity was not observed with vascular smooth muscle cells. This activity of thymidine phosphorylase was subsequently confirmed by Moghaddam et al. and Miyadera et al. (3,18).

As thymidine phosphorylase is not a mitogen for endothelial cells *in vitro*, induction of migration of endothelial cells is likely to be part of the mechanism by which this enzyme stimulates angiogenesis *in vitro*. Recruitment of inflammatory cells by thymidine phosphorylase is also likely to contribute to its angiogenic activity, as a chemotaxis response by neutrophils and monocytes to thymidine phosphorylase has also been reported (2).

Thymidine phosphorylase enhances tumour growth

Thymidine phosphorylase like the angiogenic factor, bFGF does not have a secretion signal. It is therefore important to assess the activity of thymidine phosphorylase when it is expressed intracellularly.

Ishikawa et al. transfected the cDNA for thymidine phosphorylase into a Ha-*ras* transformed 3T3 cell line, al-1 (12). Injection of these cells into nude mice resulted in tumours

the same size as the control transfected cells. Subsequent histological and cytochemical examination showed that the tumours formed with the cells overexpressing thymidine phosphorylase had a higher vascular density.

Thymidine phophorylase cDNA has also been transfected into MCF-7 cells which have the advantage over a1-1 cells of forming slow growing tumours. The PD-ECGF transfectants had a high thymidine phosphorylase activity but did not have a growth advantage *in vitro* when compared with the empty vector transfectants (3). However, when 10^7 cells were injected subcutaneously into nude mice, the thymidine phosphorylase transfectants produced larger tumours compared with the control transfectants. Histological examination of the tumours at the end of the experiment revealed that the tumour mass was carcinoma and not mouse-derived inflammatory cells infiltrating and enlarging the tumour.

Despite forming tumours that were 10 times larger than controls the vascular density of the thymidine phophorylase overexpressing tumours and control tumours was identical (see Chapter 3). It is proposed that one mechanism by which overexpression of thymidine phosphorylase in MCF-7 cells is conferring a growth advantage in nude mice but not *in vitro* may be by increasing the rate of vascularization, i.e. tumour angiogenesis. The mechanism for these observations has not yet been elucidated but a possible mode of action is proposed below. If the grafted tumour cells undergo a significant amount of necrosis, in the absence of an adequate blood supply, excess thymidine could be produced and accumulate as a result of DNA degradation. This could lead to growth arrest of cells. High concentration of thymidine leads to inhibition of ribonucleotide reductase in cells and subsequent depletion of the precursors for DNA synthesis dCDP and dCTP which are synthesized from CDP (19). Cells that have higher levels of thymidine phosphorylase are more resistant to the cytostatic activity of thymidine, as thymidine can be broken down by this enzyme to thymine and then further degraded (20). Hence, poorly vascularized MCF-7 derived tumours which are high in thymidine phosphorylase may grow faster than low thymidine phosphorylase containing tumours in the presence of cell necrosis and DNA degradation.

Mechanism of the angiogenic activity of thymidine phosphorylase

Requirement for enzyme activity

Two studies have shown that the enzyme activity of thymidine phosphorylase is required for its angiogenic activity. Haraguchi et al. and Miyadera et al. showed that the thymidine phosphorylase inhibitor 6-amino 5-chlorouracil blocked angiogenic activity of thymidine phosphorylase in the developing vascular system of the chick CAM and the gelatin sponage assay (13,14). This led to the conclusion that the enzyme activity of thymidine phosphorylase is required for its angiogenic activity.

The second study showed that enzymatic activity of thymidine phosphorylase is essential for angiogenic activity by the preparation of site-directed mutants of thymidine phosphorylase which lack enzyme activity (3,14). The mutants were analysed for enzyme activity by their rate of phosphorolysis of thymidine to thymine. The mutants were then assayed in the rat sponge model (3) or gelatin sponge implantation assay (14) for angiogenic activity and in the Boyden chamber for chemotactic activity (3).

Moghaddam *et al.* (3), targeted the mutations at sites which are conserved in the human and prokaryotic enzyme and are reported to interact with thymine/thymidine as determined by X-ray diffraction analysis of *E. coli* thymidine phosphorylase (21). Radical mutations were introduced into the recombinant enzyme by mutating in turn arginine 202 and lysine 221 to glutamic acid, and serine 217 to alanine (3). The mutants were shown to maintain a non-covalent homodimeric state and were thus assumed to have the same conformational state as the wild-type enzyme (3).

The mutants did not enhance neovascularization in the rat sponge model either at the same concentration as the wild-type enzyme or at a dose 100 times greater than that of the wild-type enzyme and it was concluded that the enzyme activity of thymidine phosphorylase was required for its angiogenic activity. Similarly, the mutants did not stimulate the migration of endothelial cells in the Boyden chamber, either at the same concentration or at 100 times higher concentration than the wild-type enzyme. The serine mutant which showed 1% of the activity of the wild-type enzyme did, however, stimulate migration of endothelial cells at a dose 1000 times that of the wild-type enzyme and the enzyme activity is required for the chemotactic activity of thymidine phosphorylase.

Miyadera *et al.* also carried out site-directed mutagenesis studies to show that the enzyme activity of thymidine phosphorylase was required for its angiogenic activity (14). Three point mutants were constructed at the sites involved in the binding of phosphate (lysine 115 to glutamine), deoxyribose (leucine 148 to arginine) and thymidine (arginine 202 to serine) according to the crystal structure of the *E. coli* enzyme. The mutants were expressed in COS-7 cells and the angiogenic activity of the cell lysate and not the purified protein was examined in the gelatin sponge assay. The mutants had lost their enzyme activity and their ability to induce blood vessels in gelatin sponges.

It is interesting to note that angiogenin-like thymidine phosphorylase is an enzyme which has angiogenic activity but does not stimulate the growth of endothelial cells. Angiogenin has ribonuclease activity, and the activity seems to be necessary but not sufficient for its angiogenic effect (22,23). In contrast ribonuclease A has no endothelial cell-promoting or angiogenic activity. More recently, angiogenin has been reported to support endothelial and fibroblast cell adhesion (24). Angiogenesis caused by angiogenin may require the induction of cell adhesion as well as ribonuclease activity. Unlike angiogenin, the enzymatic activity of thymidine phosphorylase appears to be sufficient for angiogenesis.

Thymidine is required for endothelial cell migration

The chemotactic activity of thymidine phosphorylase had been determined in the presence of 1% fetal calf serum, which contains an intrinsic nucleoside component, or in tissue culture media supplemented with nucleosides (12). The media was modified to determine whether the substrate thymidine is required for thymidine phosphorylase to induce migration of endothelial cells.

It was found that thymidine phosphorylase did not induce migration of bovine aortic endothelial cells in Dulbecco's modified Eagle's medium (DMEM) and 0.1% bovine serum albumin (BSA) if the media was not supplemented with serum. In this assay, bFGF was used as a positive control, as its chemotactic activity is independent of the presence of serum, as shown in Fig. 19.2. Thymidine phosphorylase did induce migration of endothelial cells if the media was supplemented with 1 μmol/l thymidine. Clearly, both the enzyme activity of thymidine phosphorylase and its substrate thymidine is required for its chemotactic activity and by extrapolation, angiogenic activity.

The catabolic products of the thymidine phosphorylase reaction are chemotactic and angiogenic

The catabolic products of the thymidine phosphorylase reaction, thymine and deoxyribose 1-phosphate were assayed for chemotactic activity in endothelial cells. Surprisingly, deoxyribose 1-phosphate but not thymine induced migration of bovine aortic endothelial cells in a dose-dependent manner in the absence of serum (Fig. 19.3). This excludes the possibility that 'a low local concentration of thymidine' generated by thymidine phosphorylase is the mediator of the chemotactic activity of thymidine phosphorylase, i.e. the mechanism is not by a

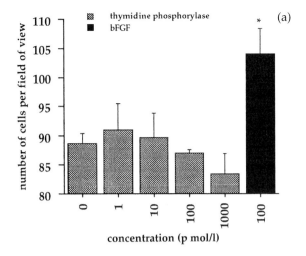

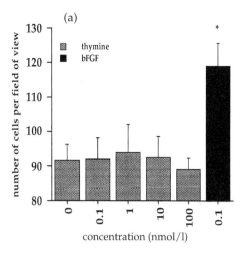

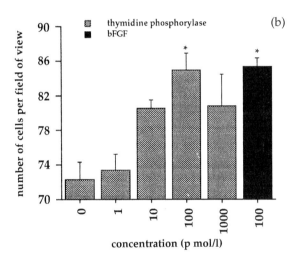

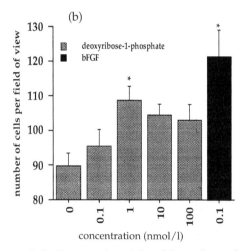

Figure 19.2. Chemotactic activity of thymidine phosphorylase in the absence of serum. Thymidine phosphorylase and basic fibroblast growth factor (bFGF) were assayed in HEPES-buffered Dulbecco's modified Eagle's medium supplemented with 0.1% bovine serum albumin in the absence (a) or the presence (b) of 1 μmol/l thymidine. Thymidine phosphorylase did not stimulate migration of endothelial cells in the absence of serum unless the media is supplemented with 1 μmol/l thymidine. * $P<0.01$, $n = 4 \pm$ SEM.

Figure 19.3. Chemotactic activity of the products of thymidine phosphorylase reaction. Thymine (a) and deoxyribose-1-phosphate (b) were assayed for chemotactic activity in the Boyden chamber in HEPES-buffered Dulbecco's modified Eagle's medium supplemented with 0.1% bovine serum albumin. Deoxyribose 1-phosphate at 1 nmol/l stimulated migration of endothelial cells in the Boyden chamber. * $P<0.01$, $n = 4 \pm$ SEM

chemorepellent response to thymidine. It is important to establish this, as thymidine phosphorylase can relieve growth inhibition of endothelial cells induced by millimolar concentrations of thymidine (5; Moghaddam and Bicknell, unpublished observations).

Haraguchi *et al.* reported that deoxyribose is also chemotactic for bovine aortic endothelial cells in the Boyden chamber at 10 μmol/l (18). The chemotactic activity of deoxyribose 1-phosphate and thymine was not reported. Deoxyribose was also reported to be angiogenic in the chick CAM assay at 50 pmol. No such activity was detected with thymidine, thymine, and deoxyribose

1-phosphate. Hence deoxyribose appears both chemotactic and angiogenic. Deoxyribose 1-phosphate is chemotactic but apparently not angiogenic in the chick CAM. It remains to be determined whether the negatively charged phosphorylated form of the sugar is biologically inactive on the CAM due to association with positively charged proteins such as albumin which would lead to rapid clearance. It is interesting that a molecule as small as 2-deoxyribose is angiogenic, but not unusal. Angiogenic activity of many small molecular weight compounds have been reported (see reference 25 for a review) but like 2-deoxyribose their mode of action is generally unknown.

Tissue distribution and levels in hyperproliferative disease

Thymidine phosphorylase activity is widespread in mammalian tissues with the highest level of activity in the liver. Other organs with significant amounts of thymidine phosphorylase activity are the spleen, blood, leucocytes, blood platelets, and keratinocytes (26,27). Immunoblotting studies have confirmed these data and shown that lymph node and lung also contain a high level of thymidine phosphorylase (28).

Pauly et al. (29–31) reported the presence of elevated levels of thymidine phosphorylase activity in plasma of patients with uncontrolled neoplastic disease as well as in ascitic fluids of tumour-bearing rats. Yoshimura et al. have reported that in three patients with either stomach, colon, or ovarian cancer, higher levels of thymidine phosphorylase were evident in the tumour samples compared with the normal control tissue counterpart (28).

Reynolds et al. have studied the expression of thymidine phosphorylase mRNA transcript in a variety of ovarian tumours by ribonuclease protection (32). A difference between the level of transcript between normal, benign, and malignant samples was found. More importantly, there was a significant correlation between the level of thymidine phosphorylase transcript and both malignancy and blood flow in the tumour tissues. Blood flow was measured by ultrasound laser Doppler flowmetry before surgery.

Breast tumours like ovarian tumours also show an elevation of thymidine phosphorylase at the mRNA and protein level (3). These results confirmed that thymidine phosphorylase expression is controlled by transcription or mRNA stability and not by translation or post-translational events.

Expression of thymidine phosphorylase in human breast tissue has been examined in detail by immunocytochemistry using a specific monoclonal antibody to thymidine phosphorylase (3). Expression in normal breast was found to be confined to inner ductal epithelial cells of mammary lobules. In breast cancers, the expression was variable both in intensity and localization. The source of thymidine phosphorylase was either the carcinoma (see Fig. 19.4a, in the plate section), infiltrating inflammatory cells (see Fig. 19.4b, in the plate section), or both. Macrophages rather than lymphocytes were more frequently the source of thymidine phosphorylase. In some tissue samples, sporadic immunostaining of tumour endothelium was also seen. Elevated immunostaining for thymidine phosphorylase in tumours compared with normal breast samples was evident. One can hypothesize that variable expression of thymidine phosphorylase may be due to induction of expression by various factors such as cytokines. Thus Eda et al. (33) have reported that thymidine phosphorylase transcription can be induced in several colon carcinoma cell lines by tumour necrosis factor (TNF) α, interferon (IFN) γ, and interleukin (IL) 1α, but not in normal fibroblasts.

Similar to breast cancers, increased vascular density has been shown to correlate well with a high incidence of metastases and a worse prognosis in bladder tumours. Thymidine phosphorylase expression is higher in bladder tumours (40-fold) compared with normal bladder and the protein was also found to be expressed differentially in the different types of bladder cancer (34). Expression of thymidine phophorylase in aggressive muscle invasive tumours was 33-fold higher than in the less aggressive superficial tumours and 260-fold higher than in normal bladders.

Asai et al. have used an ELISA assay to quantify the amount of thymidine phosphorylase protein in the synovial fluid of rheumatoid arthritis and osteoarthritis patients (35). Progression of the former is marked by extensive neovascularization. There was a significant elevation of thymidine phosphorylase immunoreactivity in the synovial fluid of rheumatoid arthritis patients compared with osteoarthritis patients.

A trend is thus becoming apparent where several hyperproliferative diseases which are dependent on new capillary formation for development have a higher level of thymidine phosphorylase compared with their control counterparts. On the other hand, proliferating lymphocytes from patients with either T-cell chronic, T-cell acute, or chronic myelogenous leukaemia have been shown to have lower thymidine phosphorylase activity than control groups (36–38). Table 19.1 lists the differential expression of thymidine phosphorylase reported in hyperproliferative disease compared with their healthy counterparts, although in many of these samples only a small number of samples were tested. From this list, it appears that the levels of both

Table 19.1. Comparison of levels of thymidine phosphorylase (TP) in human hyperproliferative disease and normal tissue counterpart

Disease type	Number of patients	Method of study	Level of TP	Reference
Psoriatic lesions	8	Enzyme activity	Elevated	47
Lung tumour	NR	Enzyme activity	Elevated	6, 48
Stomach carcinoma	1–2	Immunoblot, enzyme activity	Elevated	6, 28
Colon carcinoma	1–2	Immunoblot	Elevated	28
Ovarian carcinoma	1–2	Immunoblot	Elevated	28
T-cell acute lymphocytic leukaemia	4, 6	Enzyme activity	Decrease	20, 49
T-cell chronic lymphocytic leukaemia	2, 6–8	Enzyme activity	Decrease	37, 38
Chronic myelogenous leukaemia	6–8	Enzyme activity	Decrease	36, 38

NR, not reported

thymidine phosphorylase activity and protein are elevated in many human solid tumours.

Thymidine phosphorylase and the human endometrium

Endometrial development during the menstrual cycle involves extensive angiogenesis and is ultimately under the hormonal control of oestrogen and progesterone. Neither oestrogen nor progesterone have intrinsic angiogenic activity. Several angiogenic factors such as bFGF (39,40), transforming growth factor (TGF) β (41), and TNF-α (42) have been reported to be present in the endometrium. Interestingly, immunohistochemistry revealed that thymidine phosphorylase was unique from other angiogenic factors in that it was differentially expressed in the normal human endometrium during the menstrual cycle (Zhang L., personal communication). These findings prompted an examination of the regulation of thymidine phosphorylase expression in normal human endometrial epithelial (NEE) and stromal cells (NES). When the cells were treated with physiological doses of 17-β-oestradiol or progesterone the levels of thymidine phosphorylase remained basal. However, IFN-γ and TNF-α treatment elevated the expression of thymidine phosphorylase in NEE cells. A combination of TNF-α, IFN-γ, and IL-α resulted in a synergistic up-regulation of thymidine phosphorylase in NEE cells. Expression of thymidine phosphorylase was most strongly up-regulated by a combination of progesterone and TGF-β1 (Zhang L., Rees M., and Bicknell R., unpublished work).

The expression of thymidine phosphorylase was found to be up-regulated by physiological concentrations of IFN-γ in NES cells. If NES cells are treated with a concentration of progesterone that is considerably above physiological concentrations then an up-regulation of thymidine phosphorylase has also been reported (43).

The implications of these results are not fully understood. However, the thymidine phosphorylase promoter has oestrogen-responsive elements and whether the interaction of oestrogen with these elements is involved in endometrial angiogenesis is yet to be determined. The physiological role of thymidine phosphorylase is unknown and it is difficult to pin-point its function as more biological activities of thymidine phosphorylase are being discovered. In a recent study, gliostatin, shown to be identical to thymidine phosphorylase was demonstrated to inhibit the growth of astrocytes and astrocytoma cells (44). In addition, thymidine phosphorylase activity increases with the differentiation of keratinocytes (27,45). Considering all these facts together it is apparent that thymidine phosphorylase has varied biological functions.

A putative model for the angiogenic activity of thymidine phosphorylase

To develop a working model for the angiogenic activity of thymidine phosphorylase, several factors have to be considered. Most importantly, the enzyme is located intra-cellularly while its effects are ultimately extracellular on the nearby capillary endothelium. In solid tumours and other hyperproliferative diseases, where progression is angiogenesis dependent, elevated levels of thymidine phosphorylase are detected. In malignant breast tumours, the source of thymidine phosphorylase can be the carcinoma or stromal cells. The expression of thymidine phosphorylase in some carcinoma cells may be regulated by inflammatory cytokines (33). Thymidine phosphorylase is only angiogenic and chemotactic in the presence of its substrate thymidine. 2-deoxyribose 1-phosphate is chemotactic for endothelial cells. 2-deoxyribose is both chemotactic for endothelial cells and angiogenic. Desgranges *et al.* (46) have reported that incubation of thymidine with platelets, which contain high levels of thymidine phosphorylase, resulted in rapid appearance of thymine and 2-deoxyribose but not 2-deoxyribose 1-phosphate in the extracellular medium. The presence of a negative charge on 2-deoxyribose 1-phosphate is likely to render it impermeable to the lipid bilayer of cells. On the other hand, 2-deoxyribose formed by the action of nucleotidases in the cell is expected to cross the cellular membrane. Thus, 2-deoxyribose is the extracellular mediator of the angiogenic activity of thymidine phosphorylase. The mechanisms by which 2-deoxyribose and 2-deoxyribose 1-phosphate induce migration of endothelial cells and by which 2-deoxyribose induces angiogenesis remain to be determined.

Figure 19.5 summarizes a possible model of thymidine phosphorylase induced angiogenesis. High levels of thymidine in the cell result in its breakdown to thymine and 2-deoxyribose 1-phosphate. Dephosphorylated

2-deoxyribose 1-phosphate leaves the cell and stimulates the migration of endothelial cells. 2-deoxyribose alone is sufficient for angiogenesis. The mechanism by which this can occur has not yet been elucidated; however, it does not rule out a possible cell receptor through which this sugar molecule interacts.

Recently, expression of thymidine phosphorylase in primary human colon tumours has been shown to correlate with vascular density, invasion, metastasis, and prognosis (50,51).

A scholarly and interesting commentary by Folkman on the role of thymidine phosphorylase in tumour angiogenesis is in the same issue of *The Journal of the National Cancer Institute* (52).

Acknowledgements

The authors thank Tai-Ping D. Fan and Vivian Lees, University of Cambridge and Adrian L. Harris and Hua-Tang Zhang, University of Oxford for helpful discussions.

References

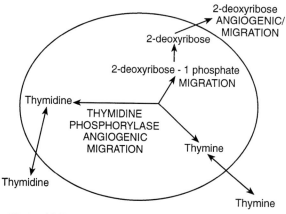

Figure 19.5. A mechanism by which thymidine phosphorylase may modulate angiogenesis. Thymidine phosphorylase expression is regulated (by cytokines) in the carcinoma or inflammatory cells. Thymidine phosphorylase is located intracellularly, while the effector molecule, deoxyribose is able to diffuse out of the cell. Thymidine and thymine, but not deoxyribose 1-phosphate are able to cross the cellular membrane.

1. Miyazono, K., Okabe, T., Urabe, A., Takaku, F., and Heldin, C. H. (1987). Purification and properties of an endothelial cell growth factor from human platelets. *J. Biol. Chem.*, **262**, 4098–103.
2. Miyazono, K. and Takaku, F. (1991). Platelet-derived endothelial cell growth factor: structure and function. *Jpn. Circ. J.*, **55**, 1022–6.
3. Moghaddam, A., Zhang, H. T., Fan, T. P., Hu, D. E., Lees, V. C., Turley, H., *et al.* (1995). Thymidine phosphorylase is angiogenic and promotes tumor growth. *Proc. Natl Acad. Sci. USA*, **92**, 998–1002.
4. Furukawa, T., Yoshimura, A., Sumizawa, T., Haraguchi, M., and Akiyama, S. I. (1992). Angiogenic factor. *Nature*, **356**, 668.
5. Finnis, C., Dodsworth, N., Pollitt, C. E., Carr, G., and Sleep, D. (1993). Thymidine phosphorylase activity of platelet-derived endothelial cell growth factor is responsible for endothelial cell mitogenicity. *Eur. J. Biochem.*, **212**, 201–10.
6. Zimmerman, M. and Seidenberg, J. (1964). Deoxyribosyl transfer I. Thymidine phosphorylase and nucleoside deoxyribosyltransferase in normal and malignant tissues. *J. Biol. Chem.*, **239**, 2618–21.
7. Gallo, R. C. and Perry, C. (1969). The enzymatic mechanism of deoxythymidine synthesis in human leukocytes. *J. Clin. Invest.*, **48**, 105–16.
8. Usuki, K., Saras, J., Waltenberger, J., Miyazono, K., Pierce, G., Thomason, A., and Heldin, C. H. (1992). Platelet-derived endothelial cell growth factor has thymidine phosphorylase activity. *Biochem. Biophys. Res. Commun.*, **184**, 1311–16.
9. Serres, F. J. (1985). *Genetic consequences of nucleotide pool imbalance*. Plenum Press, New York.
10. Schwartz, M. (1971). Thymidine phosphorylase from *Escherichia coli*. Properties and kinetics. *Eur. J. Biochem.*, **21**, 191–8.

11. Shaw, T., Smillie, R. H., Miller, A. E., and MacPhee, D. G. (1988). The role of blood platelets in nucleoside metabolism: regulation of platelet thymidine phosphorylase. *Mutat. Res.*, **200**, 117–31.

12. Ishikawa, F., Miyazono, K., Hellman, U., Drexler, H., Wernstedt, C., Hagiwara, K., *et al.* (1989). Identification of angiogenic activity and the cloning and expression of platelet-derived endothelial cell growth factor. *Nature*, **338**, 557–62.

13. Haraguchi, M., Kazutaka, M., Uemura, K., Sumizawa, T., Furukawa, T., Yamada, K., and Akiyama, S-I. (1994). Angiogenic activity of enzymes. *Nature*, **368**, 198.

14. Miyadera, K., Sumizawa, T., Haraguchi, M., Yoshida, H., Konstanty, W., Yamada, Y., and Akiyama, S. (1995). Role of thymidine phosphorylase activity in the angiogenic effect of platelet derived endothelial cell growth factor/thymidine phosphorylase. *Cancer Res.*, **55**, 1687–90.

15. Gimbrone, R. C., Leapman, S., and Folkman, J. (1974). Tumour growth neovascularisation: an experimental model using rabbit cornea. *J. Natl Cancer Inst.*, **52**, 413–27.

16. Taylor, C. M. and Weiss, J. B. (1985). Partial purification of a 5.7 K glycoprotein from bovine vitreous which inhibits both angiogenesis and collagenase activity. *Biochem. Biophys. Res. Commun.*, **133**, 911–16.

17. Lees, V. C. and Fan, T. P. D. (1994). A freeze-injured skin graft model for the quantitative study of basic fibroblast growth factor and other promoters of angiogenesis in wound healing. *Br. J. Plastic. Surg.* **47**, 349–359.

18. Haraguchi, M., Miyadera, K., Uemura, K., Sumizawa, T., Furukawa, T., Yamada, K., *et al.* (1994). Angiogenic activity of enzymes [letter]. *Nature*, **368**, 198.

19. Morris, R. N. and Fischer, G. A. (1963). Studies concerning the inhibition of cellular reproduction by deoxyribonucleosides. I. Inhibition of the synthesis of deoxycytidine by a phosphorylated derivative of thymidine. *Biochem. Biophys. Acta*, **68**, 84–92.

20. Fox, R. M., Piddington, S. K., Tripp, E. H., Dudman, N. P., and Tattersall, M. H. (1979). Thymidine sensitivity of cultured leukaemic lymphocytes. *Lancet*, **ii**, 391–3.

21. Walter, M. R., Cook, W. J., Cole, L. B., Short, S. A., Koszalka, G. W., Krenitsky, T. A., and Ealick, S. E. (1990). Three-dimensional structure of thymidine phosphorylase from *Escherichia coli* at 2.8 A resolution. *J. Biol. Chem.*, **265**, 14016–22.

22. Shapiro, R. and Vallee, B. L. (1989). Identification of functional arginines in human angiogenin by site-directed mutagenesis. *Biochemistry*, **31**, 12477–85.

23. Shapiro, R. and Vallee, B. L. (1987). Human placental ribonuclease inhibitor abolishes both angiogenic and ribonucleolytic activities of angiogenin. *Proc. Natl Acad. Sci. USA*, **84**, 2238–41.

24. Soncin, F. (1992). Angiogenin supports endothelial and fibroblast cell adhesion. *Proc. Natl Acad. Sci. USA*, **89**, 2232–6.

25. Odedra, R. and Weiss, J. B. (1991). Low molecular weight angiogenesis factors. *Pharmacol. Ther.*, **49**, 111–24.

26. Shaw, T., Smillie, R. H., and MacPhee, D. G. (1988). The role of blood platelets in nucleoside metabolism: assay, cellular location and significance of thymidine phosphorylase in human blood. *Mutat. Res.*, **200**, 99–116.

27. Fox, S. B., Moghaddam, A., Westwood, M., Turley, H., Bicknell, R., Gatler, K., and Harris, A. L. (1995). Platelet-derived endothelial cell growth factor/thymidine phosphorylase expression in normal tissues: an immunohistochemical study. *Journal of Pathology*, **176**, 183–90.

28. Yoshimura, A., Kuwazuru, Y., Furukawa, T., Yoshida, H., Yamada, K., and Akiyama, S. (1990). Purification and tissue distribution of human thymidine phosphorylase; high expression in lymphocytes, reticulocytes and tumors. *Biochim. Biophys. Acta*, **1034**, 107–13.

29. Pauly, J. L., Schuller, M. G., Zelcer, A. A., and Germain, M. J. (1977). Degradation of [³H] thymidine by a pentosyltransferase (EC 2.4.2.4) in the plasma of man and different animals. *Experientia*, **33**, 668–70.

30. Pauly, J. L., Paolini, N. S., Ebarb, R. L., and Germain, M. J. (1978). Elevated thymidine phosphorylase activity in the plasma and ascitis fluids of tumor-bearing animals. *Proc. Soc. Exp. Biol. Med.*, **157**, 262–7.

31. Pauly, J. L., Schuller, M. G., Zelcer, A. A., Kirss, T. A., Gore, S. S., and Germain, M. J. (1977). Identification and comparative analysis of thymidine phosphorylase in the plasma of healthy subjects and cancer patients. *J. Natl Cancer Inst.*, **58**, 1587–90.

32. Reynolds, K., Farzaneh, F., Collins, W. P., Campbell, S., Bourne, T. H., Lawton, F., *et al.* (1994). Correlation of ovarian malignancy with expression of platelet-derived endothelial cell growth factor. *J. Natl Cancer Inst.*, **86**, 1234–8.

33. Eda, H., Fujimoto, K., Watanabe, S., Ura, M., Hino, A., Tanaka, Y., *et al.* (1993). Cytokines induce thymidine phosphorylase expression in tumor cells and make them more susceptible to 5′-deoxy-5-fluorouridine. *Cancer Chemother. Pharmacol.*, **32**, 333–8.

34. O'Brien, T., Cranston, D., Fuggle, S., Bicknell, R., and Harris, A. L. (1995). Different angiogenic pathways characterize superficial and invasive bladder cancer. *Cancer Res.*, **55**, 510–3.

35. Asai, K., Hirano, T., Matsukawa, K., Kusada, J., Takeuchi, M., Otsuka, T., *et al.* (1993). High concentration of immunoreactive gliostatin/platelet-derived endothelial cell growth factor in synovial fluid and serum of rheumatoid arthritis. *Clin. Chim. Acta*, **218**, 1–4.

36. Vertongen, F., Fondu, P., van, d. H. B., Cauchie, C., and Mandelbaum, I. M. (1984). Thymidine kinase and thymidine phosphorylase activities in various types of leukaemia and lymphoma. *Tumour Biol.*, **5**, 303–11.

37. Gan, T. E., Hallam, L., and Van, D. W. M. (1982). Purine and pyrimidine activities in acute and chronic lymphocytic leukaemia: relation to cellular proliferative status. *Leuk. Res.*, **6**, 839–44.

38. Marsh, J. C. and Seymour, P. (1964). Thymidine catabolism by normal and leukemic human leukocytes. *J. Clin. Invest.*, **43**, 267–78.

39. Cordon, C. C., Vlodavsky, I., Haimovitz, F. A., Hicklin, D., and Fuks, Z. (1990). Expression of basic fibroblast growth factor in normal human tissues. *Lab. Invest.*, **63**, 832–40.

40. Rusnati, M., Casarotti, G., Pecorelli, S., Ragnotti, G., and Presta, M. (1990). Basic fibroblast growth factor in ovulatory cycle and postmenopausal human endometrium. *Growth Factors*, **3**, 299–307.

41. Horowitz, G. M., Scott, R. J., Drews, M. R., Navot, D., and Hofmann, G. E. (1993). Immunohistochemical localization of transforming growth factor-alpha in human endometrium, decidua, and trophoblast. *J. Clin. Endocrinol. Metab.*, **76**, 786–92.

42. Kauma, S., Matt, D., Strom, S., Eierman, D., and Turner, T. (1990). Interleukin-1 beta, human leukocyte antigen HLA-DR alpha, and transforming growth factor-beta expression in endometrium, placenta, and placental membranes. *Am. J. Obstet. Gynecol.*,

43. Osuga, Y., Toyoshima, H., Mitsuhashi, N., and Taketani, Y. (1995). The presence of platelet-derived endothelial cell growth factor in human endometrium and its characteristic expression during the menstrual cycle and early geatation period. *Hum. Reprod.*, **10**, 989–93.

44. Asai, K., Nakanishi, K., Isobe, I., Eksioglu, Y. Z., Hirano, A., Hama, K., *et al.* (1992). Neurotrophic action of gliostatin on cortical neurons. Identity of gliostatin and platelet-derived endothelial cell growth factor. *J. Biol. Chem.*, **267**, 20311–6.

45. Schwartz, P. M., Reuveni, H., and Milstone, L. M. (1988). Local and systemic implications of thymidine catabolism by human keratinocytes. *Ann. N. Y. Acad. Sci.*, **548**, 115–24.

46. Desgranges, C., Razaka, G., Rabaud, M., and Bricaud, H. (1981). Catabolism of thymidine in human blood platelets: purification and properties of thymidine phosphorylase. *Biochim. Biophys. Acta*, **654**, 211–8.

47. Hammerberg, C., Fisher, G. J., Voorhees, J. J., and Cooper, K. D. (1991). Elevated thymidine phosphorylase activity in psoriatic lesions accounts for the apparent presence of an epidermal 'growth inhibitor', but is not in itself growth inhibitory. *J. Invest. Dermatol.*, **97**, 286–90.

48. Maehara, Y., Moriguchi, S., Emi, Y., Watanabe, A., Kohnoe, S., Tsujitani, S., and Sugimachi, K. (1990). Comparison of pyrimidine nucleotide synthetic enzymes involved in 5-fluorouracil metabolism between human adenocarcinomas and squamous cell carcinomas. *Cancer*, **66**, 156–61.

49. Gan, T. E., Finch, P. D., Brumley, J. L., Hallam, L. J., and van, d. W. M. (1984). Pyrimidine and purine activities in non-Hodgkin's lymphoma. Correlation with histological status and survival. *Eur. J. Cancer Clin. Oncol.*, **20**, 361–8.

50. Takebayashi, Y., Akiyama, S., Akiba, S., Yamada, K., Miyadera, K., Sumizawa, T. *et al.* (1996). Clinicopathologic and prognostic significance of an angiogenic factor, thymidine phosphorylase, in human colorectal cancer. *J. Natl Cancer Inst.*, **88**, 1110–7.

51. Takahashi, Y., Bucana, C. D., Liu, W., Yoneda, J., Kitadai, Y., Cleary, K. R., *et al.* (1996). Platelet-derived endothelial cell growth factor in human colon cancer angiogenesis: role of infiltrating cells.

52. Folkman, J. (1996). What is the role of thymidine phosphorylase in tumour angiogenesis? *J. Natl Cancer Inst.*, **88**, 1091–2.

20. Tumour necrosis factor α and angiogenesis

Luis F. Fajardo L.-G. and Anthony C. Allison

Introduction

Tumour necrosis factor (TNF) α (cachectin) is a cytokine synthesized mainly by cells of the monocyte–macrophage lineage (1). Other sources are mast cells, T lymphocytes (CD4, CD8), natural killer cells, neutrophils, glial cells, and some tumour cells (1–3). The gene encoding TNF-α is located in chromosome 6, near the gene of a related cytokine, lymphotoxin, or TNF-β (2,4). Various stimuli induce the production of TNF, especially bacterial lipopolysaccharide (LPS). In fact TNF is a major effector of toxic shock induced by LPS (1,2,5,6). The primary gene product, pro-TNF-α, is a 26 kDa type II integral membrane protein which can be localized to plasma membrane fractions (7). Proteolytic cleavage of pro-TNF at a specific site releases 17 kDa TNF, which binds to both TNF receptors and induces a variety of responses in many cell types. More than 95% of the TNF synthesized by monocytes in response to LPS is processed and secreted. Some metalloproteinase inhibitors block pro-TNF cleavage, but the converting enzyme has not been fully characterized (8). The three-dimensional structure of TNF, determined by X-ray crystallography, shows it to be a trimer of the 17 kDa form, each subunit consisting of an anti-parallel β-sandwich (9). This cytokine, described in 1975 (10), has been sequenced, cloned, and produced by recombinant techniques: human in 1985, mouse in 1986 (11,12).

TNF acts on cells through binding two receptors, p55 and p75, which are partially homologous in their extracellular domains but have different cytoplasmic domains. Endothelial cells (EC) have both receptors (13). The role of the receptors is controversial and seems to vary according to the assays used. Interaction of TNF with the p75 receptor has been associated with cytotoxicity (14). However, mutant human TNF molecules, which bind selectively to the p55 receptor, also have cytotoxic effects on transformed cells in culture (15). Using TNF mutants with preferential binding to either p55 or to p75, it has been shown that p55 is required for EC expression of E-selectin and interleukin (IL) 8 secretion (16).

Effects of tumour necrosis factor α

Many physiological and pathological effects of TNF have been recognized and are the subject of various reviews (1,2,5,6,11,17) For the purpose of this chapter we will mention first, briefly the pathological effects, and its effects on tumours, and concentrate, below, on the functions relevant to endothelium and angiogenesis.

Pathological effects

The known pathological effects of TNF are many and include cachexia, septic shock, severe inflammatory reactions, and intravascular coagulation (5,17,18). Prolonged exposure to TNF suppresses lipoprotein lipase and other lipid enzymes resulting in lipolysis, anorexia, and cachexia (thus the name cachectin) (1). TNF is also a mediator of inflammation (19) and monoclonal antibodies against TNF are reported to have beneficial effects in rheumatoid arthritis. Elevations of blood TNF occur in Gram-negative and Gram-positive sepsis (particularly in the purpura fulminans of meningococcaemia) (20) and in cerebral malaria (both experimental and human) (21). Based on experimental data, therapy with anti-TNF antibodies has been proposed for both situations (5). Alterations of TNF have been noted in other conditions including systemic lupus erythematosus, vasculitis, sarcoidosis, leprosy, and parasitic infections (aside from malaria) (2,5) but the role of this cytokine in most of these diseases has not been established.

Effects on tumours

The name 'tumour necrosis factor' was derived from its induction of haemorrhagic necrosis in some mouse tumours (10). TNF was later found to exert direct cytotoxicity on some tumour cells and on some cell lines such as L929 fibroblasts (12), but two-thirds of tumour cells tested proved to be relatively resistant to TNF-mediated cytotoxicity (22). Nevertheless, there were hopes that recombinant TNF would be useful for cancer therapy. In fact clinical trials have been conducted (23). Unfortunately, the efficacy of the systemically administered cytokine in tumour-bearing patients proved to be very limited, while toxic effects were severe (23). However, the combination of intratumoral TNF and mild local hyperthermia produced considerable necrosis in a mouse sarcoma (RIF-1), which is otherwise TNF-resistant (24). Consistent with such experimental data, intra-arterial administration to humans, by isolated limb perfusion, of high-dose TNF together with melphalan, interferon (IFN) γ, and hyperthermia, was reported to show efficacy in otherwise unresponsive tumours (25).

These experimental and clinical findings raise questions about the mechanism(s) by which TNF exerts anti-tumour effects. As most tumour cells are relatively resistant to the cytotoxic effects of TNF (22), it has been suggested that a major effect of the cytokine is on the blood supply to tumours (5,24). Such effects could be mediated in various ways. First, TNF has direct cytotoxic effects on endothelial cells, and activates neutrophils or other effector cells that injure EC (26). Second, the procoagulant effects of TNF could induce thrombosis in blood vessels irrigating tumours. Third, TNF might inhibit angiogenesis, the formation of new microvessels, which is required for tumour growth. As described below, the latter hypothesis has been investigated in our laboratory (27–29). This subject is also relevant to the well-established relationship between angiogenesis and inflammation. In some inflammatory reactions angiogenesis can be so prominent that it is termed granulation tissue. As TNF and IL-1β are major mediators of inflammation (19), their possible role in associated angiogenesis deserves exploration.

Effects on endothelial cells

Many effects of TNF on EC have been reported. Some of the effects are reproducible in different laboratories and are generally accepted, while others are controversial. Discrepant observations can be explained, in part, by the different concentrations of TNF used and the fact that responses of microvascular EC may be different from those of human umbilical vein or bovine aorta EC (the two most common endothelial cells used for *in vitro* experiments), and other macrovascular EC. Species differences between the TNF and EC used might also have an effect because of selective receptor binding.

Induction of adhesion molecules

Like IL-1, TNF induces the expression on EC of E-selectin (ELAM-1) and ICAM-1, which increase binding of neu-

trophils, and of VCAM-1, which promotes attachment of monocytes and lymphocytes (30,31). This is an early step in leucocyte recruitment; TNF also activates neutrophils for the production of oxidants, which can damage EC (26).

Procoagulant effects

TNF acts on EC to exert a net procoagulant effect (32,33). TNF increases the expression on EC of tissue factor (thromboplastin), which, in the presence of acidic phospholipids, initiates the extrinsic pathway of blood coagulation. Small amounts of TNF induce the production of tissue-type plasminogen activator (tPA) whereas larger amounts of TNF induce the secretion of plasminogen activator inhibitor type 1 (PAI-1) resulting in opposing effects. TNF-α down-regulates thrombomodulin and thereby impairs activation of protein C. Infusion of high doses of TNF-α in dogs was found to induce microvascular thrombosis (18). Recombinant TNF-α, administered as an intravenous bolus to healthy men, induced rapid and sustained activation of the common pathway of blood coagulation, probably by the extrinsic route (33). This effect could explain thrombosis of tumour vasculature, followed by haemorrhagic necrosis. It could also contribute to the disseminated intravascular coagulation associated with septic shock (19).

Induction of prostaglandin formation

A consistent effect of TNF and IL-1β is induction of the release of PGI$_2$ (prostacyclin) by macrovascular EC and of PGE$_2$ by microvascular EC, fibroblasts and other cell types (31,34). This is partly due to induced production of the type II isoenzyme of cyclooxygenase (PGH synthase) (35). PGE$_2$ binding to EP1 receptors, and PGI$_2$ binding to IP receptors, activates adenylate cyclase and increases cyclic adenosine monophosphate levels in target cells. This inhibits the proliferation of many cell types but stimulates that of microvascular EC (34). E-type prostaglandins and stable analogues of PGI$_2$ stimulate microvascular EC proliferation and angiogenesis *in vivo* (28). A PGH synthase inhibitor, ketorolac, blocked the angiogenic effect of recombinant basic fibroblast growth factor (bFGF) *in vivo* (because it inhibited the synthesis of PGE$_2$, but did not influence the angiogenic effect of PGE$_2$), (28) (because it did not affect the already synthesized prostaglandin). Hence the angiogenic effect of bFGF is mediated by prostaglandin production, and ketorolac's inhibition of the process is specific (29). Induced prostaglandin production could explain, at least in part, the angiogenic effect of low doses of TNF.

Induction of proteinase synthesis and release

TNF and IL-1 activate the transcription of genes for neutral metalloproteinases (stromelysins, collagenases) and for the serine proteinase tPA (36). The prometallo-proteinases so produced are converted into active enzymes by several mechanisms, including the broad-spectrum serine proteinase plasmin (36). Activated stromelysins and collagenases can digest basement membranes, intercellular proteoglycans and collagen, thereby facilitating the migration of EC and the penetration of budding microvessels into connective tissues. One of the markers of migrating EC is expression of tPA (31). Thus TNF-α induction of proteinase production could contribute to angiogenesis.

Effects on endothelial cell proliferation

In human umbilical vein EC, TNF has been reported to inhibit proliferation and antagonize the mitogenic effect of bFGF (37). TNF is also reported to inhibit the proliferation of cultured capillary EC (38). However, mitogenesis of dermal, and lung microvascular EC is not inhibited by TNF (39,40). This discrepancy may be due to the different concentrations of cytokines used, or to the fact that EC from different locations vary in sensitivity to the cytostatic effects of TNF. EC of different vessels (particularly large versus capillary) are functionally and morphologically very heterogeneous (32).

Induction of class I major histocompatibility complex (MHC) gene expression

Class I MHC is expressed on EC, but at a low level. TNF increases the expression two-to fourfold over 24 h through an increase in transcription (31). IFN-γ has a synergistic effect with TNF on the class I MHC expression in EC. This could facilitate presentation of class I-restricted antigens to T cells, but is not known to affect angiogenesis.

Induction of cytokine secretion

TNF-α induces the synthesis and release by EC of several cytokines, including IL-6, IL-8, and other chemokines, granulocyte–macrophage colony-stimulating factor (GM-CSF), granulocyte colony-stimulating factor (G-CSF) and platelet-derived growth factor (PDGF) (31,32). The BB form of PDGF was reported to be chemotactic for rat brain capillary EC and to have an angiogenic effect in the chick chorioallantoic membrane (CAM) (41). In another laboratory all three forms of PDGF (AA, AB, and BB), used as recombinant proteins, were weakly angiogenic in the chick CAM (42); this effect was attributed to monocytic infiltration. It seems unlikely that PDGF is an important mediator of TNF-induced angiogenesis.

Cytotoxic effects

TNF-α has been reported to be cytotoxic for stimulated EC in vitro (38,42), especially in the presence of neutrophils (through reactive oxygen species) (26). TNF can also cause apoptosis of EC (42a) in vitro via a sphingomyelin-ceramide pathway similar to that initiated by ionizing radiation (42b). These effects may play a role in respiratory distress syndromes (26), and could also explain, at least in part, the haemorrhagic necrosis induced by TNF in some tumours. Damage to EC exposes underlying extracellular matrix that is thrombogenic, and therefore has consequences analogous to those of tissue factor activation.

Reported effects on angiogenesis

As reviewed by other contributors to this volume, adult angiogenesis is the proliferation of microvessels in the fully developed vertebrate. It involves the migration and multiplication of microvascular EC, and their arrangement into blood vessels. Angiogenic agonists and antagonists modulate one or more of these processes.

The discrepant reports about effects of TNF on EC proliferation in culture have been mentioned above. In the experiments of Sato et al. (43), TNF inhibited the formation of microvascular sprouts in vitro. However, Leibovich et al. (44) found that mouse TNF induced angiogenesis in the rat cornea. About the same time Frater-Schroder et al. (37) described a similar paradox; while TNF inhibited EC proliferation in vitro, it stimulated angiogenesis in the rabbit cornea.

Because of these different findings we decided to investigate further the effect of TNF on (in vivo) angiogenesis. Recombinant murine TNF-α was used in the mouse, thereby avoiding one source of confusion: homologous TNF binds to both p55 and p75 receptors, whereas human TNF binds only to murine p55 receptors (15). A wide range of concentrations of TNF-α was used because of the possibility that the effects of the cytokine were concentration-dependent, which proved to be the case. A quantitative angiogenesis assay developed in our laboratories (27,29) was used.

A reproducible angiogenesis assay

General description (Fig. 20.1)

The disc angiogenesis system (DAS) was based on initial observations of vascular growth in subcutaneously implanted sponges (27). After succeeding versions of the system have been tested for several years, the current DAS used (29) consists of a disc of polyvinyl alcohol foam 13 mm in diameter and 2 mm thick. The flat sides of the

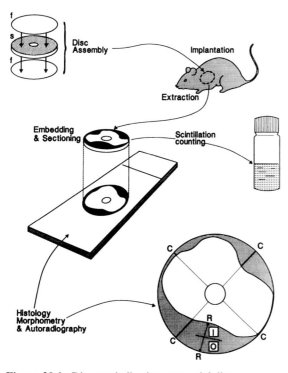

Figure 20.1. Diagram indicating sequential disc assembly, implantation, removal, embedding, sectioning, and analysis (quantitative and qualitative). See text for details of each. Reproduced, with permission, from Kowalski *et al.* (29) and the journal *Experimental and Molecular Pathology*.

discs are covered with cell-impermeable Millipore filters (orifices of less that 0.45 μm) and are sealed by no. 1 Millipore glue. This leaves only the rim (a 2 mm wide band) for penetration or exit of cells. In most studies, and prior to placement of the filters, a hole 3 mm in diameter is bored into the centre of the disc. A pellet of the same material, containing an angiogenic agonist or antagonist is coated with the acetate polymer Elvax (Dupont) and inserted in the central hole. The coating allows for slow diffusion of the contents of the pellet into the disc and surrounding tissues. Each pellet 3 mm in diameter can hold up to 20 μl of the material to be tested (29).

The discs are prepared from sterilized material and under sterile conditions in a laminar flow hood. Non-sterile discs can also be sterilized by a variety of methods, *e.g.* immersion in 100% ethanol with subsequent evaporation. The discs can tolerate dry heat up to 120°C but are damaged by boiling water (29).

Although the DAS can be implanted in many different experimental animals, mammalian and non-mammalian,

we have preferred to use mice because of their well-defined genetics. Also several recombinant mouse growth factors are available. The small size of mice is economically advantageous, especially when testing substances which are in short supply. We have preferred to use female Swiss Webster and BALB/c mice approximately 8 weeks old and weighing 20–30 g. Other investigators in various laboratories have used the DAS in rats or rabbits.

The discs are placed, subcutaneously, in the abdomen or thorax. Most often our test animals are anaesthetized by an intraperitoneal injection of ketamine hydrochloride, xylazine, and acepromazine. The shaved skin surface is bathed in 70% ethanol and a longitudinal 1.5 cm incision into the subcutis is made dorsally at the level of the thorax, at least 1 cm away from the desired location of the DAS. A subcutaneous tunnel toward the site of implantation is made with blunt scissors, and the disc is inserted after bathing the tunnel with phosphate-buffered saline. The skin wound is closed with three or four metal clips. The animals are housed then as usual with standard chow and water ad-libitum during the period of experiment which ordinarily is 2 weeks, but which can be extended or decreased as necessary. The mice tolerate well the implants and do not scratch incisions made on the dorsum or the flank (29).

After a number of days of growth, usually 14, the disc is removed following euthanasia of the animal (for instance by CO_2 narcosis). The disc is then fixed, generally in 10% formaldehyde, and embedded in paraffin or plastic. Planar sections 6 μm thick are obtained for quantitative and qualitative microscopic examination (haematoxylin and eosin), measure of total growth area (toluidine blue), scintillation counting (ten 6 μm sections without stain), etc. (Fig. 20.1). Electron microscopy, transmission, and scanning, can also be performed in such discs for qualitative assessments.

A spontaneous fibrovascular growth penetrates the disc from the rim, towards the centre, and consists of blood capillaries, fibroblasts, macrophages, and neutrophils. This spontaneous growth is modulated by angiogenic agonists and antagonists. Although the blood vessels are seen in the majority of instances, better definition of these channels is obtained from a dye, Luconyl Blue, injected intravenously or intracardially 15 min before the animal is euthanized (29) (see Fig. 20.2, in the plate section).

Quantification of angiogenesis

One of the advantages of the DAS is the ability to measure precisely vascular growth. Direct measurement of the blood vessels can be performed by various methods, including point counting on histological sections (45), the determination of intravascular volume, *e.g.* by means of radioactive isotopes (46), etc. Such methods to measure directly blood vessels are tedious and impractical when examining a large number of specimens. Therefore simpler, indirect procedures have been devised.

A comparison of the total growth area in planar sections with the area occupied by the blood vessels (the latter by means of point counting) has shown that the area occupied by blood vessels is consistently proportional to the total growth area (29). Therefore the measurement of the total growth area is in fact an accurate, indirect measurement of the area occupied by blood vessels. This total growth area can be assessed by several techniques. One of these is measuring the distance between the blood vessel closest to the centre of the disc and the peripheral edge of the disc (centripetal radial growth): the innermost blood vessel is identified and the radial distance between the 'leading' tip of such vessel and the rim of the disc is measured in centimetres, on a section projected at $100 \times$ magnification on to a horizontal surface (Fig. 20.1).

As the growth into the disc is asymmetric (probably because of the random distribution in the host subcutis of mother venules from which the new capillaries develop) it is useful to measure the radial growth at several points; *e.g.* four or eight equally spaced radii. We frequently determine the total growth by measuring the radial fibrovascular growth along two perpendicular diameters (four radii) using a projected image of a section at a $100 \times$ magnification (Fig. 20.1). The values thus obtained are averaged for each disc.

One simple and precise method of measuring total growth consists of staining 6 μm thick paraffin sections with toluidine blue to obtain a high contrast. The toluidine blue stains uniformly the area of growth and does not stain the sponge. Such sections are scanned by a camera fitted with a computer-assisted digital image analysis system which measures automatically the entire area of growth in pixels. For every experiment threshold values are standardized and the data in pixels are converted to square millimetres. This method is rapid and reproducible (29).

The above methods measure vascular growth, which results from two components: EC proliferation and EC migration. To determine the relative contribution of the former (and conversely of the latter) we have used injections of tritiated thymidine (^{3}HTdR) given to the mice, as a single bolus or in multiple doses, within the last 48 h before extraction of the disc (29). In such cases 10 serial, 6 μm thick paraffin sections are subjected to alkali solubilization and their beta radiation activity is determined in a scintillation counter. The proportion of ^{3}HTdR activity due to proliferation of endothelial cells (versus proliferation of fibroblasts or other cells) can be determined by radioautographs of the sections in which dif-

ferential counting of the labelled cells is performed. This has been established for various times of the growth period in the discs and it has shown that the maximum proliferation of cells occurs at 13 days, after which there is a progressive decrease in the number of labelled cells (29). The fibrovascular growth, however, continues up to our maximum point of observation, which is 30 days (29). Thus the DAS can discriminate between EC proliferation and EC migration.

As the DAS system is relatively inexpensive and highly reproducible, multiple discs can be used for each data point in time or dose, thereby increasing the statistical accuracy of the results and allowing dose–response studies with angiogenic or anti-angiogenic agents.

Determination of the role of tumour necrosis factor in angiogenesis

Experimental design

We have studied the effect of TNF on angiogenesis using the above described DAS method (28). In one series of experiments, discs were loaded with mouse recombinant TNF-α (mrTNF) at doses of 0.01–5000 ng (see Table 20.1a). This mrTNF was kindly provided by Drs G. Grau and P. Vassalli of the University of Geneva. The specific activity was 3×10^7 units/mg. For each dose of TNF 10 discs were prepared and placed in an equal number of female BALB/c mice 6–8 weeks old. Controls were 15 discs without any cytokine, which measured the spontaneous growth, and 11 discs containing a known angiogenic cytokine, recombinant bFGF (20 μg per disc) (Table 20.1a).

In a second series of experiments mice had, in addition to the angiogenesis discs, an osmotic minipump (Alzet 14 day, Alza, Palo Alto) placed also subcutaneously, through a different incision. Its delivering nipple was located 5 mm away from the edge of the disc. There were four groups, each of six discs (mice). In one group the minipump contained 5 μg of mrTNF (in 200 μl of phosphate-buffered saline), another had 10 μg of TNF, a third had 20 μg of TNF, and a fourth had only 200 μl of phosphate-buffered saline and acted as a control. The minipumps delivered the TNF locally (subcutaneously) at a rate of 15–60 ng/h during 14 days. None of those groups had any agonists or antagonists in the discs. The purpose of this experiment was to observe the effect of TNF delivered regionally by the osmotic pump on the spontaneous angiogenesis occurring in the disc. As a positive control six mice were fitted with discs containing 20 μg of

Table 20.1. TNF-α angiogenesis experiments

A			B		
Mice	Disc		Mice	Disc	Minipump
10	mrTNF	0.01 ng	6	—	mrTNF 5 μg
10	mrTNF	0.1 ng	6	—	mrTNF 10 μg
10	mrTNF	1.0 ng	6	—	mrTNF 20 μg
10	mrTNF	10.0 ng	6	—	PBS 200 μl
10	mrTNF	100.0 ng	6	bFGF 20 μg	PBS 200 μl
10	mrTNF	200.0 ng			
10	mrTNF	1000.0 ng			
10	mrTNF	5000.0 ng			
15	No cytokine (spontaneous growth control)				
11	bFGF	20 μg			
	(positive control)				

Two series of experiments are summarized in this table.

A (left columns): Angiogenesis discs (containing, within a centrally located pellet, mouse rTNFα in increasing amounts) were placed subcutaneously in BALB/c mice. Positive controls had bFGF instead of TNF. Spontaneous growth controls had no cytokine.

B (right columns): Mice had an angiogenesis disc and an osmotic minipump, both placed subcutaneously (diagram in Fig. 20.4). The contents of each are listed. Positive controls had bFGF in the disc, no cytokine in the minipump. Spontaneous growth controls had no cytokines but contained phosphate-buffered 0.9% NaCl (PBS) in the minipump.

TNF, tumour necrosis factor; bFGF, basic fibroblast growth factor; rTNF, recombinant TNF; mrTNF, mouse recombinant TNF.

Reproduced, with permission, from Fajardo *et al.*[28] and the *American Journal of Pathology*.

bFGF and in those animals the minipumps were loaded with 200 μl of phosphate-buffered saline (Table 20.1b).

Each of the above 136 mice was injected intraperitoneally 24, 18, and 12 h before euthanasia, with ³HTdR (specific activity 6.7 Ci/mmol). The cumulative, total dose was 200 μCi per mouse. Also each of the mice was injected as described before with the dye Luconyl Blue intracardially 15 min before euthanasia.

The data from the above-described procedures (measurements of actual growth, total area and ³HTdR incorporation) were analysed in an IBM-PC/80 computer using the RSI statistical analysis software. Having obtained a mean, standard error and standard deviation for each group of discs, comparisons of experimental and control groups were carried out using the Student's *t*-test.

Results

Figure 20.3 shows the results of the mean growth and the incorporation of ³HTdR (28). It will be noticed that TNF placed in the centre of the discs resulted in two separate and opposing effects. Concentrations of 0.01–1 ng per disc significantly stimulated angiogenesis, which was maximum at a concentration of 0.1 ng (*P* <0.01 versus spontaneous growth). As the dose of TNF was increased the angiogenic effect disappeared. Then an inhibition of

angiogenesis was observed at doses of 1–5 μg (*P* <0.01). The same effects, particularly the inhibition, were observed in the incorporation of ³HTdR.

The results of the second set of experiments can be seen in Fig. 20.4. There was a decrease in vascular growth proportional to the concentration of TNF in the pumps. Pumps containing 20 μg of TNF produced a significant decrease in angiogenesis as compared with the controls. Notice also the expected high angiogenic response to bFGF in the positive control discs. Of general interest is the fact that, regardless of the content of the disc, the one-half of the disc most proximal to the pump always had less growth than the opposite half, as illustrated in the histograms of Fig. 4.

Interpretation of results

Our results show that low doses of TNF are indeed angiogenic. Tissue concentrations in the order of 0.01–1 ng stimulate local blood vessel growth. On the other hand high concentrations, in the order of 1–5 μg, inhibit angiogenesis. It is very likely that the nanogram doses approach those concentrations that were obtained in the cornea by the above cited investigators and the microgram doses were similar to the concentrations achieved *in vitro* in other experiments. Therefore these results explain the

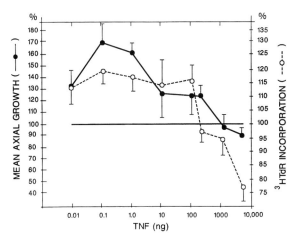

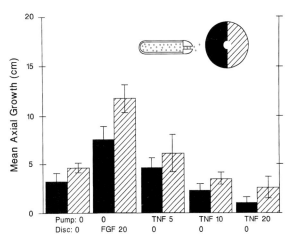

Figure 20.3. Dose-dependent bimodal effect of tumour necrosis factor (TNF) on angiogenesis. All values have been normalized in relation to the control (spontaneous growth) values, which are indicated by a straight line at the 100% level. The solid line (left scale of percentages) indicates the fibrovascular growth as measured along four axes. The broken line (right scale of percentages) indicates the incorporation of tritiated thymidine (^{3}HTdR) as measured by scintillation counting. Error bars ± SEM. The TNF contained in the centre of the discs is indicated in nanograms. Both fibrovascular growth and cell proliferation increased with the low doses of TNF and decreased with the high doses. Reproduced, with permission, from Fajardo *et al.* (28), and the *American Journal of Pathology*.

Figure 20.4. Axial growth in discs exposed to the tumour necrosis factor (TNF) released from adjacent, subcutaneous minipumps (as indicated in right upper diagram). Solid bars indicate growth in the one-half of the disc proximal to the pump, and hatched bars in the one-half distal to the pump. Legend below each set of bars indicates above the content of the minipump, and below the content of the disc, both in μg. 0 = no cytokine. Error bars = ± SEM. As expected, discs containing basic fibroblast growth factor (bFGF) had significantly greater growth than control discs (first set of bars). As in the previous experiment (Fig. 20.3.) high doses of TNF inhibited fibrovascular growth (*P*<0.01). In every group the growth was less in the side close to the minipump (solid bars) than in the opposite side. This could have been caused by the pump itself (i.e. in the controls) or by a gradient in the diffusion of TNF (i.e. in the test discs). Reproduced, with permission, from Fajardo *et al.* (28) and the *American Journal of Pathology*.

apparent contradiction of the *in vitro* versus *in vivo* observations and validate them.

Discussion

As described, low concentrations of TNF-α increase whereas high concentrations inhibit angiogenesis (28). The underlying mechanisms are unknown. However, it can be suggested that the low concentrations of TNF induce the production of PGE$_2$ and PGI$_2$, which are angiogenic (29). Furthermore, low concentrations of TNF induce the production of tPA, with activation of plasmin and neutral metalloproteinases, which facilitate penetration of microvessels into connective tissue. Higher concentrations of TNF suppress tPA production and augment that of PAI-1, thereby preventing plasmin generation and activation of metalloproteinases. TNF also induces the expression in endothelial cells of the protein B61 (a ligand for the Eck receptor protein tyrosine kinase) and the autophosphory-

lation of the latter (47). A recombinant B61 construct has been recently reported to be a chemoattractant for EC *in vitro* and to be angiogenic *in vivo*; an antibody against B61 attenuated the *in vivo* angiogenic effect of TNF but not that of bFGF (47). A separate study suggests that protein kinase C may be a mediator of the angiogenesis induced not only by TNF, but by other cytokines (48).

The inhibitory effect of high doses of TNF on angiogenesis may be due to suppression of EC proliferation and migration, or to toxic effects on EC. Following intravenous administration of TNF, or local injection of the cytokine (24), electron microscopic studies have shown EC injury. Piguet *et al.* (49) studied the results of subcutaneous perfusion of TNF-α in the mouse, at rates of 35–170 ng/h. At low doses they observed proliferation of capillaries and other stromal elements, whereas at high doses (higher than those used by us) they found necrosis of tissue. Their observations are consistent with those in our second set of experiments.

It has been suggested that the mode of delivery of TNF to EC plays a key role in their response (42). Luminal delivery, following intravenous injection of the cytokine, would induce polarized tissue factor expression and intravascular coagulation, whereas extravascular delivery, e.g. from activated monocytes, would induce opposite polar release of proteinases, facilitating degradation of extracellular matrix, EC migration, and angiogenesis (42). The observations just reviewed suggest that the concentration of TNF, rather than its mode of delivery, determines whether angiogenesis is augmented or suppressed.

Any attempt to extrapolate these results to human diseases must be made with caution. The relatively modest amounts of TNF produced by cells of monocytic lineage in local inflammatory lesions could contribute to angiogenesis, although several other cytokines might also be involved (31,42). If prostaglandins are important mediators of angiogenesis, it would be expected that cyclooxygenase inhibitors would suppress that response. An example could be chronic inflammatory periodontal disease in which angiogenesis is increased; the newly formed blood vessels are fragile, and bleed when teeth are cleaned. It can be postulated that prostaglandins mediate this angiogenesis because the inflammatory response and bleeding disappear when patients are given an oral rinse containing the cyclooxygenase inhibitor ketorolac, and alveolar bone erosion is significantly inhibited (50) (Fig. 20.5).

It would be expected from our findings that low doses of TNF stimulate angiogenesis and tumour growth. In contrast, high doses of TNF would have a procoagulant effect, damage the vasculature and suppress angiogenesis, thereby exerting anti-tumour effects. Because of the toxicity of TNF, the doses that can be administered systemically by the intravenous route are limited, and the tissue concentrations thus achieved probably correspond to our low-dose range. Therefore there would be an angiogenic, pro-tumour net effect or at least no tumour effect. Indeed such limited doses of TNF have not shown efficacy in human tumours (23).

Much higher concentrations of TNF can be administered intra-arterially by isolated limb perfusion (ILP), together with IFN-γ and melphalan (25). The objective of such therapy in a multi-centre European trial was to achieve limb salvage in patients with unresectable soft tissue sarcomas. The limb salvage rate was an excellent 90% (51). The same procedure had dramatic anti-tumour effects in stage III melanoma (52). The anti-tumour response induced by TNF was characterized by its acute onset, suggesting a rapid vascular effect. Angiograms con-

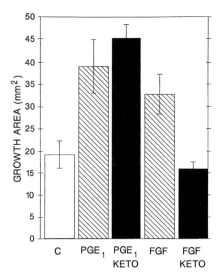

Figure 20.5. Effect of cyclooxygenase inhibitor (ketorolac) on angiogenesis. *In vitro* studies have indicated that capillary endothelial cell proliferation stimulated by fibroblast growth factor (bFGF) requires the presence of prostaglandins. As shown here in the DAS, the same occurs *in vivo*: ketorolac (4 mg/kg daily by gavage) inhibits the 14-day angiogenesis stimulated by bFGF (20 μg; last two bars), presumably because it interferes with the synthesis of new PGE. However, ketorolac does not have an effect on angiogenesis stimulated by already synthesized PGE (PGE$_1$; 75 μg in the centre of the DAS) as shown in the second and third bars. The control DAS in the first bar contained no agonist or antagonist and thus indicates spontaneous growth. C, control; PGE$_1$, prostaglandin E$_1$; FGF, basic fibroblast growth factor; KETO, ketorolac. Standard errors of means are indicated. Reproduced, with permission, from Kowalski *et al.* (29) and the journal *Experimental and Molecular Pathology*.

ducted before ILP showed hypervascularity of tumours, while 7–14 days after ILP the tumour-associated blood vessels had disappeared (52). These findings suggest that high concentrations of TNF, in combination therapy, can damage tumour vasculature while leaving intact the blood supply to normal tissues (52). Other compounds such as flavone acetic acid also damage blood vessels in tumours to a greater extent than those in normal tissues, thereby impairing tumour growth (53,54).

General lessons from our experience are the necessity for studying the effects of different doses of a cytokine, and the advisability of using homologous TNF-α because it binds to both p75 and p55 receptors. Now the experimental findings on the effects of TNF on cultured EC, on blood vessels in tumours, and on angiogenesis associated with inflammation, are becoming more consistent with clinical observations, and are opening the way to therapeutic applications.

Summary and conclusions

TNF-α, a cytokine mainly produced by macrophages, has numerous physiological and pathological effects. Prominent are its effects on EC which have at least two receptors for TNF. These effects include pro-coagulant activity, induction of adhesion molecules and prostaglandin synthesis, induction of class I MHC and EC cytotoxicity.

The role of TNF on angiogenesis has been controversial until recently. *In vitro* TNF had shown inhibition of EC proliferation and of microvascular sprouts, as well as toxicity for stimulated EC. However, in the rat and rabbit cornea human TNF had induced angiogenesis.

To clarify this paradox we have investigated the specific effect of mrTNF in 136 BALB/c mice, using the DAS. The DAS consists of a polyvinyl alcohol foam disc that is inserted subcutaneously; after 14 days of growth it is extracted and its centripetal angiogenic growth is easily and precisely quantitated. In addition, cell proliferation is measured by ^{3}HTdR incorporation.

Two sets of experiments revealed a bimodal angiogenic response to mrTNF. At low concentrations of 0.01–1 ng/disc mrTNF induced angiogenesis: both vessel growth and EC proliferation (P <0.01 as compared with spontaneous growth). At high concentrations of 1–5 μg/disc mrTNF inhibited angiogenesis (P <0.01). Subcutaneous mrTNF delivered at the high rate of 16–60 ng/h by osmotic minipumps also inhibited angiogenesis in regionally placed discs.

These results explain and validate experiments by other researchers that appeared paradoxical. They also have therapeutic implications as TNF has been used as a potential anti-cancer agent. If the tumour concentrations of systemically administered TNF are low (nanogram levels), the effect will be promotion of vessel growth and therefore of tumour growth, which may offset any direct anti-tumour effects of TNF. Indeed TNF trials in human cancers have been disappointing. Higher systemic concentrations of TNF (microgram levels) may be tumoricidal but are also toxic. However, regional perfusion of neoplasms with high doses of TNF can circumvent this problem and such modality is promising. This study emphasizes the importance of using a wide range of doses and homologous proteins in the evaluation of cytokine effects.

Acknowledgements

Supported in part by Veterans Affairs Research Funds (FAJ004) and by Syntex Research. Donna Buckley assisted in the typescript preparation.

References

1. Beutler, B. and Cerami, A. (1987). Cachectin: more than a tumor necrosis factor. *N. Engl. J. Med.*, **316**, 379–85.
2. Jaatela, M. (1991). Biologic activities and mechanisms of action of tumor necrosis factor-α/cachectin. *Lab. Invest.*, **64**, 724–42.
3. Klein, L. M., Lavker, R. M., Matis, W. L., and Murphy, G. F. (1989). Degranulation of human mast cells induces an endothelial antigen central to leukocyte adhesion. *Proc. Natl Acad. Sci. USA*, **86**, 8972–6.
4. Spies, T., Morton, C. C., Nedospasov, S. A., Fiers, W., Pious, D., Strominger, J. L. (1986). Genes for the tumor necrosis factor α and β are linked to the human major histocompatibility complex. *Proc. Natl Acad. Sci. USA*, **83**, 8699–702.
5. Fajardo, L. F. and Grau, G. E. (1991). Tumor necrosis factor in human disease. *Western J. Med.*, **154**, 88–9.
6. Tracey, K. J., Vlassara, H., and Cerami, A. (1989). Cachectin/tumor necrosis factor. *Lancet*, **i**, 1122–5.
7. Kriegler, M., Perez, C., DeFay, K., Albert, I., and Lui, S. D. (1988). A novel form of TNF/cachectin is a cell surface cytotoxic transmembrane protein: ramifications for the complex physiology of TNF. *Cell*, **53**, 45–53.
8. Gearing, A. J. H., Beckett, P., Christodoulou, M., Churchill, M., Clements, J., Davidson, A. H., *et al.* (1994). Processing of tumour necrosis factor-alpha precursor by metalloproteinases. *Nature*, **370**, 555–7.
9. Eck, M. J. and Sprang, S. R. (1989). The structure of tumor necrosis factor at 2-6A resolution. *J. Biol. Chem.*, **264**, 17595–605.
10. Carswell, E. A., Old, L. J., Kassel, R. L., Green, S., Fiore, N., and Williamson, B. (1975). An endotoxin induced serum factor that causes necrosis of tumors. *Proc. Natl Acad. Sci. USA*, **72**, 3666–70.
11. Aggarwal, B. B. and Poisik, E. (1992). Cytokines: from clone to clinic. *Arch. Biochem. Biophys.*, **292**, 335–359.
12. Sugarman, B. J., Aggarwal, B. B., Haas, P. E., Figari, I. S., Palladino, M. A., Jr., and Shepard, H. M. (1985). Recombinant human tumor necrosis factor-alpha: effects on proliferation of normal and transformed cells *in vitro*. *Science*, **230**, 943–5.
13. Shalaby, M. R., Sundan, A., Loetscher, H., Brockhaus, M., Lesslauer, W., and Espevik, T. (1990). Binding and regulation of cellular functions by monoclonal antibodies against human TNF receptors. *J. Exp. Med.*, **172**, 1517–20.
14. Heller, R. A., Song, K., Fan, N., and Chang, D. J. (1992). The p70 tumor necrosis factor receptor mediates cytotoxicity. *Cell*, **70**, 47–56.
15. Tartaglia, L. A., Goeddel, D. V. (1992). Two TNF receptors. *Immunol. Today*, **13**, 151–3.
16. Barbara, J. A., Smith, W. B., Gamble, J. R., Van Ostade, X., Vandenabeele, P., Tavernier, J., *et al.* (1994). Dissociation of TNF-α cytotoxic and proinflammatory activities by p55

receptor- and p75 receptor-selective TNF-α mutants. *EMBO J.*, **13**, 843–50.

17. Tracey, K. J. (1995). TNF and Mae West or: death from too much of a good thing. *Lancet*, **345**, 75–6.

18. Tracey, K. J., Lowry, S. F., Fahey, T. J. III, Albert, J. D., Fong, Y., Hesse, D., *et al.* (1987). Cachectin/tumor necrosis factor induces lethal shock and stress hormone responses in the dog. *Surg. Gynecol. Obstet.*, **164**, 415–22.

19. Allison, A. C., Lee, J. C., and Eugui, E. M. (1995). Pharmacological regulation of the production of the proinflammatory cytokines. TNF-α and IL-1β. In *Human cytokines: their role in disease and therapy* (ed. B. B. Aggarwal and R. K. Puri), pp. 689–713. Blackwell Science, Oxford.

20. Girardin, E., Grau, G. E., Dayer, J. M., Roux-Lombard, P., the 15 Study Group, Lambert, P-H. (1988). Tumor necrosis factor and interleukin-I in the serum of children with severe infectious purpura. *N. Engl. J. Med.*, **319**, 397–400.

21. Grau, G. E., Fajardo, L. F., Piguet, P. F., Allet, B., Lambert, P. H., and Vassalli, P. (1987). Tumor necrosis factor (cachectin) as an essential mediator in murine cerebral malaria. *Science*, **237**, 1210–12.

22. Haranaka, K. and Satoni, N. (1981). Cytotoxic activity of tumor necrosis factor (TNF) on human cancer cells *in vitro*. *J. Exp. Med.*, **51**, 191–4.

23. Hersh, E. M., Metch, B. S., Muggia, F. M., Brown, T. D., Whitehead, R. P., Budd, G. T., *et al.* (1991). Phase II studies of recombinant human tumor necrosis alpha in patients with malignant disease: a summary of the Southwest Oncology Group experience. *J. Immunother.*, **10**, 426–31.

24. Srinivasan, J. M., Fajardo, L. F., and Hahn, G. M. (1990). Mechanism of anti-tumor activity of TNF-α with hyperthermia in a TNF-α resistant tumor. *J. Natl Cancer Inst.*, **82**, 1904–10.

25. Lienard, D., Ewalenko, P., Delmotte, J. J., Renard, N., and Lejeune, F. J. (1992). High-dose recombinant tumor necrosis factor alpha in combination with interferon gamma and melphalan in isolation perfusion of the limbs for melanoma and sarcoma. *J. Clin. Oncol.*, **10**, 52–60.

26. Ward, P. A. and Varani, J. (1990). Mechanisms of neutrophil-mediated killing of endothelial cells. *J. Leukocyte Biol.*, **48**, 97–102.

27. Fajardo, L. F., Kowalski, J., Kwan, H. H., Prionas, S. D., and Allison, A. C. (1988). The disc angiogenesis system. *Lab. Invest.*, **58**, 718–24.

28. Fajardo, L. F., Kwan, H. H., Kowalski, J., Prionas, S. D., and Allison, A. C. (1992). Dual role of tumor necrosis factor-α in angiogenesis. *Am. J. Pathol.*, **140**, 539–44.

29. Kowalski, J., Kwan, H. H., Prionas, S. D., Allison, A. C., and Fajardo, L. F. (1992). Characterization and applications of the disc angiogenesis system. *Exp. Mol. Pathol.*, **56**, 1–19.

30. Gamble, J. R., Harlan, J. M., Klebanoff, S. J., and Vadas, M. A. (1985). Stimulation of the adherence of neutrophils to umbilical vein endothelium by recombinant tumor necrosis factor. *Proc. Natl Acad. Sci. USA*, **82**, 8667–71.

31. Litwin, M. S., Gamble, J. R., and Vadas, M. A. (1995). Role of cytokines in endothelial cell functions. In *Human cytokines: their role in disease and therapy* (ed. B. B. Aggarwal and R. K. Puri), pp. 101–29. Blackwell Science, Oxford.

32. Fajardo, L. F. (1989). The complexity of endothelial cells. *Am. J. Clin. Pathol.*, **92**, 241–50.

33. van der Poll, T., Büller, H. R., Ten Cate, H., Wortel, C. H., Bauer, K. A., van Deventer, S. J. H., *et al.* (1990). Activation of coagulation after administration of tumor necrosis factor to normal subjects. *N. Engl J. Med.*, **322**, 1622–9.

34. Allison, A. C. and Kowalski, W. J. (1988). Prostaglandins as transducers of proliferation signals in microvascular endothelial cells and the pharmacological control of angiogenesis. In *Vascular endothelium: receptors and transduction mechanisms* (ed. J. Catravas), pp. 33–46. Plenum Press, New York.

35. Smith, W. L., Meade, E. A., and DeWitt, D. L. (1994). Interactions of PGH synthase isozymes-1 and -2 with NSAIDs. *Ann. N. Y. Acad. Sci.*, **744**, 50–7.

36. Matrisian, L. M. (1990). Metalloproteinases and their inhibitors in matrix remodelling. *Trends Genet.*, **6**, 121–5.

37. Frater-Schroder, M., Risau, W., Hallman, P., Gautschi, R., and Bohlen, P. (1987). Tumor-necrosis factor type-a, a potent inhibitor of endothelial cell growth *in vitro*, is angiogenic *in vivo*. *Proc. Natl Acad. Sci. USA*, **84**, 5277–81.

38. Schweigerer, L., Malerstein, B., and Gospodarawicz, D. (1987). Tumor necrosis factor inhibits the proliferation of cultured capillary endothelial cells. *Biophys. Res. Commun.*, **143**, 997–1004.

39. Detman, M., Imcke, E., Ruszczak, Z., and Orfanos, C. E. (1990). Effects of recombinant tumor necrosis factor-alpha on cultured microvascular endothelial cells derived from the human dermis. *J. Invest. Dermatol.*, **95**, S219–22.

40. Meyrick, B., Christman, B., and Jesmok, G. (1991). Effects of recombinant tumor necrosis factor-alpha on cultured pulmonary artery and lung microvascular cells. *Am. J. Pathol.*, **138**, 93–101.

41. Risau, W., Drexler, H., Mironov, V., Smits, A., Siegbahn, A., Funa, K., and Heldin, C. H. (1992). Platelet-derived growth factor is angiogenic *in vivo*. *Growth Factors*, **7**, 261–6.

42. Leibovich, S. J. (1995). Role of cytokines in the process of tumor angiogenesis. In *Human cytokines: their role in cell disease and therapy* (ed. B. B. Aggarwal and R. K. Puri), pp. 539–64. Blackwell Science, Oxford.

42a. Robaye, B., Mosselmans, R., Fiers, W., Dumont, J. E., and Galand, P. (1991). Tumor necrosis factor induces apoptosis (programmed cell death) in normal endothelial cells in vitro. *Am. J. Pathol.* **138**, 447–53.

42b. Haimoritz-Friedman, A., Kan, C. C., Ehleiter, D., Persaud, R. S., McLoughlin, M., Fuks, Z., Kolesnick, R. N. (1994). Ionizing radiation acts on cellular membranes to generate ceramide and induce apoptosis. *J. Exp. Med.*, **180**, 525–35.

43. Sato, N., Fukuda, K., Nariuchi, H., and Sagara, N. (1987). Tumor necrosis factor inhibits angiogenesis in vitro. *J. Natl Cancer Inst.*, **79**, 1383–91.

44. Leibovich, S. J., Polverini, P. J., Shepard, H. M., Wiseman, D. M., Shively, V., and Nuseir, N. (1987). Macrophage-induced angiogenesis is mediated by tumor necrosis factor-a. *Nature*, **329**, 630–2.

45. Haynes, J. D. (1964). Estimation of blood vessel surface area and length in tissue. *Nature*, **201**, 425–6.

46. Mahadevan, V., Hart, I. R., and Lewis, G. P. (1989). Factors influencing blood supply in wound granuloma quantitated by a new *in vivo* technique. *Cancer Res.*, **49**, 415–19.

47. Pandey, A., Shao, H., Marks, R. M., Polverini, P. J., and Dixit, V. M. (1995). Role of B61, the ligand for the Eck receptor tyrosine kinase, in TNF-α-induced angiogenesis. *Science*, **268**, 567–9.

48. Hu, D. E. and Fan, T. P. (1995). Protein kinase C inhibitor calphostin C prevents cytokine-induced angiogenesis in the rat. *Inflammation*, **19**, 39–54.

49. Piguet, P. F., Grau, G. E., and Vassalli, P. (1990). Subcutaneous perfusion of tumor necrosis factor induces local proliferation of fibroblasts, capillaries and epidermal cells, or massive tissue necrosis. *Am. J. Pathol.*, **136**, 103–10.

50. Jeffcoat, M. K., Reddy, M. S., Buchanan, W., Goodale, M. B., Meredith, M. P., Nelson, S. L., *et al.* (1994). Ketorolac tromethamine inhibits the progression of bone loss in adult periodontitis. *J. Dent. Res.*, **73**, 126–31.

51. Eggermont, A. M. M., Schraffordt Koops, H., Kroon, B. B. R., Lienard, D., Klausner, J. M., and Lejeune, F. J. (1994). The European experience in TNFα isolated limb perfusions for nonresectable extremity soft tissue sarcomas: 90% limb salvage. *Eur. Cytokine Network*, **5**, 224–6.

52. Eggermont, A. M. M., Schraffordt Koops, H., Lienard, D., Lejeune, F., and Oudkerk, M. (1994). Destruction of tumor-associated vessels by isolated limb perfusion (ILP) with TNFα: angiographic observations in sarcoma patients. *Eur. Cytokine Network*, **5**, 222–3.

53. Bibby, M. C., Double, J. A., Loadman, P. M., and Duke, C. V. (1989). Reduction of tumor blood flow by flavone acetic acid: a possible component of therapy. *J. Natl Cancer Inst.*, **81**, 216–20.

54. Hill, S., Williams, K. D., and Denekamp, J. (1989). Vascular collapse after flavone acetic acid: a possible mechanism of its anti-tumor action. *Eur. J. Cancer Clin. Oncol.* **25**, 1419–24.

21. Pleiotrophin and related molecules

Anke M. Schulte and Anton Wellstein

Introduction

A number of polypeptide growth factors have marked affinity for the glycosaminoglycan heparin and for heparan sulphates found on cell surfaces and in the extracellular matrix (ECM). These growth factors are collectively called heparin-binding growth factors (HBGFs) and comprise distinct polypeptides such as the vascular endothelial cell growth factor (VEGF), and fibroblast growth factors (FGF) (reviewed in chapters 16, 17). FGFs are the largest group of known HBGFs comprising at least 10 different members (1) and they were the first growth factors for which heparin affinity was demonstrated (2). Several years ago a novel gene family of HBGFs was discovered that appeared biologically very closely related to FGFs but turned out to be structurally distinct from FGFs as well as from any other known growth factors. The two members of this family are pleiotrophin (PTN) and midkine (MK). They are secreted HBGFs with an apparent molecular mass of 18 and 14 kDa, respectively, and they are highly conserved between different species as well as between each other; *e.g.* the secreted portion of the human and bovine PTN protein differ by only one amino acid, and the homology between the PTN and MK proteins is on average close to 50% taking conservative amino acid replacements into account. Both proteins were original described as developmentally regulated cytokines based on their expression pattern during fetal and neonatal brain development. In addition to this, PTN as well as MK appear to participate in tumour growth and angiogenesis.

Discovery and biology of pleiotrophin

PTN was originally purified by a number of laboratories using diverse tissue sources and different names were used to describe this novel protein. Table 21.1 gives an overview of these data and includes the respective references. The protein was purified from sources as varied as bovine brain, chicken heart, human breast cancer cells, or human plasma. The common denominator in the purification protocols is heparin-affinity chromatography and this is frequently reflected in the name chosen by different laboratories (see Table 21.1). cDNAs were isolated from several of these sources as well as from a number of others including human placenta, bovine uterus, and murine osteoblastic cells (Table 21.1). Owing to its diverse activities, we decided to use the name pleiotrophin for this protein that was originally proposed by Li *et al.* (3). Protein sequence comparisons ultimately revealed that PTN belongs to a novel family of HBGFs together with the closely related protein MK (Fig. 21.1).

Protein structure of pleiotrophin

The secreted portion of the PTN protein is comprised of 135 or 136 amino acids (depending on the species) 21% of which are lysine residues (Fig. 21.1). This makes the protein very basic in nature (pK of 9.5) and explains part of its affinity for heparin and heparan sulphates. Two additional, C-terminally shortened forms of the bovine PTN protein described earlier are most likely due to protease activity during tissue extraction (4). The most distinctive feature of the PTN and of the MK protein are 10 cysteine residues, the relative positions of which are conserved between both proteins. PTN as well as MK appear to form intramolecular disulphide bridges (5,6) that generate a relatively rigid three-dimensional structure for these proteins. The disulphide bridges lend stability to the proteins with respect to physicochemical attack by changes in pH, osmolarity, or organic solvents, but make them highly sensitive to reducing conditions. Indeed, studies from our laboratory showed that PTN is resistant to 1 mol/l acetic acid, acetonitrile, and high salt concentrations, but is inactivated by reducing agents such as dithiothreitol or beta-mercaptoethanol (7). This latter feature, among many others, distinguishes PTN from FGFs, inasmuch as molecules such as FGF-1 and -2 are resistant to reducing conditions due to lack of disulphide bridges.

No major post-translational modification, other than cleavage of the secretory signal peptide, seems to take place during PTN maturation. This is based on direct

Table 21.1. Different names and sources of members of the PTN/MK gene family

Abbreviation	Name	Source	Tissue	Species	GenBank accession no.	Reference
PTN						
HARP	Heparin-affinity regulated protein	Protein	Brain	Bovine		17
HB-GAM	Heparin-binding growth-associated molecule	Protein	Heart	Chicken		6
HBGF-8	Heparin-binding growth factor-8	Protein	Uterus	Bovine		9
p18	Protein 18 kDa	Protein	Brain	Rat		8
p18	Protein 18 kDa	Protein	Brain	Bovine		5
PTN	Pleiotrophin	Protein	BCC	Human		7
PTN	Pleiotrophin	Protein	Plasma	Human		83
HB-GAM	Heparin-binding growth-associated molecule	cDNA	Brain	Rat	J05657	74
HBNF	Heparin-binding neurotrophic factor	cDNA	Brain	Rat		78
HBNF	Heparin-binding neurotrophic factor	cDNA	Brain	Human	M57399	28
OSF-1	Osteoblast-specific factor-1	cDNA	Osteoblast	Mouse	D90225	79
PTN	Pleiotrophin	cDNA	BCC	Human		7
PTN	Pleiotrophin	cDNA	Placenta	Human	X52946, U71456	3, 33
PTN	Pleiotrophin	cDNA	Uterus	Bovine	X52945	3
HG-GAM	Heparin-binding growth-associated molecule	Genomic	Liver	Mouse		82
HBNF	Heparin-binding neurotrophic factor	Genomic	Placenta	Human		83
OSF-1	Osteoblast-specific factor 1	Genomic	Liver	Mouse		40
PTN	Pleiotrophin	Genomic	Brain	Human		37
PTN	Pleiotrophin	Genomic	Placenta	Human	L33338	34, 38
PTN	Pleiotrophin	Genomic	Fibroblast	Human	U71455	33
MK						
ARAP	Amphiregulin-associated protein	Protein	BCC	Human		77
MK	Midkine	Protein	ECC	Mouse		26
MK	Midkine	cDNA	ECC	Mouse		24
MK	Midkine	cDNA	Kidney	Human		82
MK	Midkine	cDNA	Head	*X. laevis*	U06048	42
RI-HB	Retinoic acid-inducible heparin-binding	cDNA	Embryo	Chicken		76
MK	Midkine	Genomic	Placenta	Human	D90540	43
MK	Midkine	Genomic	BALB/c	Mouse	J05447	40

BCC, breast cancer cells; cDNA, cDNA library; genomic, genomic library; ECC, embryonal carcinoma cells.

amino acid sequencing of the molecule (5) as well as the molecular mass determined by mass spectrometry. The latter technique demonstrated a mass of 15 291 for PTN which was almost identical to the mass predicted from the amino acid composition (= 15 289) (6). The discrepancy between the apparent molecular mass of PTN of 18 kDa read from sodium dodecylsulphate (SDS)–polyacrylamide gels (PAGE) and the true molecular mass is probably due to its high basic amino acid content which make the protein adsorb additional SDS molecules and thus migrate slower than predicted (7).

The mature, secreted portion of PTN is very highly conserved between species (Fig. 21.1). Mouse, rat and human PTN are identical, bovine PTN has only one amino acid substitution (pro[115] → ser[115]) and chicken PTN has seven substitutions plus one amino acid deletion (ser[121]). This strong conservation indicates that the activity of the protein is very sensitive to minimal changes in its amino acid sequence that would affect its three-dimensional structure. This suggests a very rigid structure fixed by the correct positioning of the disulphide bonds in concert with other weak interactions in the molecule. In contrast with this, the secretory signal peptide diverges between species. Obviously, secretory signal peptides do not affect the activity of the 'business' portion of the growth factor but confer only a generic property to the gene product, i.e. to direct the nascent protein to the endoplasmic reticulum.

(a)
```
     hPTN    -32                        MQAQQYQQQRRKFAAAFLAFIFILAAVDTAEA    -1
     mPTN    -32                        .SS...............L.............    -1
     rPTN    -32                        .SS...............L.............    -1
     bPTN    -32                        ..TP..L........................    -1
     cPTN    n.d.
     mMK     -21                        MQHRG..LLTLA..L..LTS.V.            -1


                          x
     hPTN    +1    GKKEKPEKKVKKSDCGEWQWSVCVPTSGDCGLGTREGTRTGAECKQTMKTQ    +51
     rPTN    +1    ..................................................    +51
     mPTN    +1    ..................................................    +51
     bPTN    +1    ..................................................    +51
     cPTN    +1    .........A..............N...................T...    +51
     mMK     +1    K....VKKG---.E.S..T.GP.T.S.K...M.F....-----.GAQTQRV    +43


                          x
     hPTN    +52   RCKIPCNWKKQFGAECKYQFQAWGECDLNTALKTRTGSLKRALHNAECQKT    +102
     rPTN    +52   ..................................................    +102
     mPTN    +52   ..................................................    +102
     bPTN    +52   ..................................................    +102
     cPTN    +52   K..............................N.............    +102
     mMK     +44   H..V......E...D...K.ES..A..G..GT.A.Q.T..K.RY..Q..E.    +94


                          x
     hPTN    +103  VTISKPCGKLTKPKPQAESKKKKKEGKKQEKMLD    +136
     rPTN    +103  ................................    +136
     mPTN    +103  ................................    +136
     bPTN    +103  ..........S.....................    +136
     cPTN    +103  ..................Z.-...........B    +135
     mMK     +95   IRVT...TSK..S.TK.KKG.G.D            +118
```

(b)
```
     hMK           -22                        MQHRGFLLLTLLALLALTSAVA    -1
     mMK           -22                        ......F..A.....VV.....    -1
     cMK (RI-HB)   -21                        ..P..L...-.AL..LAAA.E.    -1
     xMK           -21                        .EL.A.CVI-..ITVLAV.SQ.    -1


                               x
     hMK           +1    KKKDK--VKKGGPGSECAEWAWGPCTPSSKDCGVGFREGTCGAQTQRIRCRV    +50
     mMK           +1    ...E.........---...S..T.............M.............VH.K.    +47
     cMK (RI-HB)   +1    A.AK.EKM..E--....QD.H....I.N.....L.Y...S..DESRKLK.KI    +50
     xMK           +1    A.NK.EKG..G--A.D.T..T...S.IFN.....A.T.....KEE.RKLK.KI    +50


                               x
     hMK           +51   PCNWKKEFGADCKYKFENWCACDCCTGTKVRQGTLKKARYNAQCQETIRVTK    +102
     mMK           +48   ................S......S....A.................    +99
     cMK (RI-HB)   +51   ......K...........S..G.SAK..V.T.S.I....L...E.E.VVY.S.    +102
     xMK           +51   L..T..A...........T.E.NAT..N...S......L...D..Q.VEA..    +102


                               x
     hMK           +103  PCTPKTKAKAKAKKGKGKD    +121
     mMK           +100  ...S...S.T.........    +118
     cMK (RI-HB)   +103  ...A.M.............    +121
     xMK           +103  ..SL...S.S.G......E    +121
```

Figure 21.1. Comparison of the amino acid sequences of (a) pleiotrophin (PTN) and (b) midkine (MK) from different species. Amino acid comparison of rat (r), mouse (m), bovine (b), *Xenopus laevis* (x) and chicken (c) MK as well as PTN to the human (h) PTN or MK sequence, respectively. The signal peptide of chicken PTN has not yet been defined (n.d.). (References for PTN: 5,6,34,39,40,74; for MK: 40,42,43,75,76). Dots represent identical amino acids in comparison with the human sequence. Hyphens indicate gaps introduced for optimal alignment and (x) mark the boundaries of the four coding exons. The conserved 10 cysteines are emphasized by bold letters.

Biological activity of pleiotrophin

Activity on neurites

The biological activity of the PTN protein was a matter of controversy between different laboratories, although neurite outgrowth-promoting activities were attributed to the protein by all reports. However, this activity was observed at concentrations varying by over 100-fold between different laboratories. PTN purified from rat brain as well as bovine brain showed neurite outgrowth activity on perinatal rat brain neurons in a range of 10 ng/ml to 1.2 μg/ml (5,8). Preparations from chicken showed neurite extension activities for chicken embryo-derived neurites by 0.5 μg/ml of protein (6). We observed neurite extension of newborn rat hippocampal neurites due to recombinant PTN from mammalian cells in the low ng/ml range (unpublished observations). This concentration range is compatible with concentrations of the protein required to exert other mitogenic effects discussed in the next section. We believe that PTN preparations that require very high concentrations (over 1 μg/ml) to observe effects on neurite outgrowth contain only a small fraction of correctly folded, biologically active protein. Alternatively this rather non-specific effect may be due to the high lysine content of PTN comparable with the effects of poly-lysine coating of dishes that serves to improve cell attachment.

Activity on fibroblasts and epithelial cells

In contrast with the neurite outgrowth activity of PTN, laboratories differ in their reports about the mitogenic activity. We reported that a purified preparation of PTN stimulates colony formation in soft agar of the epithelial cell line SW-13 and we identified PTN in this preparation by protein sequencing (7). Furthermore, PTN was purified from bovine uterus using NIH 3T3 mitogenesis as an indicator of growth factor activity (9). However, other investigators have disputed an intrinsic growth factor activity of PTN and have attributed the activities to FGFs or other growth factors contaminating the respective preparations (5,6,10,11). To resolve this controversy we expressed the human PTN cDNA in two human cell lines (adrenal carcinoma cells, SW-13; embryonal kidney cells, 293) and tested its biological activity. A point mutant cDNA with a premature translation stop codon served as a negative control in these experiments (12). We showed that PTN collected and purified from the conditioned media of transfected cells stimulated colony formation in soft agar of SW-13 epithelial cells as well as of normal rat kidney fibroblasts (NRK cells) (12). Furthermore, PTN expressed in SW-13 cells showed autocrine activity in transient trans-

fections (12,13) as well as after stable integration (12) and induced colony formation of the transfected cells in soft agar. As a reflection of the autocrine activity, non-tumorigenic SW-13 cells transfected with a PTN expression vector grew as tumours in athymic nude mice. In agreement with these results, Chauhan et al. (14) reported that expression of bovine PTN in NIH 3T3 cells induced focus formation, anchorage-independent growth, and tumour formation in nude mice. Therefore, PTN can function as an autocrine and paracrine growth factor in tumours, and exhibits transforming activity in addition to its potential role as a neurite outgrowth factor during brain development.

To address the question of biological activity of PTN in tumours in an independent manner, we used PTN-targeted ribozymes to reduce PTN mRNA in tumour cells with high endogenous levels of this growth factor and study growth factor activity released from the cells as well as phenotypic changes (13). In human melanoma cells this reduction of PTN mRNA and protein reduced the mitogenic activity secreted into the media of the cells to background. Furthermore, tumour growth and metastasis of the melanoma cells was reduced or abolished as a consequence of the PTN targeting (13,15). Experiments with anti-sense deoxyoligonucleotides as drugs and with expression of anti-sense RNA in PTN-positive cells showed the same effect and support the role of PTN in tumour growth independently (details are discussed below in the section on 'Molecular targeting of PTN', p. 284).

Endothelial cell and angiogenic activity

Originally, PTN purified from bovine brain was shown to induce mitogenesis for endothelial cells (16,17). However, these findings were challenged, as mentioned above, and some of the activities were attributed to contaminations with FGFs. We prepared recombinant human PTN from transfected human cells (see above section) and tested these preparations on human umbilical vein endothelial cells (HUVEC) as well as fetal bovine heart endothelial cells (FBHE). Both cell types were stimulated by recombinant PTN in the low ng/ml range (12). Recently D. Barritault's laboratory also demonstrated endothelial cell mitogenic activity of recombinant, purified, human PTN (18) that was produced in NIH 3T3 fibroblasts. They used bovine brain capillary cells as target cells and showed that at 1 ng/ml PTN is half-maximally effective in stimulating ^{3}H-thymidine incorporation into these cells. As a further assay, they demonstrated tube formation of endothelial cells in collagen gels by PTN. These data corroborate our findings in a similar assay testing for HUVEC tube formation in Matrigel due to addition of PTN (unpublished data). Finally, recent studies from our laboratory with human melanoma showed that reduction of PTN by ribozyme targeting reduced angiogenesis and subsequently growth of tumours *in vivo* (15).

Active and inactive forms of pleiotrophin

As mentioned above, different laboratories prepared recombinant PTN and have found different extents of bioactivity. In addition, several commercial suppliers sell recombinant PTN prepared in insect cells and, as of the writing of this chapter, none of these preparations have shown any biological activity in the low ng/ml range. In our experiments we found that recombinant PTN produced from a baculovirus vector in Sf9 insect cells was inactive and attributed that to improper formation of disulphide bonds in this expression system or post-secretion modifications of the protein in non-mammalian cells (see discussion in reference 12). On the other hand, not all preparations generated in mammalian cells appear to be equally active and discussions with numerous investigators as well as our experiments have shown that PTN produced in transfected NIH 3T3 or COS cells shows very varied activity.

A recent study from D. Barritault's laboratory could be one step in understanding this variability of activity (18). This group purified PTN from the supernatants of transfected NIH 3T3 cells and purified active material from this preparation by heparin-affinity and ion-exchange chromatography. They then went on to show that two distinct forms of PTN were eluted in two separate peaks recovered after the final purification step. A mitogenically active PTN protein showed the N-terminal sequence of NH_2-AEAGKKEKPE. In contrast with this, protein that was purified from brain and uterus or after expression in *Escherichia coli* was inactive and lacked the first three amino acids: The N-terminus was determined as NH_2-GKKEKPE. Obviously the signal peptide cleavage site is ambivalent between these two forms of the protein. They conclude that mitogenic activity of PTN is dependent on the extended protein form, whereas the 'truncated' form still possesses a partial native conformation which is sufficient to promote neurite outgrowth.

In our hands the N-terminal sequence of biologically active PTN purified from human breast cancer cells did not show the N-terminal extension (7) and was not different from the N-terminus of inactive protein generated in Sf9 insect cells (12). However, we cannot exclude that the N-terminal extension proposed by D. Barritault's laboratory was cleaved during the preparation of our active protein for amino acid sequencing. On the other hand, the loss of a few amino acids at the N-terminus may also indi-

cate further changes in the protein conformation. Our current working hypothesis is that the signal peptide cleavage site in the endoplasmic reticulum (ER) may depend on the folding of the PTN protein during translation. We hypothesize that with a co-translationally correctly folded PTN only part of the signal peptide is accessible to the signal peptidase in the ER and hydrolysis will occur at a less favoured site to yield NH_2-AEAGKKEKP as an N-terminus. However, if the folding process of the PTN protein is disturbed or cannot be carried out properly (*e.g.* in insect cells) cleavage will occur at a different site more prone to the cleavage by the signal peptidase to yield NH_2-GKKEKP as an N-terminus. As an alternative to this hypothesis, loss of the N-terminal AEA group in the PTN protein could be a symptom of an improperly folded protein that is prone to easy hydrolytic loss of this extension. It may also be argued that the loss of the AEA extension could trigger unfolding of the PTN protein and thus loss of activity. Ongoing work in our laboratory with different constructs and biochemical analysis of protein products from different systems should resolve these questions.

Receptor(s) and heparan sulphate proteoglycyan binding sites of pleiotrophin

N-syndecan

The first data that suggested specific binding of PTN to cell membranes were published by Kuo *et al.* (5). They reported binding of PTN on NIH 3T3 and PC12 rat pheochromocytoma cells with an apparent dissociation constant (K_d) of 8 nmol/l (=120 ng/ml) determined by Scatchard plot analysis. These experiments were performed with PTN that had been acid-treated during the purification procedure. In a later study a 14-fold lower K_d for PTN receptor binding on NIH 3T3 cells (0.6 nM = 10 ng/ml) was found when acid treatment was omitted during the purification procedure of the PTN ligand (19). Approximately 5000 high-affinity sites per cell were detected with this latter procedure. Gel electrophoresis with cross-linked PTN/binding site complex showed two bands of 150 kDa and 127 kDa. Competition of the complex formation was only possible with 100-fold excess of PTN but not with other known mitogenic factors — platelet-derived growth factor (PDGF), epidermal growth factor (EGF), acidic fibroblast growth factor (aFGF), basic fibroblast growth factor (bFGF), insulin — demonstrating specificity of the complex. A potent inhibitor for the receptor binding activity of PTN was identified as heparin (50% inhibition with 0.4 μg/ml of heparin). Identical binding sites were also found on NRK (normal rat kidney), SK-BR3 (human mammary adenocarcinoma), PC12 (rat pheochromocytoma), A431 (human epidermoid carcinoma), HepG2 (human hepatocellular carcinoma), and NB41A3 (mouse neuroblastoma) cells. However, it is not clear whether these binding sites represent a transmembrane signal transducing unit or a low-affinity heparan sulphate proteoglycan binding site for storage of the protein on the cell surface. Recent data show that PTN binds with a similar binding constant to N-syndecan, a heparan sulphate proteoglycan (20). In this latter study ligand-affinity chromatography was used to purify proteins directly binding to PTN. Perinatal rat brain and brain neurons served as a source of material and recombinant PTN was prepared from a baculovirus expression system in insect cells. In these experiments N-syndecan, a cell surface proteoglycan of 120 kDa was isolated and identified by immunochemical analysis and peptide sequencing. As expected, soluble heparin was a potent inhibitor of the complex formation, but also bFGF was identified as a competitor for the binding of PTN to the N-syndecan receptor.

Tyrosine and serine phosphorylation in response to pleiotrophin

Li and Deuel (21) reported that a 200 kDa protein is phosphorylated in NIH 3T3 fibroblasts and mouse neuroblastoma (NB41A3) cells 5 min after stimulation with PTN. The phosphorylation maximum was reached in the fibroblasts after 15 min using 150 ng/ml mitogenically active PTN purified from bovine uterus. For NB41A3 cells a dose-dependent response was observed between 20 and 250 ng/ml using purified PTN from rat brain. Immunoprecipitation with anti-phosphotyrosine antibodies and phosphoamino acid analysis indicated that tyrosine and serine residues are phosphorylated on the 200 kDa protein after stimulation with PTN. Still, it is not clear whether the 200 kDa phosphorylated protein is also the receptor to which PTN binds and whether other mediator molecules participate in the signal transduction. On the other hand, these results suggest that protein kinase activities are involved in transmitting the PTN signal at least in NIH 3T3 and NB41A3 cells.

In conclusion, PTN signal transduction appears to involve both heparan sulphate proteoglycans and transmembrane-acting kinases. This is similar to the paradigm demonstrated for FGF receptor signalling (1,22,23). To what extent an interaction between the heparan sulphate and PTN is required for signal transduction and how PTN initiates downstream cellular responses is not known at present.

Discovery and protein structure of midkine

The MK gene was originally discovered in mouse cDNA libraries by differential hybridization with probes generated from mRNA of retinoid acid (RA)-treated and non-treated embryonal carcinoma (EC) cells (24). MK expression was found to be increased in the first 48 h of RA-induced differentiation of EC cells. In addition, during mouse embryogenesis, MK was abundantly expressed during mid-gestation (days 8–13 of the 20 day gestation period). In contrast with this, in adult mice MK was only detectable in the kidney. The name of this protein is based on this expression pattern in *mid*-gestation and in the *kid*ney. In parallel with this, another laboratory reported the isolation of a very similar protein from chicken embryos, that was localized in basement membranes of early embryonic tissues (25). This protein was named RA-inducible, heparin-binding protein (RI-HB) and appears to be the chicken homologue of MK (Table 21.1, Fig. 21.1).

MK, like PTN, is a secreted, basic, heparin-binding protein that can be found in conditioned media of RA-treated, differentiated mouse EC cells or in 11 day old chicken embryos. SDS–PAGE analyses revealed an apparent molecular mass of 15.5 kDa (mouse) and 19 kDa (chicken) (25,26). The discrepancy between the predicted molecular mass of 13.2 kDa and the apparent mass read from the gel electrophoresis is due to the high content of basic amino acids very similar to PTN. The mature, secreted MK protein consists of 122 amino acids in human, chicken, and frog and 118 amino acids in mouse. The hydrophobic secretory signal peptide, delineated from the N-terminal sequence of the secreted chicken MK protein (25) consists of 21 or 22 amino acids depending on the species. The protein is highly conserved across different species but shows more variability between species than PTN (Fig. 21.1). However, the relative positions of all of the 10 cysteine residues are conserved between MK from different species as well as between MK and PTN. The sequence similarity between MK and PTN and the conserved positions of the cysteine residues suggests a very similar three-dimensional structure of both proteins and perhaps shared receptors.

Biological activity of midkine

MK was described by different laboratories as a protein with differentiation and mitogenic activity. Native chicken MK (27), as well as recombinant human and mouse MK protein expressed in bacteria (28) and in mammalian cells (29,30), showed neurite outgrowth-promoting activity on PC12 cells and primary neuronal cells from rat or chicken sympathetic neurons. Native mouse MK protein tested on P19 EC cells induced differentiation (31). However, like PTN, the mitogenic activity data for MK are controversial. Native mouse MK as well as chicken MK protein were described as mitogenically active on PC12 cells (27,32). Recombinant mouse MK protein was described as a weak mitogen for 10T1/2 fibroblasts and as a potent mitogen for neuroectodermal precursor cell types generated by RA treatment of 1009 EC cells. On the other hand this preparation was inactive for more mature 1009-derived neuronal cell types as well as for swiss3T3 fibroblasts (30) and NRK cells (29). Native chicken MK protein failed to show mitogenic activity for bovine epithelial lens cells (25), 3T3 fibroblasts, human and bovine umbilical vein endothelial and CC139 cells (27). Furthermore, human recombinant MK protein expressed in bacteria also failed to show mitogenic activity on aortic endothelial cells and NIH 3T3 fibroblasts (28).

Similar to the approach taken with PTN (see above), we expressed the human MK cDNA in the human adrenal carcinoma cell line SW-13 and analysed the phenotype of transiently and stably transfected cells as well as the activity of secreted proteins. Heparin-affinity purified MK harvested from the conditioned media of these transfected cells stimulated colony formation of parent SW-13 cells and proliferation of human brain and umbilical vein endothelial cells. Furthermore, SW-13 cells expressing high levels of MK grew into tumours in athymic nude mice (unpublished). This suggests a very similar activity profile for MK compared with PTN. Whether both factors share the same receptor(s) currently is unclear, but our data suggest that the overlapping activities could be driven through the same receptors.

Genomic organization of pleiotrophin

Exon/intron structure

The PTN gene in different species contains at least six exons and the open reading frame is encoded on four of these. The first exon of the open reading frame codes for the hydrophobic leader sequence and a few amino acids of the secreted protein. The second and third exon contain the two cysteine-rich regions of the protein and the fourth exon codes for the C-terminal 17 amino acids as well as for the 3′-non-translated region with the polyadenylation signal (AATAAA) (33,34). Interestingly, the coding region for the MK protein is organized along the same domains as PTN and the amino acid boundaries between the different exons are conserved (Fig. 21.1).

Pleiotrophin gene promoter(s), transcription start site(s), and 5′ exons

Different laboratories originally reported one 5′-untranslated region (5′-UTR) exon (U1) for the human PTN gene (34–36) but they differed in their predicted transcription start sites based on primer extension or S1-nuclease mapping or cDNA cloning (35–37). We detected a second, more 5′-UTR exon in this area (U2) (38) and our data suggest that the deletion analysis of a presumed promoter in this region may have been affected critically by interference with splicing events. Very recently we reported that a human endogenous retrovirus (HERV) is inserted into the human (but not the murine) PTN gene in the intron immediately upsteam of the coding region (Figure 21.2; reference 33). We demonstrated that due to this retroviral insertion, a phylogenetically new promoter is generated that drives the expression of HERV–PTN fusion transcripts with high tissue-selectivity in trophoblast-derived cells and in choriocarcinomas. The HERV-PTN fusion transcript contains a full-length coding region for the protein product and biologically active PTN protein was detected in the supernatants of trophoblast-derived choriocarcinomas. Taken together, these data suggest that alternative splicing events and/or different promoters are utilized to generate the time-dependent and tissue-specific expression patterns of PTN (37–40).

Size and chromosomal location of the pleiotrophin gene

Currently the size of the human and mouse PTN genes can only be estimated as the 5′-ends of the primary transcripts have not been defined and overlapping genomic clones for known introns have not been reported. We estimate based on restriction enzyme and hybridization analysis of genomic DNA and genomic clones that the genes span ≥50 kbp. The human PTN gene is localized on chromosome 7q33–34 (35,36), and the mouse PTN gene maps to chromosome 6, together with the same genes as human PTN (MET/TCRB, Table 21.2) (35).

Regulation of pleiotrophin gene expression

PTN is regulated in a tissue-specific and time-dependent manner during ontogenesis and appears to be up-regulated during malignant transformation. Only a few (33) regulatory regions have been defined. However, in studies of steady-state MRNA levels, induction of PTN gene expression was reported for serum-starved NIH 3t3 cells after treatment with 100 ng/ml of PDGF for 2 h (41). Furthermore, a sevenfold increase in PTN transcripts after treatment for 9 days with

Table 21.2. General characteristics of the PTN/MK gene family

Name	Species	Signal peptide	Mature protein	mRNA (kb)	Gene (kbp)	Exons	Chromosome	Loci and linkage
PTN	Human	32 aa	136 aa	~1.5	≥50	≥9	7q33–34	Between MET and TCRB
PTN	Mouse	32 aa	136 aa	~1.5	≥50	≥7	6	Between MET and TCRB
MK	Human	22 aa	122 aa	~1,2	~1.5	≥5	11p11.2	
MK	Mouse	22 aa	118 aa	~1,2	~2	≥7	2	Near Hox 4.2

aa, amino acid; kb, kilobase; kbp, kilobasepair; PTN, pleiotrophin; MK, midkine.

RA was described for the human EC cell line NT2/D1 (28). preliminary studies from our laboratory also showed that PTN MRNA is up-regulated after 3 days of RA treatment of MDA-MB 231 human breast cancer cells (unpublished). However, in other studies RA failed to induce PTN gene e- xpression in NIH 3t3 or f9 ec cells (41). Whether these effects on steady-state MRNA are direct transcriptional events will need to be assessed in future studies.

Genomic organization of midkine

Gene structure and chromosomal location of midkine

MK is a highly conserved gene between different species as far apart as human and *Xenopus laevis* (42). The MK protein is encoded on four exons that contain the same protein domains as the four exons coding for the PTN protein (Fig. 21.2, Table 21.2). However, the introns in the MK gene are much smaller resulting in a much smaller size of the gene (human MK = 1.5 kb; mouse MK = 2 kb). The human MK gene is organized in five exons and four introns (43), whereas the mouse gene consists of seven exons and only four introns (40). This apparent discrepancy in the exon/intron number of the murine MK gene is due to the fact that the second through fourth exon are not separated by in- tervening sequences but alternatively serve as introns during differential splicing into MK1, MK2, and MK3 mRNA (Fig. 21.2). MK2 is the major transcript in RA-treated EC cells (MK1 : MK2 : MK3 = 1 : 15 : 2) and the only RA-respon- sive form (26). This is most likely due to increased transcrip- tion as well as increased stability of the MK2 mRNA.

The human MK gene is located on chromosome 11p11.2 (43,44) whereas the mouse MK gene mapped to chromosome 2 near the locus Hox 4.2 (45) (Table 21.2).

Regulation of midkine gene expression

The first MK cDNA was isolated by differential screening for RA-induced genes in the clonal mouse EC cell line

HM-1. Kadomatsu *et al.* (1988) (24) reported a significant increase in MK gene expression after RA-induced dif- ferentiation of HM-1 cells into myoblasts. RA-induced expression of the MK gene was also found in F9 (mouse), and NT2/D1 (human teratocarcinoma) EC cells (28,40,41). In contrast with this, Nurcombe *et al.* (30) failed to observe this effect of RA in P19 EC and in pluripotent embryonic stem cells (ES), whereas others detected MK protein only when P19 cells were treated with RA (31). These discrepan- cies have been ascribed to differences in P19 cell sublines.

Recently, the mapping and characterization of an RA- responsive enhancer approximately 900 nucleotides upstream of the MK2 mRNA transcription start site was reported for the mouse gene (46). Transfection of an MK promoter/ CAT reporter construct in EC, F9, and HM-1 cells demonstrated a five-to 10-fold induction of CAT ac- tivity by RA after 48 h. Interestingly, cells in which RA did not affect endogenous MK gene expression also failed to show RA responsiveness of the transfected MK/CAT con- struct (PYS-2, extra-embryonic endoderm cells). Deletion mutagenesis located the RA-response element to the −1006 to −794 region and demonstrated that the element has en- hancer-like properties based on position- and orientation- independence. The core element was mapped to positions −976 to −951. Binding of an RA-receptor heterodimer (mRAR-alpha/mRXR-alpha) to this core element (−976 GGGTC<u>TGCCCC</u>GATCC<u>TGACC</u>TCTGC −951) was verified using gel shift analysis. These data suggest, that RA can directly regulate the transcription of the murine MK gene. Recently (47), the same group identified a similar DR5-type RA-responsive element in the human MK gene localized in a region highly conserved between the human and mouse (−1000 to −1016).

Common ancestry of the midkine and pleiotrophin genes

Owing to their sequence similarities and conservation across different species, it is reasonable to assume that the MK and PTN gene evolved from a common ancestor. Approximately 500 million years are discussed as the

281

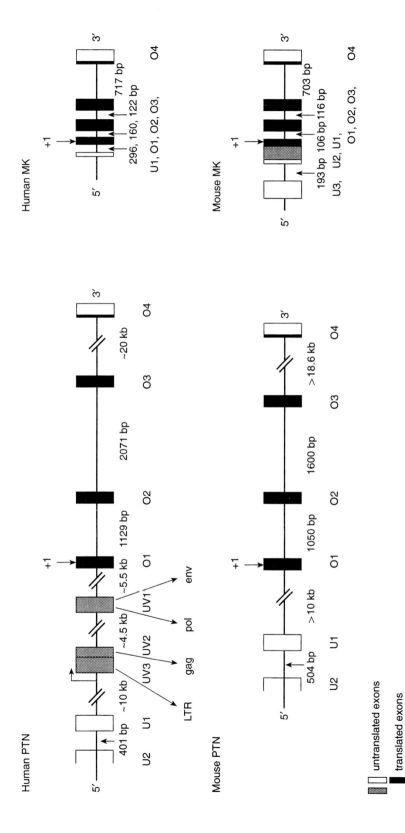

Figure 21.2. Comparison of the gene structure of pleiotrophin (PTN) and midkine (MK) in different species. Exons are represented by boxes whereas introns are depicted as lines. Translated exons are indicated by filled boxes. Open boxes indicate undefined 5'-ends. References are given in the text.

divergence time between the two genes (48). Recent discovery of an MK pseudogene in the mouse but not the human genome supports this conclusion. Based on the accumulation of nucleotide substitutions in the MK pseudogene, it appears to have been generated 19.1 million years ago and thus after the human/mouse divergence estimated at 85 million years ago.

Pleiotrophin and midkine expression during development

Nervous system

The physiological role of MK and PTN appears to be confined to different stages and tissues during development. MK is detected earlier and appears to be involved in early cell proliferation, differentiation and organogenesis in the whole rodent embryo. In contrast, the PTN gene is activated during later stages and preferentially in the brain and peripheral nervous system. In contrast to MK, PTN retains its expression in some areas of the adult rat brain, but is markedly decreased after the postnatal period (to less than 1/10). We found that PTN expression in the human adult is the highest in brain but also detectable in testis, prostate, heart, and placenta by Northern blot. Very weak signals were observed in lung, spleen, and small intestine (33). Whether the expression in the peripheral adult human tissues is limited to the peripheral nervous system or extends to the parenchyme of the different organs has not yet been studied.

The restricted expression pattern during development suggests that both cytokines play a significant part for cell growth and differentiation as well as organogenesis. The role in brain development is especially interesting as each of the factors seems to have a distinct expression pattern. Whereas expression of MK peaks in the brain in the murine mid-gestation stage (mouse embryonic days 7–11), PTN is expressed in the late embryonic to early postnatal stage (rat embryonic day 19 to postnatal day 21) (8,24). MK is expressed transiently in all murine cell lineages, whereas the expression of PTN is restricted in the rat to many, but not all neuroectodermal and mesodermal cell lineages and not expressed in endodermal, ectodermal, and trophoblast cells (49,50). Furthermore, PTN undergoes a cell-type switch in its expression pattern in the nervous system after the perinatal period which suggests that PTN has a part in maintenance of the neuronal function in the adult rat.

Comprehensive *in situ* hybridization studies in the developing and adult rat nervous system showed, that PTN is primarily expressed by neuroglial progenitor cells in the subependymal layer of the CNS during embryogenesis. During the perinatal stage, neurons as well as glial cells express PTN at high levels. Finally, in the adult brain, PTN expression is markedly reduced and restricted to specific neuronal subpopulations of the hippocampus (CA1-3 region) and the cerebral cortex (laminae II–IV). In the peripheral nervous system, PTN mRNA is detectable in ganglionic neurons during embryogenesis, whereas in the adult animal, PTN expression switches to the satellite cells of the ganglia (51,52).

Other tissues

In the 15 day embryo, only the kidney still expresses MK significantly and this expression is maintained into adulthood, although at lower levels. *In situ* hybridization studies revealed that MK expression is localized to the proximal tubules and metaplastic Bowman's epithelium, but is not expressed in other nephron segments such as glomeruli, loop of Henle, distal tubules, and collecting ducts in the kidney of adult mice (53). The chicken MK homologue RI-HB is expressed within the basement membranes in early embryonic tissues and detectable after the 18th day of embryonic life only in eye basement membranes (25). MK mRNA was also detected in adult human tissues. The intestine showed the highest levels whereas the thyroid, lung alveoli, colon, spleen, and kidney showed weaker signals (54).

In addition to brain, PTN is expressed in the basal layers of the tongue epithelium, testis, uterus (with an up-regulation during pregnancy), meninges, and iris of the adult rodent (50). As mentioned above, we found PTN expressed in Northern blots with human adult brain, but also detectable in testis, prostate, heart, and placenta and very faintly in lung, spleen, and small intestine (33, and unpublished data).

Furthermore, we studied whether PTN and MK are regulated during mammary gland development. Preliminary data show that PTN is expressed in the mammary gland of virgin mice, most likely restricted to epithelial cells. MK was not detectable. Interestingly, after a single pregnancy, PTN is permanently down-regulated in the glands. Oestrogen plus progesterone treatment was able to mimic this down-regulation whereas each hormone alone showed no effect. Thus, PTN appears to be involved in the terminal development of the female mammary gland occurring during the first pregnancy (Missner and Wellstein, unpublished).

Table 21.3. Presence of PTN and MK mRNA in different cell lines and tissues

Origin	Special characteristics	PTN	MK
Cell lines			
Breast cancer	Oestrogen receptor (ER)		
MCF-7	+	–	+
MCF-7/ADr	+	+	+
MDA-MB-231	–	+	+
MDA-MB-361	–	+	ND
MDA-MB-134	–	–	ND
MDA-MB-435	–	–	ND
MDA-MB-453	–	–	ND
MDA-MB-468	–	–	ND
SK-BR-3	–	–	ND
HS-578T	–	+	+
T47Dco	+	+	–
T47D/wt	+	–	+
ZR-75-1	+	–	ND
BT-474	–	–	ND
BT-549	–	–	ND
Prostate cancer			
PC3		+	ND
DU-145		–	ND
LNCaP		–	ND
LNCap/H26		–	ND
Cervix cancer			
ME-180	Epidermoid carcinoma	–	+
SiHa	Squamous carcinoma	+	+
Ovarian carcinoma			
A1827		+	ND
PA-1	Teratocarcinoma	+	+
A2780		–	ND
OVCAR-2,-3,-4		–	ND
Chorio carcinoma			
JEG-3		+	+
Lung cancer			
SW 900	Squamous carcinoma	+	+
NCI-H596	Adenosquamous carcinoma	–	+
NCI-H520	Squamous carcinoma	+	+
Bladder cancer			
SCaBER	Squamous carcinoma	+	+
Melanoma			
1205 LU	Metastatic melanoma	+	+
WM-852		+	+
WM-239A		+	ND
Melanocytes		–	ND
Epithelial cells			
SW 13	Adrenal cancer, non-tumorigenic	–	–

Table 21.3. *cont.*

Origin	Special characteristics	PTN	MK
Fibroblast cells			
NIH-3T3	Mouse fibroblasts	–	ND
NRK	Rat kidney fibroblasts clone 49	–	ND
Endothelial cells			
FBHE	Fetal bovine heart endothelium	–	ND
Tumour tissues:			
Human primary breast cancer		25 of 44	13 of 16
Rat carcinogen-induced mammary cancer		30 of 30	ND
Human head and neck cancer		3 of 4	4 of 4
Human brain tumours		12 of 15	5 of 15

ND, not done; +, mRNA detected; –, mRNA below detection; PTN, pleiotrophin; MK, midkine.

Pleiotrophin and midkine as tumour growth factors

Pleiotrophin

We originally purified PTN from supernatants of the highly tumorigenic human breast cancer cell line MDA-MB-231, and demonstrated that PTN present in the supernatants is an epithelial cell mitogen (7). Furthermore, we showed that expression of a human PTN cDNA can support tumour growth of non-tumorigenic SW-13 cells. SW-13/PTN cells grew into highly vascularized primary tumours when injected into a mammary fat pad (12) and recent data show that SW-13/PTN cells become metastatic in athymic nude mice (unpublished data). Similar tumour growth data were reported for NIH 3T3 cells after expression of a bovine PTN cDNA (14).

To test the potential significance of PTN gene expression for tumour growth, we analysed by Northern blot and/or RNase protection assay the PTN expression in randomly selected human breast ($n = 44$), head and neck ($n = 4$), and brain ($n = 15$) tumours as well as in 30 carcinogen-induced rat mammary carcinoma samples. We also analysed 38 cell lines of different origin and tumorigenic stage (Table 21.3) (12; and unpublished data). PTN was expressed in the majority of the breast cancer samples (60%), all of the carcinogen-induced mammary cancers, three of four head and neck cancers, and in most of the brain tumours. It is worth pointing out that in the brain tumour specimens, the PTN transcript level was much higher than in the normal brain control samples. In half of the tumorigenic cell lines of different origins we detected PTN (16 of 33), whereas in none of the non-tumorigenic or normal cells PTN mRNA was found. Melanoma cell lines belonged to the high PTN-expressing group whereas in melanocytes no PTN was detectable even by reverse transcriptase — polymerase chain reaction (RT–PCR). Interestingly, melanocytes originate form the neuroectoderm, the germ layer where PTN is highly expressed during embryonic development but down-regulated in the adult (see above). It appears that the gene becomes re-activated during malignant transformation of melanocytes.

A recent study reported a comparison of PTN expression in breast cancer specimens ($n = 23$) versus non-cancerous tissues ($n = 7$) using RT–PCR (55). PTN was detected in all of the non-cancerous tissues and in most of the cancer samples. Unfortunately, the study does not report relative amounts of transcripts and does not discuss the extreme sensitivity of RT–PCR, which can bias the assessment of the results. Furthermore, it is not clear whether the non-cancerous tissues were derived from normal areas of breast cancer surgical specimen or from other sources. Future studies with breast tissues should control for these parameters and quantitate the level of gene expression.

Another laboratory studied PTN expression in tumours by in situ hybridization. PTN was found selectively in the meningiothelial cells in 16 human benign meningiomas, and was not detectable in the stromal fibroblasts, blood vessels, and collagen bundles of meningiomas (56). Very recently, Nakagawara et al. (57) reported the expression of PTN in the majority of 72 human primary neuroblastoma samples by Northern analysis and they discuss a correlation between gene expression and less aggressive stages of the primary tumour.

Several lines of evidence suggest that PTN could contribute to the metastatic phenotype when expressed at high levels. We found that high expressors of PTN-transfected SW-13 cells form haematogenic metastases in the liver when injected intraperitoneally (unpublished data). Furthermore, the highest expressors of PTN, 1205LU human melanoma cells, form lung metastases after subcutaneous injection and immunodepletion studies showed that PTN is the major endothelial cell growth factor secreted from 1205LU melanoma cells. We selected this cell line as an additional model to study the contribution of PTN to tumour growth and metastasis. In a more non-specific approach we used the heparinoid pentosanpolysulphate (PPS) that was earlier shown to inhibit HBGFs from tumours in vivo (58). PPS blocked the stimulatory activity of PTN from melanoma cells in vitro, but did not affect the growth of the tumour cells themselves. Treatment of animals with PPS intraperitoneally did not affect subcutaneous growth of melanoma but prevented the development of lung metastases (60). In an independ-

ent series of experiments, we used molecular targeting of PTN with anti-sense deoxyoligonucleotides, anti-sense RNA, and ribozymes to elucidate the role of PTN in a more defined manner. We discuss these approaches in a separate section below (see 'Molecular targeting of PTN', p. 284).

Midkine

Comprehensive studies on the MK gene expression in human tumours were reported recently by Tsutsui et al. (54). They studied, by Northern analysis, the MK gene expression pattern in Wilms' tumour, neuroblastoma, and hepatocellular carcinoma samples as well as in xenografted tumour samples from lung, stomach, colorectal, oesophageal, and pancreatic cancer. In the majority of the samples MK transcripts were clearly identified in higher amounts than in normal control tissues. The MK gene was expressed in 70% of the tested tumour specimens (22 of 31) and was found at high levels in 50%. Expression patterns in the tumour samples appear very similar to PTN. It is worth emphasizing that MK expression is very restricted in adult normal tissues which makes this finding more significant. We have also studied MK expression in tumour samples. We detected low amounts of MK transcript in some of the brain tumour samples but not in normal brain areas. Furthermore, we found MK in the majority of breast cancer samples by Northern blot (unpublished). The breast cancer study by Garver et al. (55) discussed above, also reported the detection of MK in breast cancer samples by RT–PCR but did not detect MK in non-cancerous tissues. In addition, Nakagawara et al. (unpublished) recently described MK expression in almost all primary human neuroblastomas ($n = 72$) by Northern analysis. A very recent study correlated MK expression levels and poor outcome in patients with invasive bladder cancer (60). To our knowledge this is the first report which demonstrates that MK expression is of predictive value and suggests a direct functional role for this protein in the progression of clinical cancer.

MK is highly expressed in cell lines derived from Wilms' tumour, renal cell carcinoma, lung cancer, neuroblastoma, and stomach cancer whereas no MK transcript was detected in cells lines from Burkitt's lymphoma and T-cell leukaemia (54,55,57). Data from our laboratory on MK expression are summarized in Table 21.3.

Molecular targeting of pleiotrophin

The rationale for molecular targeting

The role of a given growth factor for tumour growth can only be assessed by specific targeting of the molecule of interest. The most feasible approach to specific targeting of a particular gene product is based on anti-sense technology (reviewed in references 61,62). In principle three different methods are useful: (i) anti-sense deoxyoligonucleotides that interfere with RNA splicing;(ii) anti-sense deoxyoligonucleotides that interfere with mRNA translation; and (iii) ribozymes that cleave defined RNA molecules. Splice inhibitors usually act by allosteric inhibition of the splicing apparatus and we are currently investigating their efficacy in targeting PTN. In addition, we are investigating phosphorothioate-based oligonucleotides that prevent translation of a specific mRNA and increase its degradation by endogenous RNases. We were able to demonstrate that such anti-sense deoxyoligonucleotides can inhibit tumour growth of some cell lines in animals (63,64). The major problem is the 'therapeutic index' for these deoxyoligonucleotides, i.e. their specific versus non-specific toxicities. The choice of a proper targeting site in the mRNA molecule appears to be the most crucial parameter for efficacy and selectivity of the anti-sense molecules used. As ribozyme targeting is a relatively new approach and was very successful in our hands, we will discuss this aspect in more detail.

Ribozyme targeting

Recently, the targeting of specific gene transcripts with ribozyme (Rz) constructs has been used successfully to inactivate gene products in cells and generate dominant-negative mutants (65–70). The principle of ribozyme targeting is that an RNA-derived RNase (the ribozyme) is targeted to a specific region in the gene transcript of interest. This is achieved by generating a catalytic core structure of the ribozyme and by targeting it to a defined substrate by virtue of anti-sense flanking sequences on either side of the catalytic core. Thus a very specific cleavage of a defined mRNA can be achieved. The principal structure of the ribozymes used by us and the predicted hybridization to one of the targeted mRNA sites in PTN is shown in Fig. 21.3 (13). One of the controls possible with this system is that the active enzyme can be point-mutated to generate only an anti-sense construct and thus distinguish between anti-sense and ribozyme activity.

One of the problems in the application of ribozymes as well as anti-sense deoxyoligonucleotides is the selection of one (or more) appropriate target site(s). To select regions in PTN for targeting by hammerhead ribozymes (66,67), we searched the predicted secondary structure of the PTN mRNA (71) for open loops that also contained the consensus sequence for ribozyme cleavage (5'-NUX sequence that is cleaved 3' of X; N is any nucleotide and X is either A, U or C) (73). From these potential sites we selected two within the open reading frame of the PTN mRNA that were 66 and 261 nucleotides downstream of the translation initiation site. Our ribozymes contain the same basic hammerhead structure designed by Haseloff and Gerlach (67) and were modified and minimized to a 22 nucleotide catalytic centre based on the mutational analysis that had shown the essential elements for a catalytically active RNA (72). As illustrated for Rz261 (see Fig. 21.3, based on reference 13), the molecule should form three double helices ('hammerhead') which meet at the targeted cleavage site. In addition, two stretches of nucleotides with the sequences 5'-CUGAXGA and 5'-GAAA (X is either A, U, or C) are required for the catalytic activity. The cleavage is directed to a specific site in the targeted RNA by two stretches of eight to 12 nucleotides each that flank the catalytic centre on its 3' and 5' side. These flanking sequences hybridize with the targeted RNA by Watson–Crick base pairing (reviewed in reference 69).

In a PTN-responsive cell line (SW-13; 7,12), co-transfection of PTN and of ribozymes specifically prevented the PTN-induced growth of the cells. A catalytically inactive, point-mutant ribozyme (72,73) was inactive in this assay (13). In human melanoma cells that constitutively express high levels of PTN mRNA, stable transfection with PTN-targeted ribozymes quenched production and secretion of PTN, inhibited colony formation of the melanoma cells in soft agar (Fig. 21.3) and prevented their growth into tumours in athymic nude mice (13). These data indicate an important part for PTN in tumour growth and show that ribozymes can be very useful tools to pinpoint the role of a growth factor. In a more recent study (15), we used a human melanoma cell line (1205LU) that expresses high levels of endogenous PTN, forms subcutaneous tumours in mice and metastasizes from the subcutaneous injection site into the lungs within 5–7 weeks (see above). Using ribozyme targeting of PTN, we were able to demonstrate that the 1205LU cell line does not depend on PTN for its growth *in vitro*. However, the cell line requires the expression of PTN for subcutaneous tumour growth and for metastasis *in vivo*. With PTN expression reduced by ribozymes, the cell line lost its tumourigenic and metastatic capacity. Similar results were obtained with the highly PTN-expressing human choriocarcinoma cell line JEG-3. Depletion of PTN mRNA to background levels diminished their invasiveness, angiogenesis, and tumourigenicity in athymic nude mice without influencing their growth *in vitro* (33).

In conclusion, these molecular targeting studies identify PTN as a rate-limiting growth factor for tumour growth and metastasis in different model cell lines. How widespread the role of this growth factor is, remains to be demonstrated. Parallel studies targeting MK are underway in our laboratory. One potential application of this approach will be the gene therapy of highly metastatic tumours expressing these growth factors.

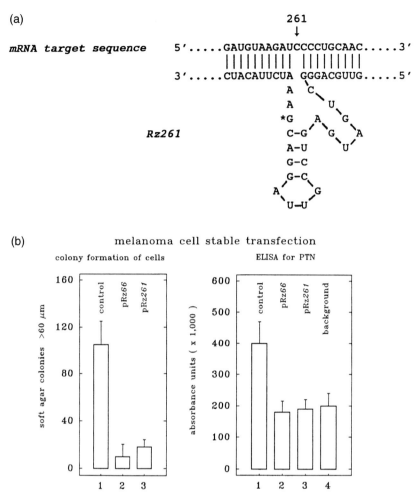

Figure 21.3. Structure and activity of pleiotrophin (PTN)-targeted ribozymes (a) Core structure and folding of the hammerhead ribozyme Rz261 are shown together with the targeted sequence in the PTN mRNA. The asterix indicates a point mutation site that will abolish enzymatic activity of the ribozyme. Details are described in (13). (b) Effect of stable transfection of PTN-positive human melanoma with PTN-targeted ribozymes. Colony formation in soft agar (left) and secretion of PTN into the media of the cells (right) are shown. Details are described in (13).

Summary and conclusions

Polypeptide growth factors contribute to the development and maintenance of normal tissues and are essential for the growth and metastasis of solid tumours. During development as well as during tumour progression these factors function as autocrine stimulators among the same cell type or as paracrine effectors supporting extension and survival of normal as well as tumorous tissue. The novel heparin-binding, polypeptide growth factors MK and PTN are highly regulated during normal development and appear to

have a number of physiological functions in the growing nervous system and in peripheral organogenesis and tissue maintenance. During malignant transformation either of the factors can be up-regulated in a number of different tumours. Overexpression studies in PTN/MK-responsive cells support their role as a tumour growth factor. Complementary with this, molecular targeting of PTN in tumour cells suggests a rate-limiting role for tumour growth and metastasis of melanoma. Whether this will be true for other tumour types is currently under investigation.

Acknowledgements

We thank the colleagues from our laboratory for sharing unpublished and preliminary data with us to make this review as up-to-date as possible: K. J. Colley (anti-sense oligodeoxynucleotides to PTN); F. Czubayko (ribozyme-targeting of PTN); S. C. Missner (hormonal regulation of PTN and MK); E. B. Sale (MK activity and gene expression). Furthermore, we thank Dr Anna Tate Riegel for critical comments during the preparation of this manuscript.

References

1. Mason, I. J. (1994). The ins and outs of fibroblast growth factors. *Cell*, **78**, 547–52.
2. Shing, Y., Folkman, J., Sullivan, R., Butterfield, C., Murray, J., and Klagsbrun, M. (1984). Heparin affinity: purification of a tumour-derived capillary endothelial cell growth factor. *Science*, **223**, 1296–1.
3. Li, Y. S., Milner, P. G., Chauhan, A. K., Watson, M. A., Hoffman, R. M., Kodner, C. M., *et al.* (1990). Cloning and expression of a developmentally regulated protein that induces mitogenic and neurite outgrowth activity. *Science*, **250**, 1690–4.
4. Böhlen, P., Müller, T., Gautschi-Sova, P., Albrecht, V., Rasool, C. G., Decker, M., *et al.* (1991). Isolation from bovine brain and structural characterization of HBNF, a heparin-binding neurotrophic factor. *Growth Factors*, **4**, 97–107.
5. Kuo, M. D., Oda, Y., Huang, J. S., and Huang, S. S. (1990). Amino acid sequence and characterization of a heparin-binding neurite-promoting factor (p18) from bovine brain. *J. Biol. Chem.*, **265**, 18749–52.
6. Hampton, B. S., Marshak, D. R., and Burgess, W. H. (1992). Structural and functional characterization of full-length heparin-binding growth associated molecule. *Mol. Biol. Cell*, **3**, 85–93.
7. Wellstein, A., Fang, W. J., Khatri, A., Lu, Y., Swain, S. S., Dickson, R. B., *et al.* (1992). A heparin-binding growth factor secreted from breast cancer cells homologous to a developmentally regulated cytokine. *J. Biol. Chem.*, **267**, 2582–7.
8. Rauvala, H. (1989). An 18-kd heparin-binding protein of developing brain that is distinct from fibroblast growth factors. *EMBO J.*, **8**, 2933–41.
9. Milner, P. G., Li, Y. S., Hoffman, R. M., Kodner, C. M., Siegel, N. R., and Deuel, T. F. (1989). A novel 17 kD heparin-binding growth factor (HBGF-8) in bovine uterus: purification and N-terminal amino acid sequence. *Biochem. Biophys. Res. Commun.*, **165**, 1096–103.
10. Takamatsu, H., Itoh, M., Kimura, M., Gospodarowicz, D., and Amann, E. (1992). Expression and purification of biologically active human OSF-1 in *Escherichia coli*. *Biochem. Biophys. Res. Commun.*, **185**, 224–30.
11. Raulo, E., Julkunen, I., Merenmies, J., Pihlaskari, R., and Rauvala, H. (1992). Secretion and biological activities of heparin-binding growth-associated molecule. *J. Biol. Chem.*, **267**, 11408–16.
12. Fang, W. J., Hartmann, N., Chow, D., Riegel, A. T., and Wellstein, A. (1992). Pleiotrophin stimulates fibroblasts, endothelial and epithelial cells, and is expressed in human cancer. *J. Biol. Chem.*, **267**, 25889–97.
13. Czubayko, F., Riegel, A. T., and Wellstein, A. (1994). Ribozyme-targeting elucidates a direct role of pleiotrophin in tumour growth. *J. Biol. Chem.*, **269**, 21358–63.
14. Chauhan, A. K., Li, Y. S., and Deuel, T. F. (1993). Pleiotrophin transforms NIH 3T3 cells and induces tumours in nude mice. *Proc. Natl Acad. Sci. USA*, **90**, 679–82.
15. Czubayko, F., Schulte, A. M., Berchem, G. J., and Wellstein, A. (1966). Melanoma angiogenesis and metastasis modulated by ribozyme targeting of the secreted growth factor pleiotrophin. *Proc. Natl Acad. Sci. USA*, **93**, 14753–8.
16. Böhlen, P., Gautschi-Sova, P., Albrecht, U., Lehmann, S., and Huber, D. (1988). Isolation and partial structural characterization of a novel heparin-binding, non FGF-like endothelial cell growth factor. *J. Cell. Biochem.*, **Suppl. 12A**, 221.
17. Courty, J., Dauchel, M. C., Caruelle, D., Perderiset, M., and Barritault, D. (1991). Mitogenic properties of a new endothelial cell growth factor related to pleiotrophin. *Biochem. Biophys. Res. Commun.*, **180**, 145–51.
18. Laaroubi, K., Delbé, J., Vacherot, F., Desgranges, P., Tardieu, M., Jaye, M., *et al.* (1994). Mitogenic and *in vitro* angiogenic activity of human recombinant heparin affin regulatory peptide. *Growth Factors*, **10**, 89–98.
19. Kuo, M. D., Huang, S. S., and Huang, J. S. (1992). Characterization of heparin-binding growth-associated factor receptor on NIH 3T3 cells. *Biochem. Biophys. Res. Commun.*, **182**, 188–94.
20. Raulo, E., Chernousov, M. A., Carey, D. J., Nolo, R., and Rauvala, H. (1994). Isolation of a neuronal cell surface receptor of heparin binding growth-associated molecule (HB-GAM). Identification as N-syndecan (syndecan-3). *J. Biol. Chem.*, **269**, 12999–3004.
21. Li, Y. S. and Deuel, T. F. (1993). Pleiotrophin stimulates tyrosine phosphorylation in NIH 3T3 and NB41A3 cells. *Biochem. Biophys. Res. Commun.*, **195**, 1089–95.
22. Aviezer, D., Hecht, D., Safran, M., Eisinger, M., David, G., and Yayon, A. (1994). Perlecan, basal lamina proteoglycan, promotes basic fibroblast growth factor-receptor binding, mitogenesis and angiogenesis. *Cell*, **79**, 1005–14.
23. Spivak-Kroizman, T., Lemmon, M. A., Kikic, I., Ladbury, J. E., Pinchasi, D., Huang, J., *et al.* (1994). Heparin-induced oligomerization of FGF molecules is responsible for FGF receptor dimerization, activation and cell proliferation. *Cell*, **79**, 1015–24.
24. Kadomatsu, K., Tomomura, M., and Muramatsu, T. (1988). cDNA cloning and sequencing of a new gene intensely expressed in early differentiation stages of embryonal carcinoma cells and in mid-gestation period of mouse embryogenesis. *Biochem. Biophys. Res. Commun.*, **151**, 1312–18.
25. Vigny, M., Raulais, D., Puzenat, N., Duprez, D., Hartmann, M. P., Jeanny, J. C., and Courtois, Y. (1989). Identification of a new heparin-binding protein localized within chick basement membranes. *Eur. J. Biochem.*, **186**, 733–40.
26. Tomomura, M., Kadomatsu, K., Matsubara, S., and Muramatsu, T. (1990). A retinoic acid-responsive gene, MK, found in the teratocarcinoma system. Heterogeneity of the transcript and the nature of the translation product. *J. Biol. Chem.*, **265**, 10765–70.
27. Raulais, D., Lagente-Chevallier, O., Guettet, C., Duprez, D., Courtois, Y., and Vigny, M. (1991). A new heparin binding

protein regulated by retinoic acid from chick embryo. *Biochem. Biophys. Res. Commun.*, **174**, 708–15.

28. Kretschmer, P. J., Fairhurst, J. L., Decker, M. M., Chan, C. P., Gluzman, Y., Böhlen, P., and Kovesdi, I. (1991). Cloning, characterization and developmental regulation of two members of a novel human gene family of neurite outgrowth-promoting proteins. *Growth Factors*, **5**, 99–114.

29. Muramatsu, H. and Muramatsu, T. (1991). Purification of recombinant midkine and examination of its biological activities: functional comparison of new heparin binding factors. *Biochem. Biophys. Res. Commun.*, **177**, 652–8.

30. Nurcombe, V., Fraser, N., Herlaar, E., and Heath, K., (1992). MK: a pluripotent embryonic stem-cell-derived neuroregulatory factor. *Development*, **116**, 1175–83.

31. Michikawa, M., Xu, R. V., Muramatsu, H., Muramatsu, T., and Kim, S. U., (1993). Midkine is a mediator of retinoid acid induced neuronal differentiation of embryonal carcinoma cells. *Biochem. Biophys. Res. Commun.*, **192**, 1312–18.

32. Tomomura, M., Kadomatsu, K., Nakamoto, M., Muramatsu, H., Kondoh, H., Imagawa, K., and Muramatsu, T. (1990). A retinoic acid responsive gene, MK, produces a secreted protein with heparin binding activity. *Biochem. Biophys. Res. Commun.*, **171**, 603–9.

33. Schulte, A. M., Lai, S., Kurtz, A., Czubayko, F., Riegel, A. T., and Wellstein, A. (1996). Human trophoblast and choriocarcinoma expression of the growth factor PTN attributable to germ-line insertion of an endogenous retrovirus. *Proc. Natl Acad. USA*, **93**, 14759–64.

34. Lai, S. P., Czubayko, F., Riegel, A. T., and Wellstein, A. (1992). Structure of the human heparin-binding growth factor gene pleiotrophin. *Biochem. Biophys. Res. Commun.*, **187**, 1113–22.

35. Li, Y. S., Hoffman, R. M., Le Beau, M. M., Espinosa, R., Jenkins, N. A., Gilbert, D. J., *et al.* (1992). Characterization of the human pleiotrophin gene. *J. Biol. Chem.*, **267**, 26011–16.

36. Milner, P. G., Shah, D., Veile, R., Donis-Keller, H., and Kumar, B. V. (1992). Cloning, nucleotide sequence and chromosome localization of the human pleiotrophin gene. *Biochemistry*, **31**, 12023–8.

37. Kretschmer, P. J., Fairhurst, J. L., Hulmes, J. D., Popjes, M. L., Böhlen, P., and Kovesdi, I. (1993). Genomic organization of the human HBNF gene and characterization of an HBNF variant protein as a splice mutant. *Biochem. Biophys. Res. Commun.*, **192**, 420–9.

38. Lai, S., Schulte, A. M., Wellstein, A., and Riegel, A. T. (1995). An additional 5′-upstream exon exists in the human pleiotrophin-encoding gene. *Gene*, **153**, 301–2.

39. Katoh, K., Takeshita, S., Sato, M., Ito, T., and Amann, E. (1992). Genomic organization of the mouse OSF-1 gene. *DNA Cell Biol.*, **11**, 735–43.

40. Matsubara, S., Tomomura, M., Kadomatsu, K., and Muramatsu, T. (1990). Structure of a retinoic acid-responsive gene, MK, which is transiently activated during the differentiation of embryonal carcinoma cells and the midgestation period of mouse embryogenesis. *J. Biol. Chem.*, **265**, 9441–3.

41. Li, Y. S., Gurrieri, M., and Deuel, T. F. (1992). Pleiotrophin gene expression is highly restricted and is regulated by platelet-derived growth factor. *Biochem. Biophys. Res. Commun.*, **184**, 427–32.

42. Fu, C., Maminta-Smith, L., Guo, C., and Deuel, T. (1994). Cloning and sequence of the *Xenopus laevis* homologue of the midkine cDNA. *Gene*, **146**, 311–12.

43. Uehara, K., Matsubara, S., Kadomatsu, K., Tsutsui, J., and Muramatsu, T. (1992). Genomic structure of human midkine (MK), a retinoic acid responsive growth/differentiation factor. *J. Biochem.*, **111**, 563–7.

44. Kaname, T., Kuwano, K., Murano, I., Uehara, K., Muramatsu, T., and Kaji, T. (1993). Midkine, a gene for prenatal differentiation and neuroregulation maps to band 11p11.2 by fluorescence *in situ*. *Genomics*, **17**, 514–15.

45. Simone-Chazottes, D., Matsubara, S., Miyauchi, T., Muramatsu, T., and Guenet, J. L. (1992). Chromosomal localization of two cell surface-associated molecules of potential importance in development: midkine (MK) and basigin (BSG). *Mamm. Genome*, **2**, 269–71.

46. Matsubara, S., Take, M., Pedraza, C., and Muramatsu, T. (1994). Mapping and characterization of a retinoid acid responsive enhancer of midkine, a novel heparin-binding growth/differentiation factor with neurotrophic activity. *J. Biochem.*, **115**, 1088–96.

47. Pedraza, C., Matsubara, S., and Muramatsu, T. (1995). A retinoic acid-responsive element in human midkine gene. *J. Biochem.*, **117**, 845–9.

48. Obama, H., Matsubara, S., Guenet, J. L., and Muramatsu, T. (1994). The midkine (MK) family of growth/differentiation factors: structure of an MK-related sequence in a pseudogene and evolutionary relationship among members of the MK family. *J. Biochem.*, **115**, 516–22.

49. Kadomatsu, K., Huang, R. P., Suganuma, T., Murata, F., and Muramatsu, T. (1990). A retinoic acid responsive gene MK found in the teratocarcinoma system is expressed in spatially and temporally controlled manner during mouse embryogenesis. *J. Cell. Biol.*, **110**, 607–16.

50. Vanderwinden, J. M., Mailleux, P., Schiffmann, S. N., and Vanderhaeghen, J. J. (1992). Cellular distribution of the new growth factor pleiotrophin (HB-GAM) mRNA in developing and adult rat tissues. *Anat. Embryol.* **186**, 387–406.

51. Wanaka, A., Carroll, S. L., and Milbrandt, J. (1993). Developmentally regulated expression of pleiotrophin, a novel heparin binding growth factor, in the nervous system of the rat. *Brain Res. Dev. Brain Res.*, **72**, 133–44.

52. Bloch, B., Normand, E., Kovesdi, I., and Böhlen, P. (1992). Expression of the HBNF (heparin-binding neurite-promoting factor) gene in the brain of fetal, neonatal and adult rat: an *in situ* hybridization study. *Brain Res. Dev. Brain Res.*, **70**, 267–278.

53. Kitamura, M., Shirasawa, T., Mitarai, T., Muramatsu, T., and Muruyama, N. (1993). A retinoid responsive cytokine gene, MK, is preferentially expressed in the proximal tubles of the kidney and human tumour cell lines. *Am. J. Pathol.*, **142**, 425–31.

54. Tsutsui, J., Kadomatsu, K., Matsubara, S., Nakagawara, A., Hamanoue, M., Takao, S., *et al.* (1993). A new family of heparin-binding growth/differentiation factors: increased midkine expression in Wilms' tumor and other human carcinomas. *Cancer Res.*, **53**, 1281–5.

55. Garver, R. I., Radford, D. M., Donis-Keller, H., Wick, M. R., and Milner, P. G. (1994). Midkine and pleiotrophin expression in normal and malignant breast tissue. *Cancer*, **74**, 1584–90.

56. Mailleux, P., Vanderwinden, J. M., and Vanderhaeghen, J. J. (1992). The new growth factor pleiotrophin (HB-GAM) mRNA is selectively present in the meningothelial cells of human meningiomas. *Neurosci. Lett.*, **142**, 31–5.

57. Nakagawara, A, Milbrandt, J., Muramatsu, T., Deuel, T. F., Zhao, H., Cnaan, A., and Brodeur, G. M. (1995). Differential expression of pleiotrophin and midkine in advanced neuroblastoma. *Cancer Res.*, **55**, 1792–7.

58. Zugmaier, G., Lippman, M. E., and Wellstein, A. (1992). Inhibition by pentosan polysulfate (PPS) of heparin-binding growth factors released from tumour cells and blockade by PPS of tumour growth in animals. *J. Natl Cancer Inst.*, **84**, 1716–24.

59. Sizmann, N., Fang, W. J., Chung, H. C., Rodeck, U., Herlyn, M., and Wellstein, A. (1996). Pleiotrophin in melanoma metastasis and inhibition by pentosanpolysulfate. *Int. J. Cancer*, (in press).

60. O'Brien, T., Cranston, D., Fuggle, S., Bicknell, R., and Harris, A. L. (1996). The angiogenic factor midkine is expressed in bladder cancer, and overexpression correlates with a poor outcome in patients with invasive cancers. *Cancer Res.*, **56**, 2515–18.

61. Stein, C. A. and Cheng, Y. C. (1993). Antisense oligonucleotides as therapeutic agents — is the bullet really magical? *Science*, **261**, 1004–12.

62. Wagner, R. W. (1994). Gene inhibition using antisense oligodeoxynucleotides. *Nature*, **372**, 333–5.

63. Colley, K. J. and Wellstein, A. (1994). Antisense oligonucleotides of pleiotrophin. *Patent Application*, **8/276, 330,**

64. Colley, K. J., Sale, E. B., Riegel, A. T., and Wellstein, A. (1995). Antisense oligonucleotides inhibit pleiotrophin action *in vitro* and *in vivo* (submitted).

65. Kruger, K., Grabowski, P. J., Zaug, A. J., Sands, J., Gottschling, D. E., and Cech, T. R. (1982). Self-splicing RNA: autoexcision and autocyclization of the ribosomal RNA intervening sequence of Tetrahymena. *Cell*, **31**, 147–57.

66. Uhlenbeck, O. C. (1987). A small catalytic oligoribonucleotide. *Nature*, **328**, 596–600.

67. Haseloff, J. and Gerlach, W. L. (1988). Simple RNA enzymes with new and highly specific endoribonuclease activities. *Nature*, **334**, 585–91.

68. Cameron, F. H. and Jennings, P. A. (1989). Specific gene suppression by engineered ribozymes in monkey cells. *Proc. Natl Acad. Sci. USA*, **86**, 9139–43.

69. Symons, R. H. (1992). Small catalytic RNAs. *Annu. Rev. Biochem.*, **61**, 641–71.

70. Pyle, A. M. (1993). Ribozymes: a distinct class of metalloenzymes. *Science*, **261**, 709–14.

71. Zuker, M. and Stiegler, P. (1981). Optimal computer folding of large RNA sequences using thermodynamics and auxiliary information. *Nucleic Acids Res.*, **9**, 133–48.

72. McCall, M. J., Hendry, P., and Jennings, P. A. (1992). Minimal sequence requirements for ribozyme activity. *Proc. Natl Acad. Sci. USA*, **89**, 5710–14.

73. Sheldon, C. C. and Symons, R. H. (1989). Mutagenesis analysis of a self-cleaving RNA. *Nucleic Acids Res.*, **17**, 5679–85.

74. Merenmies, J. and Rauvala, H. (1990). Molecular cloning of the 18-kDa growth-associated protein of developing brain. *J. Biol. Chem.*, **265**, 16721–4.

75. Tsutsui, J., Uehara, K., Kadomatsu, K., Matsubara, S., and Muramatsu, T. (1991). A new family of heparin-binding factors: strong conservation of midkine (MK) sequences between the human and the mouse. *Biochem. Biophys. Res. Commun.*, **176**, 792–7.

76. Urios, P., Duprez, D., Le Caer, J. P., Courtois, Y., Vigny, M., and Laurent, M. (1991). Molecular cloning of RI-HB, a heparin binding protein regulated by retinoic acid. *Biochem. Biophys. Res. Commun.*, **175**, 617–24.

77. Shoyab, M., McDonald, V. L., Dick, K., Modrell, B., Malik, N., and Plowman, G. (1991). Amphiregulin-associated protein: complete amino acid sequence of a protein produced by the 12-*O*-tetradecanoylphorbol-13- acetate-treated human breast adenocarcinoma cell line MCF-7. *Biochem. Biophys. Res. Commun.*, **179**, 572–8.

78. Kovesdi, I., Fairhurst, J. L., Kretschmer P. J., and Böhlen, P. (1990). Heparin-binding neurotrophic factor (HBNF) and MK, members of a new family of homologous, developmentally regulated proteins. *Biochem. Biophys. Res. Commun.*, **172**, 850–4.

79. Tezuka, K., Takeshita, S., Hakeda, Y., Kumegawa, M., Kikuno, R., and Hashimoto-Gotoh, T. (1990). Isolation of mouse and human cDNA clones encoding a protein expressed specifically in osteoblasts and brain tissues. *Biochem. Biophys. Res. Commun.*, **173**, 246–51.

80. Naito, A., Yoshikura H., and Iwamoto, A. (1992). Similarity of the genomic structure between the two members in a new family of heparin-binding factors. *Biochem. Biophys. Res. Commun.*, **183**, 701–7.

81. Kretschmer, P. J., Fairhurst, J. L., Hulmes, J. D., Popjes, M. L., Böhlen, P., and Kovesdi, I. (1993). Genomic organization of the human HBNF gene and characterization of an HBNF variant protein as a splice mutant. *Biochem. Biophys. Res. Commun.*, **192**, 420–9.

82. Tsutsui, J., Uehara, K., Kadomatsu, K., Matsubara, S., and Muramatsu, T. (1991). A new family of heparin-binding factors: Strong conservation of midkine (MK) sequences between the human and the mouse. *Biochem. Biophys. Res. Commun.*, **176**, 792–7.

83. Novotny, W. F., Maffi, T., Mehta, R. L., and Milner, P. G. (1993). Identification of novel heparin-releasable proteins, as well as cytokines midkine and pleiotrophin in human postheparin plasma. *Arterioscler. Thromb.*, **13**, 1798–805.

22. Involvement of prostanoids in angiogenesis

Enzo Spisni and Vittorio Tomasi

Introduction

Studies on angiogenesis began in the seventeenth century when Marcello Malpighi in Bologna described the development of the chick embryo. Figure 22.1 is an original drawing from Malpighi's book *De Formatione Pulli in Ovo*, as reported by Adelmann (1). Leighton, and later Folkman and collaborators, have used the chick chorioallantoic membrane (CAM) as a powerful tool with which to study the regulation of angiogenesis *in vivo*. (see Chapter 2).

This chapter will review the evidence for an involvement of arachidonic acid and its metabolites in various steps of the angiogenic process.

The arachidonate cascade

Figure 22.2 illustrates the main steps involved in the metabolism of arachidonate. Excellent reviews are available on prostanoid biosynthesis (2–4).

Prostanoids in angiogenesis: early work

The first evidence for an involvement of prostanoids in angiogenesis was reported in the late seventies. Thus, it was shown that tumours secrete prostaglandins (5), and that prostaglandins were mediators of ocular neovascularization (6).

In 1982 Ziche *et al.* showed that the interstitial fluid of some carcinomas, an ethanol extract of the tumour or neoplastic fibroblasts, induced strong angiogenic responses in the rabbit corneal assay (7). The stimulated angiogenesis was completely blocked in indomethacin treated rabbits. The tumour interstitial fluid was found to be rich in E-type prostaglandins. PGE_1 was then shown to be strongly angiogenic, much more so than PGE_2 or PGI_2 (7). PGE_2 was also independently shown to be angiogenic on the CAM

assay by Form and Auerbach in 1983 (8). Although PGI_2 was not active in the experiments of Ziche *et al.* (probably due to its well known instability) it has been shown that stable analogues of PGI_2 (*e.g.* isocarbacyclins and 7-fluoro-prostacyclin) are strongly angiogenic on the chick CAM (9,10).

It follows that the inhibition of prostaglandin H (PGH) synthase by anti-inflammatory compounds has been examined as a simple pharmacological approach to the inhibition of tumour angiogenesis. Fulton (11) showed that PGH-synthase inhibitors, such as indomethacin, can reduce the growth of malignant tumours *in vivo*. Anti-inflammatory compounds reduce the angiogenic prostanoids released by the tumour itself as well as those released from host cells within the tumour (11). We have confirmed that indomethacin is a strong inhibitor of neovascularization during development by using the CAM test (12). Nevertheless, use of anti-inflammatory agents as broad-spectrum anti-tumour agents has so far met with little success.

Recently, it has been observed that acetylsalicylic acid not only inhibits both isoforms of PGH synthase by acylation of residues present in the active site, but also acts by suppressing the gene for PGH synthase (13). In addition, acetylsalicylic acid, but not indomethacin, is a potent inhibitor of the transcription factor NF-κB which, among many other genes (14), regulates the expression of the PGH synthase 2 gene (see Table 22.1).

Arachidonic acid regulation of gene expression

It has been reported that when endothelial cells progress from a pre-confluent actively dividing phenotype to a contact-inhibited quiescent state, the stimulated release of arachidonic acid is greatly reduced (15). This is thought to be due to a modification of cellular phospholipases, in particular c-phospholipase A_2 ($cPLA_2$) activity (15,16).

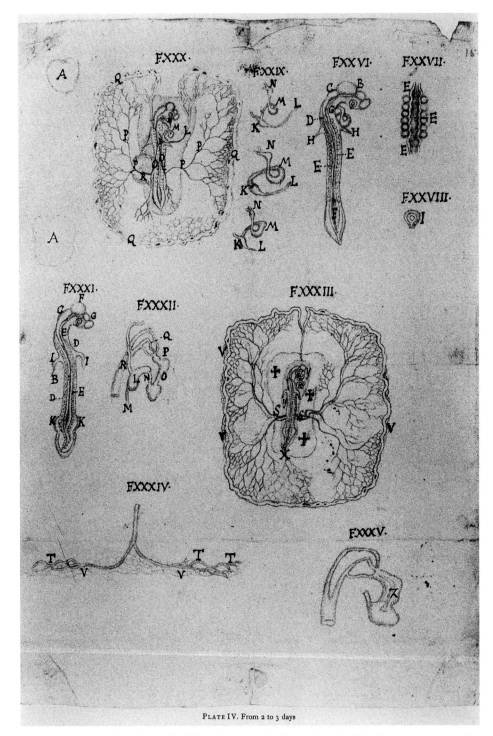

PLATE IV. From 2 to 3 days

Figure 22.1. Original drawing from Marcello Malpighi's book *De Formatione Pulli in Ovo*, as reproduced by Adelmann (1966). The figure shows the appearance of the vascular system of the chick-embryo after 2 (FXXX) or 3 (FXXXIII) days of incubation.

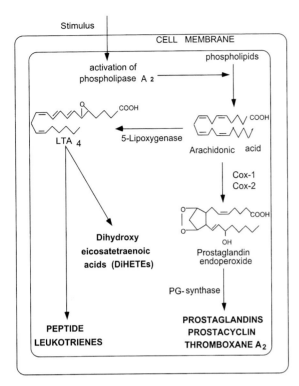

Stimulus

CELL MEMBRANE

phospholipids

activation of
phospholipase A 2

COOH

COOH

LTA 4   5-Lipoxygenase

Arachidonic acid

Cox-1
Cox-2

COOH

OH

**Dihydroxy
eicosatetraenoic
acids (DiHETEs)**

Prostaglandin
endoperoxide

PG- synthase

**PEPTIDE
LEUKOTRIENES**

**PROSTAGLANDINS
PROSTACYCLIN
THROMBOXANE A$_2$**

Figure 22.2. The arachidonate cascade: prostanoid and leukotriene biosynthesis.

Although these authors have related increased availability of arachidonate to an augmented transformation into prostanoids, other explanations may be possible. During the last few years the involvement of long-chain fatty acids in acylation processes has been intensively investigated. Saturated fatty acids appear to be involved in acylation of regulatory membrane proteins such as G proteins (and the *ras* oncogene), while long-chain unsaturated fatty acids seem to act mainly on soluble cytoplasmic proteins

(17). Examples are now discussed. The most impressive one regards the role of arachidonic acid in the modulation of heat-shock gene transcription. Morimoto and co-workers (18) have shown that arachidonate is a potent inducer of heat shock factor (HSF) which regulates heat shock genes expression. As the binding of HSF to DNA requires continuous exposure to arachidonate, it is likely that a persistent activation of cPLA$_2$ is involved (as a matter of fact the arachidonate effect is very specific). Morimoto *et al.* (18) speculate that the fatty acid activates a protein kinase C; however, it is also possible that a direct acylation of HSF occurs.

Sylvester *et al.* (19) observed that the mitogenic effect of EGF on mammary epithelial cells, was greatly potentiated after addition of arachidonate, and that indomethacin did not alter the effect of the fatty acid. Again, protein kinase C was involved as a mediator of the effect of arachidonate.

In hepatocytes an effect of a low concentration (1 μmol/l) of arachidonic acid on DNA synthesis has been reported (20). The possibility that, in this case, arachidonate is acting on liver fatty acid binding protein (L-FABP), a 14 kDa cytosolic protein which mediates the action of mitogens in liver cells (20), appears likely. Thus, this and other studies strongly suggest that arachidonate, by acylation or by binding to some proteins such as HSF or L-FAPB, induces a conformational change permitting them to translocate to the nucleus and to regulate the expression of selected genes.

If arachidonate becomes available primarily during mitogenesis of the endothelial cell, how is it to be explained that PGI$_2$ is produced almost exclusively when cells are in a contact-inhibited non-proliferating state? As we and others have shown that PGI$_2$ synthase is a constitutively expressed enzyme in human umbilical vein endothelial cells (HUVEC) (21,22), the regulation of PGI$_2$ biosynthesis must be dependent on the regulation of substrate availability and/or on the induction of the two isoforms of PGH synthase.

Table 22.1. Promoters of eicosanoid metabolizing enzyme genes (5' flanking)

Gene	AP-1/2 or PEA-3	NF-κB	SP-1	CRE	NF-IL6	TATA box	Reference
Human PGH synthase 2	1	1	1	1	1	1	63
Chicken PGH synthase 2	5	1	3	1	ND	1	64
Murine PGH synthase 1	4	–	2	1	–	ND	65
Human PGH synthase 1	4	–	1	–	–	ND	66
Human 5-lipoxygenase	2	1	Several	–	–	–	67

ND, not done.

Enzymes of prostaglandin biosynthesis

Regulation of expression of prostaglandin H synthase 1 and 2

Soon after the discovery of PGH synthase 2, a widely held hypothesis was to consider PGH synthase 1 as a constitutively expressed enzyme with 'house-keeping' functions and PGH synthase 2 as a growth factor-induced isoform, involved in cell proliferation and differentiation (23–25). This scheme, as we will show, does not apply to HUVEC and some other cells such as bone marrow-derived mast cells (21). First, when HUVEC are exposed to a potent growth factor, e.g. basic fibroblast growth factor (bFGF), despite the presence of PGI_2 synthase (21,22) and of free arachidonate (15), no PGI_2 is produced. Neither PGH synthase isoform appears to be expressed at a significant level (23). A time-course of PGH synthase induction in HUVEC by cytokines is shown in Fig. 22.3. The second point is that when bone marrow-derived mast cells are challenged with different stimuli, leading to the generation of PGD_2, both isoforms appear to be induced, at different levels, depending on the stimuli used (26). From this work a new concept is emerging, namely, that the two PGH synthase isoforms are part of a signal transduction mechanism triggered by different ligands, but having the same final effect. It will be interesting to ascertain whether the two isoforms clearly demonstrated for PGE_2 isomerase (27,28), thromboxane A_2 (TXA_2) synthase, and tentatively for PGI_2 synthase (29), are part of dichotomic signal transduction mechanism similar to that described by Murakami et al. (26).

Prostacyclin synthase

While PGH synthases have been intensively studied, much less is known about PGI_2 synthase. The enzyme has a restricted cellular distribution, being present almost exclusively in vascular endothelial cells and smooth muscle cells (29). In HUVEC the enzyme is constitutively expressed (21) and it is in vesicles uniformly distributed in the cytoplasm (see Fig. 22.4). This synthase has been difficult to purify and to characterize. Recently, two groups succeeded in obtaining the sequence of the enzyme (30,31). It was confirmed that PGI_2 synthase shows some homology with members of cytochrome P450 family; however, as the highest homology was less than 30% and the enzyme has no monooxygenase activity, PGI_2 synthase probably belongs to a family distantly related to the P450 cytochromes. The enzyme, however, shares little homology (16%) with a second possible member of the family: TxA_2 synthase (30). TxA_2 synthase and PGI_2 synthase catalyse similar reactions according to Ullrich and collaborators (31); however, in addition to homology differences, they also have a different membrane topology, the first anchored to the endoplasmic reticulum via two segments (32) but the second via one (30).

These two enzymes share an instability when challenged with the substrate PGH_2 and they are both constitutively expressed in most normal cells examined (21,33). In U937 cells, TXA_2 synthase is post-transcriptionally regulated by phorbol esters (34).

The prostaglandin I_2 receptor

All prostanoid receptors so far examined belong to the class of G protein coupled receptors. The receptors have

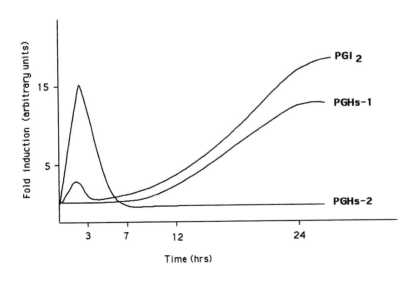

Figure 22.3. Kinetics of prostaglandin H-synthase isoform induction by cytokines (see reference 54). PGI_2 synthesis was determined as described (21).

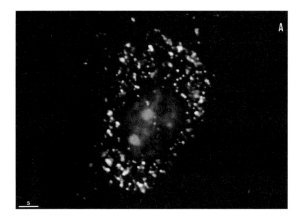

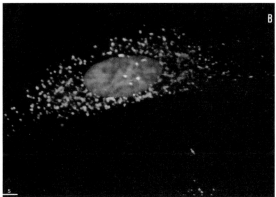

Figure 22.4. Confocal microscopy of human umbilical vein endothelial cells stained with PGI_2 synthase antibody (green) and ethidium bromide (red). Fluorescence signal from all optical sections. A differentiating cell treated with IL-1α (a) and proliferating cell treated with basic fibroblast growth factor (b) are shown.

been classified on the basis of the type of G protein involved in signal transduction and of the second messenger generated. Thus, E-prostaglandin receptors bind PGE with high affinity and activate (E_1 and E_2) or inhibit (E_3) adenylate cyclase; F-prostaglandin receptors bind $PGF_{2\alpha}$ and alter cellular calcium and inositol phosphates levels; the TxA_2 receptor couples with a member of the Gq family, the effector being phospholipase C; and, finally, the PGI_2 receptor is linked both to cyclic aderosine monophosphate (AMP) and to the generation of inositol phosphates (35–39). It is interesting that very low doses (10^{-10} mol/l) of a PGI_2 stable agonist elicit an half maximal response on cyclic AMP levels, while much higher doses (10^{-7} mol/l) are required to elicit an half maximal response in inositol

phosphate levels (39). It appears logical to speculate that while the PGI_2 receptor on platelets is exposed to low levels of ligand, much higher levels of PGI_2 are available to smooth muscle cells which can use both exogenously and endogenously produced PGI_2. Thus, the second messenger of PGI_2 receptor in platelets is likely to be mainly cyclic AMP, while in smooth-muscle cells both cyclic AMP and inositol phosphates could function as second messengers. The literature supports this possibility. Thus, Narumya and collaborators (38) have shown that alternative splicing of mRNA coding for EP_3 receptor, generates four isoforms differing in C-terminal tails and capable of coupling with different G proteins. It is possible that a similar mechanism operates for the PGI_2 receptor.

The fibroblast growth family and arachidonate metabolism in endothelial cells

Acid, basic fibroblast growth factor (aFGF) affects arachidonate metabolism differently to bFGF, and inclusion of heparin enhances the differences. Thus, Weksler (40) found that aFGF inhibited PGI_2 production in HUVEC by decreasing immunoreactive PGH synthase and PGI_2 synthase. These results do not agree with those reported by Hasegawa *et al.* (41) who found that endothelial cell growth supplement (ECGS) has no effect on PGI_2 production but is an inhibitor in the presence of heparin. It should be noted that ECGS (42) is a very crude isolate of aFGF and attributing the action of ECGS to aFGF requires caution. Heparin *per se* inhibits PGI_2-production.

This effect was also noted by others and is likely to be explained by assuming that heparin binds FGF or competes with its receptor. These observations have led Hla and Maciag to conclude that the mitogenic effect of aFGF is accompanied by a down-regulation of the gene coding for PGH synthase in HUVEC (43). bFGF, on the other hand, has no effect on PGI_2 production in HUVEC and does not modify the levels of PGI_2 synthase. According to a recent study, bFGF may regulate the conversion of arachidonic acid into lipoxygenase metabolites in HUVEC (44).

It is somewhat surprising that aFGF and bFGF have such divergent effects on arachidonic acid metabolism. The only explanation is that they interact with different cellular receptors, as suggested by Partanen *et al.* (45). A clear message emerging from these studies is that increased prostanoid biosynthesis is not essential for mitogenesis in HUVEC or other cells (25,46). A scheme summarizing these points is shown in Fig. 22.5.

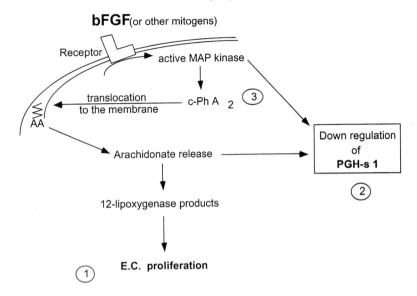

Figure 22.5. Basic fibroblast growth factor (bFGF) down-regulates prostaglandin H-I synthase but increases lipoxygenase products and cell proliferation. (1) See reference 15; (2) see references 16 and 75. EC, endothelial cell; AA, arachidonic acid; MAP, mitogen-activated protein.

Proliferation and differentiation of the endothelial cell

The control of endothelial cell differentiation

In 1986 we proposed that differentiation of human monocytes to macrophages, induced by serum, involved the induction of PGH synthase and the increased production of TxA_2 (47). Later, these findings were extended to U937 cells (48). Wu and collaborators in an elegant series of studies (46,49,50) extended this concept to endothelial cells, differentiation in this case being induced by treatment with phorbol esters. However, the most potent stimulus for HUVEC differentiation — so far identified — is interleukin 1 (IL) (51). Phorbol esters and IL-1 share the capacity to induce an early translocation of protein kinase C to the cell membrane. Maier and Ragnotti have proposed that this event is linked to expression of PGH synthase as PGH synthase mRNA accumulation is one of the first observed events (52). An alternative possibility is that IL-1 acts by decreasing the expression of high-affinity FGF-binding sites on the endothelial cell membrane (53), thus relieving the inhibitory action of aFGF on PGH synthase gene expression.

Maciag and collaborators (54) re-examining the mechanism of IL-1 action, by using a human cell line (ECV 304) concluded that the cytokine not only increases the expression of PGH synthase-2 gene, but, acting at

translational level, prolongs the half-life of the mRNA. It is interesting to note that, studying the induction of PGH synthase in U937 cells, we obtained some evidence that colony-stimulating factor 1 acts not only by regulating mRNA synthesis, but also by intervening in its translation (48).

Cell proliferation and differentiation: lipoxygenase versus cyclooxygenase

Many scattered studies in the literature point to the possibility that lipoxygenase products are involved primarily in cell proliferation, whereas cyclooxygenase products control cell differentiation. Thus, for example, Ziboh et al. (55,56) have reported that proliferating bone marrow myeloid cells release substantial amounts of arachidonate that is converted to leukotrienes. Prostanoids were also produced; however, only NDGA (but not indomethacin) inhibited proliferation (56). This finding has been confirmed using leukaemia cell lines (57). However, in normal colon cells, Craven and De Rubertis linked lipoxygenase products with cell differentiation (58).

More recently, Chang et al. (59) studied the actions of EGF on a human epidermoid carcinoma (A431 cells) and found that it induced expression of the 12-lipoxygenase mRNA concomitantly with increased cell proliferation. 12-HETE has been found to stimulate DNA synthesis in endothelial cells (60). Moreover, a careful study by D'Amore and collaborators (44) indicate that bFGF-induced endothelial cell proliferation is accompanied by a marked increase in 12-lipoxygenase products. In this study it was clearly shown that neither indomethacin nor inhibitors of 5-lipoxygenase affected cell growth. A similar mechanism may be the basis of platelet-derived growth factor-induced proliferation of smooth-muscle cells (44).

Recent data from other studies have proven conflicting. Thus, Funk et al. (61) cloned 12-lipoxygenase using human erythroleukaemia cells (HEL). Northern blots revealed that its mRNA was expressed in proliferating but not in quiescent cells. However, Izumi et al. (62) detected a small increase in 12-lipoxygenase mRNA levels during induced HEL differentiation. It is not known whether the promoter of the 12-lipoxygenase gene contains a phorbol ester-responsive element.

Promoter organization of genes coding for enzymes involved in prostanoid biosynthesis

Table 22.1 illustrates the assignment of structural motifs in the 5′-flanking regions (promoters) of the genes coding for both isoforms of PGH synthase and for 5-lipoxygenase (63–67). It is clear that the three genes are regulated by very different signals. Thus, many transcription regulators are recognized by the promoter of hPGH synthase 2, but the PGH synthase 1 gene is apparently turned on by few signals, most of which belong to the AP-PEA transcription factor family.

An unexpected characteristic of the 5-lipoxygenase promoter was the large number of sequences that recognize the SP-1 factor. As SP-1 protects from de novo methylation, the so-called 5′ CpG islands, this gene has previously been considered a housekeeping gene, that is widely expressed in tissues. However, as this is not the case, it is possible that silencer motifs detected in the promoter (67) play an important part in gene expression.

Summary and conclusions

A role for eicosanoids in tumour metastasis has been reviewed by Honn et al. (5) and more recently by Fulton (68). According to Honn and co-workers a shift in the intratumoral TxA_2/PGI_2 ratio can have profound effects on metastasis. When the ratio is high, platelets aggregate giving rise to the disseminated intravascular coagulation often characteristic of tumours that metastasize. When the ratio is low metastasis is rare. Fulton lays more emphasis on the modulation of immune system by prostanoids. This reasoning is similar to that of Tomasi et al. (69), regarding the immunosuppressive effect of PGE_2. Three main prostanoids namely, PGE_2, TxA_2, and PGI_2 are thought to be involved in different steps of tumour angiogenesis. The immunosuppressive action of PGE_2 is against T lymphocytes, natural killer cells, and perhaps monocytes and macrophages. This could partially explain why immuno-competent cells, infiltrating primary tumour and/or metastasis, are unable to mount an effective response to transformed cells (5,69). TxA_2 is produced at very high levels by stimulated monocytes and macrophages (70). We think that its main role is not to aggregate platelets (as its half-life is less than 30 s), but to function in monocyte differentiation and to act on endothelial cells following adherence (71).

PGI_2 may have angiogenic activity, as first proposed by Bicknell and Vallee while studying the mechanism of the angiogenic activity of the polypeptide angiogenin (72). The possibility that PGI_2 is involved in a more complex mechanism leading from quiescent endothelial cells to a differentiated capillary-like network of cells is a possibility that we are investigating.

Strong evidence connecting angiogenesis and PGH synthase come from studies of hypoxia-initiated angiogenesis. Keshet and co-workers (see Chapter 21) have reported that mRNA for VEGF is strongly increased in vitro and in vivo by hypoxia. Shaul et al. (73,74) in a series of studies have shown that hypoxia is a potent stimulus for the PGI_2 release in pulmonary artery endothelium. Hypoxia seems to trigger the induction of PGH synthase 1 (but not the alternative isoform) without influencing arachidonate release or PGI_2 synthase levels. This kind of specificity has been noted by Spisni et al. (21) working on IL-1α effects on PGI_2 synthase in HUVEC. Thus, it is possible that the oxygen sensor in endothelial cells is strictly coupled with a mechanism leading to the expression of genes coding for PGH synthase 1.

It would be of interest to ascertain whether a transcription factor such as NF-κB, having a broad spectrum of action within the endothelial cell and an activation mechanism dependent on the cell redox state, may be involved. Some data in the recent literature favour this possibility, but others do not. The first is that sodium salycylate, and its acetylated form, are strong inhibitors of NF-κB (14), while the second is represented by the fact that the consensus sequences for NF-κB is present in PGH synthase 2 but not in PGH synthase 1, the only form that seems to act as an oxygen sensor (see Fig. 22.6).

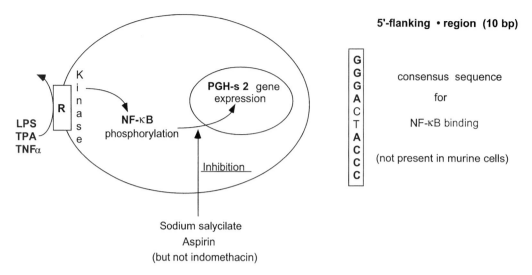

Figure 22.6. Mechanism of induction of prostaglandin H (PGH) 2 synthase in human umbilical vein endothelial cells. The promoter (5′flanking) of PGHs-1 does not contain the NF-κB consensus sequence, but contains two AP-2 and two PEA-3 motifs. LPS, lipopolysaccharide; TNF, tumour necrosis factor; TPA, phorbol myristate acetate.

References

1. Tomasi, V., Manica, F., and Spisni, E. (1990). Polypeptide growth factors and angiogenesis. *BioFactors*, **2**, 213–17.

2. Smith, W. L. and Marnett, L. J. (1991). Prostaglandin endoperoxide synthase: structure and catalysis. *Biochim. Biophys. Acta*, **1083**, 1–17.

3. Smith, W. L., Eling, T. E., Kulmacz, R. J., Marnett, L. J., and Tsai, A. (1992). Tyrosyl radicals and their role in hydroperoxide-dependent activation and inactivation of prostaglandin endoperoxide synthase. *Biochemistry*, **31**, 3–7.

4. Goppelt-Struebe, M. (1995). Regulation of prostaglandin endoperoxide synthase (cyclooxygenase) isozyme expression. *Prostaglandins Leuotrienes Essential Fatty Acids*, **52**, 213–22.

5. Honn, K. V., Bockman, R. S., and Marnett, L. J. (1981). Prostaglandin and cancer: a review of tumor initiation through tumor metastasis. *Prostaglandins*, **31**, 833–64.

6. Ben-Ezra, D. B. (1979). Neovasculogenesis. Triggering factors and possible mechanism. *Surv. Ophthalmol.*, **24**, 167–76.

7. Ziche, M., Jones, J., and Gullino, P. M. (1982). Role of prostaglandin E1 and copper in angiogenesis. *J. Natl Cancer. Inst.*, **69**, 475–81.

8. Form, D. M. and Auerbach, R. (1983). PGE2 and angiogenesis. *Proc. Soc. Exp. Biol. Med.*, **172**, 214–18.

9. Ohtsu, A., Fuji, K., and Kurozumi, S. (1988) Induction of angiogenic response by chemically stable prostacyclin analogs. *Prostaglandins Leukotrienes Essential Fatty Acids*, **33**, 35–39.

10. Kowalski, J., Kwan, H. H., Prionas, S. D., Allison, A., C., and Fajardo, L. F. (1992). Characterization and applications of the disc angiogenesis system. *Exp. Mol. Pathol.*, **56**, 1–19.

11. Fulton, A. M. (1984). Effects of indomethacin on the growth of cultured mammary tumours. *Int. J. Cancer*, **33**, 375–9.

12. Spisni, E., Manica, F., and Tomasi, V. (1992). Involvement of prostanoids in the regulation of angiogenesis by polypeptide growth factors. *Prostaglandins Leukotrienes Essential Fatty, Acids EFA*, **47**, 111–15.

13. Wu, K. K., Sanduia, R., Tsai, A., Ferhanoglu, B., and Loose-Mitchell, D. S. (1991). Aspirin inhibits interleukin 1-induced prostaglandin H synthase expression in cultured endothelial cells. *Proc. Natl Acad. Sci. USA*, **88**, 2384–7.

14. Kopp, E. and Ghosh, S. (1994). Inhibition of NF-κB by sodium salicylate and aspirin. *Science*, **265**, 956–9.

15. Whatley, R. E., Stroud, E. D., Bunting, M., Zimmerman, G. A., McIntyre, T. M., and Prescott, S. M. (1993). Growth-dependent changes in arachidonic acid release from endothelial cells are mediated by protein kinase C and changes in diacylglycerol. *J. Biol. Chem.*, **268**, 16130–8.

16. Mayer, R. J. and Marshall, L. A. (1993). New insights on mammalian phospholipase A₂(s); comparison of arachidonoyl-selective and nonselective enzymes. *FASEB J.*, **7**, 339–48.

17. Muszbek, L. and Laposata, M. (1993). Covalent modification of proteins by arachidonate and eicosapentaenoate in platelets. *J. Biol. Chem.*, **268**, 18243–8.

18. Jurivich, D. A., Sistonen, L., Sarge, K. D., and Morimoto R. I. (1994). Arachidonate is a potent modulator of human heat shock gene transcription. *Proc. Natl Acad. Sci. USA*, **91**, 2280–4.

19. Sylvester, P. W., Birkenfeld, H. P., Hosick, H. L., and Briski, K. P. (1994). Fatty acid modulation of epidermal growth factor-induced mouse mammary epithelial cell proliferation *in vitro*. *Exp. Cell Res.*, **214**, 145–53.

20. Keler, T. and Sorof, S. (1993). Growth promotion of transfected hepatoma cells by liver fatty acid binding protein. *J. Cell. Physiol.* **157**, 33–40.

21. Spisni, E., Belletti, B., Bartolini, G., Orlandi, M., and Tomasi, V. (1995). Prostacyclin (PGI2) synthase is a constitutively expressed enzyme in HUVE cells. *Exp. Cell Res.* **219**, 507–13.

22. DeWitt, D. L. and Smith, W. L. (1983). Purification of prostacyclin synthase from bovine aorta by immunoaffinity chromatography. *J. Biol. Chem.*, **258**, 3285–93.

23. Rosen, G. D., Birkenmeier, T. M., Raz, A., and Holtzman, M. J. (1989). Identification of a cyclooxygenase related gene and its potential role in prostaglandin formation. *Biochem. Biophys. Res. Commun.*, **164**, 1358–65.

24. O'Banion, M. K., Sadowski, H. B., Winn, V., and Young, D. A. (1991). A serum- and glucocorticoid-regulated 4-kilobase mRNA encodes a cyclooxygenase-related protein. *J. Biol. Chem.*, **266**, 23261–7.

25. Hla, T. and Neilson, K. (1992). Human cyclooxygenase-2 cDNA. *Proc. Natl Acad. Sci. USA*, **89**, 7384–8.

26. Murakami, M., Matsumoto, R., Austen, K. F., and Arm, J. P. (1994). Prostaglandin endoperoxide synthase-1 and -2 couple to different transmembrane stimuli to generate prostaglandin D_2 in mouse bone marrow-derived mast cells. *J. Biol. Chem.*, **269**, 22269–75.

27. Tanaka, Y., Ward, S. L., and Smith, W. L. (1987). Immunochemical and kinetic evidence for two different prostaglandin H-prostaglandin E isomerases in sheep vesicular gland microsomes. *J. Biol. Chem.*, **262**, 1374–81.

28. Ohashi, K., Ke-He, R., Kulmacz, R. J., Wu, K. K., and Wang, L. (1992). Primary structure of human thromboxane synthase determined from the cDNA sequence. *J. Biol. Chem.*, **267**, 789–93.

29. Smith, W. L. (1986). Prostaglandin biosynthesis and its compartmentation in vascular smooth muscle and endothelial cells. *Annu. Rev. Physiol.*, **48**, 251–62.

30. Pereira, B., Wu, K. K., and Wang L. H. (1994) Molecular cloning and characterization of bovine prostacyclin sinthase. *Biochem. Biophys. Res. Commun.*, **203**, 59–66.

31. Hara, S., Miyata, A., Yokoyama, C., Inoue, H., Brugger, R., Lottspeich, F., *et al.* (1994). Isolation and molecular cloning of prostacyclin synthase from bovine endothelial cells. *J. Biol. Chem.*, **269**, 19897–903.

32. Ruan, K., Li, P., Kulmacz, J., and Wu, K. (1994). Characterization of the structure and membrane interaction of NH_2-terminal domain of thromboxane A_2 synthase. *J. Biol. Chem.*, **269**, 20938–42.

33. Orlandi, M. Bartolini, G., Belletti, B., Spisni, E., and Tomasi, V. (1994). Thromboxane A_2 synthase activity in platelet free human monocytes. *Biochim. Biophys. Acta*, **1215**, 285–90.

34. Belletti, B., Spisni, E., Bartolini, G., Orlandi, M., and Tomasi, V. (1995). Post-transcriptional regulation of thromboxane A_2 synthase in U937 cells. *Biochem. Biophys. Res. Commun.*, **209**, 901–6.

35. Abramovitz, M., Boie, Y., Nguyen, T., Rushmore, T. H., Bayne, M. A., Metters, K. M., *et al.* (1994). Cloning and expression of a cDNA for the human prostanoid FP receptor. *J. Biol. Chem.*, **269**, 2632–6.

36. Kunapuli, S. P., Fen Mao, G., Bastepe, M., Liu-Chen, L. Y., Li, S., Cheung, P. P., *et al.* (1994). Cloning and expression of a prostaglandin E receptor EP_3 subtype from human erytroleukaemia cells. *Biochem. J.*, **298**, 263–7.

37. Offermanns, S., Laugwitz, K. L., Spicher, K., and Schultz, G. (1994). G proteins of the G_{12} family are activated via thromboxane A_2 and thrombin receptors in human platelets. *Proc. Natl Acad. Sci. USA*, **91**, 504–8.

38. Namba, T., Sugimoto, Y., Negishi, M., Irie, A., Ushikubi, F., Kakizuka, A., *et al.* (1993). Alternative splicing of c-terminal tail of prostaglandin E receptor subtype EP3 determines G-protein specificity. *Nature*, **365**, 166–70.

39. Katsuyama, M., Sugimoto, Y., Namba, T., Irie, A., Negishi, M., Narumiya, S., and Ichikawa, A. (1994). Cloning and

40. Weksler, B. B. (1990). Heparin and acid fibroblast growth factor interact to decrease prostacyclin synthesis in human endothelial cells by affecting both prostaglandin H synthase and prostacyclin synthase. *J. Cell. Physiol.*, **142**, 514–22.

41. Hasegawa, N., Yamamoto, M., and Yamamoto, K. (1988). Stimulation of cell growth and inhibition of prostacyclin production by heparin in human umbilical vein endothelial cells. *J. Cell. Physiol.* **137**, 603–7.

42. Maciag, T., Cerundolo, J., Ilsley, S., Kelley, P. R., and Forand, R. (1979). An endothelial cell growth factor from bovine hypothalamus: identification and partial characterization. *Proc. Natl Acad. Sci. USA*, **76**, 5674–8.

43. Hla, T. and Maciag, T. (1991). Cyclooxygenase gene expression is down regulated by heparin-binding (acidic fibroblast) growth factor-1 in human endothelial cells. *J. Biol. Chem.*, **266**, 24059–63.

44. Dethlefsen, S. M., Shepro, D., and D'Amore, P. A. (1994). Arachidonic acid metabolites in bFGF-, PDGF-, and serum stimulated vascular cell growth. *Exp. Cell. Res.*, **212**, 262–73.

45. Partanen, J., Makela, T. P., Eerola, E., Korhonen, J., Hirvonen, H., Claesson-Welsh, L., and Alitalo, K. (1991). FGFR-4, a novel acidic fibroblast growth factor receptor with a distinct expression pattern. *EMBO J.*, **10**, 1347–53.

46. Smith, C. J., Morrow, J. D., Roberts L. J., and Marnett, L. J. (1993). Differentiation of monocytoid THP-1 cells with phorbol ester induces expression of prostaglandin endoperoxide synthase-1 (COX-1). *Biochem. Biophys. Res. Commun.*, **192**, 787–93.

47. Bartolini, G., Orlandi, M., Chiricolo M., Minghetti, L., Guerrini, F., Fidan, M., *et al.* (1986). Regulation of thromboxane A2 biosynthesis in platelet-free human monocytes and the possible role of polypeptide growth factor(s) in the induction of the cyclooxygenase system. *Biochim. Biophys. Acta*, **876**, 486–93.

48. Bartolini, G., Orlandi, M., Spisni, E., Davis, J., Minghetti, L., Belletti, B., and Tomasi, V. (1995). Possible involvement of prostaglandin H synthase-1 induction in the differentiation of U937 cells. *BioFactors*, **6**, 1–8.

49. Wu, K. K., Hatzakis, H., Lo, S. S., Seong, D. C., Sanduia, S. K., and Tai, H. H. (1988). Stimulation of *de novo* synthesis of prostaglandin G/H synthase in human endothelial cells by phorbol ester. *J. Biol. Chem.*, **263**, 19043–7.

50. Fraiser-Scott, K., Hatzakis, K., Seong, D., Jones, C. M., and Wu, K. K. (1988). Influence of natural and recombinant interleukin 2 on endothelial cell arachidonate metabolism. *J. Clin. Invest.*, **82**, 1877–83.

51. Rossi, V., Breviario, F., Ghezzi, P., Dejana, E., and Mantovani, A. (1995). Prostacyclin synthesis induced in vascular cells by interleukin-1. *Science*, **229**, 174–6.

52. Maier, J. A. M., and Ragnotti, G. (1993). An oligomer targeted against protein kinase Cα prevents interleukin-1α induction of cyclooxygenase expression in human endothelial cells. *Exp. Cell Res.*, **205**, 52–8.

53. Cozzolino, F., Torcia, M., Aldinucci, D., Ziche, M., Almerigogna, F., Bani, D., and Stern, D. M. (1990). Interleukin 1 is an autocrine regulator of human endothelial cell growth. *Proc. Natl Acad. Sci. USA*, **87**, 6487–91.

54. Ristimaki, A., Garfinkel, S., Wessendorf, J., Maciag, T., and Hla, H. (1994). Induction of cyclooxygenase-2 by interleukin-1α. *J. Biol. Chem.*, **269**, 11769–75.

55. Ziboh, V. A., Miller A. M., Wu, M., Yunis, A. A., Jimenez, J., and Wong, G. (1982). Induced release and metabolism of

arachidonic acid from myeloid cells by purified colony-stimulating factor. *J. Cell Physiol.*, **113**, 67–72.

56. Ziboh, V. A., Wong, T., Wu, M., and Yunis, A. A. (1986). Modulation of colony stimulating factor-induced murine myeloid colony formation by S-peptido-lipoxygenase products. *Cancer Res.*, **46**, 600–3.

57. Tsukada, T., Nakashima, K., and Shirakawa, S. (1986). Arachidonate 5-lipoxygenase inhibitors show potent anti-proliferative effects on human leukemia cell lines. *Biochem. Biophys. Res. Commun.*, **140**, 832–6.

58. Craven, P. A. and DeRubertis, F. R. (1986). Profiles of eicosanoid production by superficial and proliferative colonic epithelial cells and sub-epithelial colonic tissue. *Prostaglandins*, **32**, 387–99.

59. Chang, W., Liu, Y., Ning, C., Suzuki, H., Yoshimoto, T., and Yamamoto, S. (1993). Induction of arachidonate 12-lipoxygenase mRNA by epidermal growth factor in A431 cells. *J. Biol. Chem.*, **268**, 18734–9.

60. Yamaja, S., Graeber, J. E., and Stuart, M. J. (1987). The mitogenic effect of 15- and 12-hydroxyeicosatetraenoic acid on endothelial cells may be mediated via diacylglycerol kinase inhibition. *J. Biol. Chem.*, **262**, 17613–22.

61. Funk, C. D., Furci, L., and FitzGerald G. A. (1990). Molecular cloning, primary structure, and expression of the human platelet/erytroleukemia cell 12-lipoxygenase. *Proc. Natl Acad. Sci. USA*, **87**, 5638–42.

62. Izumi, T., Hoshiko, S., Radmark, O., and Samuelsson, B. (1990). Cloning of the human 12-lipoxygenase. *Proc. Natl Acad. Sci. USA*, **87**, 7477–81.

63. Kosaka, T., Miyata, A., Ihara, H., Hara, S., Sugimoto, T., Takeda, O., *et al.* (1994). Characterization of the human gene (PTGS2) encoding prostaglandin-endoperoxide synthase 2. *Eur. J. Biochem.*, **221**, 889–97.

64. Xie, W., Merrill, J. R., Bradshaw, W. S., and Simmons, D. L. (1993). Structural determination and promoter analysis of the chiken mitogen-inducible prostaglandin G: H synthase gene and genetic mapping of the murine homolog. *Arch. Biochem. Biophys.*, **300**, 247–52.

65. Kraemer, S. A., Meade, E. A., and DeWitt, D. L. (1992). Prostaglandin endoperoxide synthase gene structure: identification of the transcriptional start site and 5-flanking regulatory sequences. *Arch. Biochem. Biophys.*, **293**, 391–400.

66. Wang, L., Hajibeigi, A., Xu, X., Loose-Mitchell, D., and Wu, K. K. (1993). Characterization of the promoter of human prostaglandin H synthase-1 gene. *Biochem. Biophys. Res. Commun.*, **190**, 406–11.

67. Hoshiko, S., Radmark, O., and Samuelsson, B. (1990). Characterization of the human 5-lipoxygenase gene promoter. *Proc. Natl Acad. Sci. USA*, **87**, 9073–7.

68. Fulton, A. M. (1988). The role of eicosanoids in tumor metastasis. *Prostaglandins Leukotrienes Essential Fatty Acids*, **34**, 229–237.

69. Tomasi, V., Mastacchi, R., Bartolini, G., Fadda, S., Barnabei, O., Gatto, R., *et al.* (1984). The relationships between the high production of prostaglandins by tumors and their action on lympocytes as suppressive agents. In *Genetic and phenotypic markers of tumors* (ed. S. A. Aaronson, L. Frati, and R. Verna), pp. 235–59. Plenum Press, New York.

70. Bartolini, G., Orlandi, M., Chiricolo, M., Licastro, F., Zambonelli, P., Minghetti, L., and Tomasi, V. (1990): Interleukins and interferons: yin–yang modulators of PGH synthase in human macrophages. *BioFactors*, **2**, 267–70.

71. Goldman, G., Welbourn, R., Klausner., J. M., Valeri C. R., Shepro, D., and Hechtman, H. B. (1991). Thromboxane mediates diapedesis after ischemia by activation of neutrophil adhesion receptors interacting with basally expressed intercellular adhesion molecule-1. *Circulation Res.*, **68**, 1013–19.

72. Bicknell, R. and Vallee, B. L. (1989). Angiogenin stimulates endothelial cell prostacyclin secretion by activation of phospholipase A_2 *Proc. Natl Acad. Sci. USA*, **86**, 1573–7.

73. Brannon, T. S., North, A. J., Wells, L. B., and Shaul, P. W. (1994). Prostacyclin synthesis in ovine pulmonary artery is developmentally regulated by changes in cyclooxygenase-1 gene expression. *J. Clin. Invest.*, **93**, 2230–5.

74. Shaul, P. W., Campbell, W. B., Farrar, M. A., and Magness, R. R. (1992). Oxygen modulates prostacyclin synthesis in ovine fetal pulmonary arteries by an effect on cyclo-oxygenase. *J. Clin. Invest.*, **90**, 2147–55.

75. Lin, L. L., Wartmann, M., Lin. A. Y., Knopf, J. L., Seth, A., and Davis, R. J. (1993). cPLA₂ is phosphorylated and activated by MAP kinase. *Cell*, **72**, 269–78.

23. Inhibition of tumour angiogenesis and the induction of tumour dormancy

Lars Holmgren and Roy Bicknell

Since the early 1970s when Folkman popularized the idea that tumour growth is angiogenesis-dependent and that an anti-angiogenic strategy might constitute a novel therapeutic approach for the treatment of solid tumours (1) there has been an ever increasing interest in the idea. Indeed, with the realization that anti-angiogenesis may be useful in the treatment of a number of pathologies aside from cancer (*e.g.* psoriasis, diabetic retinopathy, menorrhagia, etc.) over the last 10 years interest in the identification of a therapeutically useful anti-angiogenic compound has become intense.

A recent literature search revealed that over 200 compounds have now been reported to have anti-angiogenic activity. Many of these compounds have simply been shown to inhibit angiogenesis in one of the frequently used assays, most commonly the chick chorioallantoic membrane (CAM) assay (see Chapter 2). However, an increasing number of anti-angiogenics have been identified by focusing on individual steps in the angiogenic process as targets and then searching for inhibitors of that process. An example of the latter are the matrix metalloprotease inhibitors Batimastat (BB94) and Marimastat (BB2516) that have been identified by British Biotechnology in Oxford.

It is also true to say that for an increasing number of compounds identified using anti-angiogenesis assays, the mechanism of their anti-angiogenic activity has to a greater or lesser extent been elucidated. Examples include preferential (i.e. low-dose) inhibition of endothelial cell proliferation by AGM-1470 (a fumagillin derivative).

As already noted, angiogenesis is a complex multistep process and as such presents a number of key targets for therapeutic intervention. Examples include: (i) inhibition of the proteolytic enzymes such as the matrix metalloproteases or plasminogen activators (released by endothelial cells in response to angiogenic stimuli) that breakdown the extracellular matrix surrounding the existing capillaries; (ii) inhibition of endothelial cell migration; (iii) inhibition of endothelial cell proliferation; (iv) disruption of endothelial cell tube formation/vascular restructuring; and

(v) enhancement of tumour endothelial cell apoptosis.

The purpose of this chapter is to provide the reader with an overview of where the area of anti-angiogenesis research currently stands and what we may expect from the future. It is not our intention to review the entire anti-angiogenic literature for to do so would require a book in itself. For comprehensive reviews of the anti-angiogenic literature the interested reader is referred to the following Herblin *et al.* (2), Auerbach and Auerbach (3), Casey *et al.* (4), Fan *et al.* (15), and Bicknell and Harris (6).

Selected examples of therapeutically promising anti-angiogenics

Table 23.1 outlines targets for intervention in the angiogenic process and lists active compounds.

Inhibition of matrix metalloproteases

Among the most promising anti-cancer matrix metalloprotease inhibitors are British Biotechnologies Batimastat, the related but orally active Marimastat and various compounds such as Galardin (GM6001) being developed by Glycomed in the USA. Marimastat is currently in phase II clinical trials for advanced ovarian prostate, colon, and pancreatic cancer.

Inhibition of endothelial cell adhesion and migration

Endothelial cell migration is an important component of the angiogenic process. Migration of the endothelial cell involves complex adhesive interactions between both neighbouring endothelial cells and between endothelial cells and the extracellular matrix around them. Recent studies have identified strategies that by disrupting endothelial adhesion inhibit angiogenesis.

Table 23.1. Inhibitors of discrete targets in the angiogenesis cascade

Target	Examples of inhibitors
Activation of endothelial cells by an angiogenic signal	
Production of angiogenic factors Angiogenic (growth factor) antagonists	Glucocorticoids, gold salts, suramin, FCE 26644, xylan sulphates, pentosan polysulphate, protamine sulphate, DS-4152, PF4, HBNF, antibodies to bFGF and VEGF, bFGF receptor fragment
Receptor signal transduction	Herbimycin A, genistein, staurosporine, MDL 27032, calphostin C
Synthesis and release of degradative enzymes	Minocycline and tetracycline, derivatives, 15-deoxyspergualin, SCM-chitin III, suramin angiostatic steroids, medroxyprogesterone acetate, TIMP-1, TIMP-2, thrombospondin, cartilage-derived inhibitor, vitreous-derived inhibitor
Endothelial cell migration	Angiostatic steroids, 15-deoxyspergualin, D-penicillamine, AGM-1470, CDPGYIGSR-NH$_2$, Gly-Arg-Gly-Asp-Ser, TIMP-1, TIMP-2, thrombospondin cartilage-derived inhibitor,protamine sulphate, suramin, PF4, DS-4152, SCM-chitin III, tenascin-related peptides, eponemycin, linomide, nicardipine
Proliferation of endothelial cells	
Angiogenic (growth factor) antagonists	Suramin, FCE 26644, protamine sulphate, xylan sulphates, pentosan polysulphate, DS-4152,HAH-cortisol, PF4, HBNG, bFGF and VEGF antibodies,
Angiogenic growth factor receptor signal transduction	Herbimycin A, genistein, staurosporine, MDL-27032 calphostin C
Endothelial–preferential cytotoxic action	AGM-1470 and analogues, FR-111142, WF-16775A$_{1, 2}$
Other	Tetracycline derivatives, eponemycin, 15-deoxyspergualin, linomide, minocycline, thrombospondin, cartilage-derived collagenase inhibitor
Formation of capillary tubules and loops and their subsequent differentiation	MDL-27032, interferon γ, cyclic YIGSR peptide, AGM-1470, Gly-Arg-Gly-Asp-Ser, eponemycin, 1-deoxymannojirimycin, 15-deoxyspergualin, nicardipine
Basement membrane biosynthesis	Angiostatic steroids, proline analogues, D-penicillamine, GPA 1734, D-609, aminopropionitrile, krestin

Modified from reference 7. Agents not reviewed in this article are described in reference 7.

Antibodies that recognize the $\alpha_v\beta_3$ integrin dimer inhibit angiogenesis

It has been shown (7) that a monoclonal to the $\alpha_v\beta_3$ integrin dimer induces apoptosis of proliferating endothelial cells *in vitro* (probably by blocking endothelial cell adhesion), is anti-angiogenic *in vivo* and inhibits growth of solid tumours when they are placed on to the chick CAM. The anti-$\alpha_v\beta_3$ antibody (known as LM609), although recognizing a blocking epitope in both the chick and human $\alpha_v\beta_3$ dimer, failed to do so in the mouse dimer. Thus, in order to confirm an anti-tumour effect of the anti-

body in more conventional mouse xenograft experiments, human foreskin was xenografted into the flank of athymic mice and a carcinoma then implanted into the human skin graft. In this model the developing tumour was vascularized by endothelial cells derived from the human skin graft and the LM609 was shown to inhibit tumour growth (8).

The LM609 antibody has been humanized by the Ixsys Co. of San Diego to give the anti-angiogenic called 'Vitaxin' that it is planned to use in clinical trials against Kaposi's sarcoma, melanoma and breast carcinoma among others. High-affinity, cyclic non-RGD antagonists of the binding of the endothelial cell $\alpha_v\beta_3$ dimer to vitronectin are also being developed by Ixsys among other companies. Such compounds offer considerable promise of being future anti-angiogenic drugs.

Inhibition of endothelial cell proliferation

Inhibition of angiogenic growth factor signalling

Two main strategies have been followed here, namely: (i) antagonism of the growth factor – growth factor receptor interaction, and (ii) antagonism of signal transduction by the growth factor receptor after growth factor binding to the receptor. Examples of the former include suramin (9), pentosan polysulphate (10), and related polyanions (11) that bind tightly to a number of angiogenic growth factors such as the fibroblast growth factors and vascular endothelial growth factor (VEGF). Binding of the polyanion to the growth factor blocks binding of the latter to their cognate receptors. The latter strategy includes tyrosine kinase inhibitors such as genistein (12). In view of the apparent importance of VEGF in tumour angiogenesis, specific low molecular weight inhibitors of VEGF receptor (KDR and *flt*-1) signal transduction offer particular promise as anti-angiogenics, but none have yet been described. Dominant negative receptors such as the truncated KDR receptor that has been delivered to endothelium by retrovirus to inhibit xenografted glioblastoma growth (13; and see Chapter 1) also fall within this targeting strategy.

Preferential inhibition of endothelial cell proliferation

Anti-angiogenics of interest here include the fumagillin derivatives known as the angioinhibins, particularly the compound AGM-1470 (14). These compounds preferentially hold endothelial cells cytostatic at concentrations several orders of magnitude less than they do cells of other lineages. The mechanism of action of AGM-1470 and why it is far more potent in the inhibition of endothelial cell proliferation than that of other cell types is still unclear; although there is some evidence that AGM-1470 may interact with endothelial cell cyclins (15).

Stimulation of tumour endothelial cell apoptosis

The proteolytic fragment of plasminogen named angiostatin was recently identified as a naturally occurring inhibitor of angiogenesis (16). Angiostatin is one of several naturally occurring inhibitors of angiogenesis and it will now be discussed in some detail.

Negative regulators of angiogenesis: angiostatin

Tumorigenesis is a multistep process involving not only an increase in cell proliferation but often also a decrease in cell death (apoptosis). Apoptosis is characterized by the rapid elimination of single cells in an environment of living cells (17). Activation of cell death programmes can be triggered by exogenous signals such as the FAS-ligand or tumour necrosis factor alpha which bind high-affinity receptors that mediate the death signal or by depletion of survival signals normally required by the cell to block activation of a default cell death programme (18,19). Apoptosis is a normal process occurring during embryonic development, in neural cells during neural development, and between developing digits during limb bud formation. In adults, apoptosis plays an important part in the maintenance of tissue homeostasis; in the human small intestine alone, approximately 10^9 cells apoptose every hour and are sloughed off into the lumen of the gut (20,21).

The finding that some transforming oncogenes not only stimulate proliferation, but also trigger apoptosis, has shown that the signalling pathways mediating these events are tightly coupled (22–25). For a tumour to progress it is therefore necessary that activation of cell suicide is inhibited. This may be accomplished through the up-regulation of apoptosis-suppressor molecules, for example, bcl-2 (26,27).

Another pathway is the inactivation of p53, the latter which plays a pivotal role in the decision to undergo apoptosis. For example, the simian virus 40 large T oncoprotein does not only stimulate proliferation but also prevent apoptosis by complexing with p53 (28). These are examples of intracellular events that modulate cell survival in response to an increased proliferative potential. Equally important, however, is the ability of the tumour to manipulate its extracellular environment to ensure that tumour cell proliferation results in an increase in cell number and tumour volume.

A crucial step during tumour progression is the switch to an angiogenic phenotype (29). Indirect evidence for this has been accumulated in several model systems for example; mouse sarcoma tumour pieces implanted under the skin, rat sarcoma tumours grown on the chick CAM and V2 carcinoma implanted in the avascular rabbit cornea (30–32). In all these experiments, the tumours grow no larger than a few millimetres in size until vascularized by host vessels. V2 carcinoma cells implanted in the vitreous of the eye remain dormant for up to 10 weeks with no or little growth (33). Once the tumours attach to the retina they vascularized and expanded 19 000-fold in mass over 2 weeks. The escape from dormancy was thus directly correlated to the time of onset of angiogenesis.

The escape from dormancy by induction of angiogenesis has been studied in Lewis lung carcinoma (LLC) and T241 fibrosarcoma mouse model systems. In these model systems the presence of a primary tumour maintained metastases in a dormant phase. However, surgical removal of the primary tumour resulted in rapid growth of metastases in the lungs (34). Dormant metastases formed perivascular cuffs around pre-existing lung venules and three-dimensional analyses of the blood vessels indicating that these tumours were indeed avascular. Removal of the primary tumour resulted in extensive angiogenesis within 5 days of the operation.

Neovascularization resulted in rapid growth of the metastases but did not alter the cell proliferation rate. Growth of new blood vessels did, however, affect the survival rate of the tumour cells. DNA fragmentation is a hallmark of apoptosis and can be detected *in situ* by terminal transferase labelling of 3′DNA ends (35,36). In dormant metastases, approximately 7% of the tumour cells exhibited fragmented DNA as determined by the terminal transferase method. In vascularized metastases the corresponding percentage dropped to 2%. The removal of apoptotic cells is very rapid (1–2 h), which means that a 3–4-fold change in the apoptotic index will have a substantial impact on the rate of tumour growth (37,38).

The molecular mechanism by which the primary tumour suppresses angiogenesis of its metastases has been elucidated. That the anti-metastatic activity was mediated by a circulating inhibitor was suggested by the following: (i) angiogenesis was systemically suppressed: (ii) serum from tumour-bearing animals contained activity that inhibited endothelial cell proliferation *in vitro*; and (iii) serum from tumour-bearing mice also contained anti-metastatic activity *in vivo* (34). This factor was purified from serum as well as urine from tumour-bearing mice, and sequencing analysis revealed a 98% homology to plasminogen. This fragment, named angiostatin, inhibits endothelial cell proliferation *in vitro* and angiogenesis *in vivo* (34). Angiostatin treatment of mice with LLC lung metastases shows that an angiogenesis inhibitor mimics the effect of the primary tumour in maintaining the dormant phase of the lung metastases. Angiostatin suppresses angiogenesis and maintains a high index of apoptosis in the tumours. Angiostatin is not only effective in treating metastases from mouse tumours, for systemic treatment of established subcutaneous PC3 human prostate tumours in severe combined immune deficient mice for

30 days resulted in regression of tumour mass. Residual tumours remained as perivascular cuffs in the dermal mesenchyme, and could only be detected by histology (O'Reilly, Holmgren, Chen, and Folkman, unpublished data). A fivefold higher incidence of apoptosis was detected in the angiostatin-treated tumours when compared with saline-treated controls, whereas no effect on tumour cell proliferation could be detected. Treatment of tumour cells with angiostatin *in vitro* showed no effect on either proliferation or apoptosis indicating that this effect is indirectly caused by the inhibition of neovascularization. This indirect effect on tumour cell apoptosis is not restricted to treatment with angiostatin. Similar effects on tumour apoptosis *in vivo* have been detected after treatment with TNP 470 (previously AGM-1470) in LLC lung metastases (34). Early treatment of mice in a transgenic β-cell tumour model with a combination of TNP-470, minocycline and alpha/beta interferon markedly inhibited tumour growth but did not prevent tumour formation. The apoptotic index was doubled in treated animals whereas the proliferation index was similar to that of controls (39). In conclusion, these studies suggest that the main effect controlling angiogenesis in tumours is elevating the incidence of cell death by apoptosis. Dormancy or homeostasis is achieved when the tumours reach an equilibrium where cell generation is balanced by cell death.

What are factors that control tumour cell apoptosis when access to blood supply is restricted? Previous studies show that one vessel can support a tumour mass of approximately 250–300 mm in diameter. This is supposedly the diffusion range of factor(s) required for tumour cell survival. The induction of angiogenesis may promote tumour growth via increased perfusion of molecules present in the circulation; however, paracrine interaction with factors produced by infiltrating endothelial cells may also be of importance.

Endothelial cells have been shown to produce a number of growth factors such as platelet-derived growth factor, insulin-like growth factor (IGF) 1, heparin-binding epidermal growth factor, and interleukin 6, some or all of which may promote tumour growth. Transformation of cells may result in increased dependency on either high serum concentration or the presence of such growth factor. For example, fibroblasts transformed by c-*myc* require the presence of high serum or IGF-1 levels to avoid apoptosis (23,40). Neovascularization may increase the availability of survival factors either present in the circulation, or produced directly by endothelial cells or both (42,43).

In vivo nuclear magnetic resonance spectroscopy studies have shown that tumour metabolism is dependent on blood flow. Controlling the access to circulating glucose and oxygen may be one way by which anti-angiogenic therapy controls tumour growth. In a model system where tumours were perfused *in vitro*, it was shown that the tumour energy status is dependent on the perfusing glucose concentration (44). However, lowering oxygen levels has little or no effect on tumour energy levels. High glucose metabolism has long been recognized as a distinguishing characteristic of tumour cells. Oncogenes such as *src*, *ras*, and *myc* have been shown to increase the uptake and metabolism of glucose (45,46). The transport of glucose into the cell represents a rate-limiting step in the regulation of its metabolism. Indeed, interleukin -3 has now been shown to block apoptosis by stimulating glucose transport (47). It is therefore possible that some tumours are not only dependent on the rate of glucose perfusion, but are also dependent on growth factors that stimulate uptake of glucose. Oxygen is also a potential modulator of tumour apoptosis. Hypoxia induces apoptosis in Rat1 fibroblast cells transformed by the *myc* oncogene. However, tumour cells acquire resistance to hypoxia by either inactivation of p53 or overexpression of bcl-2 (48). Taken together, there are several different pathways and molecules that may influence tumour cell survival.

Metastasis is the major cause of mortality in cancer patients (49). In many cases the metastatic disease is not detectable by clinical methods at the time of diagnosis, but metastases recur after treatment of the primary tumour. In some cancers such as melanoma and breast cancer, metastases may remain dormant for several years until relapse occurs., Clinical studies have shown that the extensive lag time until recurrence is not explained by a slower growth rate. In some breast cancer patients, for example, the rate of growth of previously dormant local recurrences follows that of the original tumour (50). In melanoma patients who relapse years after removal of the primary tumour, the survival rate is not significantly different than that of patients who relapse within months (51). These studies support a model of biphasic growth of tumours in which the tumours are under growth restraint during dormancy which the tumour escapes from during relapse. Exactly how this growth restraint is maintained in patients is not known. The studies of angiogenic control of dormancy in mouse lung metastases suggests a potential mechanism of tumour dormancy in patients. In the absence of neovascularization, the tumour cells are in an equilibrium of proliferation balanced by apoptosis. This state is stable over longer periods as shown by studies of B16F10 melanoma lung metastases that remain dormant for months (34).

Micrometastases may escape dormancy by increasing their angiogenic potential. This may be achieved by at least two mechanisms: the removal of a circulating inhibitor (*e.g.* removal of a primary tumour resulting in the disappearance of circulating angiostatin), or a subset of

tumour cells within the micrometastases may switch to an angiogenic phenotype. Proliferation without growth in dormant metastases could over time generate mutations or genetic alterations necessary for such a switch to occur. An important question yet to be answered is whether the recurrent metastases in cancer patients have been proliferating during the dormant phase. This question could possibly be answered by analysing the accumulated mutations or divergence of microsatellite repeats during long-term dormancy in cancer patients who are deficient in DNA repair enzymes.

In conclusion, deeper understanding of the mechanisms behind tumour dormancy is of importance as it could lead to development of new therapies aiming to extend the period of tumour quiescence. Owing to the low toxicity, anti-angiogenic therapy may be applied for this purpose to control the growth of residual cancer disease. This may not lead to cure but would prolong the asymptomatic phase of the disease and potentially be combined with other treatments such as immunotherapy.

Acknowledgements

L. H. is supported by grants from the Swedish Cancer Society and the Jeannska Foundation. R. B. is supported by the Imperial Cancer Research Fund.

References

1. Folkman, J. (1971). Tumour angiogenesis: therapeutic implications. *N. Eng. J. Med.*, **285**, 1182–6.
2. Herblin, W. F., Brem, S., Fan, T. P., and Gross, J. L. (1994). Recent advances in angiogenesis inhibitors. *Exp. Opin. Ther. Patents*, **4**, 641–54.
3. Auerbach, W. and Auerbach, R. (1994). Angiogenesis inhibition: a review. *Pharmacol. Ther.*, **63**, 265–311.
4. Casey, R., Li, W. W., and Li, V. W. (1995). Angiogenesis in malignancy. *Future Oncol.*, **1**, 185–200,
5. Fan, T. P. D., Jaggar, R., and Bicknell, R. (1995). Controlling the vasculature: angiogenesis, anti-angiogenesis and vascular targeting of gene therapy. *Trends Pharmacol. Sci.*, **16**, 57–60.
6. Bicknell, R. and Harris, A. L. (1996). Mechanisms and therapeutic implications of angiogenesis. *Curr. Opin. Oncol.*, **8**, 60–5.
7. Brooks, P. C., Montgomery, A. M., Rosenfeld, M., Reisfeld, R. A., Hu, T., Klier, G., and Cheresh, D. A. (1994). Integrin alpha v beta 3 antagonists promote tumor regression by inducing apoptosis of angiogenic blood vessels. *Cell*, **79**, 1157–64.
8. Brooks, P. C., Stromblad, S., Klemke, R., Visscher, D., Sarkar, F. H., and Chenesh, D. A. (1995). Antiintegrin $\alpha_v \beta_3$ blocks human breast cancer growth and angiogenesis in human skin. *J. Clin. Invest.*, **96**, 1815–22.
9. Gagliardi, A., Hadd, H., and Collins, D. C. (1992). Inhibition of angiogenesis by suramin. *Cancer Res.*, **52**, 5073–5.

10. Wellstein, A., Zugmaier, G., Califano, J. A., Kern, F., Paik, S., and Lippman, M. E. (1991). Tumour growth dependent on Kaposi's sarcoma-derived fibroblast growth factor inhibited by pentosan polysulphate. *J. Natl Cancer Inst.*, **83**, 716–20.

11. Braddock, P. S., Hu, D. E., Fan, T. P. D., Stratford, I. J., Harris, A. L., and Bicknell, R. (1994). A structure-activity analysis of antagonism of the growth factor and angiogenic activity of basic fibroblast growth factor by suramin and related polyanions. *Br. J. Cancer*, **69**, 890–8.

12. Fotsis, T., Pepper, M., Adlercreutz, H., Fleischmann, G., Hase, T., Montesano, R., and Schweigerer, L. (1993). Genistein, a dietary-derived inhibitor of *in vitro* angiogenesis. *Proc. Natl Acad. Sci. USA*, **90**, 2690–4.

13. Millauer, B., Shawver, L. K., Plate, K. H., Risau, W., and Ullrich, A. (1994). Glioblastoma growth inhibited *in vivo* by a dominant-negative FLK-1 mutant. *Nature*, **367**, 576–9.

14. Ingber, D., Fujita, T., Kishimoto, S., Sudo, K., Kanamaru, T., Brem, H., and Folkman, J. (1990). Synthetic analogues of fumagillin that inhibit angiogenesis and suppress tumour growth. *Nature*, **348**, 555–7.

15. Abe, J. I., Zhou, W., Takuwa, N., Taguchi, J. I., Kurokawa, K., Kumada, M., and Takuwa, Y. (1994). A fumagillin derivative angiogenesis inhibitor, AGM-1470, inhibits activation of cyclin-dependent kinases and phosphorylation of retinoblastoma gene product but not protein tyrosyl phosphorylation or protooncogene expression in vascular endothelial cells. *Cancer Res.*, **54**, 3407–12.

16. O'Reilly, M. S., Holmgren, L., Shing, Y., Chen, C., Rosenthal, R. A., Moses, M., *et al.* (1994). Angiostatin: a novel angiogenesis inhibitor that mediates the suppression of metastases of a Lewis lung carcinoma. *Cell*, **79**, 315–28.

17. Kerr, J. F. K., Wyllie, A. H., and Currie, A. H. (1972). Apoptosis, a basic biological phenonemon with a wider implication in tissue kinetics. *Br. J. Cancer*, **26**, 239–45.

18. Nagata, S. and Golstein, P. (1995). The Fas death factor. *Science*, **267**, 144–50.

19. Raff, M. C. (1992). Social controls on cell survival and cell death. *Nature*, **356**, 397–400.

20. Wyllie, A. H. (1992). Apoptosis and the regulation of cell numbers in normal and neoplastic tissue: an overview. *Cancer Metastasis Rev.*, **11**, 95–103.

21. Potten, C. S. (1992). The significance of spontaneous and induced apoptosis in the gastrointestinal tract of mice. *Cancer Metastasis Rev.*, **11**, 179–95.

22. White, E., Cipriani, R., Sabattini, P., and Denton, A. (1991). Adenovirus E1B 19-kilodalton protein overcomes the cytotoxicity of E1A proteins. *J. Virol.*, **65**, 2968–78.

23. Evan, G. I., Wyllie, A. H., Gilbert, C. S., Littlewood, T. D., Land, H., Brooks, M., *et al.* (1992). Induction of apoptosis in fibroblasts by c-myc protein. *Cell*, **69**, 119–28.

24. Dedera, D. A., Waller, K. E., LeBrun, D. P., Sen-Majumdar, A., Stevens, M. E., Barsh, G. S., and Cleary, M. L. (1993). Chimeric homeobox gene *E2A-PBX1* induces proliferation, apoptosis and malignant lymphomas in transgenic mice. *Cell*, **74**, 833–43.

25. Harrington, E. A., Fanidi, A., and Evan, G. I. (1994). Oncogenes and cell death. *Curr. Opin. Gen. Dev.*, **4**, 120–9.

26. Hockenberry, D. M., Zutter, M., Hickey, W., Nahm, M., and Korsmeyer, S. J. (1990). Bcl-2 is an inner mitochondrial membrane protein that blocks cell death. *Nature*, **348**, 334–6.

27. Bissonnette, R. P., Echeverri, F., Mahboudi, A., and Green, D. R. (1992). Apoptotic cell death induced by c-myc is inhibited by bcl-2. *Nature*, **359**, 552–3.

28. Libermann, D. A., Hoffman, B., and Steinman, R. A. (1995). Molecular controls of growth arrest and apoptosis: p53-dependent and independent pathways. *Oncogene*, **11**, 199–210.

29. Folkman, J., Watson, K., Ingber, D., and Hanahan, D. (1989). Induction of angiogenesis during the transition from hyperplasia to neoplasia. *Nature*, **339**, 58–61.

30. Algire, G. H. and Chalkley, H. W. (1945). Vascular reactions of normal and malignant tissues *in vivo* of mice to wounds and to normal and neoplastic transplants. *J. Natl Cancer Inst.*, **6**, 73–85.

31. Knighton, D., Ausprunk, D., Tapper, D., and Folkman, J. (1977). Studies of the avascular and vascular phases of tumor growth in the chick embryo. *Br. J. Cancer*, **35**, 347–56.

32. Gimbrone, M. A. J., Cotran, R. S., and Folkman, J. (1974). Tumor growth and neovascularization: an experimental model using rabbit cornea. *J. Natl Cancer Inst.*, **52**, 413–27.

33. Brem, S., Brem, H., Folkman, J., Finkelstein, D., and Patz, A. (1976). Prolonged tumor dormancy by prevention of vascularization in the vitreous. *Cancer Res.*, **36**, 2807–12.

34. Holmgren, L., O'Reilly, M. S., and Folkman, J. (1995). Dormancy of micrometastases: balanced proliferation and apoptosis in the presence of angiogenesis suppression. *Nature Med.*, **1**, 149–53.

35. Wyllie, A. H. (1980). Glucocortoid-induced thymocyte apoptosis is associated with endogenous endonuclease activation. *Nature*, **284**, 555–6.

36. Gavrieli, Y., Sherman, Y., and Ben-Sasson, S. A. (1992). Identification of programmed cell death *in situ* via specific labeling of nuclear DNA fragmentation. *J. Cell Biol.*, **119**, 493–501.

37. Bursch, W., Paffe, S., Putz, B., Barthel, S., and Schulte-Hermann, R. (1990). Determination of the length of the histological stages of apoptosis in normal liver and altered hepatic foci of rats. *Carcinogenesis*, **11**, 847–53.

38. Barres, B. A., Hart, I. K., Coles, H. S. R., Burne, J. F., Voyvodic, J. T., Richardson, W. D., and Raff, M. C. (1992). Cell death and control of cell survival in the oligonucleotide lineage. *Cell*, **70**, 31–46.

39. Parangi, S., O'Reilly, M. S., Christofori, G., Holmgren, L., Grosfeld, J., Folkman, J., and Hanahan, D. (1996). Anti-angiogenic therapy of transgenic mice impairs *de novo* tumor growth. *Proc. Natl Acad. Sci. USA*, **93**, 2002–7.

40. Harrington, E. A., Bennett, M. R., Fanidi, A., and Evan, G. I. (1994). c-myc-induced apoptosis in fibroblasts is inhibited by specific cytokines. *EMBO J.*, **13**, 3286–10.

41. Resnicoff, M., Abraham, D., Yutanawiboonchai, W., Rotman, H. L., Kajstura, J., Rubin, R., *et al.* (1995). The insulin-like growth factor 1 receptor protects tumor cells from apoptosis *in vivo*. *Cancer Res.*, **55**, 2463–9.

42. Nicosia, R. F., Tchao, R., and Leighton, J. (1983). Angiogenesis-dependent tumor spread in reinforced fibrin clot culture. *Cancer Res.*, **43**, 2159–66.

43. Hamada, J., Cavanagh, P. G., Lotan, O., and Nicolson, G. L. (1992). Separable growth and migration factors for large-cell lymphoma cells secreted by microvascular endothelial cells derived form target organs for metastasis. *Br. J. Cancer*, **66**, 349–54.

44. Eskey, J. C., Koretsky, A. P., Domach, M. M., and Jain, R. K. (1993). Role of oxygen vs. glucose in energy metabolism in a mammary carcinoma perfused *ex vivo*: Direct measurement by p31 NMR. *Proc. Natl Acad. Sci. USA*, **90**, 2646–50.

45. Flier, J. S., Mueckler, M. M., Usher, P., and Lodish, H. F. (1987). Elevated levels of glucose transport and transporter messenger RNA are induced by ras or src oncogenes. *Science*, **235**, 1492–5.

46. Valera, A., Pujol, A., Gregori, X., Riu, E., Visa, J., and Bosch, F. (1995). Evidence from transgenic mice that myc regulates hepatic glycosis. *FASEB J.*, **9**, 1067–78.

47. Kan, O., Baldwin, S. A., and Whetton, A. D. (1994). Apoptosis is regulated by the rate of glucose transport in an IL-3-dependent haemopoietic cell line. *Biochem. Soc. Trans.*, **22**, 102–3.

48. Graeber, T. G., Osmanian, C., Jacks, T., Housman, D. E., Koch, C. J., Lowe, S. W., and Giaccia, A. J. (1996). Hypoxia-mediated selection of cells with diminished apoptotic potential in solid tumours. *Nature*, **370**, 88–91.

49. Fidler, I. J. (1991). Cancer metastasis. *Br. Med. Bull.*, **47**, 157–77.

50. Demicheli, R., Terenziani, M., Valagussa, P., Moliterni, A., Zambetti, M., and Bonadonna, G. (1994). Local recurrences following mastectomy: support for the concept of tumor dormancy. *J. Natl Cancer Inst.*, **86**, 45–8.

51. Crowley, N. J. and Seigler, H. F. (1992). Relationship between disease-free interval and survival in patients with recurrent melanoma. *Arch. Surg.*, **127**, 1303–8.

24. Endothelial cells transformed by polyomavirus middle T oncogene: a model for haemangiomas and other vascular tumours

Michael S. Pepper, Fabienne Tacchini-Cottier, T. Kanaga Sabapathy, Roberto Montesano, and Erwin F. Wagner

Introduction

The establishment of a functional vascular system is an absolute requirement for the growth of normal and neoplastic tissues. However, like all other systems in the living organism, cells of the vascular system are susceptible to genetic and epigenetic changes which may ultimately lead to tumour formation. Recent studies on the endothelial cell-specific transforming ability of the polyoma virus middle T oncogene have defined a model for the study of endothelial cell tumours. The purpose of this chapter is to summarize these studies, and to place them in the context of what is known about the pathogenesis of vascular tumours in humans.

Blood vessels are formed by two processes: (i) vasculogenesis, in which a primary capillary plexus is formed from endothelial cells which differentiate *in situ* from mesodermal precursors, and (ii) angiogenesis, the formation of new capillary blood vessels by a process of sprouting from pre-existing vessels (reviewed in reference 1). While both processes are required for formation of the vascular system during embryonic development, neovascularization which occurs in postnatal life is attributed to angiogenesis. Physiological angiogenesis thus occurs in female reproductive organs, during the wound healing process, and in response to the tissue hypoxia associated with vessel occlusion. Much of our interest in angiogenesis comes from the notion that for solid tumours to grow beyond a critical size, they must recruit endothelial cells from the surrounding stroma to form their own endogenous microcirculation (2). Angiogenesis is also an important element in the pathophysiology of inflammatory arthritis (*e.g.* rheumatoid arthritis), ocular neovascularization (*e.g.* diabetic proliferative retinopathy), and haemangiomas of infancy and childhood (one of the major themes of this chapter).

Vascular morphogenesis is characterized by alterations in at least three endothelial cell functions: (i) modulation of interactions with the extracellular matrix, which requires alterations of cell–matrix contacts and the production of matrix-degrading proteolytic enzymes; (ii) an initial increase and a subsequent decrease in locomotion (migration), which allows the cells to translocate towards the angiogenic stimulus and to stop once they reach their destination; and (iii) an increase in proliferation, which provides new cells for the growing and elongating vessel, and a subsequent return to the quiescent state once the vessel is formed. Together, these cellular functions contribute to the process of capillary morphogenesis, i.e. the formation of three-dimensional patent tube-like structures.

Endothelial activation status is determined by a balance between positive and negative regulators: in activated (angiogenic) endothelium, positive regulators predominate, whereas endothelial quiescence is achieved and maintained by the dominance of negative regulators. The most thoroughly characterized positive regulators are vascular endothelial growth factor (VEGF) and acidic and basic fibroblast growth factors (aFGF, bFGF). Although VEGF and FGFs are angiogenic, much controversy still exists as to whether or not the FGFs are relevant to the endogenous control of angiogenesis *in vivo*. In contrast to VEGF and FGF which are mitogenic for endothelial cells, transforming growth factor β (TGF-β) and tumour necrosis factor α (TNF-α) inhibit endothelial cell growth *in vitro*, and have therefore been considered as direct-acting negative regulators. However, both TGF-β and TNF-α are angiogenic *in vivo*, and in this context are considered to be indirect positive regulators. Other cytokines which regulate angiogenesis *in vivo* include interleukins (IL-1, IL-6, and IL-8), hepatocyte growth factor, epidermal growth factor/TGF-α, platelet-derived growth factor BB, interferons, and colony-stimulating factors. Finally, angiogenesis can be regulated by a variety of other factors including hypoxia, enzymes (angiogenin, platelet-derived endothelial cell growth factor/thymidine phosphorylase), chemokines (*e.g.* platelet factor 4), extracellular matrix components or fragments thereof (*e.g.* thrombospondin), prostaglandins, adipocyte lipids, and copper ions (reviewed in references 3–5).

Human vascular endothelial cell tumours constitute a broad spectrum of lesions which can be classified according to two major criteria: (i) the relative number of well-differentiated vascular channels, and (ii) the association of endothelial cell proliferation with vascular channel formation (6). Benign lesions are characterized by a predominance of well-differentiated endothelial-lined vascular channels, in which the high levels of endothelial cell proliferation are part of the angiogenic process which is responsible for neovessel formation. In contrast, frankly malignant lesions are highly cellular with scant numbers of poorly developed vascular channels, in which the high levels of endothelial cell proliferation are associated with an increase in tumour cell mass rather than with the formation of well-differentiated and functional neovessels.

Vascular endothelial cell tumours in humans

Haemangiomas are the classic example of benign endothelial cell tumours. Although commonly present in the skin, they may occur in virtually any location in the body. Haemangiomas are extremely common. They occur most frequently in infancy and childhood, and constitute 7% of all benign tumours during this period. Macroscopically, they vary in size from a few millimetres to several centimetres, they may be elevated above the surface, and they are frequently bright red or blue in colour (see Fig. 24.1a, in the plate section). Juvenile (or 'strawberry') haemangiomas grow rapidly in the first year of life, and more than 80% involute spontaneously over the next 5–10 years. Three phases can be identified in the life cycle of these haemangiomas: (i) the proliferative phase; (ii) the phase of involution; and (iii) the post-involution (or involuted) phase (7). Immunohistochemical analysis of cell prolifera-

tion in the three phases has revealed high levels of pericyte and endothelial cell proliferation in the proliferative phase, with proliferation being virtually undetectable during and after the phase of involution. The marked reduction in staining for endothelial cell markers [CD31, von Willebrand factor (vWF)] in the post-involution phase, is indicative of the high-vessel density in the tumour and reflects a return to normal vessel density after involution (7). Histologically, two forms of haemangioma can be recognized, capillary and cavernous. Capillary haemangiomas are composed of tightly packed aggregates of thin-walled vessels which are characteristically heterogeneous in size, varying from capillaries to post-capillary and larger venules. The vessels are separated by scant connective tissue containing stromal cells with plump nuclei. Haemangiomas may be lobulated and surrounded by a pseudo-capsule (see Fig. 24.1b-f, in the plate section). Cavernous haemangiomas consist of larger or cavernous vascular spaces which are also separated by scant connective tissue stroma (6,8). Haemangioma endothelial cells express classical endothelial cell markers such as vWF, CD31/PECAM-1, CD34, *Ulex europaeus* agglutinin-1 lectin and VE-cadherin (7,9–13). Of three endothelial cell activation-dependent adhesion molecules, E-selectin, VCAM-1, and ICAM-1, only moderate staining for the latter has been observed in haemangiomas (12). Alpha-actin-positive cells (pericytes and smooth muscle cells) are present in close apposition to endothelial cells, and are most prominent in vessels of larger diameter (M. S. Pepper, unpublished observation). Although these cells are seen in all phases of the life cycle of juvenile haemangiomas, they are present at a significantly higher density during the phase of involution, suggesting that they may be causally involved in the process of vessel regression which occurs during this phase (7). A variant of juvenile haemangiomas has been described in which areas of spindle cells form slit-like vascular spaces similar to those described in Kaposi's sarcoma (14).

Frankly malignant endothelial tumours are rare, with only a minor proportion arising in pre-existing benign tumours. Angiosarcoma and Kaposi's sarcoma are the most frequent malignant endothelial tumours, with the incidence of the latter having increased sharply to almost endemic proportions as a consequence of its association with AIDS. Angiosarcomas display widely varying degrees of differentiation, from those that contain clearly recognizable vascular channels to those which are undifferentiated and contain few recognizable vessels. Central necrosis and haemorrhage are frequent. These tumours are characterized by local invasion and distant metastatic spread, and are frequently a cause of death. Kaposi's sarcoma, which behaves as an opportunistic tumour, also comprises a heterogeneous spectrum of lesions. One form has features of both a simple haemangioma and granulation tissue, and is characterized by thin-walled, dilated vascular spaces with interstitial inflammatory cells and haemosiderin deposition. Other forms of the tumour, in which vascular spaces are less prominent, are highly cellular and contain characteristic spindle-shaped stromal cells which delimit irregular slit-like spaces filled with red blood cells. Although they may be widely disseminated, Kaposi's sarcoma lesions are infrequently a cause of death (6,8).

PymT induces vascular endothelial cell tumours in rodents

It is generally accepted that tumorigenesis is a multistep process which requires several genetic alterations, and which is often characterized by long latency periods between the initiating event and the appearance of the tumour. The study of tumour formation can be facilitated by the use of selected viral oncogenes which are capable of rapidly transforming specific target tissues *in vivo* in a single-step manner, i.e. without the need for additional genetic events. The polyomavirus middle T antigen appears to be an example of a such a transforming viral oncogene. The polyomaviruses are members of the papovavirus group of DNA viruses. Two polyomaviruses have been isolated, one from mouse and one from hamster. Each encodes three proteins involved in cellular transformation in the 'early' region of their genome. These tumour (or T) antigens are called large, middle, and small. Of the three antigens, middle T (PymT) carries the cellular transforming activity. Large T is involved in viral replication and is capable of immortalizing primary cells to continuous growth in culture, while small T increases the efficiency of cellular transformation. The three proteins of the 'early' region therefore cooperate to transform primary cells in culture. Under normal circumstances, the virus does not induce tumours in its natural host. Its name derives from the observation that infection of neonatal or immunosuppressed rodents results in transformation of epithelial, connective tissue, and endothelial cells, giving rise to carcinomas, sarcomas, and cavernous endothelial cell tumours, the so-called 'polyomavirus tumour constellation' (reviewed in references 15,16).

PymT is membrane associated and possesses no intrinsic activity, but induces transformation by interacting with and changing the activity of several cellular proteins involved in signal transduction. These include at least three Src family tyrosine kinases, namely Src, Fyn, and Yes, the 85 kDa regulatory subunit of phosphatidyl inositol 3-kinase, the regulatory and catalytic subunits the serine/threonine phosphatase 2A, the Src homologous and collagen (Shc) family of adaptor proteins, growth factor receptor-binding protein 2 (Grb2), and 14-3-3 proteins (reviewed in references 15,16). PymT acts as a constitutively activated truncated receptor, and is unique in its ability to form complexes with the Src family of kinases. The gene product of the viral PymT oncogene has no known cellular homologue.

The transforming ability of PymT has been studied *in vivo* in two ways: (i) infection of newborn and adult animals with viruses engineered to express PymT, and (ii) the generation of transgenic and chimeric mice in which PymT is expressed from a variety of promoters. From these studies it appears that endothelial cells are the primary target of PymT's transforming ability *in vivo* (17–19). The specificity of PymT for endothelial cells may be due to the extraordinarily rapid kinetics with which this cellular compartment is transformed. The rapidity of transformation suggests that it does not require cooperation with any other mutagenic event to elicit tumour formation. Although transformation of other cell types may occur, the latency period is considerably longer, and this suggests that multiple steps are required. Tumour formation in non-endothelial cells is probably confined to situations in which expression of PymT in endothelial cells has been excluded. In contrast to PymT, tumorigenicity seen with the entire 'early' region of polyomavirus is not restricted to endothelium, while the constellation of tumours seen with the whole polyomavirus is even broader (reviewed in reference 16).

Based on the definition of a 'tumour' in Churchill's (20) and Dorland's (21) *Illustrated medical dictionaries* as 'a new expanding growth of tissue due to a progressive, uncontrolled proliferation of cells', the notion of tumour will be used to describe PymT-induced lesions throughout this chapter. Tumours are further defined as benign if they remain localized to the site of origin. Malignant lesions are characterized (i) by local invasion of neighbouring tissues, and (ii) by spread via lymphatic or blood circulations to other tissues or organs, resulting in the formation of secondary growths or metastatic tumours. With few exceptions (22), tumours induced by PymT-transformed endothelial cells are usually not invasive or metastatic. Some authors have therefore followed the convention of attaching the suffix '-oma' to the cell type of origin to indicate that PymT-induced tumours are benign. As the endothelial cell is the primary target in these lesions, non-metastatic PymT-induced vascular tumours have been referred to as endotheliomas.

Transformation by PymT facilitates the establishment of permanent endothelial cell lines

Knowledge of the molecular alterations which occur in endothelial cells upon exposure to an angiogenic stimulus is at present limited in part by the fact that endothelial cells are notoriously difficult to culture. Fortuitously, PymT transformation has become a very useful tool for generating permanent endothelial cell lines (reviewed in reference 1). These cells have been derived (i) by subculture from primary tumours, or (ii) following transduction of primary endothelial cells *in vitro*. In contrast to primary endothelial cells, PymT-transformed endothelial cells have the potential to grow indefinitely. Because of their growth advantage over other PymT expressing cell types, PymT-transformed endothelial cells can easily be derived from heterogeneous cultures containing non-endothelial cells, and in contrast to most primary endothelial cells, PymT-transformed endothelial cells can easily be cloned (19,22–26).

Williams *et al.* (19,27) isolated the first series of PymT-transformed endothelial cells from primary tumours in chimeric mouse embryos and virus-infected neonatal mice, and called these End cells. The cells are named according to their origin: sEnd.1 from a *s*kin (*s*ubcutaneous) tumour in a 3-week-old outbred ICR mouse; tEnd.1 from a *t*hymic tumour in the same mouse; eEnd.1 and eEnd.2 from mid-gestation chimeric *e*mbryos, in which the parental ES cells were derived from a male 129/Sv mouse. bEnd.1, bEnd.3, and bEnd.4 cell lines were obtained by transducing primary BALB/c mouse brain endothelial cells with a PymT-expressing retrovirus (23). A single polyomavirus-transformed endothelial cell line, Py-4-1 has also been isolated from a 13-week transgenic mouse of the strain Py-4 (24). The Py-4 strain carries the complete polyoma early region and was established in B6D2 mice. Py-4 mice develop multiple endothelial cell tumours with 100% penetrance at 6–8 weeks of age. These mice also develop osteosarcomas and lymphangiomas. Py-4-1 cells were labelled with fluorescent acetylated low-density lipoprotein (LDL) and were isolated by two subsequent rounds of cell sorting. They express all three polyoma T antigens and do not form colonies in soft agar (28). Transduction with PymT has also been employed in the isolation of endothelial cells from trypsin-dissociated organs of 15 day C57BL/6 mouse embryos. Stable lines have been obtained from whole embryo (E10V), heart (H.End.FB and H5V), and brain (B.End.FB and B9V) (22,29).

PymT-transformed endothelial cells retain important features of differentiated endothelium, including expression of proteins characteristic for endothelial cells (vWF, CD31/PECAM-1, MECA-32), internalization of acetylated LDL, expression of VEGF receptor 2 (VEGFR-2 or Flk-1), and the formation of capillary-like tubes when cultured in appropriate three-dimensional conditions *in vitro* (see below) (19,22–27). PymT-transformed endothelial cells also express a series of cytokines (including IL-6) either constitutively or upon stimulation with IL-1, TNF-α, or endotoxin. IL-1 and TNF-α promote procoagulant activity and platelet-activating factor synthesis in End cells (30). IL-1 modulates the adhesive properties of PymT-transformed endothelial cells for monocytes and tumour cells, while TNF-α induces cellular adhesion molecules (E-selectin, P-selectin, ICAM-1, and VCAM-1) on the surface of different PymT-transformed endothelial cell lines with kinetics similar to those reported for primary human and mouse endothelial cells (30–32; F. Tacchini-Cottier and M. S. Pepper, unpublished data). These findings indicate that PymT-transformed endothelial cells retain important endothelial-specific properties.

Host age appears to determine the ease with which PymT-expressing endothelial cells can be isolated from primary tumours. End cells (which express only PymT) can be isolated with relative ease from embryonic and newborn mouse tissues. Isolation of PymT-expressing endothelial cells from adult mice is difficult. When successful, these cells could only be propagated for a few passages before senescence (19,27). In contrast, isolation of PymT-expressing endothelial cells from adult mice is possible if all three Py antigens are expressed. This suggests that PymT's transforming ability is sufficient to generate endothelial cell lines from embryo and neonatal mice, but that cooperation between all three T antigens appears to be required to establish cell lines from adult mice (24).

General characteristics of endothelioma formation *in vivo*

Primary and PymT-transformed endothelial cell-induced tumour formation

Tumours can be induced either by PymT itself (primary tumours) or following subcutaneous or intraperitoneal injection of transformed endothelial cell lines expressing PymT. For the sake of convenience, tumours induced by injection of PymT-transformed endothelial cells will be referred to as 'secondary' tumours (Fig. 24.2). It is crucial that secondary tumours are clearly distinguished from lesions that develop following haematogenous or lymphatic seeding of cells from an existing tumour. The latter are true metastatic lesions, and will be referred to as such throughout this chapter. As it is difficult to determine whether mice with primary lesions develop true metastases, the term 'endothelioma' will be reserved for secondary lesions. Furthermore, 'endothelioma' will be used for secondary tumours which are non-metastatic (i.e. those induced by End cells).

Primary tumours are induced (i) in normal animals (mice, chickens) following infection with retroviruses engineered to express PymT, and (ii) in PymT transgenic and chimeric mice. Primary tumours develop in multiple organs in a non-specific manner, i.e. this depends on the site at which disseminated virus interacts with endothelial cells (17,19). Thus, injection of virus into the tail vein of adult mice results in the formation of multiple vascular tumours in organs remote from the site of injection (19). Similarly, primary tumours develop at multiple sites in transgenic and chimeric mice expressing PymT. In transgenic mice in which constitutive expression of PymT is driven by its own (18) or a heterologous (33) promoter, the effects of the transgene are dominant and exhibit 100%

penetrance. Primary tumours are most frequently observed in highly vascular organs such as lung and liver, and are transplantable (18). Chimeric mice have been produced from blastocyst injection of embryonic stem cells infected with a retrovirus in which PymT expression was driven by the thymidine kinase gene promoter (19). Development was arrested at mid-gestation, immediately after the appearance of endothelial cells (vasculogenesis). This was principally due to the formation of haemorrhagic cysts in both embryonic and extra-embryonic tissues. Yolk sac and fetal tumours were transplantable into syngeneic hosts.

Secondary tumours are induced following injection of PymT-transformed endothelial cells (isolated as described above) either subcutaneously or intraperitoneally into a variety of syngeneic or non-syngeneic hosts including avian embryos and newborn and adult mice and rats (19,22,24,27). Tumours induced by PymT-transformed endothelial cells are specific for this cell type: non-transformed endothelial cells or PymT-transformed non-endothelial cells (fibroblasts, embryonal carcinoma, and ES (embryonic stem) cells) are not capable of eliciting this

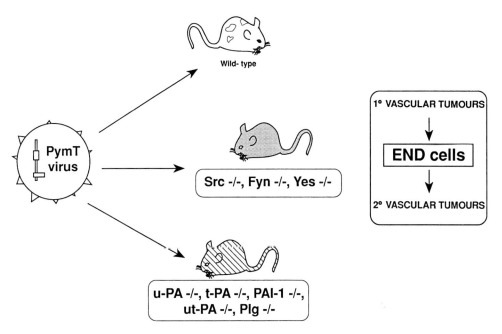

Figure 24.2. Primary and secondary tumour induction in wild-type and gene-inactivation mice. Primary tumours are induced following injection of a PymT-expressing retrovirus into wild-type, Src-family kinase (Src, Fyn, Yes)-deficient and protease (uPA and tPA (utPA)), plasminogen)/protease inhibitor (PAI-1)-deficient mice. Endothelial cells isolated from primary tumours are called End cells. Upon re-injection of these cells into mice, non-metastatic lesions form at the site of injection. These lesions are called endotheliomas to reflect their benign characteristics. These lesions are also referred to as 'secondary' tumours. They should, however, be clearly distinguished from metastatic lesions, which with few exceptions are usually not observed with PymT-transformed endothelial cell-induced secondary tumours (see text for details).

tumour type (19,27). Although End and Py-4-1 cell-induced tumours are not usually disseminated beyond the site of injection (18,19,27,34,35; F. Tacchini-Cottier and M. S. Pepper, unpublished observation), the occurrence of true metastases has been reported with H5V cells (22). The reasons for the differences in metastatic potential between End/Py-4-1 and H5V cells is not known.

Tumours which result from PymT itself (primary tumours) or following injection of established PymT-transformed endothelial cell lines (secondary tumours) are morphologically indistinguishable. Essentially, these tumours consist of large blood-filled cavernous or cystic structures (see Fig. 24.3a, in the plate section) (36,17–19,27). The nature of the cells lining these haemorrhagic cysts is not entirely clear, although a discontinuous layer of flattened vWF-positive (and presumably endothelial) cells has been observed in some cases (27) but not in others (22). A prominent feature of endotheliomas in the early phase of tumour growth prior to cyst formation, is massive hemorrhage, which may completely disrupt normal tissue architecture at the site of injection (see Fig. 24.3b, in the plate section). Secondary tumours are characterized by an intense inflammatory reaction, which is more prominent in immunocompetent (syngeneic) than in immunodeficient mice. The peritumoral granulation tissue contains monocytes, lymphocytes, and myofibroblast-like cells as well as a prominent neovascular response (22,27; M. S. Pepper, unpublished observation) (see Fig. 24.3c, in the plate section). Kaposi's sarcoma-like regions containing spindle-shaped cells have been observed at the tumour periphery (22; M. S. Pepper, unpublished observation). Metastatic tumours, when observed, exhibit morphological features which are similar to the tumours from which they were derived, although peritumoral inflammation is less prominent (22). Secondary tumours induced by injection of PymT-transformed endothelial cells into the peritoneal cavity of newborn or adult mice form well circumscribed blood-filled cavernous structures of varying diameter which are lined by a monolayer of flattened cells (Fig. 24.4b,d, in the plate section). The cavities of these tumours are frequently subdivided into multiple compartments by thin septa which originate from the tumour wall (Fig. 24.6b).

Phases of tumour growth

Based on growth characteristics and systemic functional consequences, it is possible to distinguish early and late phases of tumour growth. The early phase is characterized by haemorrhaging and recruitment of host cells (see below). The late phase is characterized by rapid expansion of haemorrhagic cysts which leads to alterations in sys-temic parameters including reduction in platelet count and haematocrit, splenomegaly, and extramedullary haematopoiesis (Kasabach–Merritt syndrome) (37). The level of endothelial cell proliferation and the extent to which the tumour is comprised of PymT-transformed endothelial cells have not been clearly established, and may differ significantly in the two phases of tumour growth (see below). Evidence for the importance of End cell proliferation in the formation of secondary tumours comes from the following observation. When End cells are injected subcutaneously into adult syngeneic hosts, tumours develop rapidly and form stable lesions which persist for up to 3 months without obvious negative consequences to the host. These tumours can be transplanted. However, when End cells are pretreated with the mitosis inhibitor mitomycin C, following an initial phase of tumour growth there is almost complete regression after 3 weeks. Furthermore, these tumours are not transplantable. Finally, although mitomycin C-treated End cells also induce endotheliomas in avian embryos, tumour formation is delayed and more localized than when embryos are injected with untreated End cells (27). Taken together, these observations point to the importance of End cell proliferation in endothelioma development.

A consistent pattern of tumour growth, regression, and regrowth has been observed upon injection of some PymT-transformed endothelial cell lines such as H5V into syngeneic hosts (22,38). The phase of regression has been interpreted as a transient phase of growth retardation concomitant with the development of effective host immunity, as has been observed with many experimental tumours.

Death in embryos and neonates occurs primarily from haemorrhaging, whereas adult animals die from sequestration of erythrocytes and platelets which leads to severe anaemia and thrombocytopenia.

Tumour growth is dependent on host age and immune status

With respect to the growth of primary tumours, this is most rapid (i.e. shortest latency period) when ES cells are used to derive chimeric mice; development in these mice is arrested in mid-gestation, immediately after the appearance of endothelial cells (19). Injection of a PymT retroviral construct into chicks (wing webs) and newborn mice (peritoneal cavity) results in rapidly growing tumours after 2–6 weeks (17,19). Injection of virus into the tail vein of adult mice results in the formation of disseminated vascular tumours after 4–6 weeks (19). Tumours develop in adult transgenic mice with a latency of 2 months to 1 year (18,33).

The growth of secondary tumours is also dependent on the age of the target animals. Following injection into avian embryos and newborn mice (27), End cell lines cause extensive disruption of the vasculature and haemorrhaging within 18 h to 4 days. Most chick and quail embryos die 2 days after injection, and syngeneic newborn mice succumb within 1–2 weeks. In adult mice, endotheliomas are relatively stable structures which may persist for months without adverse effects to the animal. Thus, when End cells (which only express PymT) are injected subcutaneously into syngeneic adult mice, only 50% die. The remaining half form stable tumours after about 1 week of rapid growth, which persist for up to 3 months with no increase in size. Upon serial subcutaneous transplantation, these tumours lose their potential to induce tumours (27). Injection of Py-4-1 cells (which express all three T antigens) into syngeneic adult hosts or nude mice results in the formation of tumours which are always fatal to the host within 3–10 weeks, depending on the number of cells injected (24). Tumour growth characteristics following subcutaneous injection of H5V cells into syngeneic adult mice is strictly dependent on the number of cells injected (22). High doses (5×10^6 cells) induce tumours after 2–3 days, and 100% of mice succumb with a mean survival time of 55 days. With an intermediate dose of cells (1×10^6 cells), tumours grow for 10 days, regress in 80% of mice after 20 days, and reappear after 35–40 days in 80% of mice. With a low dose of cells (2×10^5 cells), tumours appear in only 50% of mice, undergo regression, and reappear in only 30%.

Tumour formation is also dependent on the immune status of the host. Tumorigenicity of PymT-transformed endothelial cells is reduced in non-syngeneic animals and is accentuated in immunocompromised hosts. Thus, although the early phase of End cell-induced endothelioma formation is similar in syngeneic and non-syngeneic animals, tumours regress in the latter over a period of 3 weeks, presumably due to rejection by the host immune system (27). In immunodepressed (nude, irradiated, or anti-T-cell antibody-treated) mice, H5V-cell induced tumour growth is more rapid, subcutaneous metastatic lesions are observed, and regression is seen less frequently than in immunocompetent mice. Immunoneutralization with monoclonal antibodies completely abrogates rejection seen with a low dose of H5V cells in syngeneic mice. Similarly, immunocompetent syngeneic mice which survive an intermediate dose of cells, are completely resistant to a second challenge of cells (22).

Host cell recruitment

Tumours develop rapidly after injection of PymT-transformed endothelial cells. This suggests that recruited host cells are an important component of these tumours. Early phase host cell recruitment has been extensively studied in tumours induced by subcutaneous injection of End cells. The first indication that host cells may contribute to endothelioma formation came from experiments using an isoenzyme marker (glucose phosphate isomerase 1: Gpi-1). Injection of sEnd. 1 cells derived from outbred ICR mice homozygous for the Gpi-1^b allele into 126/Sv mice homozygous for the Gpi-1^a allele displayed only the Gpi-1^a isoenzyme. A second line of evidence came from the use of mitomycin C-treated End cells, which are unable to proliferate and have a short life span. Under these conditions, the vast majority of tumour tissue in adult syngeneic and non-syngeneic mice was host derived. Similarly, using mitomycin C-arrested [^{3}H]thymidine-labelled End cells, it was shown that only 1–5% of cells in newborn and adult mice were injected cells (27). These [^{3}H]thymidine-labelled cells were found at regular intervals along the inner wall of the haemorrhagic cysts, as well as in morphologically normal capillaries surrounding the tumours. This suggests that End cells can integrate into normal host blood vessels. However, the degree to which End cells contribute to the total endothelial cell population in endotheliomas and surrounding host vessels has not been described. A third line of evidence came from experiments using a quail endothelial cell-specific antibody MB1. It was shown that tumours induced by injection of End cells into quail embryos were predominantly of quail origin (27). To assess proliferation during recruitment in the early phase, 5-bromo-2′-deoxyuridine (BrdU) was administered to newborn rats which had been injected with End cells. Only 1–2% of nuclei were labelled with BrdU, suggesting that the cells which form the tumour are not proliferating (27). As peritumoral inflammation is prominent during the early phase of endothelioma development, inflammatory leucocytes may constitute an important proportion of non-proliferating recruited host cells. Taken together, these findings indicate that in the early phase, End cell-induced tumours are formed primarily by recruitment of host cells (endothelial and non-endothelial) to the site of injection, and that this involves mainly cell migration with relatively low levels of proliferation.

Using H5V cells, it has been reported that approximately 5% of total tumour DNA is derived from injected cells (22). However, these authors give no indication as to what percentage of tumour cells are endothelial in nature, nor do they indicate what percentage of tumour-associated endothelial cells are of H5V origin. Therefore the extent to which host endothelial and non-endothelial cells (inflammatory cells, fibroblasts, myofibroblasts, smooth muscle cells) contribute to these lesions is not known. In contrast to the End and H5V cell lines, mitomycin C-treated Py-4-1 cells do not form tumours upon injection into syngeneic hosts (24). A possible reason for differences between End and Py-4-1 cells might be the age of the mice from which the cells were isolated (Py-4-1 cells are from adult mice, End cells from embryo or neonatal mice).

The following is a working hypothesis for the early phase of secondary tumour formation. Following subcutaneous injection into embryos or neonates, PymT-transformed endothelial cells invade and integrate into host blood vessels leading to their rupture and subsequent haemorrhage. This in turn is followed by rapid recruitment of host endothelial and non-endothelial cells. Recruited endothelial cells form new capillary blood vessels which feed the growing cystic tumour. Recruitment is dependent on the continuous presence of PymT-transformed endothelial cells and mainly involves host cell migration with low levels of proliferation. The signal for host endothelial cell recruitment is not known, but may originate from the injected PymT-transformed cells (possibly a cell-associated non-diffusible factor) or from the intense inflammatory reaction observed at the periphery of the haemorrhagic cysts. Newly formed feeder vessels at the tumour periphery contribute to further rapid cyst expansion. These mechanisms pertain to the early phase of tumour growth. Mechanisms responsible for growth in the late phase have not been extensively studied. It is likely that in addition to host cell recruitment, proliferating PymT-transformed endothelial cells themselves contribute significantly to tumour expansion during this phase.

Do PymT-transformed endothelial cells produce a soluble tumour-inducing factor? Using End cell co-cultures or conditioned medium, Williams et al. (27) were unable to detect mitogenic activity for non-transformed endothelial cells. Conditioned medium was tested in the presence or absence of heparin or bFGF to assess potential interactions between angiogenic factors and co-factors. Similarly, End cell conditioned medium and cell lysates lacked angiogenic activity in vivo, and live cells separated from host tissue by a nitrocellulose filter were unable to induce tumour formation (27). Using an in vitro model of angiogenesis which assays for both endothelial cell invasion and capillary morphogenesis (tube formation) (39), we have been unable to detect angiogenic activity in conditioned medium from four End cell lines. In these experiments, conditioned medium was analysed in the absence or presence of bFGF or VEGF to assess for possible synergism between these factors (40). Likewise, co-culture of End cells with non-transformed endothelial cells did not induce an angiogenic phenotype in the latter (R. Montesano and M. S. Pepper, unpublished data). It is interesting to note that End cells express VEGF mRNA in vivo and in vitro (27; S. Wizigmann-Voos et al., unpublished data). Why then does End cell VEGF not synergize with bFGF in the in vitro angiogenesis assay? If End cell VEGF is indeed required for endothelioma formation in vivo, one possibility might be that End cells produce the higher molecular weight VEGF isoforms which rapidly associate with the cell surface and extracellular matrix following secretion, and which are therefore undetectable in conditioned medium (41,42).

Taraboletti et al. (43) have partially characterized a PymT-transformed endothelial cell-derived motility factor (EDMF). Conditioned medium from these cells induces chemotaxis (increased directional migration), chemoinvasion (which requires basement membrane degradation), and haptotaxis (in which the attractant provides both the stimulus and the substrate for migration) but not chemokinesis (increase in random migration) of a variety of non-transformed endothelial cells. A frequently used in vivo assay of angiogenesis involves subcutaneous implantation of a Matrigel pellet to which angiogenesis-regulating factors are added (44). Incorporation of eEnd.1 cell supernatant together with heparin into a Matrigel pellet strongly increased the angiogenic response when compared with the response seen with heparin alone (43). Preliminary characterization of EDMF suggests that the factor is a heparin-binding protein whose conformation requires disulphide bonding for activity. Size exclusion chromatography indicates the presence of two peaks of activity, one with a molecular weight of 40–65 000 and the other with an M_r greater than 200 000. EDMF elutes from heparin sepharose with 0.65 mol/l NaCl, which suggests that it is not bFGF (which requires at least 1.0 mol/l Nacl). VEGF is undetectable by enzyme-linked immunosorbent assay, and EDMF activity could not be inhibited by antibodies to VEGF (43).

Is host cell recruitment a feature of vascular tumours in humans? With respect to haemangiomas, there is at present no evidence to suggest that this may be the case. However, the precise nature of Kaposi's sarcoma remains an enigma, and recruitment may well be an important component. Thus, when Kaposi's sarcoma-like lesions were induced in nude mice following injection of human AIDS–Kaposi's sarcoma (AIDS-KS) cells (see below), chromosomal analysis of proliferating cells in these lesions showed that they were all of mouse (i.e. host) origin, implying the existence of a recruitment process. Taken together with the observations on host cell recruitment in PymT-induced tumours, these observations suggest that certain vascular tumours may be sustained by a minor proportion of transformed cells (22).

An *in vitro* model of endothelioma formation

To study the autonomous morphogenetic behaviour of End cells, an in vitro model was developed (23). This consists

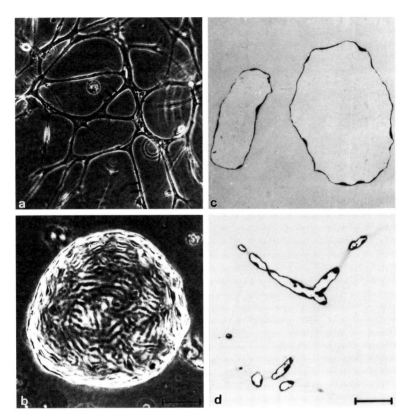

Figure 24.5. Morphogenetic behaviour of normal mouse brain endothelial cells (BECs) and PymT-expressing endothelioma (End) cells grown within three-dimensional fibrin gels. (a) Phase contrast view of a network of branching and anastomosing cords formed by primary mouse BECs; fine slit-like lumina are indicated by the small arrows. (b) Phase contrast view of a spherical cyst formed by End cells. In this picture, the focus is approximately at the equatorial plane of the cyst. The cells lining the floor and the roof of the cavity appear blurred in the centre of the cyst. (c) Semi-thin section showing the formation of a cavernous cyst lined by a continuous monolayer of flattened endothelial cells. (d) Semi-thin section of PymT-expressing endothelial cells grown in the presence of Trasylol, an inhibitor of serine proteases; the cells have formed branching tubules resembling capillary blood vessels. Bars: (a), (b) = 100 μm; (c), (d) = 250 μm. (From Montesano *et al.*, 1990. With copyright permission from Cell Press.)

of growing End cells in suspension in three-dimensional fibrin gels. In fibrin gels, End cells proliferate rapidly, and after 10–14 days form large cystic structures lined by a monolayer of endothelial cells (Fig. 24.5b,c). These cyst-like structures are strikingly reminiscent of the cavernous endotheliomas which develop *in vivo*. Under the same experimental conditions, non-transformed endothelial cells from a variety of species and organs form elongated branching tube-like structures (Fig. 24.5a); in no instance are cyst-like structures seen.

A consistent finding in endotheliomas which develop after intraperitoneal injection of End cells, is the presence of multiple thin septae which originate from the tumour periphery (Fig. 24.6b). The presence of these structures suggests that large cysts may have arisen by confluence of

multiple smaller cysts. This hypothesis is illustrated schematically in Fig. 24.6c. Evidence for the formation of large cysts from multiple smaller cysts has come from *in vitro* observations in the fibrin gel system (Fig. 24.6a). At a time point intermediate between the formation of small, well-defined cysts and complete lysis of the fibrin gel, numerous large elongated and interconnecting cyst-like structures can be observed. These structures arise by progressive fibrinolysis and confluence of multiple smaller cysts. The fibrin gel model, in which normal vascular morphogenesis is disrupted, i.e. formation of endothelial-lined cyst-like rather than tube-like structures, provides a powerful model for investigating endothelial-dependent mechanisms of PymT-induced endothelial cell tumour formation *in vitro*.

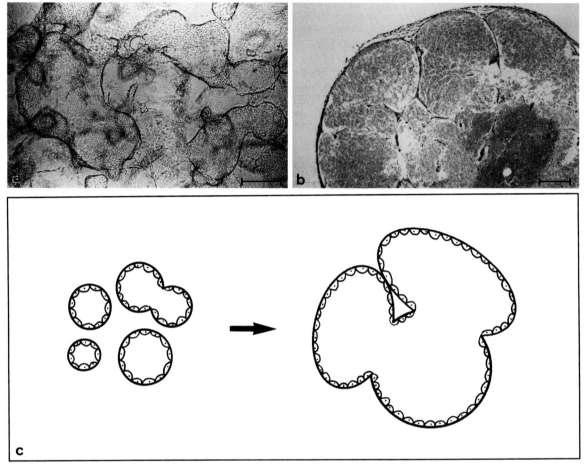

Figure 24.6. End cell cyst formation *in vitro* and endothelioma formation *in vivo*: a unifying hypothesis on formation of large cysts from multiple smaller cysts. (a) Phase contrast view of a fibrin gel at a time point intermediate between the formation of small, well-defined cysts (Fig. 24.4b, c) and complete lysis of the fibrin gel. Large irregular and interconnecting cysts can be observed. These structures arise by progressive fibrinolysis and the confluence of multiple smaller cysts. (b) A consistent finding in endotheliomas which develop after intraperitoneal injection of End cells, is the presence of multiple thin septa which originate from the periphery of the cyst. The presence of these structures suggests that large cysts may have arisen by confluence of multiple smaller cysts. Magnification in (b) is the same as in Figs 24.1 (c–e), 24.2. (b, c), and 24.3 (a, b). (c) Schematic illustration of this hypothesis. Bars: (a) = 400 μm; (b) = 150 μm.

Molecular mechanisms of endothelioma formation

Requirement for Src-related kinases in PymT-mediated endothelial cell transformation

Activation of Src-related kinases, Src, Fyn, and Yes, is believed to be an important component of PymT-induced endothelial cell transformation. The availability of mice in which individual kinase genes have been inactivated has made it possible to analyse the requirement for these kinases in PymT-induced tumour formation (Fig. 24.2) (26,45). Primary tumour formation following inoculation with a PymT-transducing retrovirus in newborn mice lacking either *src* or *fyn* is indistinguishable from tumours induced in wild-type mice, both with respect to morphological features and kinetics of induction. Similarly, the frequency of tumour formation in Src- and Fyn-deficient mice varies according to the age of the pups at the time of injection, as seen in wild-type mice. Thus primary tumours develop rapidly in mice injected within 8–12 days after birth, whereas mice injected between 16 and 20 days after birth fail almost completely to respond to the virus. In contrast, primary tumour formation in Yes-deficient mice inoculated with virus within 10 days after birth is characterized by a 32% reduction in tumour number and a significant increase (more than twofold) in the latency period (26). The reduced efficiency of transformation in Yes-deficient mice suggests that this kinase plays a major part in the oncogenic process. It is, however, possible that additional PymT-binding proteins are also involved in the transformation function of PymT (Fig. 24.7A). The availability of double knockout mice for *src* and *yes* or *src* and *fyn* in which the total PymT-associated kinase activity is further reduced, will allow a better definition of the role of the known Src-family kinases in the process of PymT-mediated transformation and the control of endothelial cell growth.

Transformed endothelial cell lines have been derived from primary endotheliomas in kinase-deficient mice (26). These cells display morphological features indistinguishable from wild-type cells, and like the latter express the VEGFR-2 (Flk-1) gene. Biochemical analysis in kinase-deficient End cells of complexes between PymT and the Src-related kinases indicates that in cells lacking a single Src-family kinase member, the remaining kinases do not compensate for its absence by increased binding to PymT or by elevating kinase activity. Thus, complex formation between PymT and a particular Src-related kinase is not influenced by the presence or absence of other kinase family members. This suggests that the remaining PymT-associated kinase activity is sufficient to reach the threshold level necessary for endothelial cell transformation (Fig. 24.7B). It is also possible that other as yet undefined PymT-binding proteins are required for transformation (Fig. 24.7A). Kinase-deficient End cells are fully transformed as shown by their ability to induce tumours upon injection into newborn and adult mice. However, unlike what is seen with primary tumours, kinase-deficient End cells do not differ in their tumorigenic properties when compared with End cell lines established from wild-type mice.

It has been observed that Yes is responsible for a significant proportion (at least 50%) of PymT-associated kinase activity in transformed wild-type End cells (26). Taken together with the observation that primary endothelioma formation was reduced in Yes-deficient mice, this suggests that Yes is the most important of the three kinases in primary endothelioma formation. Reasons for the differences in behaviour between viral-induced primary tumours in kinase-deficient mice and secondary tumours induced by injection of kinase-deficient End cells, are not known. These findings none the less suggest that the rate-limiting step is the formation of the primary tumour, and that subsequent immortalization events in the derivation and tumorigenicity of End cell lines are independent of the kinases Src, Fyn, and Yes. These findings also point to the possibility that Yes may be an important component of the signal transduction pathway leading to proliferation of normal endothelial cells (26).

Cell–extracellular matrix interactions

The extracellular matrix is an intricate and complex network of proteinaceous fibres and other macromolecules, which as in all other tissues, is likely to have profound influences on endothelial cell function and tissue architecture in vascular tumours. Immunohistochemical analysis has revealed that major components of the vascular basement membrane, namely collagen type IV, laminin, and fibronectin are correctly expressed and organized in haemangiomas and other vascular tumours (12,13). Marked reactivity for laminin type 2 (merosin) was seen in juvenile capillary haemangiomas. Vitronectin was observed in intravascular thrombi, and tenascin was present in the intercapillary stroma of haemangiomas, as has been described for normal tissues. Like blood vessels in many normal tissues, endothelial cells in haemangiomas and other vascular tumours are positive for β_1, β_3, β_4, α_1, α_2, α_3, α_5, α_6, and α_v integrin subunits, although a decrease in β_3, β_4, and, α_v subunits is seen in malignant vascular tumours, especially angiosarcomas (12,46).

PymT-transformed endothelial cells have been studied with respect to extracellular matrix production and cell–matrix adhesion. End cells constitutively synthesize and secrete basement membrane proteins laminin, entactin (nidogen), and collagen type IV. However, unlike non-transformed endothelial cells, fibronectin, or thrombospondin-1 (TSP-1) are virtually undetectable in End and Py-4-1 cells, although TSP-1 can be increased by exogenously added TGF-β1 (47,48). End and Py-4-1 cells also synthesize SPARC (secreted protein, acidic and rich in cysteine) (47,48), which is a secreted anti-adhesive glycoprotein that binds to collagens produced by endothelial cells, but does not itself become incorporated into their matrix. End cell-derived SPARC alters the morphology and growth pattern of non-transformed endothelial cell lines. However, comparison of End and non- transformed endothelial cells, revealed no significant differences in levels of SPARC, and SPARC expression was unaffected following exposure to TGF-β1 (47,48). End cells also demonstrate an altered pattern of adhesion and spreading on laminin when compared with non-transformed endothelial cells (49).

Could alterations in the adhesive capacity of PymT-transformed endothelial cells or their profile of secreted

PymT-kinase complexes in endothelial cell transformation

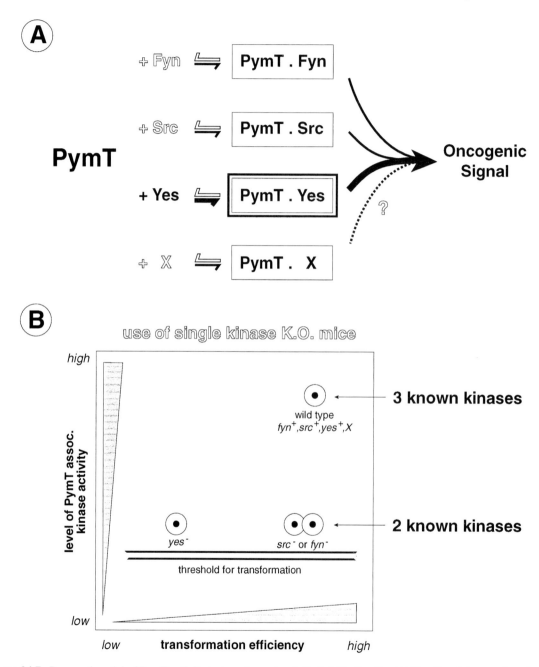

Figure 24.7. Proposed model of PymT activity in transformed endothelial (End) cells. (A) PymT activity as a function of its association with the three known Src-family tyrosine kinases, Src, Fyn, and Yes, and possibly with other as yet unidentified tyrosine kinases (X). (B) End cells lacking one of the Src-family genes contain reduced levels of PymT-associated kinase activity. This activity is none the less still above the threshold required for transformation of endothelial cells, even in Yes-deficient mice where the transformation efficiency is markedly reduced. K.O., Knockout (mice).

matrix components *in vitro* be associated with endothelioma formation *in vivo*? One possibility might be related to thrombospondin. The thrombospondins are a multigene family of modular glycoproteins involved in the regulation of a variety of cellular functions, and thrombospondin and fragments thereof are potent inhibitors of angiogenesis *in vivo* (reviewed in reference 50). To determine whether the lack of expression of thrompospondin by PymT-transformed endothelial cells (47,48) might be related to their tumorigenicity, bEnd.3 cells were transfected with an expression vector containing the entire coding region of human TSP-1 (35). *In vitro*, cells expressing TSP-1 had a slower growth rate, reached a much lower saturation density, and displayed a more cobble-stone-like morphology which is typical of nontransformed endothelial cells. These effects occurred independently of alterations in TGF-β1 activity (35), and were consistent with the observation that exogenously added thrombospondin inhibits End cell proliferation *in vitro* (48). In addition, fibrinolytic activity of bEnd.3 cells was decreased in TSP-1 transfectants, both as a consequence of a reduction in urokinase-type plasminogen activator (uPA) as well as an increase in PA inhibitor-1 (PAI-1). Finally, *in vivo* tumorigenicity of these cells was markedly reduced upon subcutaneous injection into nude mice, as manifested both by a reduction in tumour incidence and an increase in tumour latency. Histologically, the injection sites of TSP-1 transfectants showed necrotic cells surrounded by a fibrous capsule (35). Alterations in growth rate, adhesive properties, and extracellular proteolytic activity may all contribute to the inhibitory effect of TSP-1 on secondary endothelioma formation.

Matrix-degrading proteolytic enzymes

Many biological processes such as cell migration, morphogenesis, and tissue remodelling (including growth and involution) require tightly controlled extracellular proteolysis. With respect to angiogenesis, basement membrane degradation, extracellular matrix invasion, and lumen formation are proteolytically mediated events. Extracellular proteolysis also regulates cytokine activity, and one of the consequences of proteolysis is the generation of a variety of matrix degradation products, many of which themselves have biological activity. A number of enzyme systems have been implicated. In view of the variety of substrates, some of which (*e.g.* the fibrillar collagens) are resistant to broad-spectrum proteases, this diversity is not surprising. However, many of the relevant enzymes belong to one of two families: the serine proteases, in particular the plasminogen activator (PA)/plasmin system, and the matrix metalloproteinases (MMPs). It has been clearly established that angiogenesis is dependent on MMP activity, which

suggests that MMPs are likely to be key therapeutic targets in anti-angiogenesis therapy. The role of the PA–plasmin system, although more extensively studied in the context of angiogenesis, is less clearly defined (reviewed in reference 51). Thus mice lacking either plasminogen or both uPA and tissue-type PA (tPA) are viable and fertile, which demonstrates that developmental and physiological angiogenesis can occur in the absence of these enzymes (52–54). *In vitro* studies on the PA–plasmin system have none the less given rise to the notion that it is the net balance between protease and protease inhibitor activity at the cell surface which determines the morphogenetic behaviour of endothelial cells (55).

Expression of type IV collagenase, tissue inhibitor of metalloproteinases-1 (TIMP-1) and uPA has been studied in human juvenile haemangiomas (7). Type IV collagenase immunoreactivity was detected in the cytoplasm of endothelial cells and pericytes in the proliferative phase only. uPA immunoreactivity was detected in the cytoplasm and nuclei of endothelial cells and pericytes, and was most abundant during the phases of proliferation and involution. In contrast, TIMP-1 staining was not observed during the proliferative phase, but was present at high levels in the cytoplasm of pericytes during the phase of involution. Type IV collagenase and TIMP-1 might therefore serve as useful markers of the phases of proliferation and involution, respectively. The expression of uPA during the phases of proliferation and involution suggests that this enzyme is important both for cell migration during haemangioma growth, as well as for tissue remodelling events which occur during involution.

With regard to MMPs and endothelioma formation, Taraboletti *et al.* (34) have demonstrated that growth of tumours induced by injection of PymT-transformed endothelial cells can be inhibited by the hydroxamic acid-based peptide derivative Batimastat (also known as BB94 and produced by British Biotech Pharmaceuticals Ltd, Oxford, UK). Batimastat inhibits collagenase, stromelysin, and gelatinases A and B with IC_{50}s of 4, 20, 4, and 2 nmol/l, respectively. Daily local injection of the inhibitor at the site of eEnd.1 cell injection increased tumour doubling time approximately twofold. The effect of the inhibitor was dose-dependent. Inhibition of tumour growth lasted as long as Batimastat was given, and when treatment was stopped, the tumours resumed a pattern of growth similar to that seen in controls. Histologically, treated tumours consisted of solid cellular aggregates that circumscribed small-medium blood-filled spaces. Subcutaneous haemorrhage was rarely observed in treated animals. Angiogenesis induced by subcutaneous implantation of a Matrigel pellet containing eEnd.1 cell supernatant and heparin was significantly inhibited by Batimastat. The effect of Batimastat on EDMF-induced HUVE cell motility and invasion was analysed *in vitro* using a Boyden chamber. Motility, assayed as chemotaxis or haptotaxis in the absence of Matrigel, was unaffected by Batimastat. In contrast, Batimastat almost completely inhibited HUVE cell chemoinvasion of Matrigel, which requires active digestion of the matrix substrate by invading cells. EDMF also stimulates MMP production by endothelial cells (34). As host cell recruitement is important in the early phase of tumour formation, it is possible that Batimastat might inhibit tumour growth by inhibiting EDMF-induced MMP activity in invading recruited host cells.

With regard to the PA–plasmin system, transformed endothelial cells (End, Py-4-1, and EOMA; see below) display increased PA activity when compared with non-transformed endothelial cells, which can be accounted for both by an increase in uPA and in some cell lines by a concomitant decrease in PAI-1 (Figs 24.8 and 24.9) (23,56,57). The mechanism for this increase is not known, although it has been shown that PymT increases uPA gene activation without influencing uPA mRNA stability (57). Taken together with the observation that transformed endothelial cells form cyst-like structures when embedded in fibrin gels (see above), these findings demonstrate that excessive proteolysis is associated with aberrant vascular morphogenesis. *In vitro* cyst formation can be inhibited to varying degrees under the following circumstances: (i) by addition of serine protease inhibitors, either by broad-spectrum inhibitors such as Trasylol, ε-amino-caproic acid or soya bean trypsin inhibitor, which inhibit plasmin but not PAs, or by the specific plasmin inhibitor α_2-antiplasmin; (ii) by depletion of plasminogen from serum; (iii) by the addition of neutralizing antibodies to murine uPA; (iv) by the addition of recombinant human PAI-2; and (v) by the addition of a peptide corresponding to the receptor binding region of mouse uPA which competitively inhibits the binding of uPA to its receptor (23,56; M. S. Pepper *et al.*, unpublished observations). The morphology of the resulting structures varies from small cysts to star-shaped structures apparently devoid of a lumen. The most striking alteration in morphogenesis in fibrin gels is observed upon addition of broad-spectrum serine protease inhibitors to End cells (23); under these conditions, the cells form a branching network of capillary-like tubes (Fig. 24.6d). These results demonstrate that the excessive proteolytic activity of transformed endothelial cells results in the formation of endothelial-lined cysts, and is therefore not compatible with normal capillary morphogenesis. Reduction of this activity by inhibiting plasmin restores normal morphogenetic properties, i.e. the formation of capillary-like tubes, to these cells. Taken together, these findings implicate increased PA–plasmin-mediated proteolysis in aberrant vascular morphogenesis *in vitro*.

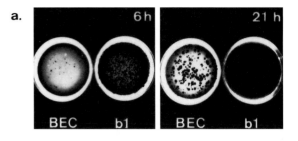

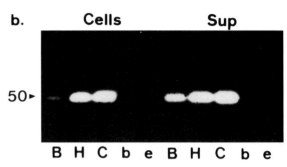

Figure 24.8. Plasminogen activator (PA) plaque assay and reverse zymography. (a) Plaque assay for the detection of PA activity. Under dark field illumination, large plaques of plasminogen-dependent casein lysis are seen around individual PymT-transformed primary mouse brain endothelial cells (bEnd.1 = b1) after 6 h, at which stage lysis around normal mouse brain endothelial cells (BEC) is barely visible. After 21 h, bEnd.1 overlays are completely lysed, whereas plaques of lysis now become clearly visible around BECs. No lysis of the casein substrate was observed when plasminogen was omitted from the overlay (M. S. Pepper, unpublished observation). (b) Reverse zymographic analysis for PAI-1. Endothelial cell-derived PAI-1 (50 kDa) is present in the cell extracts (cells) and culture supernatants (sup) of normal endothelial cells derived from the bovine adrenal cortex (B), human umbilical vein (H) and calf pulmonary artery (C). In contrast, no PAI-1 is detectable in bEnd.1 cells or in endothelial cells isolated from PymT-induced endotheliomas in midgestation chimeric mice (eEnd.2 = e) (From Montesano *et al.*, 1990. With copyright permission from Cell Press.)

Based on these *in vitro* observations, we hypothesized that PA–plasmin activity might also mediate endothelioma formation *in vivo*. The availability of uPA-/-, tPA-/-, PAI-1-/-, and plasminogen-/- mice has allowed us to test this directly (Fig. 24.2). Essentially, primary tumour formation is virtually unaffected in the different genotypes. However, in secondary tumours induced by injection of wild-type End cells, tumour incidence and latency

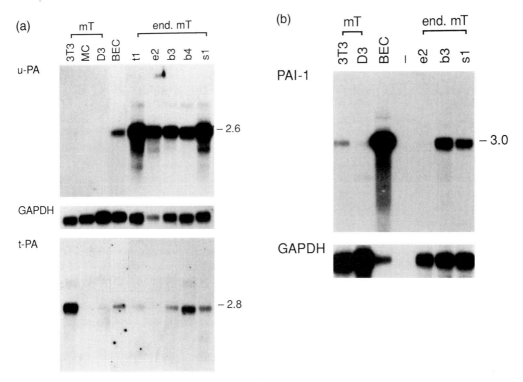

Figure 24.9. Northern blots of urokinase plasminogen activator (uPA), tissue-type plasminogen (tPA), and plasminogen activator inhibitor 1 (PAI) mRNA in End cells. (a) Expression of uPA and tPA mRNA in NIH 3T3 fibroblasts (3T3), IL-3 dependent bone marrow-derived mast cells (MC), and embryonic stem cells ES-D3 (D3) transduced with a PymT-containing retrovirus was compared with expression in non-transformed primary brain endothelial cells (BEC) and four PymT-transformed endothelial cell lines (end.mT). By northern analysis, uPA mRNA was undetectable in PymT-transformed non-endothelial cells, and was greatly increased in all PymT-transformed endothelial cells when compared with BEC. GAPDH (glyceraldehyde-3-phosphate dehydrogenase) was used as an internal control to determine the amount of RNA loaded per lane. Differences in tPA expression between the different cell lines was unremarkable. (b) Samples in (a) were assessed for PAI-1 mRNA expression. Relative to BEC, PAI-1 mRMA was markedly reduced in PymT-transformed endothelial cell lines. (From Montesano *et al.*, 1990. With copyright permission from Cell Press.)

are increased in uPA-/- and uPA/tPA-/- mice. Tumour incidence and latency are also increased when uPA-/- and uPA/tPA-/- End cells derived from tumour-bearing protease knockout mice are injected into wild-type mice, (E. F. Wagner *et al.* manuscript submitted). These genetic studies show that absence of components of the PA–plasmin system reduce secondary tumour growth *in vivo*. They do not, however, address the issue of restoration of normal capillary morphogenesis by reduction of protease activity.

With respect to the *in vitro* behaviour of End cells derived from the protease knockout mice, two general conclusions can be drawn. First, there is marked heterogeneity between clones with a single genotype (see also reference 31, for basal and induced cytokine production by different End cell lines), and second, while PA activity is necessary, it does not appear to be sufficient for cyst formation, i.e.

the 'balance' is a poor predictor of behaviour in fibrin gels in which other factors such as cell–cell or cell–matrix adhesion may be dominant (M. S. Pepper, E. F. Wagner, unpublished observations).

Cytokines

bFGF and VEGF immunoreactivity have been reported in human juvenile haemangiomas (7). VEGF was localized predominantly to the cytoplasm of endothelial cells and pericytes during the phase of proliferation; staining was not seen during the phase of involution. Similarly, although bFGF was detected in the cytoplasm of endothelial cells during all phases of the haemangioma life cycle, levels were highest during the proliferative phase and lowest during the period following complete involution.

The pattern of VEGF expression suggests a role for this endothelial-specific mitogen during haemangioma growth, and co-expression of bFGF during the same period raises the possibility that these two cytokines may be acting synergistically (40).

With respect to endotheliomas, End cells express VEGF mRNA *in vivo* and *in vitro* (27; S. Wizigmann-Voos *et al.*, unpublished data). The observation that these cells also express VEGFR-2 *in vitro* (26), suggests that VEGF might stimulate End cell proliferation in an autocrine manner. PymT-transformed endothelial cells express a number of other cytokines including IL-6, macrophage colony-stimulating factor (M-CSF), granulocyte–macrophage colony-stimulating factor (GM-CSF), and monocyte chemotactic cytokines (MCP-1 and Gro-α) either constitutively or upon stimulation with IL-1, TNF-α, or endotoxin (30). Basal and endotoxin- or IL-1-stimulated IL-6 production is also increased by IL-10 (58). IL-1 effects appear to be mediated via the type 1 IL-receptor (59). Finally, PymT-transformed endothelial cells proliferate and migrate in response to granulocyte colony-stimulating factor (G-CSF), and express transcripts for the G-CSF receptor (29). It remains to be determined whether the capacity of PymT-transformed endothelial cells to produce and respond to cytokines that act on inflammatory, endothelial, and other stromal cells is important during tumour induction *in vivo*.

Studies on juvenile haemangiomas in humans have revealed that the number of mast cells is higher in the phases of growth and involution than in the post-involution phase or in normal skin (7,60–62). The signals responsible for changes in mast cell density have recently been explored. Conditioned medium from the transformed EOMA cell line (see below) but not from non-transformed endothelial cells stimulates the proliferation of cultured mast cells, and this activity could be inhibited with a neutralizing antibody specific for stem cell factor (SCF). Both PymT-transformed endothelial cells (End and Py-4-1 cells) and EOMA cells express SCF (63).

Nitric oxide

Nitric oxide (NO) is a soluble free radical gas produced by endothelial and other cell types. NO synthesis is dependent on the enzyme NO synthase (NOS). As the *in vivo* half-life of NO is only a matter of seconds, the gas acts only on cells in close proximity to where it is produced, and this accounts for the specificity of its action. Endothelial-derived NO participates in the regulation of vascular smooth muscle tone, and is believed to be the endothelium-derived relaxing factor (EDRF) which mediates smooth muscle cell relaxation and consequently vaso-

dilatation. Endothelial cell NOS (eNOS; calcium-dependent) is believed to be involved in maintaining a basal level of vasodilatation, while inducible NOS (iNOS; calcium-independent) is thought to mediate the hypotension associated with septic shock. Endothelial NO also inhibits platelet aggregation and adhesion, and decreases smooth muscle cell proliferation. Many other functions in a variety of other cell types have been attributed to NO (reviewed in references 64,65). PymT-transformed endothelial cells contain up to 200-fold more NOS activity than non-transformed controls, and express both eNOS and iNOS (66). A soluble factor derived from PymT-transformed endothelial cells increases calcium-independent eNOS activity by 300–800-fold in non-transformed HUVE cells. Preliminary characterization indicates that this factor is an anionic protein. With regard to tumour formation, administration of the NOS inhibitor L-canavanine to mice injected with H5V cells significantly reduced tumour volume and markedly diminished the occurrence of tumour relapse which is typically seen with these cells (66). Although these findings raise the interesting possibility that NO may contribute to the characteristic cavernous nature of PymT-induced tumours, they imply that contractile NO-responsive cells (such as smooth muscle cells) must be present in the wall of these tumours. To date, however, evidence to support this assumption is lacking.

Other models of vascular tumour formation

In addition to the PymT model, a number of animal models have been used to study vascular tumour growth. A few representative models will be described. In the first, v-*src* was introduced into stage 24 chick embryo limb buds using replication-defective retroviral vectors (67). Approximately 60% of injected limb buds developed macroscopic vascular lesions which were first visible 5 days after injection. Histologically, the lesions were haemorrhagic cysts, and invasive neoplastic mesenchymal tissue was frequently seen in close association with the cysts. Presumptive endothelial cells were rarely positive for vWF. The lesions showed extensive expression of pp60[v-src], alluding to the direct involvement of the oncoprotein. These lesions may arise by a mechanism related to that required for PymT-induced tumour formation.

A second model has been developed from a spontaneously occurring haemangioendothelioma that arose in the subcutaneous mid-dorsum of a 129/J mouse (68). When cell suspensions derived from this tumour are transplanted subcutaneously into syngeneic mice, rapidly growing vascular tumours form with high efficiency. If tumour suspension is injected intraperitoneally, diffuse seeding results in the formation of multiple tumour foci; the tumour nodules involve the peritoneal surface without penetrating the organs. In no instance were metastases found beyond the site of injection, i.e. depending on the injection site, the tumour either remained in its subcutaneous localization or was confined to the peritoneal cavity. Histologically, these tumours are composed of immature endothelial cells with extensive atypia. Vascular spaces are poorly organized and incompletely lined by endothelium. Animals seldom survive beyond 3 weeks after appearance of the tumours, and death is associated with the development of severe anaemia and thrombocytopenia (Kasabach–Merritt syndrome) (68,69). A single cell line named EOMA has been derived from this transplantable tumour (70). EOMA cells retain many characteristics of endothelial cells, and when implanted subcutaneously into syngeneic mice induce large rapidly growing haemangioendotheliomas, which if left untreated are fatal (70,71). Host cell recruitment has not been studied in this model.

A third model employs a transformed endothelial cells line, F-2, derived from a tumour that arose in the skin of a nude mouse exposed to ultraviolet (UV) B light (72). This cell line retains many characteristics of endothelium, and induces the formation of haemorrhagic cyst-like tumours after subcutaneous inoculation into allogenic or syngeneic nude mice (73). UV irradiation has also been reported to induce the formation of cystic or cavernous haemorrhagic lesions in the skin of hairless mice (74). A fourth model utilizes cell lines derived from angiosarcomas which develop selectively in the livers of adult BALB/c mice exposed to 1,2-dimethylhydrazine dihydrochloride. These tumours contain hyperproliferative foci composed of endothelial cells with vascular lumina of various sizes (75). D10 and D14 are cell lines derived from separate tumours, which have a spindle-shaped morphology and display transformed characteristics *in vitro*. Further characterization as to the endothelial nature of these cells has not been described. When inoculated subcutaneously into syngeneic mice at high doses (10^7 cells), these cells induced tumours which undergo complete involution after 5–6 weeks. Histologically, D10-induced tumours display features of Kaposi's sarcoma, namely spindle-shaped cells with fine capillary networks. D14-induced tumours are largely undifferentiated (76). A fifth model uses bovine aortic endothelial cells transformed *in vitro* with benzo(*a*)pyrene (77). Upon injection into nude mice, only clones which grew in multilayers *in vitro* (and not those which grew as monolayers) developed into highly vascular nodular tumours. Depending on the number of population dou-

blings *in vitro* prior to injection, some tumours either persisted for 2–3 weeks and then regressed, while rapid growth continued unabated in others. Histologically, the tumours were composed of aggregates of mesenchymal cells interspersed with capillary-sized vessels, and were diagnosed as haemangioendotheliomas. Karyotypic analysis of cells explanted from rapidly growing tumours revealed that they were all of bovine origin. Reinjection of explanted cells into nude mice induced tumour formation.

A number of cell lines with endothelial characteristics have also been established from biopsied Kaposi's sarcoma lesions, from associated pleural or peritoneal effusions, and from peripheral blood of patients with this tumour (78–86). Most of these cell lines grow for short periods in culture, require exogenously added growth factors, and induce transient non-metastatic lesions in immunodeficient mice. For example, when spindle-shaped AIDS-KS cells, which retain some properties of endothelial cells (*e.g.* binding sites for the lectin *Ulex europaeus*, uptake of acetylated LDL), but not others (*e.g.* vWF), are inoculated subcutaneously into nude mice, haemorrhagic vascular lesions develop at the site of injection (80). These lesions, which are reminiscent of Kaposi's sarcoma, increase in size until day 6 and then gradually regress. No metastases were observed. The expansion of these lesions is dependent on a process of recruitment similar to that seen in the early phase of secondary endothelioma formation. In contrast to these and most other Kaposi's sarcoma-derived cells, two cell lines have been established which grow autonomously, display a transformed phenotype *in vitro*, and produce malignant tumours when injected into nude mice. The first is the human KS SLK cell line (82) which originated from a classical (non-HIV-associated) Kaposi's sarcoma lesion. These cells have an epitheliod rather than spindle-shaped morphology and express endothelial cell markers (*e.g.* vWF, *Ulex europaeus* positivity, CD31 and CD34). KS SLK cells form colonies *in vitro* when embedded in methylcellulose, and induce tumours in nude mice which appear 2–3 weeks after inoculation. All tumour-bearing animals die after 6 weeks, and the histological pattern of the lesions after autopsy resembles the classic light microscopic features of the original Kaposi's sarcoma lesions. No metastases were noted, and the tumours are transplantable. High levels of uPA antigen were detected in the culture supernatant of these cells (82,85). The second transformed cell line, KS Y-1, was established from a mononuclear cell suspension isolated from the pleural effusion associated with a pulmonary lesion in a patient with AIDS (86). These cells express endothelial markers (CD31, CD43, endoglin) and form colonies *in vitro* when embedded in methylcellulose. When injected into nude mice, these cells induce rapidly growing solid and metastatic tumours.

Although continuous lines of endothelial cells from human haemangiomas have not been reported, cultured haemangioma cells with endothelial-like morphology and *in vitro* growth characteristics typical of endothelial cells have been described (87). These cells organized into tube-like structures after 1–2 months in culture. When haemangioma-derived tissue fragments were embedded in three-dimensional fibrin clots, cells grew out rapidly into the surrounding fibrin gel to form tubular structures after 5 days (87). Finally, conditioned medium from cultures of cells (uncharacterized) derived from human haemangiomas has been used to establish primary cultures of normal endothelial cells (88).

Transformed endothelial cells as targets for novel therapeutic agents

With the possible exception of interferon (IFN) α (89,90), which inhibits angiogenesis both *in vivo* and *in vitro* (91–93), there is at present no effective treatment for life-threatening juvenile haemangiomas. With respect to Kaposi's sarcoma, a variety of local and systemic approaches have been used, depending on the extent of the disease, and IFN-α has proved to be effective in the treatment of some patients (reviewed in reference 94). Studies using the PymT-transformed endothelial, EOMA and AIDS–KS cell models have recently been used to assess the effect of cytokines and novel angiogenesis inhibitors on vascular tumour formation in mice.

Dong *et al.* (38) have recently demonstrated that IFN-γ and TGF-β1 significantly delay H5V-induced tumour growth and increase survival time in syngeneic hosts. However, very little effect was seen with these cytokines in nude mice. Both IFN-γ (38) and TGF-β1 (38,48) decrease PymT-transformed endothelial cell proliferation *in vitro*. These cytokines also reduce the activity of phosphatidylinositol-3-kinase and the production of phosphatidylinositol 3,4-biphosphate, without modifying the tyrosine kinase activity associated with PymT (38). Similarly, TGF-β1 decreases net PA-mediated proteolytic activity of bEnd.1 cells in a dose-dependent manner, although cyst formation in fibrin gels was unaffected by TGF-β1 up to a concentration of 10 ng/ml (M. S. Pepper and R. Montesano, unpublished observations). These results demonstrate that although IFN-γ and TGF-β1 have direct anti-proliferative activity on PymT-transformed endothelial cells *in vitro* (and at least in the case of TGF-β1, anti-proteolytic activity and induction of TSP-1; see

above), the anti-tumour activity *in vivo* is largely dependent on intact T-cell-mediated immunity. With respect to other cytokines, IFN-α and TNF-α had marginal anti-proliferative activity *in vitro*, and did not affect tumour growth *in vivo* (38). Similarly, IFN-α (up to 100 000 IU/ml) does not alter bEnd.1 cell behaviour in three-dimensional fibrin gels or PA-mediated proteolysis *in vitro* (M. S. Pepper, unpublished observation). Other cytokines including IL-1, IL-2, IL-4, IL-6, IL-13, IFN-β, leukaemia inhibitory factor, oncostatin M and GM-CSF did not affect PymT-transformed endothelial cell growth *in vitro* (38). It is interesting to note that in contrast to End cells, TGF-β1 had no effect on Py-4-1 cell proliferation (48).

The novel angiogenesis inhibitor TNP-470 (also known as AGM-1470), which is a synthetic analogue of the antibiotic fumagillin, and which inhibits endothelial cell proliferation *in vitro* at several orders of magnitude lower than for other cell types (95), has recently been shown to inhibit EOMA-induced haemangioendothelioma growth *in vivo* (71).

Nude mouse models, which utilize Kaposi's sarcoma-derived non-transformed and transformed cells, have been used for the identification of novel therapeutic agents. A sulphated polysaccharide-peptidoglycan compound (SP-PG), a naturally occurring bacterial cell wall product, has been reported to inhibit AIDS–KS cell growth *in vitro* (96). This effect is more potent on AIDS–KS than HUVE cells, and is endothelial cell specific. SP-PG inhibits AIDS–KS cell-induced angiogenesis in the CAM and in nude mice, and this effect is potentiated by tetrahydrocortisone in the CAM. Surprisingly, IFN-α did not inhibit angiogenesis in the CAM assay, and only a partial inhibitory effect was observed in nude mice. Anti-sense oligonucleotides directed against bFGF mRNA inhibit AIDS–KS cell induced Kaposi's sarcoma-like lesions in nude mice (97). These effects are specific, and are due to inhibition of synthesis of bFGF by AIDS–KS cells. bFGF is required for AIDS–KS cell proliferation and for the induction of angiogenesis by these cells, and bFGF and the HIV Tat protein (which is released from infected T cells) synergize to induce Kaposi's sarcoma-like lesions in nude mice (98). Angiogenesis induced *in vivo* by conditioned medium from Kaposi's sarcoma-derived cells can be inhibited by exogenously added recombinant TIMP-2 (99). Finally, the β-chain of human chorionic gonadotrophin (β-hCG, a pregnancy hormone) has been identified as an inhibitor of Kaposi's sarcoma formation in nude mice (86). This finding resulted from the observation that Kaposi's sarcoma is more frequent in males and may regress during pregnancy. Using the transformed KS-Y-1 cell line, it was observed that in contrast to male and non-pregnant female mice, metastatic tumours did not develop in mice inoculated in the early stages of pregnancy. β-hCG levels are highest during early pregnancy, and sera obtained from humans and mice in the early stages of pregnancy were inhibitory in *in vitro* proliferation and clonogenic assays. This could be mimicked by native hCG and β-hCG. Pretreatment of KS-Y-1 cells with hCG or administration of hCG to nude mice inhibited the development of metastatic tumours.

Summary and conclusions

The purpose of this chapter has been to review the PymT-transformed endothelial cell model in the context of vascular tumour pathogenesis in humans. Although this model has provided a large amount of information on the mechanisms and consequences of vascular tumour growth, its relevance to the pathogenesis of haemangiomas and Kaposi's sarcoma needs to be clearly defined. Thus, from a morphological point of view, there are significant differences between human haemangiomas and PymT-induced cavernous endotheliomas. In the latter, the ratio of lumen diameter to vessel wall thickness greatly exceeds that of normal vessels (Fig. 24.4b,d), whereas haemangiomas consist of a very dense network of capillaries and venules of essentially normal diameter (Figs 24.1b–f and 24.4a,b). The PymT model may be closer morphologically to cavernous than to capillary haemangiomas. A second major difference is that endothelial cell transformation does not appear to occur in haemangiomas, as at least in the case of juvenile haemangiomas, spontaneous involution occurs in more than 80% of cases. And third, there is at present no evidence for host cell recruitment in haemangioma pathogenesis. Based on the phenomenon of host cell recruitment and on the presence of spindle cells in the walls of tumours induced by PymT-transformed endothelial cells, it has been suggested that the PymT model may be relevant to the pathogenesis of Kaposi's sarcoma. However, there are important morphological differences between these two lesions, the most important of which is the absence of large haemorrhagic cysts in the latter.

None the less, although there may be some question as to the precise morphological resemblance, the PymT model does serve as a good *functional model* of haemangiomas for the following reasons: (1) the tumours are endothelial specific and organ non-specific; (ii) there appears to be rapid uncontrolled endothelial cell proliferation, although the extent to which proliferation of host and PymT-expressing endothelial cells contribute to tumour formation remains to be established; (iii) there is fre-

quently involvement (including compression) of vital organs; and (iv) mice develop many features of the Kasabach–Merritt syndrome, which includes sequestration of platelets and other blood components as well as splenomegaly. In addition, the study of tumour formation, in which PymT acts as a constitutively activated truncated receptor, may provide a powerful tool for understanding the intracellular signal transduction pathways which control proliferation in normal endothelial cells in response to well defined angiogenic cytokines such as VEGF and bFGF.

A number of important issues concerning PymT-induced vascular tumour formation remain to be resolved. First, the precise nature of the cellular components of these lesions needs to be defined both in the early and late phases of tumour development. The nature of the peritumoral 'inflammatory' cells and the cells that line the haemorrhagic cysts has not been elucidated. In addition, if cells lining the cysts of secondary tumours are indeed endothelial in nature, what proportion are derived from injected PymT-transformed endothelial cells? The same question can be asked for endothelial cells of neovessels in the peritumoral region. Second, the notion of cellular transformation has been used extensively to describe the phenotype of PymT-expressing endothelial cells, and it is abundantly clear that PymT-induced lesions are lethal to a variety of host species. But do PymT-expressing endothelial cells meet the criteria which are traditionally used to define the transformed phenotype? For example, it has not been clearly established whether these cells are capable of anchorage-independent growth. The third and perhaps most important question relates to cell proliferation. As has been clearly described above, host cell recruitment is of major importance in the early phase of PymT vascular tumour formation. What has not been established is whether tumour growth (cyst expansion) is dependent on uncontrolled proliferation of endothelial and non-endothelial cells, particularly in the late phase. For if one considers the initial definition of tumour as 'a new expanding growth of tissue due to a progressive, uncontrolled proliferation of cells', and host cell recruitment rather that cell proliferation is the major mechanism of tumour expansion in both early and late phases, are we justified in referring to non-metastatic PymT-induced lesions as 'tumours'? Or should we expand our definition of vascular tumours to include lesions in which a minimal number of transformed cells can induce tumour growth primarily as a consequence of host cell recruitment?

It will be interesting in the future to determine what accounts for differences in behaviour and resulting morphology between the mouse PymT model and haemangiomas in humans. One important difference might be related to the stimulus for endothelial cell proliferation. In the case of endotheliomas, the primary stimulus is clearly intrinsic. In the case of haemangiomas, the origin of the primary stimulus is not known. Thus there may be a primary defect in the endothelial cells of rapidly growing new vessels, which either allows them to grow auto-nomously or renders them more sensitive to incoming signals from cytokines and other angiogenic stimuli. Immunohistochemical analyses have revealed no sig-nificant differences in the expression of endothelial markers, basement membrane composition and activation-dependent adhesion molecules between normal endothelial cells and endothelial cells of haemangiomas. It would be interesting, however, to know whether tyrosine kinase receptors of angiogenic cytokines are aberrantly ex-pressed, or whether levels of thrombospondin are reduced in endothelial cells in rapidly growing haemangiomas. Alternatively, the primary defect in haemangiomas might be in the stromal cells, which either intrinsically or in response to environmental signals such as hypoxia, are induced to synthesize increased levels of cytokines and other angiogenic stimuli. For example, immuno-reactivity for VEGF and bFGF is increased in the pro-liferative phase of juvenile haemangiomas. Co-expression of these two well characterized angiogenic cytokines, and the observation that they synergize in the induction of angiogenesis *in vivo* and *in vitro* (reviewed in reference 5), suggests that they are likely to be key regulators. Differences in the number of mast cells and in α-actin-positive cells in the different phases of the life cycle of juvenile haemangiomas, points to a possible role for these cell types in the pathogenesis of human vascular tumours.

In conclusion, there is at present no animal model which faithfully recapitulates human haemangioma patho-physiology. Of the animal models which utilize trans-formed endothelial cells, the PymT model has been the most extensively characterized. Although as indicated above, this model serves as a good functional model for haemangiomas, interpretation of morphological para-meters should be undertaken with care. Further studies are required to determine the relevance of the PymT model to the pathogenesis of Kaposi's sarcoma, although it is unlikely that this model will supersede models which use AIDS–KS and other Kaposi's sarcoma-derived cells. Based on our knowledge of the mechanisms of angiogenesis and of PymT-induced endothelial cell transformation and tumour formation, a primary ob-jective for future studies should be to focus on the identification of novel inhibitors of vascular tumour growth.

Acknowledgements

We would like to thank Drs Friedemann Kiefer, Lelio Orci, Werner Risau, and Lothar Schweigerer for their encouragement and valuable contributions to our work, the Dermatology Clinic, Geneva University Hospital for assistance in obtaining and preparing the material shown in Figs 24.1 and 24.4, and C. Di Sanza, B. Favri, I. Fetka, J-P. Gerber, U. Möhle-Steinlein, M. Quayzin and J. Rial for technical assistance. Work performed in the authors' laboratories has been supported by the Swiss National Science Foundation, the Juvenile Diabetes Foundation (International) and the Sir Jules Thorn Charitable Overseas Trust.

References

1. Wagner, E. F. and Risau, W. (1994). Oncogenes in the study of endothelial cell growth and differentiation. *Semin. Cancer Biol.*, **5**, 137–45.

2. Folkman, J. (1974). Tumor angiogenesis. *Adv. Cancer Res.*, **19**, 331–58.

3. Folkman, J. and Klagsbrun, M. (1987). Angiogenic factors. *Science*, **235**, 442–7.

4. Leek, R. D., Harris, A. L., and Lewis, C. E. (1994). Cytokine networks in solid human tumors: regulation of angiogenesis. *J. Leukocyte Biol.*, **56**, 423–35.

5. Pepper, M. S., Mandriota, S., Vassalli, J-D., Orci, L., and Montesano, R. (1996). Angiogenesis regulating cytokines: activities and interactions. In *Current topics in microbiology and immunology: attempts to understand metastasis for-mation*. Vol. **213/II** (ed. U. Günthert and W. Birchmeier) pp. 31–67, Springer-Verlag, Berlin.

6. Cotran, R. S., Kumar, V., and Robbins, S. L. (1994). Blood vessels. In *Robbins pathologic basis of disease*, 5th edn, pp. 506–12. W. B. Saunders Company, Philadelphia.

7. Takahashi, K., Mulliken, J. B., Kozakewich, H. P. W., Rogers, R. A., Folkman, J., and Ezekowitz, R. A. B. (1994). Cellular markers that distinguish the phases of hemangioma during infancy and childhood. *J. Clin. Invest.*, **93**, 2357–64.

8. Benditt, E. P. and Schwartz, S. M. (1994). Blood vessels. In *Pathology*, 2nd edn (ed. E. Rubin and J. L. Farber), pp. 497–500. J. B. Lippincott, Philadelphia.

9. Parums, D. V., Cordell, J. L., Micklem, K., Heryet, A. R., Gatter, K. C., and Mason, D. Y. (1990). JC70: a new monoclonal antibody that detects vascular endothelium associated antigen on routinely processed tissue sections. *J. Clin. Pathol.*, **43**, 752–57.

10. Pearson, J. M. and Mc William, L. J. (1990). A light micro-scopical, immunohistochemical, and ultrastructural com-parison of hemangiomata and lymphangiomata. *Ultrastruct. Pathol.*, **14**, 497–504.

11. Kuzu, I., Bicknell, R., Harris, A. L., Jones, M., Gatter, K. C., and Mason, D. Y. (1992). Heterogeneity of vascular endo-thelial cells with relevance to diagnosis of vascular tumours. *J. Clin. Pathol.*, **45**, 143–8.

12. Martin-Padura, I., de Castellarnau C., Uccini, S., Pilozzi, E., Natalia, P. G., Nicotra, M. R., *et al.* (1995). Expression of

VE (vascular endothelial)–cadherin and other endothelial-specific markers in hemangiomas. *J. Pathol.*, **175**, 51–7.

13. Suthipintawong, C., Leong, A. S-Y., and Vinyuvat, S. (1995). A comparative study of immunomarkers for lymphangiomas and hemangiomas. *Appl. Immunohistochem.*, **3**, 239–44.

14. Niedt, G. W., Greco, M. A., Blanc, W. A., and Knowles, D. M. (1989). Hemangioma with Kaposi's sarcoma-like features: report of two cases. *Pediatric Pathol.*, **9**, 567–75.

15. Brizuela, L., Olcese, L. M., and Courtneidge, S. A. (1994). Transformation by middle T antigens. *Semin. Virol.*, **5**, 381–9.

16. Kiefer, F., Courtneidge, S. A., and Wagner, E. F. (1994). Oncogenic properties of the middle T antigens of polyomavirus. *Adv. Cancer Res.*, **64**, 125–57.

17. Kornbluth, S., Cross, F. R., Harbison, M., and Hanafusa, H. (1986). Transformation of chicken embryo fibroblasts and tumor induction by the middle T antigen of polyomavirus carried in an avian retroviral vector. *Mol. Cell. Biol.*, **6**, 1545–51.

18. Bautch, V. L., Toda, S., Hassell, J. A., and Hanahan, D. (1987). Endothelial cell tumors develop in transgenic mice carrying polyoma virus middle T oncogene. *Cell*, **51**, 529–38.

19. Williams, R. L., Courtneidge, S. A., and Wagner, E. F. (1988). Embryonic lethalities and endothelial tumors in chimeric mice expressing polyoma virus middle T oncogene. *Cell*, **52**, 121–31.

20. (1989). *Churchill's illustrated medical dictionary*, p. 2011. Churchill Livingstone, New York.

21. (1994). *Dorland's illustrated medical dictionary*, 28th edn, pp. 1761–2. W. B. Saunders, Philadelphia.

22. Garlanda, C., Parravicini, C., Sironi, M., de Rossi, M., Wainstok de Calmanovici, R., Carozzi, F., *et al.* (1994). Progressive growth in immunodeficient mice and host cell recruitment by mouse endothelial cells transformed by polyoma middle-sized T antigen: implications for the pathogenesis of opportunistic vascular tumors. *Proc. Natl Acad. Sci. USA*, **91**, 7291–5.

23. Montesano, R., Pepper, M. S., Möhle-Steinlein, U., Risau, W., Wagner, E. F., and Orci, L. (1990). Increased proteolytic activity is responsible for the aberrant morphogenetic behavior of endothelial cells expressing middle T oncogene. *Cell*, **62**, 435–45.

24. Dubois, N. A., Kolpack, L. C., Wang, R., Azizkhan, R. G., and Bautch, V. L. (1991). Isolation and characterization of an established endothelial cell line from transgenic mouse hemangiomas. *Exp. Cell Res.*, **196**, 302–13.

25. Vecchi, A., Garlanda, C., Lampugnani, M. G., Resnati, M., Matteucci, C., Stoppacciaro, A., *et al.* (1994). Monoclonal antibodies specific for endothelial cells of mouse blood vessels. Their application in the identification of adult and embryonic endothelium. *Eur. J. Cell Biol.*, **63**, 247–54.

26. Kiefer, F., Anhauser, I., Soriano, P., Aguzzi, A., Courtneidge, S. A., and Wagner, E. F. (1994). Endothelial cell transformation by the polyomavirus middle T antigen in mice lacking Src-related kinases. *Curr. Biol.*, **4**, 100–9.

27. Williams, R. L., Risau, W., Zerwes, H-G., Drexler, H., Aguzzi, A., and Wagner E. F. (1989). Endothelioma cells expressing the polyoma middle T oncogene induce hemangiomas by host cell recruitment. *Cell*, **57**, 1053–63.

28. Wang, R. and Bautch, V. L. (1991). The polyomavirus early region gene in transgenic mice causes vascular and bone tumors. *J. Virol.*, **65**, 5174–83.

29. Bocchietto, E., Guglielmetti, A., Silvagno, F., Taraboletti, G., Pescarmona, G. P., Mantovani, A., and Bussolino, F. (1993). Proliferative and migratory responses of murine microvascular endothelial cells to granulocyte-colony-stimulating factor. *J. Cell. Physiol.*, **155**, 89–95.

30. Bussolino, F., de Rossi, M., Sica, A., Colotta, F., Wang, J. M., Bocchietto, E., *et al.* (1991). Murine endothelioma cell lines transformed by polyoma middle T oncogene as target for and producers of cytokines. *J. Immunol.*, **147**, 2122–29.

31. Hahne, M., Jäger, U., Isenmann, S., Hallmann, R., and Vestweber, D. (1993). Five tumor necrosis factor-inducible cell adhesion mechanisms on the surface of mouse endothelioma cells mediate the binding of leukocytes. *J. Cell Biol.*, **121**, 655–64.

32. Heyward, S. A., Dubois-Stringfellow, N., Rapoport, R., and Bautch, V. L. (1995). Expression and inducibility of vascular adhesion receptors in development. *FASEB J.*, **9**, 956–62.

33. Wagner, E. F., Williams, R. L., and Rüther U. (1989). c-*fos* and polyoma middle T oncogene expression in transgenic mice and embryonal stem cell chimeras. In *Cell to cell signals in mammalian development*, NATO ASI Series, Vol. H26 (ed. S. W. Laat *et al.*), pp. 301–10. Springer-Verlag, Berlin.

34. Taraboletti, G., Garofalo, A., Belotti, D., Drudis, T., Borsotti, P., Scanziani, E., *et al.* (1995). Inhibition of angiogenesis and murine hemangioma growth by Batimastat, a synthetic inhibitor of matrix metalloproteinases. *J. Natl Cancer Inst.*, **87**, 293–8.

35. Sheibani, N. and Frazier, W. A. (1995). Thrombospondin 1 expression in transformed endothelial cells restores a normal phenotype and suppresses their tumorigenesis. *Proc. Natl Acad. Sci. USA*, **92**, 6788–92.

36. Defendi, V. and Lehman, J. M. (1964). The nature of the hemorrhagic lesions induced by polyoma virus in hamsters. *Cancer Res.*, **24**, 329–43.

37. Dubois-Stringfellow, N., Kolpack-Martindale, L., Bautch, V. L., and Azizkhan, R. G. (1994). Mice with hemangiomas induced by transgenic endothelial cells. A model for the Kasabach-Merritt syndrome. *Am. J. Pathol.*, **144**, 796–806.

38. Dong, Q. G., Graziani, A., Garlanda, C., Wainstok de Calmanovici, R., Arese, M., Soldi, R., *et al.* (1996). Antitumor activity of cytokines against mouse opportunistic vascular tumors. *Int. J. Cancer*, **65**, 700–8.

39. Montesano, R. and Orci, L. (1985). Tumor-promoting phorbol esters induce angiogenesis *in vitro*. *Cell*, **42**, 469–77.

40. Pepper, M. S., Ferrara, N., Orci, L., and Montesano, R. (1992). Potent synergism between vascular endothelial growth factor and basic fibroblast growth factor in the induction of angiogenesis *in vitro*. *Biochem. Biophys. Res. Commun.*, **189**, 824–31.

41. Houck, K. A., Leung, D. W., Rowland, A. M., Winer, J., and Ferrara, N. (1992). Dual regulation of vascular endothelial growth factor bioavailability by genetic and proteolytic mechanisms. *J. Biol. Chem.*, **267**, 26031–37.

42. Park J. E., Keller, G-A., and Ferrara, N. (1993). The vascular endothelial growth factor (VEGF) isoforms: differential deposition into the subepithelial extracellular matrix and bioavailability of extracellular matrix-bound VEGF. *Mol. Biol. Cell*, **4**, 1317–26.

43. Taraboletti, G., Belotti, D., Dejana, E., Mantovani, A., and Giavazzi, R. (1993). Endothelial cell migration and invasiveness are induced by a soluble factor produced by murine

endothelioma cells transformed by polyoma virus middle T oncogene. *Cancer Res.*, **53**, 3812–16.

44. Passaniti, A., Taylor, R. M., Pili, R., Guo, Y., Long, P. V., Haney, J. A., *et al.* (1992). A simple, quantitative method for assessing angiogenesis and anti-angiogenic agents using reconstituted basement membrane, heparin, and fibroblast growth factor. *Lab. Invest.*, **67**, 519–28.

45. Thomas, J. E., Aguzzi, A., Soriano, P., Wagner, E. F., and Brugge, J. S. (1993). Induction of tumor formation and cell transformation by polyoma middle T antigen in the absence of Src. *Oncogene*, **8**, 2521–9.

46. Mechtersheimer, G., Barth, T., Hartschuh, W., Lehnert, T., and Möller, P. (1994). *In situ* expression of β1, β3 and β4 integrin subunits in non-neoplastic endothelium and vascular tumours. *Virchows Archiv.*, **425**, 375–84.

47. Sage, E. H. (1992). Secretion of SPARC by endothelial cells transformed by polyoma middle T oncogene inhibits the growth of normal endothelial cells *in vitro*. *Biochem. Cell. Biol.*, **70**, 579–92.

48. RayChaudhury, A., Frazier, W. A., and D'Amore, P. A. (1994). Comparison of normal and tumorigenic endothelial cells: differences in thrombospondin production and responses to transforming growth factor-beta. *J. Cell Sci.*, **107**, 39–46.

49. Aumailley, M., Timpl, R., and Risau, W. (1991). Differences in laminin fragment interactions of normal and transformed endothelial cells. *Exp. Cell Res.*, **196**, 177–83.

50. Volpert, O. V., Stellmach, V., and Bouck, N. (1995). The modulation of thrombospondin and other naturally occurring inhibitors of angiogenesis during tumor progression. *Breast Cancer Res. Treatment*, **36**, 119–26.

51. Pepper, M. S., Montesano, R., Mandriota, S., Orci, L., and Vassalli, J-D. (1996). Angiogenesis: a paradigm for balanced extracellular proteolysis during cell migration and morphogenesis. *Enzyme protein*, **49**, 138–62.

52. Carmeliet, P., Schoonjans, L., Kleckens, L., Ream, B., Degan, J., Bronson, R., *et al.* (1994). Physiological consequences of loss of plasminogen activator gene function in mice. *Nature*, **368**, 419–24.

53. Bugge, T. H., Flick, M. J., Daugherty, C. C., and Degan, J. L. (1995). Plasminogen deficiency causes severe thrombosis but is compatible with development and reproduction. *Genes Dev.*, **9**, 794–807.

54. Ploplis, V. A., Carmeliet, P., Vazirzadeh, S., Van Vlaenderen, I., Moons, L., Plow, E. F., and Collen, D. (1995). Effects of disruption of the plasminogen gene on thrombosis, growth, and health in mice. *Circulation*, **92**, 2585–93.

55. Pepper, M. S. and Montesano, R. (1990). Proteolytic balance and capillary morphogenesis. *Cell Differ. Dev.*, **32**, 319–28.

56. Dubois-Stringfellow, N., Jonczyk, J., and Bautch, V. L. (1994). Perturbations in the fibrinolytic pathway abolish cyst formation but not capillary-like organization of cultured murine endothelial cells. *Blood*, **83**, 3206–17.

57. Besser, D., Urich, M., Sakaue, M., Messerschmitt, A., Ballmer-Hofer K., and Nagamine, Y. (1995). Urokinase-type plasminogen activator gene regulation by polyomavirus middle-T antigen. *Oncogene*, **11**, 2383–91.

58. Sironi, M., Mu/noz, C., Pollicino, T., Siboni, A., Sciacca, F. L., Bernasconi, S., *et al.* (1993). Divergent effects of interleukin-10 on cytokine production by mononuclear phagocytes and endothelial cells. *Eur. J. Immunol.*, **23**, 2692–5.

59. Boraschi, D., Rambaldi, A., Sica, A., Ghiara, P., Colotta, F., Wang, J. M., *et al.* (1991). Endothelial cells express the interleukin-1 receptor type I. *Blood*, **78**, 1262–7.

60. Glowacki, J. and Mulliken, J. B. (1982). Mast cells in hemangiomas and vascular malformations. *Pediatrics*, **70**, 48–51.

61. Pasyk, K. A., Cherry, G. W., Grabb, W. C., and Sasaki, G. H. (1984). Quantitative evaluation of mast cells in cellularly dynamic and adynamic vascular malformations. *Plast. Reconstr. Surg.*, **73**, 69–77.

62. Dethlefsen, S. M., Mulliken, J., and Glowacki, J. (1986). An ultrastructural study of mast cell interactions in hemangiomas. *Ultrastruct. Pathol.*, **10**, 175–83.

63. Meininger, C. J., Brightman, S. E., Kelly, K. A., and Zetter, B. R. (1995). Increased stem cell factor release by hemangioma-derived endothelial cells. *Lab. Invest.*, **72**, 166–73.

64. Moncada, S., Palmer, R. M. J., and Higgs, E. A. (1991). Nitric oxide: physiology, pathophysiology, and pharmacology. *Pharmacol. Rev.*, **43**, 109–42.

65. Billiar, T. R. (1995). Nitric oxide. Novel biology with clinical relevance. *Ann. Surg.*, **221**, 339–49.

66. Ghio, D., Arese, M., Todde, R., Vecchi, A., Silvagno, F., Costamagna, C., *et al.*, (1995). Middle T antigen-transformed endothelial cells exhibit an increased activity of nitric oxide synthase. *J. Exp. Med.*, **181**, 9–19.

67. Stoker, A. W., Hatier, C., and Bissell, M. J. (1990). The embryonic environment strongly attenuates v-*src* oncogenesis in mesenchymal and epithelial tissues, but not in endothelial. *J. Cell Biol.*, **111**, 217–28.

68. Hoak, J. C., Warner, E. D., Cheng, H. F., Fry, G. L., and Hankenson, R. R. (1971). Hemangioma with thrombocytopenia and microangiopathic anemia (Kasabach-Merritt syndrome): an animal model. *J. Lab. Clin. Med.*, **77**, 941–50.

69. Warner, E. D., Hoak, J. C., and Fry, G. L. (1971). Hemangioma, thrombocytopenia, and anemia. The Kasabach-Merritt syndrome in an animal model. *Arch. Pathol.*, **91**, 523–8.

70. Obeso, J., Weber, J., and Auerbach, R. (1990). A hemangioendothelioma-derived cell line: its use as a model for the study of endothelial cell biology. *Lab. Invest.*, **63**, 259–69.

71. O'Reilly, M. S., Brem, H., and Folkman, J. (1995). Treatment of murine hemangioendotheliomas with the angiogenesis inhibitor AGM-1470. *J. Pediatric Surg.*, **30**, 325–30.

72. Toda, K-I., Tsujioka, K., Maruguchi, Y., Ishii, K., Miyachi, Y., Kuribayashi, K., and Imamura, S. (1990). Establishment and characterization of a tumorigenic murine vascular endothelial cell line (F-2). *Cancer Res.*, **50**, 5526–30.

73. Toda, K-I., Miyachi, Y., Kuribayashi, K., and Imamura, S. (1986). Decreased NK activity of nude mice receiving long-term ultraviolet irradiation: in relation to tumor induction. *J. Clin. Lab. Immunol.*, **20**, 129–31.

74. Gallagher, C. H., Canfield, P. J., Greenoak, G. E., and Reeve, V. E. (1984). Characterization and histogenesis of tumors in the hairless mouse produced by low-dosage incremental ultraviolet radiation. *J. Invest. Dermatol.*, **83**, 169–74.

75. Sato, N., Kaku, T., Dempo, K., and Kikuchi, K. (1984). The relationship of colonic carcinogenesis and hepatic vascular tumors induced by subcutaneously injected 1,2-dimethylhydrazine dihydrochloride in specific pathogen free mice. *Cancer Lett.*, **24**, 213–20.

76. Sato, N., Sato, T., Takahashi, S., and Kikuchi, K. (1986). Establishment of murine endothelial cell lines that develop angiosarcomas *in vivo*: brief demonstration of a proposed animal model for Kaposi's sarcoma. *Cancer Res.*, **46**, 362–6.

77. Grinspan, J. B., Mueller, S. N., and Levine, E. M. (1983). Bovine endothelial cells transformed *in vitro* by benzo(*a*)pyrene. *J. Cell. Physiol.*, **114**, 328–38.

78. Nakamura, S., Salahuddin, S. Z., Biberfeld, P., Ensoli, B., Markham, P. D., Wong-Staal, F., and Gallo, R. C. (1988). Kaposi's sarcoma cells: long-term culture with growth factor from retrovirus-infected CD4 + T cells. *Science*, **242**, 426–30.

79. Roth, W. K., Werner, S., Risau, W., Remberger, K., and Hofschneider P. H. (1988). Cultured, AIDS-related Kaposi's sarcoma cells express endothelial cell markers and are weakly malignant *in vitro*. *Int. J. Cancer*, **42**, 767–73.

80. Salahuddin, S. Z., Nakamura, S., Biberfeld, P., Kaplan, M. H., Markham, P. D., Larsson, L., and Gallo, R. C. (1988). Angiogenic properties of Kaposi's sarcoma-derived cells after long-term culture *in vitro*. *Science*, **242**, 430–3.

81. Ensoli, B., Nakamura, S., Salahuddin, S. Z., Biberfeld, P., Larsson, L., Beaver, B., *et al.* (1989). AIDS–Kaposi's sarcoma-derived cells express cytokines with autocrine and paracrine growth effects. *Science*, **243**, 223–6.

82. Siegal, B., Levinton-Kriss, S., Schiffer, A., Sayar, J., Engelberg, I., Vonsover, A., *et al.* (1990). Kaposi's sarcoma in immunosuppression. Possibly the result of a dual viral infection. *Cancer*, **65**, 492–8.

83. Corbeil, J., Evans, L. A., Vasak, E., Cooper, D. A., and Penny, R. (1991). Culture and properties of cells derived from Kaposi sarcoma. *J. Immunol.*, **146**, 2972–6.

84. Browning, P. J., Sechler, J. M. G., Kaplan, M., Washington, R. H., Gendelman, R., Yarchoan, R., *et al.* (1994). Identification and culture of Kaposi's sarcoma-like spindle cells from the peripheral blood of human immunodeficiency virus-1-infected individuals and normal controls. *Blood*, **84**, 2711–20.

85. Herndier, B. G., Werner, A., Arnstein, P., Abbey, N. W., Demartis, F., Cohen, R. L., *et al.* (1994). Characterization of a human Kaposi's sarcoma cell line that induces angiogenic tumors in animals. *AIDS*, **8**, 575–81.

86. Lunardi-Iskandar, Y., Bryant, J. L., Zeman, R. A., Lam, V. H., Samaniego, F., Besnier, J. M., *et al.* (1995). Tumorigenesis and metastasis of neoplastic Kaposi's sarcoma cell line in immunodeficient mice blocked by a human pregnancy hormone. *Nature*, **375**, 64–8.

87. Mulliken, J. B., Zetter, B. R., and Folkman, J. (1982). *In vitro* characteristics of endothelium from hemangiomas and vascular malformations. *Surgery*, **92**, 348–53.

88. Berard M., Carrier, J. L., Baudin, B., and Drouet, L. (1992). Culture of porcine brain capillary endothelial cells: improvement using human hemangioma-conditioned medium. *J. Tissue Culture Methods*, **14**, 101–6.

89. Orchard, P. J., Smith, C. M., Woods, W. G., Day, D. L., Dehner, L. P., and Shapiro, R. (1989). Treatment of hemangioendotheliomas with alpha interferon. *Lancet*, **ii**, 565–7.

90. Ezekowitz, R. A. B., Mulliken, J. B., and Folkman, J. (1992). Interferon alfa-2a therapy for life-threatening hemangiomas of infancy. *N. Engl. J. Med.*, **326**, 1456–63.

91. Sidkey, Y. A. and Borden, E. C. (1987). Inhibition of angiogenesis by interferons: effects of tumor- and lymphocyte-induced vascular responses. *Cancer Res.*, **47**, 5155–61.

92. Majewski, S., Szmurlo, A., Marczak, M., Jablonska, S., and Bollag, W. (1994). Synergistic effect of retinoids and interferon α on tumor-induced angiogenesis: anti-angiogenic effect on HPV-harbouring tumor cell lines. *Int. J. Cancer*, **57**, 81–5.

93. Pepper, M. S., Vassalli, J.-D., Wilks, J. W., Schweigerer, L., Orci, L., and Montesano, R. (1994). Modulation of microvascular endothelial cell proteolytic properties by inhibitors of angiogenesis. *J. Cell. Biochem.*, **55**, 419–34.

94. Safai, B., Bason, M., Friedman-Birnbaum, R., and Nisce, L. (1990). Interferon in the treatment of AIDS-associated Kaposi's sarcoma: the American experience. *J. Invest. Dermatol.*, **95**, 166–9S.

95. Ingber D., Fujita, T., Kishimoto, S., Sudo, K., Kanamaru, T., Brem, H., and Folkman, J. (1990). Synthetic analogues of fumagillin that inhibit angiogenesis and tumour growth. *Nature*, **348**, 555–7.

96. Nakamura, S., Sakurada, S., Salahuddin, S. Z., Osada, Y., Tanaka, N. G., Sakamoto, N., *et al.* (1992). Inhibition of development of Kaposi's sarcoma-related lesions by a bacterial cell wall complex. *Science*, **255**, 1437–40.

97. Ensoli, B., Markham, P., Kao, V., Barillari, G., Fiorelli, V., Gendelman, R., *et al.* (1994). Block of AIDS–Kaposi's sarcoma (KS) cell growth, angiogenesis, and lesion formation in nude mice by antisense oligonucleotide targeting basic fibroblast growth factor. *J. Clin. Invest.*, **94**, 1736–46.

98. Ensoli, B., Gendelman, R., Markham, Fiorelli, V., Colombini, S., Raffeld, M., Cafaro, A., *et al.* (1994). Synergy between basic fibroblast growth factor and HIV-1 Tat protein in induction of Kaposi's sarcoma. *Nature*, **371**, 674–80.

99. Albini, A., Fontanini, G., Masiello, L., Tacchetti, C., Bigini, D., Luzzi, P., *et al.* (1994). Angiogenic potential *in vivo* by Kaposi's sarcoma cell-free supernatants and HIV-1 *tat* product: inhibition of KS-like lesions by tissue inhibitor of metalloproteinase-2. *AIDS*, **8**, 1237–44.

25. Development of the embryonic vascular system

Paul E. Young and Laurence A. Lasky

Introduction

Establishment of the vascular system is a critical step in the development of the vertebrate embryo. Numerous mutations and gene knockouts that indirectly compromise the ability of the mammalian embryo to establish and maintain an embryonic and/or yolk sac vasculature frequently result in early embryonic lethality (for review, see reference 1). As the embryo develops bulk and the various organ primordia appear and become organized, it is essential that all cells within a tissue mass receive an adequate supply of oxygen and nutrients and an efficient means of clearing waste products.

Studies indicate that the endothelial cells which constitute the inner lining of all blood vessels in fact are responsible for the positioning and patterning of the vasculature during development (2–4). As endothelial cells differentiate from the mesoderm following gastrulation early in development, they proliferate and interconnect into cords and channels in the precise locations of future blood vessels. Once these patterns have been established and the lumens of the vessels have been formed, the endothelium becomes invested with a basement membrane, smooth muscle cells, and other characteristics of the vasculature (3–6).

The development and establishment of the vascular endothelial system involves two distinct processes: vasculogenesis and angiogenesis (2,7,8). Vasculogenesis represents the *de novo* differentiation of endothelial cell precursors, or angioblasts, from mesoderm, followed by the subsequent migration, adhesion, maturation, and interconnection of these cells into cords and tubes that form the endothelial monolayer of the blood vessel (8,11). This process typifies the development of several of the major blood vessels of the embryo such as the dorsal aortae and posterior cardinal veins (2,10), as well as the initial vasculature of the embryonic yolk sac (11,12). Angiogenesis involves the branching off and subsequent proliferation of endothelial sprouts from pre-existing vessels into avascular areas, such as occurs during the formation of the intersomitic vessels and during the vascularization of the brain

(2,8). Angiogenesis does not involve additional differentiation of endothelial cells from pluripotent progenitors, but rather the reorganization and/or elaboration of an existing vascular network in response to some angiogenic factor or stimulus. Much attention has been focused on elucidating the physiology and mechanisms of angiogenesis, as this process characterizes various pathological conditions of the adult organism, such as diabetic retinopathy and arthritis, and particularly the vascularization and metastases of tumours (13–15), the subject of this compendium. Although it has not yet been clinically observed, researchers believe that it will not be entirely surprising if some form of postnatal vasculogenesis may also participate in the development of tumours (16).

Current models suggest that a common bipotential precursor cell termed the haemangioblast gives rise to both endothelial and haematopoietic cell lineages (17,18). This is based primarily upon shared antigenic markers present on both early endothelial cells and blood stem cells (9,19–20) and the simultaneous temporal and spatial appearance of endothelial and haematopoietic cells in the blood islands (11). Blood islands are observed in the vertebrate yolk sac and represent the first sites of embryonic haematopoiesis and the first appearance of endothelial cells during development. They are believed to arise from haemangioblasts that differentiate from mesodermal mesenchyme following gastrulation. These haemangioblasts proliferate and undergo additional differentiation to give rise to clusters of cells consisting of haematopoietic stem cells at their centre and early endothelial cells or endothelial cell precursors called angioblasts at their periphery.

Much of our current understanding of vertebrate embryonic vascular development has been derived from avian studies (2,10). This has been due to several reasons, including the relative accessibility of avian embryos to study, the relative ease and ability to perform *in vitro* experimental manipulations and tissue grafting during avian development, and the existence of antigenic markers that identify the early endothelial cell lineage during avian development. This stands in marked contrast to the difficulties of the mammalian system posed by such factors as the intrauterine development of the embryo, the difficulty of reproducing developmental conditions *in vitro*, and the paucity of markers that reliably identify endothelial cells during embryogenesis. A detailed understanding of mammalian vasculogenesis and angiogenesis is desirable, and will contribute to the analysis of the phenotypes of animals derived from homologous gene disruption and will directly facilitate the analysis of human vascular development.

Morphological studies of vascular development: light and electron microscopic analysis

Experiments conducted by Reagen (21) first demonstrated that the blood vessels of the embryo originate within the body proper and not through passive invasion from the yolk sac vasculature. The early work of Sabin (22) provided some of the best early descriptions of avian vascular development, and were based upon light microscopic observations on living blastodiscs explanted *in vitro*. These studies described the formation of capillary plexi through the coming together of small vessels, the fusion of these vessels into syncytia, the formation of the lumen of early blood vessels by liquefaction of the innermost cells, the gradual enlargement of vessels along major vascular routes, and the anastomosing of vessels in the area pellucida and area opaca. Dense luminal contents that were observed during early embryonic development were believed to represent a breakdown product of the disintegrating angioblasts (6,22).

Later ultrastructural studies using both scanning and transmission electron microscopy confirmed and extended these findings (5,6,10,23). Such studies have particularly focused on vasculogenesis and the *in situ* assembly of differentiated endothelial cells, such as during the development of the dorsal aorta and posterior cardinal veins, the yolk sac vasculature, and during blood island formation (5,10,23,24). They have generally supported Sabin's early work (22) and have similarly demonstrated that early blood vessels initially appear as cords or clusters of cells that with continued development form a lumen near the centre of the cell mass. However, they did not find support for the syncytial nature of early mesodermal clusters (blood islands) nor for the concept of liquefaction involved in lumen formation as all endothelial cells appeared to remain intact. Instead, some studies suggested that polarized secretion and increases in hydrostatic forces could result in blood vessel lumen formation (5,6).

Ultrastructural studies were unable to identify early endothelial cell precursors (haemangioblasts) upon the basis of morphology or subcellular features (5). Instead, the mesodermal cell population appeared morphologically homogeneous until the appearance of defined endothelial cells. Other studies focused on the identification of the earliest recognizable morphological specializations involved in the specification of haematopoietic versus endothelial lineages (11).

Electron microscopic analysis of the development of the chick embryonic myocardium suggested that blood vessels do not develop *de novo* within this tissue, but rather via the angiogenic invasion by the external vasculature (6). It was noted that the myocardium was characterized by extensive intracellular spaces prior to the onset of vascularization, and that these spaces are possibly necessary to provide channels for the uninhibited growth of angiogenic capillaries. This would suggest that angiogenesis of the heart involves a concerted interplay of the myocardial tissue and the angiogenic vessels, rather than the simple invasion of the heart muscular layer by vascular elements (6).

A combination of scanning and transmission electron microscopy verified that vasculogenesis accounts for the formation of primitive blood vessels, such as the vitelline vessels, the dorsal aorta, and the cardinal vein (25,26). The development of these vessels does not involve sprouting from pre-existing angioblastic cords, but instead the vessels are formed from connections between pre-existing cords by newly developing angioblasts. These studies have also addressed the canalization of the early endothelial tubes, and have similarly found no support for the theory of liquefaction. However, these studies have also argued against any contribution of polarized secretion in the expansion of the vascular cavity. Secretory organelles were not characteristically abundant in endothelial cells, and the single endothelial layer lining early blood vessels was marked by holes and clefts along its wall, that would fail to contain and rather would leak any fluids secreted into the prospective lumenal space. These researchers suggest that lumen formation involves the expansion of intracellular space within endothelial masses and the active enclosure of this space by attenuated endothelial cells.

Initial attempts to detect endothelial cells in the developing embryo

Researchers have attempted to develop labelling techniques that would facilitate the analysis of the vasculature and permit the unambiguous detection of endothelial cells and endothelial precursors in the developing embryo. Several studies have injected dyes and inks into the embryonic circulation (12) to analyse vessel development and brain an-giogenesis. Such injection studies have been limited in their usefulness during early stages of vascularization, when de-veloping vessels have narrow lumina or none at all (27). Other studies have attempted to exploit the differential bio-chemical properties of endothelium as a labelling tool (28).

Some studies have attempted to take advantage of transgenic technology to analyse mammalian vascular development in mice (29,30). In particular, the use of endothelial cell lineage-specific promoters from such genes as the tie-2 receptor tyrosine kinase (for more information, see below) has permitted preliminary low-resolution views of the developing vasculature (30). However, transgenic animals carrying tie-2 promoter/lac-z fusion constructs failed to direct lac-z expression to all vascular endothelial cells, the lac-z expression levels depended greatly upon the developmental stage of the embryo under examination, and the lac-z expression ap-peared to be highly sensitive to other inductive influences. For example, the primitive vasculature of *in vitro* derived embryoid bodies failed to express lac-z under the control of the tie-2 promoter.

Development of antibody probes and fluorescent markers for endothelial cells in the embryo

Studies on vascular development took a great step forward with the development of antibodies that could specifically recognize endothelial cells during embryonic develop-ment. Investigators had expressed the need for an endothe-lial cell marker that could unambiguously identify presumptive endothelial cells just as they segregate from the mesoderm and begin organizing into angioblastic cords during early vasculogenesis (25). Two of the first anti-bodies developed, anti-QH1 and anti-MB1, were both monoclonals that specifically detected quail endothelial and haematopoietic cells during development (9,20). To date, the precise molecular identity of the QH-1/MB-1 antigenic determinant remains unknown (31).

A number of studies have used these antibody probes to document vascular development during early quail em-bryogenesis (2,9). These studies have documented the origins of such avian vascular structures as the vitelline vessels, the dorsal aortae, the aortic arches, the carotid ar-teries, the cephalic capillary plexus, the vertebral arteries, the intersomitic vessels, and the cardinal veins. Other anti-body probes have also been generated against endothelial cells from avian embryos and have confirmed the observa-tions obtained from these earlier experiments (32).

The QH1/MB1 epitopes are expressed soon after pre-sumptive endothelial cells, or angioblasts, begin to dif-ferentiate from the lateral plate mesoderm. Therefore, these studies have permitted the analysis of the behaviour and movements of angioblasts prior to their incorporation into angioblastic cords and vessel rudiments. They demon-strate during vasculogenesis that angioblasts migrate over the surface of the mesoderm as individual cells or as clus-ters termed angiogenic islets, until they recognize a par-ticular stimulus that causes them to become sedentary and contribute to a particular blood vessel (2). Additionally, these studies demonstrate that presumptive endothelial cells arising at angiogenic sites become segregated for sep-arate developmental fates and follow divergent migratory pathways that result in their contribution to distinct endothelial structures. For example, common pools of angioblasts segregate to give rise to either heart endo-cardium or dorsal aorta, and similarly to either dorsal aorta or the cardinal veins.

Attempts to analyse endothelial development in mammals have been hampered by a lack of suitable probes. Antibodies that recognize specific proteins expressed by adult or cultured endothelial cells, such as von Willebrand's factor, have failed to identify reliably endothelial cells in embryos (8,33). Similarly, the use of such endothelial-specific markers such as the uptake of Dil-Ac-LDL have met with little success (33). However, a recent study used affinity-purified antibodies against CD34 to identify successfully endothelial cells in all developing vessels and capillaries of the mouse embryo. The specificity of the antibody and the use of confocal micro-scopy combine to provide the most thorough immuno-fluorescent analysis of mammalian vascular development in the literature. This antibody could label vessels under-going both vasculogenesis and angiogenesis and even appeared to identify potentially haemangioblasts as they emerged in the yolk sac shortly following gastrulation. This study is particularly interesting, in that it identifies elaborate filopodial processes associated with the tips of angiogenic vessels and describes a morphological structure associated with the growing tips of embryonic vessels that resembles the growth cones of neurons (34). It is therefore not unreasonable to suggest that during embryonic angio-genesis, blood vessels and vascular patterns are established through a pathfinding process similar to that observed during neurogenesis.

It is tempting to speculate that capillary pathfinding may be a complex multistep process similar to that involved in the extravasation of leukocytes during inflammation and lymphocyte recirculation during immune surveillance (35). In this model, capillary pathfinding would involve an initial step wherein the endothelial growth cone participates in low-affinity interactions with the surrounding embryonic tissues and matrix, in a manner analogous to the interactions between selectins and their carbohydrate ligands during the rolling step of leukcocyte extravasation. Interestingly, *in vitro* studies have indicated a role for selectins in capillary morphogenesis (36); however, the significance and relevance of such studies to embryonic vascular development is difficult to determine, as mice carrying homozygous disruptions of their selectin loci fail to exhibit significant embryonic developmental defects (37,38). Studies using other knockout mice have, however, demonstrated a requirement for glycosylation in normal blood vessel development (39). In this model, endothelial cells would then activate signalling pathways upon encountering gradients of molecules that specify the location of blood vessels in the surrounding tissues, that induce the expression of higher-affinity receptor/ligand combinations (*e.g.* integrins) that would stabilize the positioning of endothelial cells. Indeed, antibody blocking experiments demonstrate the requirement for $\alpha_v\beta_3$ integrins (an endothelial cell receptor for von Willebrand's factor, fibrinogen, and fibronectin) and β_1 integrins during embryonic vasculogenesis, neovascularization, and angiogenesis (40,41). Immunofluorescence verifies that an increase in the levels of $\alpha_v\beta_3$ expression on capillaries is linked to the induction of angiogenesis (41).

Other studies have attempted to identify immunological markers that could differentiate between endothelial cells that line the capillaries of different organs (42,43). Perhaps organ-specific determinants expressed on the endothelial cell surface may play important parts in the differences in vascular pattern established in the various organs during development.

Avian chimeras determine the relative contributions of vasculogenesis and angiogenesis to organ vascularization

One advantage of the avian system is the ability to construct quail/chick chimeric embryos *in vitro* using tissue grafting techniques (*e.g.* reference 44). In such experiments, a tissue fragment or organ from one species of embryo is transplanted and grafted to a region of the embryo of the other species. The cells from the donor and host species can be distinguished from one another based upon the morphology of the nuclear heterochromatin (45) or by the species-specific expression of antigenic determinants. Following a set time of development after grafting, one can examine the chimeric embryo and determine the relative influence of the host embryo upon the

development of the donor tissue fragment, and vice versa.

Investigators have used this technique to establish the degree to which various organs undergo vasculogenesis and/or angiogenesis during avian embryogenesis (*e.g.* reference 46) This has been accomplished through the use of the two antibodies that recognize MB1 and QH1 (10,19), the antigenic determinants specifically expressed by quail endothelial and haematopoietic cells. Because of the species-specificity of these monoclonal antibodies, blood vessels that are MB1 or QH1 positive that appear within a grafted organ rudiment must be of quail origin. Therefore, if a quail embryonic organ that was grafted to a chicken embryo later contains MB1/QH1 positive endothelial cells, then vascularization of that organ must involve vasculogenesis (i.e. the vessels of that organ are, at least in part, derived from endogenous endothelial cell precursors or angioblasts). Likewise, if a chicken organ that was grafted to a quail embryo upon later inspection contains MB1/QH1 positive endothelial cells, then the organ must have undergone angiogenesis (i.e. must have been invaded by blood vessels from the host quail embryo). Of course, for the unambiguous interpretation of such experiments, all organs must be removed from donor embryos and grafted into hosts at a time in development prior to the establishment of endothelial cells within that organ.

These experiments demonstrate that particular organs such as brain, kidney, and limb bud appear to establish their vasculature exclusively through angiogenesis (44, 46–48,49–51). These organs do not undergo vasculogenesis, at least in this experimental system. In contrast, certain organs like lung and pancreas establish blood vessels via vasculogenesis (46) and do not undergo appreciable exogenous angiogenesis. As a generalization, it appears that the capacities of the two embryonic mesodermal layers are different — namely, only the splanchnopleural layer (mesoderm associated with endoderm) produces endothelial cells, while the somatopleural layer (mesoderm associated with ectoderm) becomes colonized by extrinsic endothelial cell precursors (18,46). Such differences in the ability of embryonic organs to participate in vasculogenic/angiogenic processes suggest interesting organ-specific differences in the expression of factors capable of inducing endothelial cell differentiation and proliferation. Chimeric studies have also demonstrated that during vasculogenesis, angioblasts migrate along defined pathways through restricted points of entry to establish blood vessels in the embryo (8). The precise molecular nature of the positional or environmental cues that are recognized during such migrations remain unknown.

Studies on chimeric embryos have also been used to analyse the development of the blood–brain barrier (20,47). The blood–brain barrier represents morphological and biochemical specializations of blood vessels within brain tissue that ensure blood-borne solutes cannot passively diffuse between cells, but rather must pass through them in order to enter the brain. Endothelial cells that display blood–brain barrier characteristics are connected by tight junctions, lack fenestrae, display reduced levels of vesicular transport, have elevated mitochondrial density, and express high levels of several enzymes not significantly present in non-neural capillaries, including alkaline phosphatase and cholinesterase. Transplantation studies have demonstrated that host-derived blood vessels from non-neuronal sources (*e.g.* gut) will develop functional, structural, and histochemical features of capillaries with a blood–brain barrier once they have invaded and vascularized donor brain tissue following angiogenesis (20,47). Therefore, brain tissue, or the neural environment provides some signals or factors capable of inducing blood–brain specializations. However, the precise identity of such factors or even those cells that produce such factors remains unknown. Interestingly, such neural signals can even reprogramme the species-specificity of the observed blood–brain barrier characteristics. For example, when chick gut endothelial cells invade quail embryonic brain tissue, not only do they develop blood–brain barrier characteristics, but they even develop blood–brain barrier characteristics of quail brain capillaries (i.e. elevated mitochondrial density, cholinesterase expression) that are never observed in normal chick brain capillaries during embryogenesis (47).

Chimeric studies have provided conclusive support for the pluripotency of mesoderm and endothelial cells to form a variety of vessels (8). Mesodermal or endothelial cells from donor embryos derived from regions that would typically give rise to a specific blood vessel (*e.g.* dorsal aorta) will contribute or give rise to vessels that are characteristic of their newly transplanted location (*e.g.* endocardium). Therefore, no inherent programme exists within these cells that restricts or specifies the development of particular vascular structures. Rather, the local environment appears to dictate the precise arrangement and specialization of vascular morphogenesis.

Role of the extracellular matrix on development of the vascular endothelial network

Both vasculogenesis and angiogenesis involve extensive endothelial cell migration (8,48). It is likely that such migrations are controlled or directed by cell substrate adhesion molecules present in the embryonic extracellular matrix (ECM). Curiously, early ultrastructural studies failed to identify a significant ECM surrounding the vessel wall during the early stages of vasculogenesis (5). A later study demonstrated that the earliest vascular ECM components appear prior to the onset of circulation, when presumptive endothelial cells have delaminated from the central cell clusters of blood islands (24). This matrix underwent further elaboration, including the appearance of glycosaminoglycans and collagen fibrils, coincident with the cyto differentiation of both layers of the developing vessel wall (endothelium and smooth muscle). This led to the suggestion that the appearance and composition of the ECM may act as an inducing stimulus for vessel differentiation.

Later immunofluorescence studies specifically analysed dynamic changes in the distribution of fibronectin and laminin during chick embryonic development (48,49). They demonstrated that in the embryo, blood vessels develop and migrate within a matrix rich in fibronectin. Even the blood islands are surrounded by fibronectin. Shortly after vessels have been established, endothelial cells begin to express laminin in increasing amounts. During mammalian brain angiogenesis, laminin is detected along the borders of capillary sprouts, but is absent at the leading edge surrounding the filopodial processes (48,49). This suggests that laminin is only produced by mature vessels and may stabilize such vessels following their formation, and again argues for the dynamic nature of the leading edge or 'growth cone' of angiogenic vessels. The signals that trigger laminin expression in maturing endothelial cells are unknown.

Gene disruption experiments verify a role for fibronectin in vascular development. Homozygous disruptions of the fibronectin locus result in embryonic lethality and are characterized by defects in normal vascular development (50). Such embryos develop erythroblasts and endothelial cells that are arranged into vascular structures, so there does not appear to be a defect in the haemangioblast-derived differentiation pathways. Similarly, deletion of the locus for the α_5 integrin subunit that participates in the $\alpha_5\beta_1$ receptor for the RGD cell adhesion site of fibronectin also results in embryonic lethality and aberrant vascular development, albeit less severe than that observed for fibronectin deficiency (51). This slightly attenuated phenotype may be attributed to the fact that several other integrins can also function as fibronectin receptors.

Biochemical and molecular approaches to the study of embryonic angiogenesis and vasculogenesis

Several studies have attempted to isolate factors involved in promoting embryonic angiogenesis (*e.g.* references 52).

It is believed that the identification of such angiogenic factors will help elucidate angiogenesis that ccompanies tumour neovascularization and other adult pathological conditions. Following studies on chimeric avian embryos that demonstrated the angiogenic-promoting activity of brain and kidney (46–49) researchers have biochemically purified molecular factors from embryonic organ extracts that induce endothelial cell proliferation *in vitro* (53,54).

There has been particular interest placed on the analysis of the expression of the angiogenic factor VEGF (vascular endothelial growth factor) during embryogenesis (for review, reference 58). Results from *in situ* hybridization strongly suggest that VEGF plays a part during embryonic angiogenesis (56,57). Specifically, VEGF is expressed in cells of the ventricular epithelium of the developing rodent brain at times coincident with the initiation of angiogenic activity. During brain angiogenesis, capillaries sprout off from the perineural plexus at the pial surface of the brain and grow radially inwards towards the ventricular surface as they invade the neuroepithelium. Filopodial processes at the leading edge of these capillaries are uniformly oriented towards the ventricular epithelium. Therefore, the results are consistent with a model wherein VEGF expressed by cells of the ventricular epithelium establishes a gradient that is recognized by receptors present on endothelial cells or filopodia of endothelial sprouts, and that directs and contributes to their inward migration and proliferation. A role for VEGF as an angiogenic growth factor for fetal blood vessels is further substantiated by the identification of high levels of VEGF mRNA in the early embryonic kidney, which also undergoes vascularization by angiogenesis (56).

Several studies have attempted to isolate receptors expressed by endothelial cells that are responsible for the recognition and interpretation of angiogenic stimuli. Various lines of evidence have suggested that at least some such receptors may be associated with tyrosine kinase activity. Molecular attempts to clone such receptors via degenerate polymerase chain reaction based upon conserved domains of the receptor tyrosine kinase family have identified various novel endothelial-specific RTKs expressed during embryonic vascular development, including flt-1 and flk-1 (58–60), and the tek/tie receptors (61–65). Binding studies have demonstrated that flt-1/flk-1 is the receptor for VEGF (66,67). *In situ* analysis of the expression of these various receptors during development has provided some low resolution views of the vascular system during mammalian development (59–61,64–66). These studies have also demonstrated expression of these receptors in putative haemangioblasts/angioblasts prior to their incorporation into blood vessels and have suggested that these receptors may play a part in vasculogenesis and

endothelial differentiation (60,65). Gene disruption experiments provide some support for this concept, as animals that carry homozygous deletions in the tek/tie locus develop fewer endothelial cells than do their wild-type littermates (67). However, these animals still are capable of appreciable endothelial cell differentiation and vascular formation.

Other research attempts have attempted to establish *in vitro* models of vasculogenesis/angiogenesis that could be used for the isolation of novel factors that control endothelial development. One system involves the dissociation of quail blastodisc cells at stages prior to endothelial differentiation (69,70). When grown under normal conditions, such cultures fail to develop endothelial cells (33), in particular as judged by the absence of labelling with MB1/QH1 monoclonal antibodies (69). However, similar cultures readily develop endothelial cells as early as 3 days following dissociation when treated with acidic or basic fibroblast growth factor (aFGF or bFGF). Such results are difficult to interpret, as previous studies have failed to identify the endothelial cell expression of receptors for fibroblast growth factor in developing embryos by *in situ* analysis (71,72).

Other researchers have attempted to analyse mammalian vascular development through the use of *in vitro* differentiated embryoid bodies (7,73). Undifferentiated, pluripotent embryonic stem cells derived from the inner cell mass of preimplantation blastocysts will spontaneously undergo differentiation to form embryoid bodies (EBs) in culture following the removal of leukaemia inhibitory factor (LIF) from the culture media (74). These EBs develop a variety of differentiated terminal cell types and structures, including blood islands, endothelial cells, haematopoietic cells, and cardiac muscle (74). Studies indicate that the blood islands structurally resemble blood islands formed in the yolk sac *in vivo*, and that additional endothelial cells are arranged into cords and channels and resemble a primitive vasculature, albeit highly unorganized (7,73,74). The efficiency and frequency of blood island formation by EBs appears dependent upon culture conditions, such as the inclusion of human cord blood serum (74), and presumably reflects a dependence upon exogenous factors. However, the formation of a primitive vasculature within EBs appears less dependent upon complex culture conditions, and can readily occur with the use of fetal calf serum (73).

Other researchers have focused their efforts on the identification of novel *in vitro* assays for the identification of angiogenic factors and angiogenic activity. One study has modified the standard chick chorioallantoic membrane assay (CAM) in an attempt to quantify angiogenesis and angiogenic inhibitors for the chick embryo (75).

Future directions and perspectives: verification of the haemangioblast model

As mentioned, current models suggest that endothelial cells originate from a bipotential precursor cell capable of giving rise to both endothelial and haematopoietic cells in the embryo (17,18). Recent attempts to verify specifically the existence of the haemangioblast have been difficult to control adequately and have been inconclusive (76,77). The haemangioblast model makes important predictions, not only about vascular development, but about embryonic haematopoiesis as well. Whereas vasculogenesis is somewhat widespread in the early embryo, haematopoiesis is confined to only very few select areas (i.e. the blood islands of the yolk sac and the para-aortic region, or AGM (78). If indeed all endothelial and haematopoietic cells share a common precursor cell, then the developmental choice between the two prospective cell fates must be highly regulated and not merely a stochastic event. Factors must be required to influence directly at least haematopoietic cell differentiation and must be expressed by a very limited inducing cell population within presumptive haematopoietic loci. Otherwise, all areas of the embryo that undergo vasculogenesis would also develop haematopoietic foci. Alternatively, different inductive factors or influences may act earlier in development upon the mesodermal cell population to determine the differentiation of either haemangioblasts (bipotential precursors) or angioblasts.

Some researchers have suggested that endodermal cells produce factors that influence endothelial cell differentiation (e.g. references 46,79,80). Such factors were diffusible and affected the differentiation of both endothelial and haematopoietic cells, suggesting that they could exert their influence on the presumptive haemangioblast (79). Ultrastructural studies demonstrate that early blood vessels possess an incomplete basement membrane that would permit 'communication' between endothelial cells and endoderm during development (11).

As mentioned previously, homozygous disruption of the fibronectin locus results in embronic lethality and aberrant vascular morphogenesis (50). Close inspection of mutant embryos reveals a significant separation of the mesodermal and endodermal cell layers, particularly visible in the yolk sac. It is possible that such morphological disruptions interfere with normal signalling or induction pathways between the endodermal and mesodermal cell layers that contribute to the defects in vascular development.

Relevance of embryonic angiogenesis to adult tumour angiogenesis

Angiogenesis that accompanies the neovascularization of tumours is a complex process (14,15,52,80). It involves several steps, including the secretion of proteases, the breakdown of basement membranes, the release of angiogenic factors, and the stimulation of endothelial cell migration (15).

The extent to which embryonic angiogenesis parallels tumour angiogenesis depends upon the tissue under examination. For example, embryonic brain angiogenesis appears to follow a similar progression. During the initial steps of vascular invasion into the neuroectoderm, endothelial sprouts dissolve the underlying cortical basal lamina and subsequently penetrate into neural tissue (27,48,49,82–84). However, in contrast, capillaries were never observed to penetrate a basement membrane at any stage during angiogenesis of the embryonic kidney (48,49,85).

During normal embryonic development, angiogenesis is a highly regulated process, both temporally and spatially. Endothelial cells sprout along defined pathways, at precise times in development, for brief periods of time, after which such angiogenic growth is completely inhibited. In contrast, angiogenesis that accompanies tumour neovascularization is a disregulated process, that probably represents a subversion of the normal angiogenesis that typifies embryogenesis.

Update: spring 1997

Since this chapter was written, gene inactivation of VEGF and its receptors flt-1 and flk-1 have shown that VEGF plays a critical role in vasculogenesis. Thus, homozygous mutants inactivating flt-1 (86) or flk-1/KDR (87) and even heterozygous inactivation of the VEGF gene (88,89) are all lethal with either little or no vasculogenesis and in the case of the flk-1/KDR gene knockout without the appearance of blood islands (87).

References

1. Copp, A. J. (1995). Death before birth: clues from gene knockouts and mutations. TIG, **11**, 87–93.
2. Coffin, J. D. and Poole, T. J. (1988). Embryonic vascular development: immunohistochemical identification of the origin and subsequent morphogenesis of the major vessel primordia in quail embryos. *Development*, **102**, 735–48.

3. Nakamura, H. (1988). Electron microscopic study of the prenatal development of the thoracic aorta in the rat. *Am. J. Anat.*, **181**, 406–18.
4. Schwartz, S. M., Heimark, R. L., and Majesky, M. W. (1990). Developmental mechanisms underlying pathology of arteries. *Physiol. Rev.*, **70**, 1177–209.
5. Gonzalez-Crussi, F. (1971). Vasculogenesis in the chick embryo. An ultrastructural study. *Am. J. Anat.*, **130**, 441–60.
6. Manasek, F. J. (1971). The ultrastructure of embryonic myocardial blood vessels. *Dev. Biol.*, **26**, 42–54.
7. Risau, W., Sariola, H., Zerwes, H., Sasse, J., Ekblom, P., Kemler, R., and Doetschman, T. (1988). Vasculogenesis and angiogenesis in embryonic-stem-cell-derived embryoid bodies. *Development*, **102**, 471–8.
8. Coffin, J. D. and Poole, T. J. (1991). Endothelial cell origin and migration in embryonic heart and cranial blood vessel development. *Anat. Rec.*, **231**, 383–95.
9. Coffin, J. D., Harrison, J., Schwartz, S., and Heimark, R. (1991). Angioblast differentiation and morphogenesis of the vascular endothelium in the mouse embryo. *Dev. Biol.*, **148**, 51–62.
10. Pardanaud, L., Altmann, C., Kitos, P., Dieterlen-Lievre, F., and Buck, C. A. (1987). Vasculogenesis in the early quail blastodisc as studied with a monoclonal antibody recognizing endothelial cells. *Development*, **100**, 339–49.
11. Haar, J. L. and Ackerman, G. A. (1971). A phase and electron microscopic study of vasculogenesis and erythropoiesis in the yolk sac of the mouse. *Anat. Rec.*, **170**, 199–224.
12. Houser, J. W., Ackerman, G. A., and Knouff, R. A. (1961). Vasculogenesis and erythropoiesis in the living yolk sac of the chick embryo. *Anat. Rec.*
13. Ausprunk, D. H., Knighton, D. R., and Folkman, J. (1975). Vascularization of normal and neoplastic tissues grafted to the chick chorioallantois: role of host and preexisting graft blood vessels. *Am. J. Pathol.*, **79**, 597–618.
14. Folkman, J. (1985). Tumor angiogenesis. *Adv. Cancer Res.*, **43**, 175–203.
15. Folkman, J. and Shing, Y. (1992). Angiogenesis. *J. Biol. Chem.*, **267**, 10931–4.
16. Folkman, J. (1995). Angiogenesis in cancer, vascular, rheumatoid, and other disease. *Nature Med.*, **1**, 27–31.
17. His, W. (1900). Lecithoblast und angioblast der wirbelthiere. *Abhandl. K. S. Ges. Wiss. Math. Phys.*, **22**, 171–328.
18. Dieterlen-Lievre, F., Luton, D., and Pardanaud, L. (1994). Embryology of the endothelial network: is there an hemangioblastic anlage? In *Angiogenesis: molecular biology, clinical aspects* (ed. M. E. Maragoudakis *et al.*) pp. 1–8.
19. Peault, B. M., Thiery, J-P., and LeDouarin, N. M. (1983). Surface marker for hemopoietic and endothelial cell lineages in quail that is defined by a monoclonal antibody. *Proc. Natl Acad. Sci. USA*, **80**, 2976–80.
20. Risau, W., Hallmann, R., Albrecht, U., and Henke-Fahle, S. (1986). Brain induces the expression of an early cell surface marker for blood–brain barrier-specific endothelium. *EMBO J.*, **5**, 3179–83.
21. Reagan, F. P. (1915). Vascularization phenomena in fragments of embryonic bodies completely isolated from yolk-sac blastoderm. *Anat. Rec.*, **9**, 329–41.
22. Sabin, F. (1920). Studies on the origin of the blood vessels and of red blood corpuscles as seen in the living blastoderm of chick during the second day of incubation.
23. Meier, S. (1980). Development of the chick embryo mesoblast: pronephros, lateral plate, and early vasculature. *J. Embryol. Exp. Morphol.*, **55**, 291–306.
24. Murphy, M. E. and Carlson, E. C. (1978). An ultrastructural study of developing extracellular matrix in vitelline blood vessels of the early chick embryo. *Am. J. Anat.*, **151**, 345–76.
25. Hirakow, R. and Hiruma, T. (1981). Scanning electron microscopic study on the development of primitive blood vessels in chick embryos at the early somite-stage. *Anat. Embryol.*, **163**, 299–306.
26. Hirakow, R. and Hiruma, T. (1983). TEM-studies on development and canalization of the dorsal aorta in the chick embryo. *Anat. Embryol.*, **166**, 307–15.
27. Nakao, T., Ishizawa, A., and Ogawa, R. (1988). Observations of vascularization in the spinal cord of mouse embryos, with special reference to development of boundary membranes and perivascular spaces. *Anat. Rec.*, **221**, 663–77.
28. McLeod, D. S., Lutty, G. A., Wajer, S. D., and Flower, R. W. (1987). Visualization of a developing vasculature. *Microvasc. Res.*, **33**, 257–69.
29. Kadokawa, Y., Suemori, H., and Nakatsuji, N. (1990). Cell lineage analyses of epithelia and blood vessels in chimeric mouse embryos by use of an embryonic stem cell line expressing the b-galactosidase gene. *Cell Differ. Dev.*, **29**, 187–94.
30. Schlaeger, T. M., Qin, Y., Fujiwara, Y., Magram, J., and Sato, T. N. (1995). Vascular endothelial cell lineage-specific promoter in transgenic mice. *Development*, **121**, 1089–98.
31. Labastie, M., Poole, T. J., Peault, B. M., and LeDouarin, N. M. (1986). MB1, a quail leukocyte–endothelium antigen: partial characterization of the cell surface and secreted forms in cultured endothelial cells. *Proc. Natl Acad. Sci. USA*, **83**, 9016–20.
32. Aoyama, H., Asamoto, K., Nojyo, Y., and Kinutani, M. (1992). Monoclonal antibodies specific to quail embryo tissues: their epitopes in the developing quail embryo and their applications to identification of quail cells in quail-chick chimeras. *J. Histochem. Cytochem.*, **40**, 1769–77.
33. Yablonka-Reuveni, Z. (1989). The emergence of the endothelial cell lineage in the chick embryo can be detected by uptake of acetylated low density lipoprotein and the presence of a von Willebrand-like factor. *Dev. Biol.*, **132**, 230–40.
34. Zheng, J., Felder, M., Connor, J., and Poo, M. (1994). Turning of nerve growth cones induced by neurotransmitters. *Nature*, **368**, 140.
35. Lasky, L. A. (1992). Selectins: interpreters of cell-specific carbohydrate information during inflammation. *Science*, **258**, 964–9.
36. Nguyen, M., Strubel, N. A., and Bischoff, J. (1993). A role for sialyl Lewis-X/A glycoconjugates in capillary morphogenesis. *Nature*, **365**, 267–9.
37. Mayadas, T. N., Johnson, R. C., Rayburn, H., Hynes, R. O., and Wagner, D. D. (1993). Leukocyte rolling and extravasation are severaly compromised in P-selectin-deficient mice. *Cell*, **74**, 541–54.
38. Arbones, M. L., Ord, D. C., Ley, K., Ratech, H., Maynard-Curry, C., Otten, G., *et al.* (1994). Lymphocyte homing and leukocyte rolling and migration are impaired in L-selectin-deficient mice. *Immunity*, **1**, 247–60.
39. Metzler, M., Gertz, A., Sarkar, M., Schachter, H., Schrader, J. W., and Marth, J. D. (1994). Complex asparagine-linked oligosaccharides are required for morphogenic events during post-implantation development. *EMBO J.*, **13**, 2056–65.
40. Drake, C. J., Davis, L. A., and Little, C. D. (1992). Antibodies to b1-integrins cause alterations of aortic vasculogenesis, *in vivo*. *Dev. Dyn.*, **193**, 83–91.

41. Brooks, P. C., Clark, R. A. F., and Cheresh, D. A. (1994). Requirement of vascular integrin $\alpha_v\beta_3$ for angiogenesis. *Science*, **264**, 569–71.

42. Auerbach, R., Alby, L., Morrissey, L. W., Tu, M., and Joseph, J. (1985). Expression of organ-specific antigens on capillary endothelial cells. *Microvasc. Res.*, **29**, 401–11.

43. Gumkowski, F., Kaminska, G., Kaminski, M., Morrisey, L. W., and Auerbach, R. (1987). Heterogeneity of mouse vascular endothelium: *in vitro* studies of lymphatic, large blood vessel and microvascular endothelial cells. *Blood Vessels*, **24**, 11–23.

44. Sariola, H. (1985). Interspecies chimeras: an experimental approach for studies on embryonic angiogenesis. *Med. Biol.*, **63**, 43–65.

45. Le Douarin, N. M. (1973). A biological cell labeling technique and its use in experimental embryology. *Dev. Biol.*, **30**, 217–22.

46. Pardanaud, L., Yassine, F., and Dieterlen-Lievre, F. (1989). Relationship between vasculogenesis, angiogenesis, and haemopoiesis during avain ontogeny. *Development*, **105**, 473–85.

47. Stewart, P. A. and Wiley, M. J. (1981). Developing nervous tissue induces formation of blood–brain barrier characteristics in invading endothelial cells: a study using quali-chick transplantation chimeras. *Dev. Biol.*, **84**, 183–92.

48. Ekblom, P., Sariola, H., Karkinen-Jaaskelainen, M., and Saxen, L. (1982). The origin of the glomerular endothelium. *Cell Differ.*, **11**, 35–9.

49. Risau, W. and Lemmon, V. (1988). Changes in the vascular extracellular matrix during embryonic vasculogenesis and angiogenesis. *Dev. Biol.*, **125**, 441–50.

50. George, E. L., Georges-Labouesse, E. N., Patel-King, R. S., Rayburn, H., and Hynes, R. O. (1993). Defects in mesoderm, neural tube and vascular development in mouse embryos lacking fibronectin. *Development*, **119**, 1079–91.

51. Yang, J. T., Rayburn, H., and Hynes, R. O. (1993). Embryonic mesodermal defects in a5 integrin-deficient mice. *Development*, **119**, 1093–105.

52. Folkman, J. and Klagsbrun, M. (1987). Angiogenic factors. *Science*, **235**, 442–7.

53. Risau, W. (1986). Developing brain produces an angiogenic factor. *Proc. Natl Acad. Sci. USA*, **83**, 3855–9.

54. Risau, W. and Ekblom, P. (1986). Production of a heparin-binding angiogenesis factor by the embryonic kidney. *J. Cell Biol.*, **103**, 1101–7.

55. Ferrara, N. (1993). Vascular endothelial growth factor. *TCM*, **3**, 244–50.

56. Breier, G., Albrecht, U., Sterrer, S., and Risau, W. (1992). Expression of vascular endothelial growth factor during embryonic angiogenesis and endothelial cell differentiation. *Development*, **114**, 521–32.

57. Jakeman, L. B., Armanini, M., Phillips, H. S., and Ferrara, N. (1993). Developmental expression of binding sites and messenger ribonucleic acid for vascular endothelial growth factor suggests a role for this protein in vasculogenesis and angiogenesis. *Endocrinology*, **133**, 848–59.

58. Matthews, W., Jordan, C. T., Gavin, M., Jenkins, N. A., Copeland, N. G., and Lemischka, I. R. (1991). A receptor tyrosine kinase cDNA isolated from a population of enriched primitive hematopoietic cells and exhibiting close genetic linkage to *c-kit*. *Proc. Natl Acad. Sci. USA*, **88**, 9026–30.

59. Oelrichs, R. B., Reid, H. H., Bernard, O., Ziemiecki, A., and Wilks, A. F. (1993). NYK/FLK-1: A putative receptor protein tyrosine kinase isolated from E10 embryonic neuroepithelium is expressed in endothelial cells of the developing embryo. *Oncogene*, **8**, 11–18.

60. Yamaguchi, T. P., Dumont, D. J., Conlon, R. A., Breitman, M. L., and Rossant, J. (1993). Flk-1, an flt-related receptor tyrosine kinase is an early marker for endothelial cell precursors. *Development*, **118**, 489–98.

61. Dumont, D. J., Yamaguchi, T. P., Conlon, R. A., Rossant, J., and Breitman, M. L. (1992). Tek, a novel tyrosine kinase gene located on mouse chromosome 4, is expressed in endothelial cells and their presumptive precursors. *Oncogene*, **7**, 1471–80.

62. Partanen, J., Armstrong, E., Makela, T. P., Korhonen, J., Sandberg, M., Renkonen, R., *et al.* (1992). A novel endothelial cell surface receptor tyrosine kinase with extracellular epidermal growth factor homology domains. *Mol. Cell. Biol.*, **12**, 1698–707.

63. Dumont, D. J., Gradwohl, G. J., Fong, G-H., Auerbach, R., and Breitman, M. L. (1993). The endothelial-specific receptor tyrosine kinase, tek, is a member of a new subfamily of receptors. *Oncogene*, **8**, 1293–301.

64. Korhonen, J., Polvi, A., Partanen, J., and Alitalo, K. (1994). The mouse tie receptor tyrosine kinase gene: expression during embryonic angiogenesis. *Oncogene*, **9**, 395–403.

65. Sato, T. N., Qin, Y., Kozak, C. A., and Audus, K. L. (1993). Tie-1 and tie-2 define another class of putative receptor tyrosine kinase genes expressed in early embryonic vascular system. *Proc. Natl Acad. Sci. USA.*, **90**, 9355–8.

66. Millauer, B., Wizigmann-Voos, S., Schnurch, H., Martinez, R., Moller, N. P. H., Risau, W., and Ullrich, A. (1993). High affinity VEGF binding and developmental expression suggest flk-1 as a major regulator of vasculogenesis and angiogenesis. *Cell*, **72**, 835–46.

67. Quinn, T. P., Peters, K. G., DeVries, C., Ferrara, N., and Williams, L. T. (1993). Fetal liver kinase 1 is a receptor for vascular endothelial growth factor and is selectively expressed in vascular endothelium. *Proc Natl Acad. Sci. USA*, **90**, 7533–7.

68. Dumont, D. J., Gradwohl, G., Fong, G. H., Puri, M. C., Gertsenstein, M., Auerbach, A., and Breitman, M. L. (1994). Dominant-negative and targeted null mutations in the endothelial receptor tyrosine kinase, tek, reveal a critical role in vasculogenesis of the embryo. *Genes Dev.*, **8**, 1897–909.

69. Flamme, I. and Risau, W. (1992). Induction of vasculogenesis and hematopoiesis *in vitro*. *Development*, **116**, 435–9.

70. Flamme, I., Baranowski, A., and Risau, W. (1993). A new model of vasculogenesis and angiogenesis *in vitro* as compared with vascular growth in the avian area vasculosa. *Anat. Rec.*, **237**, 49–57.

71. Heuer, J. G., vonBartheld, C. S., Kinoshita, Y., Evers, P. C., and Bothwell, M. (1990). Alternating phases of FGF receptor and NGF receptor expression in the developing chicken nervous system. *Neuron*, **5**, 283–96.

72. Peters, K. G., Werner, S., Chen, G., and Williams, L. T. (1992). Two FGF receptor genes are differentially expressed in epithelial and mesenchymal tissues during limb formation and organogenesis in the mouse. *Development*, **114**, 233–43.

73. Wang, R., Clark, R., and Bautch, V. L. (1992). Embryonic stem cell-derived cystic embryoid bodies form vascular channels: an *in vitro* model of blood vessel development. *Development*, **114**, 303–16.

74. Doetschman, T. C., Eistetter, H., Katz, M., Schmidt, W., and Kemler, R. (1985). The *in vitro* development of blastocyst-

derived embryonic stem cell lines: formation of visceral yolk sac, blood islands, and myocardium. *J. Embryol. Exp. Morphol.*, **87**, 27–45.

75. Nguyen, M., Shing, Y., and Folkman, J. (1994). Quantitation of angiogenesis and antiangiogenesis in the chick embryo chorioallantoic membrane. *Microvasc. Res.*, **47**, 31–40.

76. Huang, S. and Terstappen, L. W. M. M. (1992). Formation of haematopoietic microenvironment and haematopoietic stem cells from single human bone marrow stem cells. *Nature*, **360**, 745–9.

77. Huang, S. and Terstappen, L. W. M. M. (1994). Correction: formation of haematopoietic microenvironment and haematopoietic stem cells from single human bone marrow stem cells. *Nature*, **368**, 664.

78. Dieterlen-Lievre, F. and Martin, C. (1981). Diffuse intra-embryonic hemopoiesis in normal and chimeric avian development. *Dev. Biol.*, **88**, 180–91.

79. Miura, Y. and Wilt, F. H. (1969). Tissue interaction and the formation of the first erythroblasts of the chick embryo. *Dev. Biol.*, **19**, 201–11.

80. Folkman, J. and Haudenschild, C. (1980). Angiogenesis in vitro. *Nature*, **288**, 551–6.

81. Flamme, I. (1989). Is extraembryonic angiogenesis in the chick embryo controlled by the endoderm? A morphological study. *Anat. Embryol.*, **180**, 259–72.

82. Feeney, J. F., Jr., and Watterson, R. L. (1946). The development of the vascular pattern within the walls of the central nervous system of the chick embryo. *J. Morphol.*, **78**, 231–303.

83. Marin-Padilla, M. (1985). Early vascularization of the embryonic cerebral cortex: Golgi and electron microscopic studies. *J. Comp. Neurol.*, **241**, 237–49.

84. Roncali, L., Ribatti, D., and Ambrosi, G. (1985). Ultra-structural basis of the vessel wall differentiation in the chick embryo optic tectum. *J. Submicrosc. Cytol.*, **17**, 83–8.

85. Sariola, H., Peault, B., LeDouarin, N. M., Buck, C. A., Dieterlen, F., and Saxen, L. (1984). Extracellular matrix and capillary ingrowth in interspecies chimeric kidneys. *Cell Differ.*, **15**, 43–52.

86. Fong, G. H., Rossant, J., Gertsenstein, M., and Breitman, M. L. (1966). Role of the flt-1 receptor tyrosine kinase in regulating the assembly of vascular endothelium. *Nature*, **376**, 66–70.

87. Shalaby, F., Rossant, J., Yamaguchi, T. P., Gertsenstein, M., Wu, X.-F., Breitman, M. L., and Schuh, A. C. (1995). Failure of blood-island formation and vasculogenesis in flk-1 deficient mice. *Nature*, **376**, 62–6.

88. Carmeliet, P., Ferreira, V., Breier, G., Pollefeyt, S., Kieckens, L., Gertsenstein, M., *et al.* (1996). Abnormal blood vessel development and lethality in embryos lacking a single VEGF allele. *Nature*, **380**, 435–9.

89. Ferrara, N., Carver-Moore, K., Chen, H., Dowd, M., Lu, L., O'Shea, K. S., *et al.* (1996). Heterozygous embryonic lethality induced by targeted inactivation of the VEGF gene. *Nature*, **380**, 439–42.

26. Targeting the tumour endothelium using specific antibodies

Elaine J. Derbyshire and Philip E. Thorpe

Introduction

Monoclonal antibodies have been considered for many years as a means to deliver cytotoxic agents specifically to tumour cells. While the approach has proved promising in clinical trials of leukaemia and lymphoma (1,2), the results of antibody trials in solid tumours, which account for 90% of malignancies (3), have so far been disappointing (4,5).

The main reason for the lack of therapeutic efficacy of antibody conjugates in solid tumours is the resistance of the tumour to penetration by macromolecules (6–8). In studies with radiolabelled antibodies, typically only 0.001–0.01% of the injected dose localizes to each gram of solid tumour in humans (9,10). The poor penetration of antibodies into solid tumours is due to several factors (reviewed in references 7,11). First, antibody in the circulation must travel across the endothelial cell layer and often through dense fibrous stroma before encountering the tumour cells. Secondly, the dense packing of tumour cells and tight junctions between epithelial tumour cells hinder transport of the antibody within the tumour mass. Thirdly, the absence of lymphatics within the tumour contributes to the build up of a high interstitial pressure which opposes the influx of molecules into the tumour core. Fourthly, the antibody entering the tumour becomes absorbed to the perivascular regions by the first tumour cells encountered, leaving none to reach tumour cells at sites further from the blood vessels (12).

A solution to the poor penetration of antibody conjugates into solid tumours would be to attack the endothelial cells in the tumour instead of the tumour cells themselves, as first proposed by Juliana Denekamp (13). Specific killing of vascular endothelial cells within the tumour should cause denudation of the endothelial lining. Platelets and coagulation factors in the blood then become activated on the exposed basal lamina leading to the formation of an occlusive thrombus within the affected vessels (14). The tumour cells that rely on these vessels for obtaining their oxygen and nutrients should then die away

Vascular targeting has a number of advantages over direct tumour cell targeting. First, the endothelial cells are directly accessible to intravenously injected antibody in the circulation, circumventing the need for tumour penetration (6,15). Secondly, there is an in-built amplification mechanism in that the occlusion of each individual capillary should lead to the death of thousands of tumour cells which rely on that capillary for deriving their oxygen and nutrients necessary for survival (16). Thirdly, it is possible that only a minority of endothelial cells within a capillary need to be killed to cause complete occlusion of the vessel. Hence, not all endothelial cells in the tumour need express the target antigen. Fourthly, a single vascular targeting agent should be suitable for targeting most or all types of solid tumours as they rely on similar types of vessels expressing similar migration or proliferation-linked cell surface determinants. Fifthly, endothelial cells are genetically stable and so should not mutate to become resistant to the therapy, as tumour cells often do.

Differences between the vasculature of tumours and normal tissues

There are numerous reports of anatomical, morphological and behavioural differences between blood vessels in tumours and normal tissues (reviewed in references 7,16,17) which suggest that antigenic differences also exist which will provide targets for vascular targeting agents.

Initially, a tumour acquires its nutritional supply from existing normal vessels. These vessels become incorporated into the expanding tumour mass but they do not adequately meet the nutritional needs of the growing tumour. Metabolites, catabolites, and specific angiogenic factors act as stimulants for angiogenesis, the formation of new blood vessels (18). The newly formed vessels are usually hyperpermeable, thin-walled capillaries or sinusoids with a basement membrane but no smooth muscle layer or enervation (16). During angiogenesis, endothelial cells from small venules or capillaries closest to the angiogenic stimulus degrade their underlying basement membrane and start to migrate towards the angiogenic stimulus. The endothelial cells behind the migratory cells proliferate so that the new capillary sprout can elongate. A new basement membrane is then synthesized, individual sprouts join with each other and blood flow begins (19,20). Thus during angiogenesis, migration of endothelial cells could expose previously inaccessible abluminal proteins to circulating vascular targeting agents (21) or could require the expression of new molecules that mediate tissue degradation or cellular locomotion. Similarly, because endothelial cells in solid tumours proliferate at a rate 50–200 times greater than do endothelial cells in normal tissues (22), proliferation-linked determinants could serve as markers for tumour endothelium. In addition, it is possible that tumour-derived angiogenic growth factors could directly induce new cell surface molecules on the local vasculature. Angiogenesis is not, however, unique to tumour growth. It takes place during a variety of normal and pathological processes such as wound healing, inflammatory arthritis, atherosclerosis, and diabetic retinopathy (23–26). Therefore, initiation of vascular targeting therapy against migration or proliferation-linked markers must be performed with caution, especially in the elderly.

Although the sequential events of capillary formation are similar regardless of how angiogenesis is induced, tumours impose modifications on a new capillary bed which differ from that in non-neoplastic tissues and which may result in markers with greater specificity for tumour vasculature (27). Tumours often contain giant capillaries, vessels with blind endings, arteriovenous shunts, and blood may even flow from one venule to another (17). The chaotic arrangement of the tumour vessels, together with suboptimal intercapillary spacing for nutrient provision and physical compression of tumour vessels by the tumour cells themselves, result in areas of hypoxia and tumour necrosis. Hypoxia is more prevalent in tumours than it is in other pathological conditions, including arthritis, atherosclerosis, and diabetic retinopathy. Tumour endothelial cells might therefore contain a greater abundance of hypoxia-generated molecules than do endothelial cells in non-malignant sites of tissue repair. One such molecule is vascular endothelial growth factor (VEGF), which concentrates on tumour endothelial cells (28). In addition, the already inadequate blood supply to tumours may be more easily compromised than the blood supply to normal tissues by thrombosis induced by vascular targeting agents.

Hypercoagulability is common in cancer (29). Newly formed capillaries lack the features of mature endothelium which may be important in controlling coagulation (16).

Also, tumour cells produce soluble substances such as VEGF and interleukin 1 that can induce procoagulant activity on the surface of local endothelial cells (30–33). Thus, thrombosis-linked determinants may be preferentially expressed on the tumour vasculature.

Validation of the vascular targeting approach in mice

Mouse model

We first set out to demonstrate the principle of vascular targeting in a mouse model (6,34). A murine neuroblastoma cell line (C1300 Mu γ), transfected with the murine interferon *gamma* gene, was injected subcutaneously into BALB/c nu/nu mice. The interferon *gamma* secreted by the tumour cells induced the expression of class II antigens of the major histocompatibility complex on the tumour vascular endothelial cells. Vascular endothelial cells in normal mouse tissues do not express class II antigens unless activated by interferon *gamma* and so the class II antigen acted as a tumour vasculature specific marker in this model.

Targeting ricin A-chain to the tumour vasculature

Immunotoxins, prepared by linking the A-chain of the toxin ricin to monoclonal antibodies, selectively kill cells expressing the relevant target antigens at their surfaces by irreversibly inactivating ribosomes and inhibiting protein synthesis (35). A single intravenous injection of an anti-class II ricin A-chain immunotoxin into mice bearing large (≥1 cm in diameter) solid tumours induced potent, dose-dependent anti-tumour effects (Fig. 26.1). Tumours regressed, usually completely, although in all cases, mice later relapsed with progressively growing tumour at the original site of tumour growth. In contrast, an anti-tumour cell immunotoxin directed against the class I antigens of the tumour allograft only destroyed those tumour cells close to blood vessels and had little effect on tumour growth. The vascular targeting and direct tumour cell targeting approaches were complementary as, when both immunotoxins were used in combination, improved anti-tumour effects were achieved: 60% of animals treated with the combination cleared their tumours and remained disease-free (Fig. 26.2).

A study of the time courses of the events in the tumours of mice treated with the anti-class II immunotoxin confirmed that vascular endothelial cell destruction was the first visible event and that tumour necrosis occurred

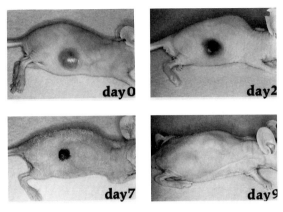

Figure 26.1. Gross appearance of subcutaneous tumours in mice treated with an immunotoxin directed against tumour vasculature. Mice bearing solid C1300 Muγ tumours were treated with an immunotoxin that was specific for the class II antigens which were induced on the tumour endothelial cells by interferon *gamma* secreted by the tumour. Before treatment (day 0), tumours were pink/purple, indicating florid vascularization. Two days after treatment, massive intratumoral haemorrhage caused a blackened discoloration, and by day 7 the tumour mass had largely collapsed into a scabrous tissue plug, which later dropped off to reveal a white, avascular nodule of dead tumour tissue (day 9). Representative mice at different stages of therapy are shown

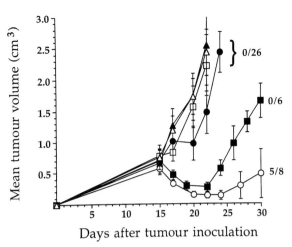

Figure 26.2. Regressions of solid tumours induced by an anti-tumour endothelial cell immunotoxin. C1300 Muγ tumour-bearing mice were given intravenous injections of 40 μg of anti-class II.dgA (■) directed against the tumour endothelial cells or 100 μg of anti-class I.dgA (●) directed against the tumour cells themselves. Other mice received a combination of 20 μg anti-class II.dgA plus 50 μg anti-class I.dgA (○), 100 μg of an isotype-matched control immunotoxin (△) or phosphate-buffered saline (▲). Error bars indicate the standard error of the mean. Also indicated: percentage of permanent complete remissions.

secondarily. The first loss of endothelial cells occurred about 2 h after injection of the immunotoxin (Fig. 26.3). Degeneration of the endothelial cell layer induced platelet adhesion and fibrin deposition. By 6 h, many blood vessels in the tumour were occluded with thrombi and were stripped of their endothelial cell lining. At this time, the tumour cells were morphologically unchanged. By 24 h, all vessels contained mature thrombi and the surrounding tumour cells had pyknotic nuclei. By 48 h, widespread tumour necrosis had occurred, followed by autolysis and the physical collapse of the tumour mass.

TEC-11: a candidate for vascular targeting in humans

From the above studies, it appears that vascular targeting is a valid and powerful approach to the therapy of solid tumours. This prompted us to search for tumour vasculature selective markers in humans so that the approach can be extended to humans.

TEC-11 antibody

TEC-11 is a mouse monoclonal antibody of the immunoglobulin (Ig)M class which was raised by immunizing BALB/c mice with human umbilical vein endothelial cells (HUVEC) (41). The HUVEC were proliferating and migrating at the time they were used for immunization and had been cultured in the presence of conditioned media from a human colorectal carcinoma cell line to emulate the tumour microenvironment. Hybridoma supernatants were screened in three steps: first, for reactivity with proliferating HUVEC cell surface antigens; secondly, for lack of reactivity with quiescent HUVEC in frozen sections of human umbilical vein by immuno-histochemistry; and thirdly, for reactivity with endothelial cells in frozen sections of human malignant but not normal tissue.

Immunoprecipitation studies and flow cytometric analysis of murine L-cells transfected with human endoglin indicated that TEC-11 recognized endoglin. Endoglin is an essential component of the transforming growth factor (TGF) β receptor system on human endothelial cells binding TGF-β1 and TGF-β3 with high affinity ($K_D = 50$ pM)

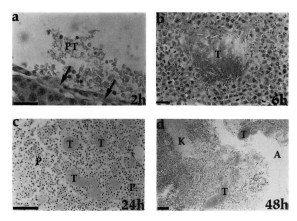

Figure 26.3. Time course of vascular thrombosis and tumour necrosis after administration of anti-tumour endothelial cell immunotoxins. (a) Two hours: a few endothelial cells had become denuded with exposure of the underlying subendothelial extracellular matrix (arrows). Platelet (PT) adhesion and aggregation on the damaged areas was visible. (b) Six hours: many vessels had become completely occluded by mature fibrin thrombi (T). (c)Twenty-four hours: all vessels were thrombotic and surrounding tumour cells had pyknotic nuclei (P). (d) Forty-eight hours: tumour necrosis had advanced and areas of pyknosis, karyolysis (K), and autolysis (A) were apparent. Hematoxylin and eosin stain. (Bars: a and b, 15 μm; c and d, 60 μm).

Table 26.1. Reactivity of TEC-11 with vascular endothelial cells in neoplastic tissues

Tumour	n	TEC-11
Angiosarcoma	1	+++*
Breast carcinoma	12	++/+++
Cecum carcinoma	1	+++
Colon carcinoma	3	+++
Hodgkin's disease	11	+++
Lymphoma	2	+
Lung carcinoma	1	++
Melanoma	1	++
Osteosarcoma	1	++
Ovarian carcinoma	1	++
Parotid tumor	3	+++
Pharyngeal carcinoma	2	++
Rectosigmoid carcinoma	6	+++

* Staining intensity was strong (+++), moderate (++) or weak (+).

(42). It is a dimeric glycoprotein composed of two 95 kDa disulphide-linked subunits whose primary sequence is known (43) and against which monoclonal antibodies have previously been raised (44–47). Endoglin is expressed on human endothelial cells, fetal syncytiotrophoblast (45), some macrophages (46), immature erythroid cells (47), and some leukaemic and haemopoietic cell lines (44–47). Its expression on dermal endothelium has been shown to be up-regulated in several chronic inflammatory skin lesions (48).

TEC-11 binding to malignant and normal human tissues

TEC-11 produced moderate to strong staining of vascular endothelial cells in a panel of frozen sections of miscellaneous human malignant tumours (Table 26.1). This panel included an extensive series of breast, rectosigmoid, and Hodgkin's tumours. The only human tumours whose vascular endothelial cells were weakly stained by TEC-11 were two cases of non-Hodgkin's B-cell lymphoma.

In most tumour samples, 80–100% of endothelial cells which stained with the positive control marker for endo-

thelial cells (anti-von Willebrand's factor antibody) were also stained by TEC-11. Often, TEC-11 stained capillaries more uniformly than did the anti-von Willebrand's factor antibody. TEC-11 stained the cytoplasm and luminal plasma membranes of endothelial cells in capillaries and venules, but did not stain arterioles.

In contrast to the strong staining of endothelial cells in the majority of malignant human tissues, TEC-11 demonstrated weak or undetectable staining of endothelial cells in the majority of frozen sections of normal human tissues (Table 26.2). The exceptions were adrenals, placenta, and lymphoid organs in which the endothelial cells showed moderate staining.

The marked difference in intensity of staining between endothelial cells in malignant and normal tissue by TEC-11 is exemplified in Fig. 26.4 where a sample of parotid tumour and associated histologically normal parotid gland from the same tissue section are stained with TEC-11 and compared. Vessels in the normal glandular tissue section are stained whereas all capillaries and venules stained strongly in the adjacent malignant tumour. By contrast, the anti-von Willebrand's factor antibody stained vessels in the normal and malignant areas with equal intensity.

A study of TEC-11 binding to a series of breast tissues at different stages of neoplastic progression revealed that TEC-11 binding became up-regulated on endothelial cells at approximately the stage at which breast tumours become invasive. Vessels in benign fibroadenomas, low-grade hyperplastic lesions, and early carcinoma *in situ* showed little or no reactivity with TEC-11 (Fig. 26.5). In contrast, all vessels in sections of invasive breast carcino-

Table 26.2. Reactivity of TEC-11 with endothelial cells in non-neoplastic tissues

Normal tissue	TEC-11	Normal tissue	TEC-11
Digestive		Lymphoid	
Colon	+*	Spleen	++
Gall-bladder	+	Thymus	++
Jejunum	–	Tonsil	++
Liver	+/–		
Pancreas	–	Endocrine	
Parotid	+/–	Adrenal	++
Salivary gland	+	Parathyroid	+
Stomach	+/–	Thyroid	+/–
Reproductive		Respiratory	
Breast	–	Lung	–
Cervix	–†		
Ovary	–	Nervous	
Placenta	++	Brain cortex	–
Prostate	+/–	Brain stem	–
Testis	+	Cerebellum	–
Uterus	+	Cranial nerve	–
Vagina	–		
Urinary		Integumentary	
Bladder	–	Skin	–
Kidney	+		

* Staining intensity was moderate (++), weak (+), or negative (–). In all cases, staining of endothelium was negative (–) with isotype-matched control antibodies.

†Veins and venules in cervix were ++; capillaries and arterioles were –.

mas stained strongly with TEC-11. Vessels in breast tumours of all histological grades stained strongly with anti-von Willebrand's Factor antibody.

Several authors have previously reported stronger staining of endothelial cells in normal organs, especially kidney, liver (44–48), and umbilical cord (44), with anti-endoglin antibodies than we observed with TEC-11. The possibility that TEC-11, unlike the other antibodies, recognizes an isoform of endoglin which is manufactured selectively by endothelial cells in tumours, was discounted by our finding that three different anti-endoglin antibodies (TEC-11, TEC-4, 44G4) directed against different epitopes showed the same selectivity for tumour vasculature. The discrepancies between the present and prior reports probably reflect differences in the sensitivity of the immunohistochemical staining techniques employed. In the present study, staining conditions were selected to give the best differential between the staining of endothelial cells in normal and malignant tissues.

Correlation between TEC-11 binding and endothelial cell proliferation

TEC-11 binding to the surface of HUVEC at different stages of growth was analysed by flow cytometry. Subconfluent HUVEC bound uniformly high levels of TEC-11, but when the same cells were grown to confluence and allowed to become partially quiescent over a further 3–6 days, an additional population of cells emerged which bound approximately five times less TEC-11. When the two populations in the confluent culture were sorted from each other and separated into zones in dot plots according to standard criteria, virtually all the cells binding low levels of TEC-11 were assigned to the G_0 (non-cycling) fraction whereas 15% and 5% of the cells binding high levels of TEC-11 were located in the G_1 (activated) and S + G_2/M (proliferating) fractions respectively. This result indicates that endoglin is up-regulated on dividing HUVEC and becomes down-regulated again as the cells become quiescent. However, the finding that the majority of cells binding TEC-11 at high levels were also in G_0, suggests that cell surface endoglin is long-lived and is maintained at high levels in cells that have divided and subsequently enter a non-cycling state.

The discovery that endoglin is a proliferation-linked marker explains the stronger staining of endothelial cells in malignant tissues which proliferate at a rates up to 50–200 times greater than endothelial cells in most normal tissues (49). It also explains why endothelial cells in non-Hodgkin's B-cell lymphoma were weakly stained by TEC-11 because, unlike carcinomas and non-lymphoid sarcomas, such lymphomas appear to grow by infiltrating existing vascular tracts rather than inducing new blood vessel growth (49).

Selective toxicity of a TEC-11 immunotoxin to proliferating human umbilical vein endothelial cells

An immunotoxin was prepared by linking TEC-11 to ricin A-chain. TEC-11.ricin A-chain was potently toxic to proliferating subconfluent cultures of HUVEC, reducing [³H]leucine incorporation by 50% at a concentration of 7.5×10^{-11} mol/l (Fig. 26.6). In contrast, the immunotoxin was 3000-fold less potent against partially quiescent confluent cultures inhibiting [³H]leucine incorporation by only 30% at 1×10^{-7} mol/l. TEC-11.ricin A-chain was no more toxic to the confluent cultures than was an isotype-matched control immunotoxin of irrelevant specificity, indicating that no toxicity was mediated through TEC-11 binding to the confluent cells. Proliferating and confluent HUVEC cultures were equally sensitive to ricin.

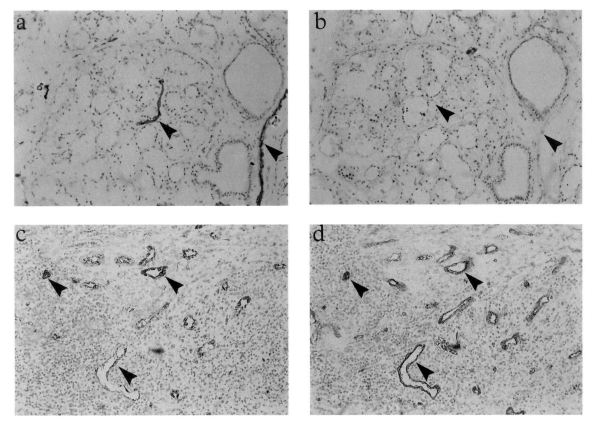

Figure 26.4. Stronger binding of TEC-11 to vessels in malignant parotid tumour as compared with adjacent normal parotid tissue. Frozen tissue sections of normal parotid gland (a,b) and adjacent parotid tumour (c,d) stained with anti-von Willebrand's factor antibody, F8/86 (a,c), or TEC-11 (b,d). Numerous blood vessels are stained strongly by F8/86 in both tissues, whereas strong TEC-11 labelling is only seen in the malignant sample. Antibody binding was detected with biotinylated F (ab')$_2$ rabbit anti-mouse IgG (F8/86) or IgM (TEC-11) and SABC-HRP with AEC substrate and haematoxylin counter staining.

The selective toxicity of TEC-11.ricin A-chain against proliferating HUVEC may be explained in part by the higher levels of TEC-11 bound by proliferating HUVEC compared with confluent cells. However, the small difference in levels of TEC-11 bound by the two cell populations (less than fivefold) is unlikely to account for the 3000-fold difference in susceptibility to intoxication unless there is a threshold amount of immunotoxin that must bind before cytotoxicity occurs. It is likely that aspects of the proliferative response other than antigen density are important in TEC-11.ricin A-chain-mediated cytotoxicity as has been found with of other immunotoxins against different cell types (36–40). It is possible that TEC-11.ricin A-chain is routed differently in proliferating and confluent HUVEC. Proliferating HUVEC may internalize the immunotoxin more rapidly or extensively, or internalize it by a pathway that avoids lysosomal degradation and favours A-chain translocation to the cytosol, where the A-chain has its toxic action.

It is conceivable that an anti-endoglin immunotoxin would have clinical utility as quiescent endothelial cells in normal tissue may be unharmed by the immunotoxin, although they express endoglin at low levels. In contrast, dividing endothelial cells in the tumour, which express higher levels of endoglin would be effectively killed.

Other antigens preferentially expressed in tumour vasculature

The perfect antibody for vascular targeting of solid tumours would: (i) recognize a high proportion of tumour

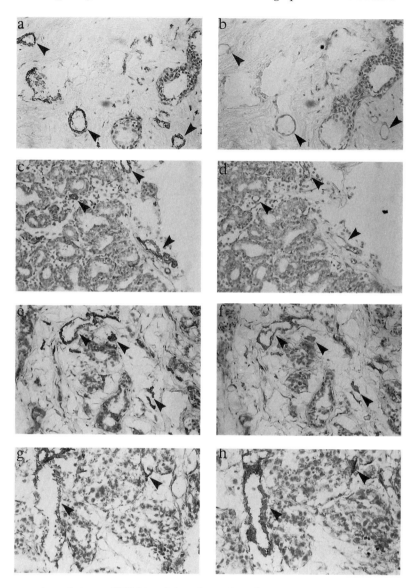

Figure 26.5. Correspondence between TEC-11 staining of vessels and tumour progression in human breast tissues. Frozen tissue sections of benign fibroadenoma (a,b), lobular hyperplasia (c,d), or invasive breast carcinoma (e–h) stained with anti-von Willebrand's factor antibody, F8/86 (a,c,e,g) or TEC-11 (b,d,f,h). Numerous blood vessels are stained strongly by F8/86 in tumours of all histological grades whereas TEC-11 staining is very weak in the premalignant samples (b,d), increasing to heavy labelling in the frank carcinomas (f,h). Antibody binding was detected as in the legend in Fig. 26.4.

vascular endothelial cells in diverse solid tumours, and (ii) show no cross-reactivity with endothelial cells, or other cells, in normal tissues. The search for tumour vasculature specific antibodies is a relatively young field and to date no antibodies have been found which meet both criteria. However, a number of antigens in addition to endoglin have been reported to show preferential expression in tumour vascular endothelial cells and these are described below.

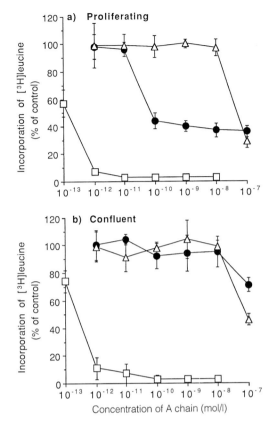

Figure 26.6. Selective toxicity of TEC-11-ricin A-chain to proliferation human umbilical vein endothelial cells (HUVECs). (a) Proliferating and (b) confluent HUVEC cultures prepared in 96-well plates were treated for 24 h at 37°C with TEC-11-recin A-chain (●), an isotype-matched control immunotoxin (△), or with ricin (□), and for a further 24 h in the presence of 1 μCi of [³H]leucine. The results are expressed as the mean and standard deviation of triplicate determinations of [³H]leucine incorporation as a percentage of untreated control cultures.

EN 7/44 antigen

In 1986, Hagemeier *et al.* described the first monoclonal antibody selective for human tumour vasculature (50). The antibody EN 7/44 of the IgM class, was raised by immunizing mice with cell suspensions of capillary-rich fragments of mammary carcinomas. EN 7/44 detects an antigen of 30.5 kDa expressed in about 50% of cultured HUVEC and in endothelial cells from placenta, acute inflammatory and immune reactions, and tumours *in vivo*. The antibody does not detectably stain non-endothelial tissues. A few capillary buds and small venules stained

with EN 7/44 in normal proliferating tissues such as colon and foreskin. In some tumours, especially carcinomas, EN 7/44 stained large vessels, venules and veins, and sometimes small arteries. In most tumours, the strongest reactions were seen with the capillary buds which contained migrating and proliferating endothelial cells. Although the antigen was weakly expressed at the surface of tumour vascular endothelial cells, its expression appeared mainly restricted to the cytoplasm, limiting its use as a vascular target.

Endosialin

Monoclonal antibody FB5 of the IgG2a isotype, was raised against cultured human fetal fibroblasts and detects a novel cell surface antigen, endosialin (51). Endosialin has a molecular mass of 165 kDa comprised of a 95 kDa core polypeptide and highly sialyated O-linked oligosaccharides and is encoded by a gene located on chromosome 11q13–qter. FB5 detects endothelial cells in 67% of human tumours whereas normal blood vessels and other adult tissues tested lacked detectable endosialin. There was considerable variability between tumours in the number of FB5-positive vessels, ranging from a small subset of capillaries to virtually the entire capillary bed. No discernible parameter distinguished the degree of FB5 reactivity within the tumour. FB5 also reacted with cultured fibroblasts and neuroblastoma cell lines. No reactivity was detected against other tumour types or with HUVEC even after activation with cytokines. FB5 is rapidly internalized into endosialin expressing cells and so is a candidate for the vascular targeting of agents, such as ricin A-chain, which have intracellular sites of action.

E-9 antigen

E-9 is an IgG1 monoclonal antibody which was raised against cultured HUVEC and detects an antigen of 170 kDa under non-reducing conditions and 96 kDa under reducing conditions (52). The antigen recognized by E-9 was detected in vascular endothelial cells of all tumours, fetal organs, and inflamed tissues examined. Some staining of normal endothelium was seen, but the intensity was weaker than in tumours, with the exception of tonsil. E-9 is now known to recognize endoglin (53). However, the antigens recognized by E-9 and TEC-11 appear to be differently distributed because the endothelium of placenta was reported not to stain with E-9. It is possible that there are epitope differences between endoglin in different locations and that E-9 and TEC-11 distinguish between these.

BC-1 antigen

Monoclonal antibody BC-1, raised against fibronectin from the culture medium of simian virus 40-transformed human fibroblasts, reacts with an isoform of fibronectin that is produced almost exclusively by transformed cells (54). The epitope recognized by BC-1 is unmasked in molecules containing the ED-B sequence of fibronectin. In normal adult tissues, BC-1 staining was limited to the superficial synovial cells, the intima of some ovarian vessels, scattered areas of the ovarian interstitium and isolated areas of the basement membranes of the celomic epithelium, and to areas of the myometrium. In contrast, BC-1 extensively stained fetal tissue and about 38% of human tumours tested were BC-1 positive. Within a given tumour type, the incidence of BC-1 positive tumours was variable and no correlation was found with the degree of differentiation or the tumour histotype. In almost all the positive tumours, BC-1 staining was confined to the tumour interstitium surrounding tumour cell nests. A frequent feature was staining in the vascular intima which was never seen in normal adult tissues with the exception of some ovarian vessels. It is not clear whether tumour vascular endothelial cells manufacture the fibronectin isoform recognized by BC-1 or whether they bind BC-1 positive fibronectin manufactured by tumour cells or surrounding mesenchymal cells. However, a recent immunohistochemical study identified intense BC-1 staining in the cytoplasm of endothelial cells in glioblastoma multiforme and anaplastic astrocytoma, whereas there was no staining associated with the tumour cells (55). This suggests that the BC-1-positive fibronectin isoform may well be produced in the tumour vascular endothelial cells.

TP-1 and TP-3 antigen

The monoclonal antibodies TP-1 and TP-3 raised against cells from a human osteosarcoma xenograft, bind to two different epitopes on the same osteosarcoma-associated antigen (56). The antigen is a monomeric peptide with a molecular mass of approximately 80 kDa which is restricted to some subgroups of human sarcomas especially osteosarcomas. The two antibodies show the same staining profile. Staining of normal tissues was limited to clusters of cells in the adrenal medulla and in proximal kidney tubules, and to placental capillaries. However, budding capillaries in most tumours stained with the antibodies.

Integrins

The integrin $\alpha_v\beta_3$ has been identified as a marker of angiogenic vascular tissue. The integrin was found to be expressed on blood vessels in human wound granulation tissue but not in normal skin, and it showed a fourfold increase in expression during angiogenesis on the chick chorioallantoic membrane (CAM) (57).

The monoclonal antibody LM609, which binds to $\alpha_v\beta_3$ inhibited tumour-induced and basic fibroblast growth factor (bFGF)-induced angiogenesis on the CAM after intravenous injection (58). After induction of angiogenesis, endothelial cells enter the cell cycle and express increased levels of $\alpha_v\beta_3$. LM609 antagonizes the binding of $\alpha_v\beta_3$ to extracellular matrix components. This inhibits the interaction of stimulated endothelial cells with the extracellular matrix and causes apoptosis in the endothelial cells undergoing angiogenesis (58).

Antibodies against integrins may bind selectively to dividing endothelial cells in human tumours for two reasons: (i) the integrins may be expressed more abundantly on dividing compared with resting endothelial cells as is the case for $\alpha_v\beta_3$, and (ii) endothelial cells undergoing angiogenesis depolarize and detach from the underlying basement membrane in order to migrate towards the angiogenic stimulus (19). Integrins such as the fibronectin receptor, which are concentrated on the abluminal cell surface in quiescent cells, become expressed on the luminal surface of the dividing endothelial cells (21) where they are accessible to intravenously injected antibodies. In this regard, anti-fibronectin receptor immunotoxins are more toxic to sparse cultures of proliferating endothelial cells than to quiescent, confluent cultures (59).

Vascular endothelial growth factor

Vascular endothelial growth factor (VEGF), also known as vascular permeability factor, is a dimeric M_r 34 000–42 000 glycoprotein that is secreted by many tumour cells, probably as a response to hypoxia (60). The molecule is an endothelial cell-specific mitogen and enhances vascular permeability, both properties being important in the neovascularization of solid tumours (61).

Dvorak and colleagues raised polyclonal antibodies to the amino terminus of VEGF and found that they uniformly and intensely stained the endothelial cells immediately adjacent to tumour cells as well as the tumour cells themselves. In contrast, endothelial cells in normal tissue more than 0.5 mm away from the tumour did not stain (28). VEGF mRNA is localized to tumour cells and is absent from endothelial cells. By contrast, the mRNA for the VEGF receptors (Flt and KDR) is restricted to endothelium (61). These findings indicate that VEGF synthesized by the tumour cells is secreted, binds to VEGF receptors on adjacent endothelial cells, and is accumulated within these tumour vessels. VEGF may therefore provide a target for tumour vasculature imaging or antibody-directed therapy.

Tie receptor tyrosine kinase

Tie-1 is the protein product of a recently described receptor tyrosine kinase cDNA (62). The Tie-1 receptor tyrosine kinase, and the related receptor Tie-2, possess two extracellular immunoglobulin homology domains, three epidermal growth factor domains and then three fibronectin type II domains closest to the transmembrane domain (62). In humans, *tie* mRNA is abundantly expressed in neovascular endothelial cells of metastatic melanoma cells undergoing tumour angiogenesis. In contrast, very weak Tie signals were obtained from endothelial cells in vessels of normal adult skin (63). The *tie* genes are abundantly expressed in vascular endothelial cells during embryonic development as well as in some megakaryoblastic and erythroleukaemia cell lines in culture (62). In adult mice, enhanced *tie* mRNA expression is found in newly formed capillaries in hormone-induced, maturing ovarian folicles, and in granulation tissue of skin wounds (64).

Brain tumour vascular markers

Several markers are selectively induced in blood vessels in astrocytomas and glioblastoma lesions, including the antigen recognized by the PAL-E antibody (65) and the receptors for VEGF (28) and Platelet-derived growth factor (66). All three antigens are found in normal vasculature outside the brain (65,67,68) suggesting that, in brain tumours, the highly differentiated endothelial cells which make up the normal blood–brain barrier assume the differentiation state of vessels normally found in the periphery. Up-regulation of VEGF receptors occurs in tumour blood vessels giving marked differences between VEGF receptor density on brain tumors versus normal brain tissue.

Clinical applications

Diagnosis

Antibodies that detect endothelial proliferation antigens may be useful in determining the angiogenic status of tumours, which may help in choosing appropriate treatment. Studies in breast (69,70), bladder (71), and cervical carcinomas (72) have revealed that high vessel density or tumour angiogenic activity strongly correlate with risk of metastasis and poor prognosis and so could be used to determine when aggressive postoperative therapy is warranted. Diagnosis in these cases requires laborious enumeration of capillaries stained with pan-endothelial cell markers (69,70) or the use of complex *in vivo* assays

of angiogenesis (71). Both these procedures could be replaced by a simple and fast immunohistochemical staining of tumour sections using antibodies which detect endothelial proliferation antigens, such as endoglin.

Imaging

Tumour vascular selective antibodies should be useful for imaging tumours. Antigens expressed on the luminal surface of tumour vascular endothelial cells are freely accessible to circulating antibody and could give very rapid and intense imaging of tumours, overcoming the problem of poor tumour penetration with anti-tumour cell antibodies. Kennel *et al.* compared the localization of a tumour-specific antibody with an antibody reactive with a marker expressed on the luminal membrane of mouse lung endothelial cells (15). Maximum uptake values of 3.5% of the injected dose per gram (ID/g) were reported in solid tumours by comparison with 276% ID/g in lung endothelium (15). Furthermore, antibody accumulation in solid tumours is slow, with maximum levels being achieved as long as 7 days after anti-tumour cell antibody injection (15) whereas saturation of endothelial-binding sites can be achieved within 1 h of anti-endothelial cell antibody injection (6,15). Therefore, injection of antibody at a concentration slightly lower than that required for antigen saturation would be likely to result in the rapid binding of most of the antibody, leaving little in the circulation. IgM antibodies may be preferable to those of the IgG class because their large size limits extravasation, minimizing background at extravascular sites.

Although the concept of using antibodies against vascular markers for imaging has not been tested *in vivo* for tumours so far, the concept has been demonstrated for the imaging of localized inflammatory tissue using an anti-E-selectin antibody (73).

Therapy

The most exciting application of tumour vasculature-selective antibodies is in the therapy of solid tumours in humans. A key advantage of this approach is that the endothelial cells which line the blood vessels of solid tumours are freely accessible to vascular targeting agents, whereas the majority of tumour cells are inaccessible. Therefore, they are capable of inducing major anti-tumour effects even in large solid tumours. Vascular targeting agents demonstrate powerful anti-tumour effects because there is an in-built amplification mechanism in that the occlusion of each individual capillary leads to the death of thousands of tumour cells which rely on that capillary for deriving their oxygen and nutrients.

We demonstrated in our mouse model that the principle of vascular targeting is valid. We showed that specific killing of tumour vascular endothelial cells by ricin A-chain induces coagulation of tumour blood vessels leading to major tumour regressions (34). The vascular targeting approach is complementary to existing therapies as cytotoxic agents which act on dividing tumour cells at the growing edge of the tumour mass are relatively ineffective against hypoxic tumour cells in the centre of solid tumours. In contrast, vascular targeting agents destroy tumours from the inside-out and may miss the dividing tumour cells on the outside of the tumour which derive their oxygen and nutrients from vasculature which is less affected by the tumour and so may not express the tumour-associated markers.

It is likely that tumour vasculature markers will be expressed on the vasculature of some normal or non-malignant pathological tissues. As ricin A-chain is toxic to both dividing and non-dividing cells, it is critical to assess whether cross-reactivity with endothelium in normal tissues can be tolerated. There are several reasons why some cross-reactivity might be tolerated. First, the level of target antigen expression in normal endothelium may be below a threshold level required to bind sufficient immunoconjugate to initiate endothelial cell killing. Secondly, the internalization route of a given immunotoxin may differ between dividing endothelial cells in tumours and quiescent endothelial cells in normal tissues rendering the latter refractory to the toxic effects of the cytotoxic moiety. This appears to be the case for the anti-endoglin immunotoxin, TEC-11. ricin A-chain. Thirdly, there is little vascular redundancy in solid tumours as tumour cell proliferation and viability are rate-limited by the supply of oxygen and nutrients. Therefore, tumour cell killing may occur under conditions where normal tissues survive. In the event of unacceptable cross-reactivities of anti-tumour vasculature antibodies precluding the use of toxins, short-path radioisotopes or chemotherapeutic drugs, which have selectivity for dividing cells, should be considered to minimize damage to non-dividing normal tissues.

In addition to agents which cause killing of endothelial cells in the tumour vasculature, there are other agents that could have therapeutic activity in solid tumours. We have obtained coagulation of tumour vasculature and major tumour regressions in mice by treating them with a vascular targeting agent containing an engineered form of the human coagulation-inducing protein, tissue factor (74). Alternatively, cytokines or chemokines targeted to the surface of tumour endothelial cells could increase leucocyte adhesion and extravasation selectively at the tumour site, which is at present inefficient and limits the efficacy of cellular immunotherapeutic strategies. Endothelial cells are amenable to genetic modification in situ, so it may be possible to use antibodies to target DNA to tumour endothelial cells and confer pro-inflammatory, immunoregulatory, or tumour growth regulatory activities upon them.

Summary and conclusions

An attractive strategy for the therapy of solid tumours would be to target cytotoxic agents or host effectors to the endothelial cells of the tumour vasculature rather than to the tumour cells themselves. The key advantage of this approach is that endothelial cells are freely accessible to intravenously injected antibody conjugates whereas the tumour cells are, for the most part, inaccessible. Also, endothelial cells are similar in different tumours, making it feasible to develop a single reagent for treating numerous types of cancer.

We have demonstrated the vascular targeting approach to be valid in a mouse model in which class II antigens of the major histocompatibility complex were experimentally induced selectively on the tumour vascular endothelial cells. Targeting of ricin A-chain to class II-expressing tumour endothelial cells caused denudation of the tumour endothelial lining (34). Once exposed to the underlying basal lamina, coagulation factors and platelets lead to the formation of an occlusive thrombus, depriving the tumour cells of their oxygen and nutrients, and eventually leading to tumour cell death.

In order to apply the approach to humans, antibodies are needed that selectively recognize human tumour vasculature. The field of vascular targeting is relatively young and although no monoclonal antibodies have been found which show complete tumour endothelial cell specificity some preferentially recognize endothelial cells within tumours compared with endothelial cells in normal tissue. One such antibody, raised in this laboratory, is TEC-11, which recognizes endoglin (41). Endoglin is an endothelial cell proliferation marker that is up-regulated on endothelial cells in miscellaneous human solid tumours. TEC-11 could be useful for the diagnosis and therapy of human cancer. First, it might be used to distinguish between histologically indistinct benign and malignant lesions to determine when aggressive postoperative therapy is appropriate. Secondly, TEC-11 might be useful for imaging tumours in cancer patients. Thirdly, the antibody might be useful for targeting a cytotoxic agent to the tumour vasculature. Endoglin is present at moderately high levels on the vascular endothelium in certain vital normal tissues and so the cytotoxic agent used should not be damaging to the quiescent endothelium at those sites.

Short-path radioisotopes or DNA-synthesis inhibitors might not damage quiescent endothelium in normal tissues, yet destroy the tumour vascular bed when delivered to the dividing tumour endothelium. Ricin A-chain might also be used since TEC-11.ricin A chain was potently toxic to dividing endothelial cells but non-toxic to quiescent endothelial cells.

Acknowledgement

We would like to thank Karen Schiller for preparing the manuscript.

References

1. Lowder, J. N., Meeker, T. C., Campbell, M., Garcia, C. F., Gralow, J., Miller, R. A., *et al.* (1987). Studies on B lymphoid tumors treated with monoclonal anti-idiotype antibodies: Correlation with clinical responses. *Blood*, **69**, 199–210.
2. Vitetta, E. S., Stone, M., Amlot, P., Fay, J., May, R., Till, M., *et al.* (1991). A Phase I immunotoxin trial in patients with B cell lymphoma. *Cancer Res.*, **15**, 4052–8.
3. Shockley, T. R., Lin, K., Nagy, J. A., Tompkins, R. G., Dvorak, H. F., and Yarmush, M. L. (1991). Penetration of tumor tissue by antibodies and other immunoproteins. *Ann. N. Y. Acad. Sci.*, **617**, 367–82.
4. Byers, V. S. and Baldwin, R. W. (1988). Therapeutic strategies with monoclonal antibodies and immunoconjugates. *Immunology*, **65**, 329–35.
5. Vaickus, L. and Foon, K. A. (1991). Overview of monoclonal antibodies in the diagnosis and therapy of cancer. *Cancer Invest.*, **9**, 195–209.
6. Burrows, F. J., Watanabe, Y., and Thorpe, P. E. (1992). A murine model for antibody-directed targeting of vascular endothelial cells in solid tumors. *Cancer Res.*, **52**, 5954–62.
7. Dvorak, H. F., Nagy, J. A., and Dvorak, A. M. (1991). Structure of solid tumors and their vasculature: implications for therapy with monoclonal antibodies. *Cancer Cells*, **3**, 77–85.
8. Baxter, L. T. and Jain, R. K. (1991). Transport of fluid and macromolecules in tumors. *Microcirc. Res.*, **41**, 5–23.
9. Sands, H. (1988). Radioimmunoconjugates: an overview of problems and promises. *Antibody Immunoconj. Radiopharm.*, **1**, 213–26.
10. Epenetos, A. A., Snook, D., Durbin, H., Johnson, P. M., and Taylor-Papadimitriou, J. (1986). Limitations of radiolabeled monoclonal antibodies for localization of human neoplasms. *Cancer Res.*, **46**, 3183–91.
11. Jain, R. K. (1994). Barriers to drug delivery in solid tumors. *Sci. Am.*, **271**, 58–65.
12. Juweid, M., Neumann, R., Paik, C., Perez-Bacete, M. J., Sato, J., van Osdol, W., and Weinstein, J. N. (1992). Micropharmacology of monoclonal antibodies in solid tumors; direct experimental evidence for a binding site barrier. *Cancer Res.*, **52**, 5144–53.
13. Denekamp, J. (1984). Vasculature as a target for tumour therapy. *Prog. Appl. Microcirc.*, **4**, 28–38.
14. Jaffe, E. A. (1984). *Biology of endothelial cells*. Martinus Nijhoff, Boston.
15. Kennel, S. J., Falcioni, R., and Wesley, J. W. (1991). Microdistribution of specific rat monoclonal antibodies to mouse tissues and human tumor xenografts. *Cancer Res.*, **51**, 1529–36.
16. Denekamp, J. (1990). Vascular attack as a therapeutic strategy for cancer. *Cancer Metastasis Rev.*, **9**, 267–82.
17. Jain, R. K. (1988). Determinants of tumour blood flow: a review. *Cancer Res.*, **48**, 2641–58.
18. Folkman, J. and Klagsbrun, M. (1987). Angiogenic factors. *Science*, **235**, 442–6.
19. Folkman, J. (1985). Angiogenesis and its inhibitors. In *Important advances in oncology*, Part I. (ed. V. T. DeVita, S. Hellman, and S. A. Rosenberg), pp. 42–62. J. B. Lippincott, Philadelphia.
20. Folkman, J. (1985). Tumor angiogenesis. *Adv. Cancer Res.*, **43**, 175–230.
21. Gospodarowicz, D., Greenburg, G., Vlodavsky, I., Alvarado, J., and Johnson, L. K. (1979). The identification and localization of fibronectin in cultured corneal endothelial cells: cell surface polarity and physiological implications. *Exp. Eye Res.*, **29**, 485–509.
22. Hobson, B. and Denekamp, J. (1984). Endothelial proliferation in tumours and normal tissues: continuous labelling studies. *Br. J Cancer*, **49**, 405–13.
23. Arnold, F. and West, D. C. (1991). Angiogenesis in wound healing. *Pharmacol. Ther.*, **52**, 407–22.
24. Brown, R. A. and Weiss, J. B. (1988). Neovascularization and its role in the osteoarthritic process. *Ann. Rheum. Dis.*, **47**, 881–5.
25. Kahlon, R., Shapero, J., and Gotlieb, A. I. (1992). Angiogenesis in atherosclerosis. *Can. J. Cardiol.*, **8**, 60–4.
26. Gartner, S. and Henkind, P. (1978). Neovascularization of the iris (rubeosis iridis). *Surv. Ophthalmol.*, **22**, 291–312.
27. Folkman, J. and Brem, H. (1992). Angiogenesis and inflammation. In *Inflammation: basic principles and clinical correlates*, 2nd edn (ed. J. I. Gallin, I. M. Goldstein, and R. Synderman), pp. 821–39. Raven Press, New York.
28. Dvorak, H. F., Sioussat, T. M., Brown, L. F., Berse, B., Nagy, J. A., Sotrel, A., *et al.* (1991). Distribution of vascular permeability factor (vascular endothelial growth factor) in tumors — concentration in tumor blood vessels. *J. Exp. Med.*, **174**, 1275–8.
29. Sack, G. M., Levin, J., and Bell, W. R. (1977). Trousseau's syndrome and other manifestations of chronic disseminated coagulopathy in patients with neoplasms: clinical, pathophysiologic and therapeutic features. *Medicine*, **56**, 1–37.
30. Connolly, D. T. (1991). Vascular permeability factor: A unique regulator of blood vessel function. *J. Cell. Biochem.*, **47**, 219–23.
31. Burrows, F. J., Haskard, D. O., Hart, I. R., Marshall, J. F., Selkirk, S., Poole, S., and Thorpe, P. E. (1991). Influence of tumor-derived interleukin-1 on melanoma–endothelial cell interactions *in vitro. Cancer Res.*, **51**, 4768–75.
32. Murray, J. C., Clauss, M., Thurston, G., and Stern, D. (1991). Tumour-derived factors which induce endothelial tissue factor and enhance the procoagulant response to TNF. *Int. J. Radiat. Biol.*, **60**, 273–7.
33. Nawroth, P. P., Bank, I., Handley, D., Cassimeris, J., Chess, L., and Stern, D. (1986). Tumor necrosis factor/cachectin interacts with endothelial cell receptors to induce release of interleukin 1. *J. Exp. Med.*, **163**, 1363–75.

34. Burrows, F. J. and Thorpe, P. E. (1993). Eradication of large solid tumors in mice with an immunotoxin directed against tumor vasculature. *Proc. Natl Acad. Sci. USA*, **90**, 8996–9600.

35. Vitetta, E. S., Thorpe, P. E., and Uhr, J. W. (1993). Immunotoxins: magic bullets or misguided missiles. *Immunol. Today*, **14**, 148–54.

36. Fulcher, S., Lui, G. M., Houston, L. L., Ramakrishnan, S., Burris, T., Polansky, J., and Alvarado, J. (1988). Use of immunotoxin to inhibit proliferating human corneal endothelium. *Invest. Ophthalmol. Visual Sci.*, **29**, 755–9.

37. Wilkerson, M., Fulcher, S., Shields, M. B., Foulks, G. N., Hatchell, D. L., and Houston, L. L. (1992). Inhibition of human subconjunctival fibroblast proliferation by immunotoxin. *Invest. Ophthalmol. Visual Sci.*, **33**, 2293–8.

38. Fulcher, S., Lui, G., Houston, L. L., Ramakrishnan, S., Burris, T., Polansky, J., and Alvarado, J. (1992). Inhibition of human corneal epithelium with immunotoxin 454A12-rRA. *Cornea*, **11**, 413–17.

39. Jaffe, G. J., Earnest, K., Fulcher, S., Lui, G. M., and Houston, L. L. (1990). Antitransferrin receptor immunotoxin inhibits proliferating human retinal pigment epithelial cells. *Arch. Ophthalmol.*, **108**, 1163–8.

40. Davis, A. A., Whidby, D. E., Privette, T., Houston, L. L., and Hunt, R. C. (1990). Selective inhibition of growing pigment epithelial cells by a receptor-directed immunotoxin. *Invest. Ophthalmol. Visual Sci.*, **31**, 2514–2519.

41. Burrows, F. J., Derbyshire, E. J., Tazzari, P. L., Amlot, P.., Gazdar, A. F., King, S. W., *et al.* (1995). Endoglin is an endothelial cell proliferation marker that is upregulated in tumor vasculature. *Clin. Cancer Res.*, **1**, 1623–34.

42. Cheifetz, S., Bellon, T., Cales, C., Vera, S., Bernabeu, C., Massague, J., and Letarte, M. (1992). Endoglin is a component of the transforming growth factor-beta receptor system in human endothelial cells. *J. Biol. Chem.*, **267**, 19027–30.

43. Gougos, A. and Letarte, M. (1990). Primary structure of endoglin an RGD-containing glycoprotein of human endothelial cells. *J. Biol. Chem.*, **265**, 8361–4.

44. Gougos, A. and Letarte, M. (1988). Identification of a human endothelial cell antigen with monoclonal antibody 44G4 produced against a pre-B leukemic cell line. *J. Immunol.*, **141**, 1925–33.

45. Gougos, A., St Jacques, S., Greaves, A., O'Connell, P. J., d'Apice, A. J. F., Buhring, H. J., *et al.* (1992). Identification of distinct epitopes of endoglin an RGD-containing glycoprotein of endothelial cells, leukemic cells and syncitiotrophoblasts. *Int. Immunol*, **4**, 83–92.

46. O'Connell, P. J., McKenzie, A., Fisicaro, N., Rockman, S. P., Pearse, M. J., and d'Apice, A. J. F. (1992). Endoglin: a 180-kD endothelial cell and macrophage restricted differentiation molecule. *Clin Exp. Immunol*, **90**, 154–9.

47. Buhring, H. J., Muller, C. A., Letarte, M., Gougos, A., Saalmuller, A., van Agthoven, A. J., and Busch, F. W. (1991). Endoglin is expressed on a subpopulation of immature erythroid cells or normal bone marrow. *Leukemia*, **5**, 841–7.

48. Westphal, J. R., Willems, H. W., Schalkwijk, C. J., Ruiter, D. J., and deWaal, R. M. (1993). A new 180-kDa dermal endothelial cell activation antigen: *in vitro* and *in situ* characteristics. *J. Invest. Dermatol.*, **100**, 27–34.

49. Denekamp, J. and Hobson, B. (1982). Endothelial cell proliferation in experimental tumours. *Br. J. Cancer*, **461**, 711–20.

50. Hagemeier, H. H., Vollmer, E., Goerdt, S., Schulze-Osthoff, K., and Sorg, C. (1986). A monoclonal antibody reacting with endothelial cells of budding vessels in tumours and inflammatory tissues and non-reactive with normal adult tissues. *Int. J. Cancer*, **38**, 481–8.

51. Rettig, W. J., Garinchesa, P., Healey, J. H., Su, S. L., Jaffe, E. A., and Old, L. J. (1992). Identification of endosialin, a cell surface glycoprotein of vascular endothelial cells in human cancer. *Proc. Natl Acad. Sci. USA*, **89**, 10832–6.

52. Wang, J. M., Kumar, S., Pye, D., Vanagthoven, A. J., Krupinski, J., and Hunter, R. D. (1993). A monoclonal antibody detect heterogeneity in vascular endothelium of tumours and normal tissues. *Int. J. Cancer*, **54**, 363–70.

53. Letarte, M., Greaves, A., and Vera, S. (1995). CD105 (endoglin) cluster report. In *Leukocyte typing V: white cell differentiation antigens* (ed. S. F. Schlossman, L. Boumsell, W. Gilks, J. Harlan, T. Kishimoto, C. Morimoto, *et al.*, pp. 1756–9. Oxford University Press, Oxford.

54. Carnemolla, B., Balza, E., Siri, A., Zardi, L., Nicotra, M. R., Bigotti, A., and Natali, P. G. (1989). A tumor-associated fibronectin isoform generated by alternative splicing of messenger RNA precursors. *J. Cell Biol.*, **108**, 1139–48.

55. Castellani, P., Viale, G., Dorcaratto, A., Nicolo, G., Kaczmarek, J., Querze, G., and Zardi, L. (1994). The fibronectin isoform containing the ED-B oncofetal domain: a marker of angiogenesis. *Int. J. Cancer*, **59**, 612–18.

56. Bruland, O. S., Fodstad, O., Stenwig, A. E., and Pihl, A. (1988). Expression and characteristics of a novel human osteosarcoma-associated cell surface antigen. *Cancer Res.*, **48**, 5302–9.

57. Brooks, P. C., Clark, R. A., and Cheresh, D. A. (1994). Requirement of vascular integrin $\alpha_v\beta_3$ for angiogenesis. *Science*, **264**, 569–71.

58. Brooks, P. C., Montgomery, A. M. P., Rosenfeld, M., Reisfeld, R. A., Hu, T., Klier, G., and Cheresh, D. A. (1994). Integrin $\alpha_v\beta_3$ antagonists promote tumor regression by inducing apoptosis of angiogenic blood vessels. *Cell*, **79**, 1157–64.

59. Thorpe, P. E., Wallace, P. M., Knyba, R. E., Watson, G. J., Mahadevan, V. A., Land, H., *et al.* (1985). Selective killing of proliferating vascular endothelial cells by an anti-fibronectin receptor immunotoxin. *Int. J. Radiat. Biol.*, **60**, 24A.

60. Shweiki, D., Itin, A., Soffer, D., and Keshet, E. (1992). Vascular endothelial growth factor induced by hypoxia may mediate hypoxia-initiated angiogenesis. *Nature*, **359**, 843–5.

61. Senger, D. R., Vandewater, L., Brown, L. F., Nagy, J. A., Yeo, K-T., Yeo, T-K., *et al.* (1993). Vascular permeability factor (VPF, VEGF) in tumor biology. *Cancer Metastasis Rev.*, **12**, 303–24.

62. Partanen, J., Armstrong, E., Makela, T. P., Korhonen, J., Sandberg, M., Renkonen, R., *et al.* (1992). A novel endothelial cell surface receptor tyrosine kinase with extracellular epidermal growth factor homology domains. *Mol. Cell. Biol.*, **12**, 1698–707.

63. Kaipainen, A., Vlaykova, T., Hatva, E., Bohling, T., Jekunen, A., Pyrhonen, S., and Alitalo, K. (1994). Enhanced expression of the tie receptor tyrosine kinase messenger RNA in the vascular endothelium metastatic melanomas. *Cancer Res.*, **54**, 6571–7.

64. Korhonen, J., Partanen, J., Armstrong, E., Vaahtokari, A., Elenius, K., Jalkanen, M., and Alitalo, K. (1992). Enhanced expression of the tie receptor kinase in endothelial cells during neovascularization. *Blood*, **80**, 2548–55.

65. Schlingemann, R. O., Dingjan, G. M., Emeis, J. J., Block, J., Warnaar, S. O., and Ruiter, D. J. (1985). Monoclonal antibody PAL-E specific for endothelium. *Lab. Invest.*, **52**, 71–6.

66. Plate, K. H., Breier, G., Farrell, C. L., and Risau, W. (1992). Platelet-derived growth factor receptor-beta is induced during tumor development and upregulated during tumor progression in endothelial cells in human gliomas. *Lab. Invest.*, **67**, 529–34.

67. Franklin, W. A., Christison, W. H., Colley, M., Montag, A. G., Stephens, J. K., and Hart, C. E. (1990). *In situ* distribution of the alpha-subunit of platelet-derived growth factor receptor in nonneoplastic tissue and in soft tissue tumors. *Cancer Res.*, **50**, 6344–8.

68. Jakeman, L. B., Winer, J., Bennett, G. L., Altar, A., and Ferrara, N. (1992). Binding sites for vascular endothelial growth factor are localized on endothelial cells in adult rat tissues. *J. Clin. Invest.*, **89**, 244–53.

69. Weidner, N., Folkman, J., Pozza, F., Bevilacqua, P., Allred, E. N., Moore, D. H., *et al.* (1992). Tumor angiogenesis — a new significant and independent prognostic indicator in early-stage breast carcinoma. *J. Natl Cancer Inst.*, **84**, 1875–87.

70. Horak, E. R., Leek, R., Klenk, N., Lejeune, S., Smith, K., Stuart, N., *et al.* (1992). Angiogenesis, assessed by platelet endothelial cell adhesion molecule antibodies, as indicator of node metastases and survival in breast cancer. *Lancet*, **340**, 1120–4.

71. Chodak, G. W., Haudenschild, C., Gittes, R. F., and Folkman, J. (1980). Angiogenic activity as a marker of neoplastic and preneoplastic lesions of the human bladder. *Ann. Surg.*, **192**, 762–71.

72. Sillman, F., Boyce, J., and Fruchter, R. (1981). The significance of atypical vessels and neovascularization in cervical neoplasia. *Am. J. Obstet. Gynecol.*, **139**, 154–9.

73. Keelan, E. T. M., Harrison, A. A., Chapman, P. T., Binns, R. M., Peters, A. M., and Haskard, D. O. (1994). Imaging vascular endothelial activation — an approach using radio-labeled monoclonal antibodies against the endothelial cell adhesion molecule e-selectin. *J. Nucl. Med.*, **35**, 276–81.

74. Huang, X., Molema, G., King, S., Watkins, L., Edgington, T. S., and Thorpe, P. E. (1997). Tumor infarction in mice by antibody-directed targeting of tissue factor to tumor vasculature. *Science* (in press).

27. Vascular targeting of anti-cancer gene therapy

Rhys T. Jaggar and Roy Bicknell

Introduction

In anti-cancer gene therapy we have the opportunity to be destructive rather than correctional and for this reason anti-cancer studies are likely to comprise a major area of gene therapy research in the near future. Nevertheless, there are many problems to be surmounted. Foremost among these is that of delivery of the gene to the cell in which function of the gene product is required. The cells of the vascular endothelium are some of the most accessible in the body, comprising a single monolayer which are all in intimate contact with the blood. This makes vascular targeting of gene delivery systems a particularly appealing strategy.

Approaches to vascular targeting as an anti-cancer strategy have attempted to exploit differences between tumour and normal vasculature in order to target therapies to a tumour (1,2). It has been shown by others to be an effective anti-tumour strategy in animal models (3; and Chapter 26). Vascular targeting should be distinguished from the inhibition of angiogenesis, as the former aims to destroy the tumour vasculature directly via a variety of cytotoxic agents, whereas the latter involves inhibition of endothelial migration and proliferation.

In this article, we aim to identify potentially useful toxic gene products, discuss the advantages and limitations of the delivery systems for DNA encoding such gene products, and consider the usage of such targeting agents in combination with other techniques of cancer therapy.

Destructive approaches

One of the major considerations in any gene therapy research programme is the nature of the gene to be delivered. Toxicity for proliferating endothelium is a desirable characteristic of a vascular targeting approach to anti-cancer gene therapy.

Tumour necrosis factor alpha

One molecule which displays such a characteristic is tumour necrosis factor (TNF) α. TNF-α, also termed cachectin, was originally identified as a molecule produced by activated macrophages, which eradicates the methA sarcoma very efficiently from mice by the induction of haemorrhagic necrosis after caudal vein administration of recombinant human TNF-α to tumour-bearing animals (4). It is a 17 kDa homotrimeric polypeptide, which is secreted from cells after cleavage of a plasma membrane-associated 26 kDa propolypeptide. TNF-α is toxic to proliferating, but not quiescent, microvascular endothelial cells *in vitro* (5,6). This cytotoxicity may be due to induction of apoptosis (7). Paradoxically, low doses of TNF-α stimulate angiogenesis in several angiogenesis assays, including the rat and rabbit corneas (8,9).

A more detailed study has indicated that TNF-α stimulates angiogenesis at low concentration, while inhibiting the process at high concentrations (Chapter 14). Whether such anomalous results arise from using recombinant TNF-α across species is unclear, indicating that it may be difficult to perform relevant animal experiments using human TNF-α gene therapies prior to use in human clinical trials.

Local administration of high doses of purified TNF-α protein by isolated limb perfusion elicts rapid necrosis of metastasized melanoma when used in combination with interferon γ and melphalan. This has permitted the salvage of limbs of patients with unrespectable soft tissue tumours (10).

Interestingly, when a human adenocarcinoma was xenografted into nude mice, tumour growth could be reduced when the animals were treated by intravenous administration of group B *Streptococcus* B toxin (GBS toxin) (11). The tumours in treated animals showed evidence of haemorrhagic necrosis. GBS toxin has been shown to bind to the tumour vasculature. The treatment induces TNF-α within 1 h *in vivo*, which suggests, but does not prove, that TNF-α is a mediator of the vascular destruction induced by GBS toxin.

Unfortunately, systemic delivery of TNF-α for treatment of human cancer is not an option due to toxic shock or severe cachexia/weight loss (hence the term cachectin). Thus for the treatment of metastases or non-accessible primary tumours, gene therapy by delivery of TNF-α expression vectors to either tumours cells or tumour endothelium is an attractive strategy. Due to the toxic nature of the protein, it will be necessary to incorporate inducible or regulatory elements, possibly at the transcriptional level, so that strict control is placed upon TNF-α expression in human patients.

Pro-drug activating systems

An alternative to TNF-α is targeting of pro-drug activating enzymes to the vasculature. The two best known systems of pro-drug activating enzymes are herpes simplex virus thymidine kinase (HSV tk) activating ganciclovir (12) and *Escherichia coli* cytosine deaminase (CD) which converts 5-fluorocytosine to 5-fluorouracil (13). These are particularly attractive for systemic delivery, as toxic side-effects may be reversed upon withdrawal of pro-drug. Such systems have been shown to eradicate tumour cell lines transfected with the pro-drug activating gene (14) and to have an anti-tumour effect when the gene is delivered via retroviral vectors to tumours *in vivo* (15).

Such destructive methods are said to demonstrate a 'by-stander effect', in that expression of the gene in a subset of cells leads to destruction of many adjacent cells not expressing the gene (16). The mechanism of action is a combination of intercell drug transfer (termed metabolic cooperation) via tight junctions, gap junctions, and immunological activation (see reference 17 for a discussion of this phenomenon).

As yet, no detailed experiments have been carried out which compare the efficacy of different therapeutic genes using identical delivery systems in tumour models. It is thus not yet clear whether any one of the systems being put forward will actually be more efficacious than others in therapeutic applications.

Dosage requirements

Although pharmacology has, until recently, been a neglected aspect of the gene therapy research effort, it is important to consider at the outset what doses might be required using a given route of administration for a succesful therapy, and whether such doses can be achieved using available technology.

If one assumes that an average adult is 70 kg, there will be 10^{13}–10^{14} cells in the body for an average cell of 10 μm diameter. If one assumes that approximately 1% of these cells are endothelial cells, then there will be 10^{11}–10^{12} endothelial cells in the body. For a tumour of 1–10 cm^3 there will be 10^9–10^{10} tumour cells and therefore 10^7–10^8 non-neoplastic endothelial cells within the tumour.

Two important points are apparent from this analysis: first, that tumour endothelial cells are outnumbered approximately 1000 times by normal endothelium; and secondly, that for a dose of one drug molecule/tumour endothelial cell, a minimum of 10^7 molecules would be required, even assuming a completely tumour-specific delivery and a 100% efficiency of delivery. In the short term, there appears to be no method available which will achieve completely selective delivery to tumour endothelium; it is thus likely that doses well in excess of 10^7

Table 27.1. Comparison of current production capabilities for different gene therapy delivery systems. This table shows a comparison of the current position (mid-1995). However, in a rapidly moving field, it may already be out of date when this edition appears. Estimation of cost is not included for this production.

Delivery system	Current manufacturing capability	Number of copies of gene
Naked plasmid DNA/liposome encapsidated DNA/DNA linked to ligands	10 mg to 10 g DNA from one bacterial production run in 2–500 ml sterile saline solution	10^{14}–10^{17}, dividable into suitable aliquots for therapy
Conventional retrovirus	10^9–10^{11} virus particles in several litres of culture medium	10^6–10^7 per ml of supernatant
VSV G pseudotyped retrovirus	10^9–10^{11} virus particles in several ml of culture medium	10^8–10^9 per ml of supernatant
Retroviruses grown in capillary bed production units	10^9–10^{11} virus particles in several hundred ml of culture medium	10^7–10^8 per ml of supernatant
Adenovirus	10^{12}–10^{15} virus particles in 1–1000 ml	10^{11}–10^{12} per ml of virus preparation
Adeno-associated virus	10^{10}–10^{14} virus particles in 1–1000 ml	10^{10}–10^{11} per ml of virus preparation

molecules will be required, due to non-specific delivery to normal endothelium and blood cells and due to the clearance of the therapeutic agent from the blood. Most conservative estimates indicate that approximately 10^{11}–10^{13} copies of an untargeted therapeutic gene may well be required for a useful clinical dose in humans, although actual experience in trials may modify this figure. Table 27.1 shows easily achievable doses using current expression systems. Further discussion of the implications of these figures are to be found in the next section.

Animal models

With the currently available viral titres it should be feasible to examine the efficacy of viral targeting in tumour models that are perfused by a single vessel. Thus, following similar arguments to those above, if 1% of the cells in a mouse are endothelium this will be about 10^9 cells. In a moderately sized xenografted tumour there will be about 10^7 endothelial cells and delivery of 10^8–10^9 virions should achieve effective viral transduction. Several models have been developed that result in tumours that are perfused by a single vessel, *e.g.* growth of tumour after implantation in the ovary.

Methods of delivery and current limitations

Seven major methods of DNA delivery are being evaluated for gene therapy at present. These are:

(1)   naked plasmid DNA;

(2)   plasmid DNA encapsidated within liposomes;

(3)   DNA electrostatically linked to molecules such as growth factors or transferrin;

(4)   retroviral particles;

(5)   adenoviral particles; (AAV)

(6)   adeno-associated viral (AAV) particles;

(7)   herpesvirus particles.

(Other methods such as the use of Sendai virus, Vaccinia virus, and microprojectiles are also being considered and doubtless, vectors based on novel viruses will continue to be developed.) Herpesvirus vectors have been studied with particular emphasis to the brain, and will not be further discussed here, despite their great potential for many gene therapy applications. Of the remaining six, each method has advantages, each has limitations. This section will examine the progress made with each delivery system

toward the goal of gene therapy in general; the following section will consider their usefulness for vascular targeting and indicate the areas where progress must be made before clinically useful reagents will become available.

Naked plasmid DNA or DNA encapsidated within liposomes

The delivery of genes using simple plasmid DNA, perhaps within liposomes, has many theoretical attractions.

1. Preparation of such DNA in large quantities is technically simple and validation procedures for high-grade pharmaceutical production are relatively inexpensive (T. Seddon, ICRF Production Unit, personal communication) (18).

2. The transcription regulatory signals controlling expression of the therapeutic gene may be analysed accurately in tissue culture and animal model systems prior to human clinical trials, without the possible complications of enhancer elements found in viral delivery systems.

3. Production of a large number of plasmid constructs is relatively simple, as is screening of such constructs in tissue culture or animal model systems for the most efficacious candidate plasmid.

4. Large numbers of lipid formulations may be analysed rapidly for the optimization of the delivery vehicle.

5. Possible health hazards appear, at least at present, to pose fewer problems than those of viral vectors for use in the treatment of humans.

Following a number of demonstrations in animal models of effective gene expression after direct injection of DNA into tumours (19,20), clinical trials using direct injection of liposome-encapsidated DNA have now been undertaken in the USA for the treatment of cutaneous melanoma (21) and approval has been granted in the UK for a trial co-ordinated by the ICRF in Oxford for direct intratumoral injection of naked DNA into melanomas (A. L. Harris, personal communication).

The lipid used in the US study is a formulation termed DCChol/DOPE, originally characterized by Gao and Huang (22). This is a cationic liposome with greater stability than other cationic formulations, which fuses very efficiently with the plasma membranes of cells. It may therefore be of use for local administration or for inhalation by cystic fibrosis patients (23) (clinical trials are currently underway in the US and UK), but is likely to be of less use for systemic delivery, as its half life in the blood is very short, due to uptake by cells of the spleen.

An improved formulation, DIMRE/DOPE, which fa-cilitates more efficient gene transfer than DCChol *in vitro* and leads to more effective anti-tumour effects when delivering the (foreign) H-2K^d allele of the major histo-compatibility complex (MHC), has also recently been sub-jected to toxicity studies in animals with no harmful side-effects (24). This formulation is now ready to be used in the near future in clinical trials.

A third cationic lipid formulation, DOTMA/DOPE has been reported to allow effective delivery to a variety of tissues, following intravenous delivery (25), but this for-mulation has not yet been developed further for clinical work.

Other anionic formulations, such as the 'stealth' lipo-somes (26) have been specifically engineered to increase their circulation time in the blood. Encapsidation of drugs such as doxorubicin into these liposomes has led to a more effective anti-tumour effect than with drug alone or drug encapsidated in conventional cationic liposome formula-tions (27). No reports of gene delivery using this com-pound, however, have yet appeared in the literature, suggesting that fusion of such liposomes to cell mem-branes may not be as efficient as the cationic formulations.

Several companies in the USA are actively searching for improved lipid formulations and these may be available at the time of printing.

The biggest challenge to systemic delivery by this method involves the targeting of gene expression to specific tissues. A recent survey of liposome formulations has indicated that preferential targeting to either lung or liver following systemic delivery is achievable (28) with specific lipid mixtures, which may be of great utility in the targeting of tumour metastases. However, these data are yet to be published or confirmed.

Another possible method of targeting involves the incorporation of antibodies which recognize tissue- or tumour-specific cell-surface antigens. Using radioactive indium, Holmberg *et al.* (29) have demonstrated that lipo-somes containing an antibody which recognizes pul-monary endothelium (34A), localize efficiently to the lung. However, as yet, no successful delivery of a gene using such 'immunoliposomes' has been reported, so it is unclear whether effective uptake of DNA is yet possible by such a method.

One of the biggest favourable attributes for the liposome strategy is the relative lack of immunogenicity of either DNA or the liposomes themselves, hence the optimism over its use for long-term replacement strategies such as cystic fibrosis treatment. Of great interest for clinicians is the observation that liposome-mediated gene transfer is stimulated by prior exposure of tumour cells in culture to the chemotherapeutic agent cis-platin (30), an observation

confirmed by a response in a patient in a clinical trial who had been treated with cis-platin prior to liposome-mediated gene transfer (31). Whether the incorporation of proteins for tissue-specific targeting will result in an adverse immune response is a key question.

It appears at present that balancing favourable phar-macokinetic properties of liposomes with effective fusion to target tissues and subsequent gene expression following systemic delivery is not particularly easy to achieve. For further progress using this approach, it may well be necessary to:

(1) use targeting molecules which stimulate subsequent endocytosis of the liposome following binding to target tissues,

(2) to incorporate methods for preventing DNA degrada-tion in endosomes after fusion to target cells.

DNA physically linked to biological ligands

The linking of DNA to ligands which bind to cell-surface receptors is an attractive approach to gene therapy. Ligands might be growth factors, single-chain antibodies or molecules such as the iron-binding protein transferrin. The main aim is to target DNA to specific cell types using the conjugating ligand. However, the approach must satisfy the following requirements:

(1) ligand-receptor binding must lead to subsequent endocytosis, thus limiting the number of potentially useful systems;

(2) destruction of the complex in the endosome following endocytosis must be avoided;

(3) transport of the DNA from the cytoplasm to the nucleus must occur, unless specific systems which allow cytoplasmic transcription (such as Vaccinia or Sindbis virus) are incorporated into the delivery vehicle

Two systems which satisfy these criteria are now de-scribed.

Transferrinfection

Development of varieties of the so-called 'transferr-infection' protocol has to date been quite successful; this originally involved the conjugation of DNA to the iron-binding molecule transferrin via a poly-lysine or pro-tamine adaptor (32,33). The efficiency of gene expression in tissue culture cells was augmented up to 2000-fold by the addition of a replication-incompetent adenovirus, that possesses mechanisms which disrupt endosome function

(34). The method has been generalized by linking DNA directly to adenovirus particles via a polylysine–streptavidin–biotin complex, or by the use of antibodies to a mutagenized epitope of the adenoviral hexon structural protein (35).

In order to develop tissue-specific targeting using this method, an antibody to the adenoviral fibre protein, which inhibits virus-receptor-mediated entry, has been isolated. When this antibody was added to poly-lysine-linked adenovirus, and the virus-antibody combination was conjugated to transferrin–DNA complexes, no effect on subsequent gene expression was observed, indicating that uptake via the transferrin receptor pathway is unaffected. To date, this system has not yet incorporated a tissue-specific receptor.

Transferrinfection has been used succesfully with large DNA molecules, which is perhaps useful in the gene replacement strategies for some inherited disorders where large genes or intronic sequences may be required (36).

To date, protracted expression in tissue culture cells of a gene product has not been demonstrated following this method of delivery, although generation of stable transfectants producing recombinant retroviruses has been reported recently (37). Furthermore, transfection of primary fibroblasts with factor VIII followed by implantation into mice allowed expression for only 24–48 h (38). The sustained expression of genes both *in vitro* and *in vivo* thus represents a major challenge in the development of this area of research.

It is unclear as yet what the reason for this loss of expression is. It may be associated with cellular responses to infection, whereby mechanisms may exist within cells for the rapid transcriptional down-regulation of any DNA which enters cells. Whether the adenoviruses have also acquired mechanisms to counter such a response, is as yet unclear. Alternatively, it may be that necessary transcriptional control sequences are not present in the particular constructs used. Therefore, further basic research may be necessary to allow such an approach to lead to long-term gene expression, although it is not clear yet whether this will be a problem for anti-cancer gene therapy.

Asialoglycoprotein-linked delivery to liver

In 1987, Wu and Wu (39) showed that coupling of DNA to an asialoglycoprotein (one which carries a galactose sugar as the terminal sugar moiety) via a poly-lysine molecule allowed efficient delivery of DNA to hepatocytes and subsequent expression of the reporter gene chloramphenicol acetyltransferase (CAT) in experimental rats. In further studies, they showed that the use of a liver-specific promoter, that of mouse albumin, allowed expression of CAT for 72 h post-treatment, and for at least 11 weeks if rats were subjected to partial hepatectomy prior to treatment (40). A similar result was obtained when delivering the human albumin gene to rats or the low-density lipoprotein (LDL) receptor to Watanabe rabbits using albumin promoters (41,42). Interestingly, DNA was retained without replicating or integrating into the host chromosome (43).

A recent study has indicated that the formulation of the DNA/poly-lysine conjugate may have an effect on the persistence of transgene expression (44). Using high ratios of DNA/poly-lysine (100:1 to 100:4), expression is limited to 2 or 3 days, in the absence of partial hepatectomy. However, using ratios of DNA/poly-lysine of 1:1, expression is increased to up to 140 days without partial hepatectomy. It is proposed that such increases result from improved efficiency of nuclear transport as the nuclear localization sequences are usually runs of five to six basic amino acids such as lysine) and increased resistance to degradation.

As yet, however, no physiological levels of liver-specific proteins have been delivered. This may be due to the design of the expression vectors, lacking sequences required for long-term, high-level expression in hepatocytes, or it may reflect a low efficiency of gene transduction.

These two methods of delivery have a number of theoretical advantages:

(1) the conjugation processes appear to be technically simple and are amenable to large-scale screening for optimal formulations for individual applications;

(2) there is no apparent size limitation to DNA size, unlike the viral transduction systems;

(3) the various means for targeting (cell-surface receptors for the ligand and transcriptional control signals within the therapeutic plasmid) may well have no effect on one another, as they will be located on distinct parts of the targeting vehicle

Work in the area of long-term gene expression will be required to increase the usefulness of this delivery method.

From the above discussions it would appear clear that an attempt to incorporate the tissue-targeting approaches of ligand-bound DNA with the liposome formulations described in the previous section may be of great benefit in yielding further improvements in specific gene delivery. Alternatively, coupling of DNA to cell-type specific molecules may be a worthwhile avenue of research. A recent report (45) coupling DNA to antibodies to the T-cell-specific CD3 antigen (a component of the T-cell receptor), which led *in vivo* to transduction efficiencies of up to 50% in T-cell lines, demonstrates the potential feasibility of the approach.

Retroviruses

Retroviruses are single-stranded RNA viruses which replicate via a double-stranded DNA intermediate (the *provirus*) which integrates into the genome of the infected cell. Retroviruses appear to require cell division for the integration of the proviral DNA form into the host cell. This may allow a certain level of selectivity of delivery *in vivo*, although as yet, no detailed knowledge concerning infection of non-dividing cells subsequently stimulated to divide at some indeterminate time post-infection is available.

There are three key issues to address concerning use of retroviral vectors in *in vivo* gene therapy.

1. First, that for systemic treatment of, for example, cancer by intravenous or intraperitoneal injection, technical advances may be required to increase deliverable viral titres by an order of 1–100 000.

2. Secondly, that the viral particles should ideally be made more resistant to the actions of human complement, which rapidly inactivates particles derived from most currently used vector systems.

3. Finally, that safety and ethical issues pertaining to stable retroviral integration into a human patient, particularly with regard to insertional mutagenesis, and germ-line infection/transmission in cases where the treated person is of child-bearing age or younger, must be evaluated prior to human clinical trials.

Retroviral vector production: packaging cells and virus production

The principles of retroviral vector packaging are shown in Fig. 27.1. A packaging cell line normally expresses all the necessary retroviral proteins (*gag*, *pol*, and *env*), but con-

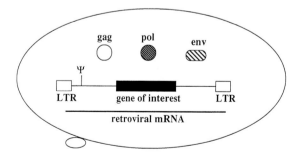

Figure 27.1. For explanation see text.

tains no packageable viral RNA. A retroviral vector, when stably transfected into a packaging cell line, produces a retroviral RNA which can be packaged, but which contains no coding sequence for retroviral proteins. The vectors normally carry a selectable marker such as *neo*, *puro*, or *gpt*, but vectors devoid of such markers have been developed. Table 27.2 summarizes the methods of packaging developed to date and achievable titres.

One major advantage of retroviral vectors is that no virus-specific proteins are produced, and hence no problems with immune responses to vector proteins are likely to occur.

Of prime concern in the vector production process is the generation, through recombination events, of replication competent retroviruses (RCRs), which are able to undergo multiple rounds of replication and infection of the host cells. This leads to multiple random integration events within host cells, which may contribute towards the development of cancer, as has been shown in the classic studies using, among others, Moloney murine leukaemia virus (MoMuLV), mouse mammary tumour virus (MMTV), feline leukaemia virus (46–48). Hence, of paramount importance for gene therapy applications are packaging systems in which generation of RCR does not occur.

This problem has been dealt with with some success in the packaging systems ΨCRE and ΨCRIP (49) and even more effectively in the systems GP+E86 and GP+env am12 (50,51), by the separation of the gag+pol and env coding sequences on to distinct plasmids. In the latter two cases, at least three independent recombination events are required for the generation of RCR using these packaging systems. As yet, no reports of RCR resulting from virus packaged from these lines have appeared in the literature.

The highest viral titres achieved using these traditional vectors and packaging lines is ≈ 1–4×10^7 colony-forming units/ml (c.f.u./ml) (52) although more usually, titres of 10^5–10^6 are achieved.

Retroviral vectors have recently been constructed, which do not carry a selectable marker gene; this increases the coding capacity of the vector for gene(s) of interest. In particular, the MFG vector developed in Richard Mulligan's laboratory is now being used succesfully by many researchers. This vector, which allows fusion of the coding sequence of interest to the naturally occurring gag initiatior methionine codon, has been used successfully for the high-level expression of many genes. Briefly, retroviral vectors are co-transfected into a packaging cell line with a *neo* expression plasmid and putative high producer clones are selected on the basis of expression of the gene of interest. Titring viruses produced in this way is perhaps more irksome, requiring a quantitative Southern blotting protocol, but is by no means difficult.

Table 27.2. Comparison of titres, infectivity of human cells, and specificity of transgene expression using retroviral vectors systems currently under study

Type of vector retroviral	Currently achievable titre/c.f.u. per ml	Infection of human cells; tissue specificity of expression
Constitutive expression of a transgene:		
Wild-type vector		
Amphotropic MoMuLV (52)	10^6–10^7	Yes; none
Spleen necrosis virus (64)	5×10^5–10^6	Yes/no; none
Reticuloendotheliosis virus A (65)	10^5–10^7	No; none
Gibbon ape leukaemia virus (67)	10^5–10^7	Yes; none
Self-inactivating vector		
MoMuLV (80–82)	10^3–10^5	Yes; none
Spleen necrosis virus (64)	5×10^5	Yes; none
Tissue-specific promoter directing expression		
anti-sense to LTR driventranscription:		
MoMULV wild-type vector (78,79)	10^3–10^5	Yes; increased specificity of expression
SIN MoMuLV vector (140)	10^3–10^5	Yes; absolute specificity of expression
Modified envelope protein carrying		
tissue-specific epitope:		
Ecotropic MoMuLV (120)	10^1–10^2	Only infect cells carrying appropriate receptor
Spleen necrosis virus (70)	10^1–5×10^2	Only infect cells carrying appropriate receptor

More recently, a highly efficient transient transfection procedure has been developed for the generation of recombinant retroviruses (53). This has the safety advantage that long-term passaging of virus-producing cells in tissue culture is unecessary and thus greatly reduces risk for the generation of RCR. It is also possible to package toxic gene products within retroviral particles, of great interest for anti-cancer research. The packaging line is derived from the adenovirus-transformed 293 kidney cell which had been transfected with a temperature-sensitive simian virus 40 T antigen (293 T1 cells), subsequently transfected with the retroviral protein expression vectors used for the generation of ψCRIP (the final producer cell line was termed BOSC 23). Fifty to 90% of cells are transfectable in a transient assay and virus particles are harvested from the medium 72–96 h later. The disadvantage of such a system is that the transient transfection procedure is difficult to standardize and characterization of viruses produced in this manner is more difficult.

One potential advantage of the retrovirus system is that envelope proteins from different viruses may be used to *pseudotype* the viruses. A transient transfection system has recently been used by Yee *et al.* (54) for pseudotyping MoMuLV retroviral vectors with the vesicular stomatitis virus G (VSV) G protein, using a 293 cell line transfected with *gag* and *pol-*, but not the *env* gene, as the packaging cell line (termed 293 GP).

The great advantage of this system is that viruses pseudotyped with VSV G are concentratable by up to 1000-fold by ultracentrifugation, unlike conventional retroviruses, which become non-infective following such treatment. As yet, it has not been possible to develop packaging lines which stably express VSV G, as stable expression of this protein, even at low levels, is toxic to most cells. The development of a non-leaky inducible expression system for VSV G would be a key technical advance in this method of packaging. A cell line capable of packaging an individual retroviral vector, which utilizes a tetracycline-inducible VSV G expression system has recently been reported (55), but this is not a generalized packaging line for VSV G pseudotyped vectors.

The highest titres reported using these transient transfection protocols is of the order of 5×10^6 c.f.u./ml for the BOSC 23 system and 1–2×10^9 c.f.u./ml for the VSV G pseudotyping system (after concentration by ultracentrifugation).

Another recent report indicates that the method of transfection of DNA into producer cells may affect the subsequent titres of virus produced (37). Using the transferrinfection procedure, high titres of virus following transient transfection were obtainable. Also, following stable transfection, titres produced were up to 25-fold higher as compared with stable transfectants generated by either calcium phosphate co-precipitation or infection with an ecotropic retrovirus. The highest titres reported were $1–2 \times 10^7$ c.f.u./ml. The reason for these improved titres may be a high copy number of transfected DNA copies integrating into the chromosomes of the recipient producer cell line.

A recent report has indicated the first shift towards industrial production of retroviruses (56). It was reported that culturing cells at 32°C improves viral titre five-to six fold and processing the viral supernatant using a pellicon tangential flow concentration system increases titre by 25-fold. Lyophilization of vectors without loss of infectivity was achieved, an important corollary for clinical grade material. The highest titre reported in the paper, using conventional amphotropic packaging systems such as the PA317 cell line, was 2×10^8 c.f.u./ml. In an unpublished meeting report (Keystone Symposium Gene Therapy Meeting abstract), artificial capillary cell production systems (Cellco Inc.) were used to increase titres of virus 25-fold; this was due to increased cell density in the cell culture environment. Undoubtedly, the next 5 years will see further research into production technology, leading to higher achievable viral titres as the demand for retroviral material increases.

Polycistronic vectors

In prokaryotes, the transcriptional unit (the *operon*) often encodes more than one polypeptide which are translated equally efficiently. In eukaryotes, it was believed for many years that only one polypeptide product was derived from a single RNA. Recently, however, it has emerged from the study of the picornaviruses (57) that polycistronic RNAs do also exist in eukaryotes. The translation of the second open reading frame (ORF) is made possible by the presence of specific RNA sequences which constitute an *internal ribosome entry site* (IRES) (58). A second approach to the development of polycistronic vectors based on proximity has also been reported (59).

Retroviral vectors have been developed recently which carry such IRES sequences (60), and viruses containing two IRESs have also been reported, allowing the expression of a selectable marker and two gene products. This is of particular interest for the expression of heterodimeric or -trimeric proteins such as interleukin (IL) 12 (61) or in situations where one wishes to coexpress two physiologically synergistic polypeptides, such as TNF-α

and interferon γ, or combinations of cytokines such as granulocyte– macrophage colony-stimulating factor and IL-2.

Such retroviruses give similar titres to more conventional monocistronic vectors, indicating that the IRES sequences do not affect retroviral packaging or replication. Whether co-ordinate expression of two genes by this method may be coupled to non-long-terminal repeat (non-LTR), tissue-specific or inducible promoters successfully is a question of major importance in future vector design.

Different retroviral vector systems

To date, the vast majority of retroviral vectors have been based on the MoMuLV. This has possibly had more to do with technological ease than long-term considerations of human gene therapy applications, as amphotropic particles, which are able to infect human cells, have been readily produced using MoMuLV-based systems. Unfortunately, MoMuLV particles are inactivated by human serum (62), although not by cerebrospinal fluid (63). However, a great deal of useful information has emerged from this system, which will be applicable in other systems.

Most other vector systems so far developed involve reticuloendotheliosis viruses (REVs) such as spleen necrosis virus (64) or REV-A (65; reviewed in reference 66); or gibbon ape leukaemia virus (GALV) (67). Of these virus packaging systems, GALV is able to infect human cells, while results with SNV and REV-A are as yet unclear: some workers report infectivity of human cells while others find minimal infectivity (68–70). Titres are no better, and often worse, than those achieved using the MoMuLV V systems. Nevertheless, continuous exposure of poultry workers to such viruses has led neither to any human pathology or to antibodies being raised against the virus, indicating their potential safety as vectors. Two lines of work indicate possible methods for utilizing these viruses as gene therapy vectors. Work using SNV vectors pseudotyped with bovine leukaemia virus indicates that transfer to bovine cells was possible, although inefficient (71), which may lead to alternative methods of delivery to human cells. Also, MoMuLV-based vectors may be packaged using REV-based packaging lines (66), which may allow the use of well characterized vectors in this packaging system.

Inability to infect human cells may prove to be an advantage, if engineering of envelope proteins to express novel epitopes allows effective targeting of viruses to specific cell types (for a first attempt at such work, see references 69 and 70), as uptake of virus by non-target tissues would be eliminated. However, the susceptibility of such viruses to human serum may preclude their successful use in *in vivo* human gene therapy applications.

Undoubtedly, novel viral vector systems will be developed in the future. HIV-based vectors are being developed for delivery to CD4+ T cells (e.g. reference 72). The human foamy viruses offer great potential (reviewed in reference 73), although further research is necessary in areas of suspected foamy-virus-associated human pathology before the latter will be acceptable as a gene therapy vehicle, while packaging systems must be developed before feasibility studies may be undertaken *in vitro* and in animal model systems. Finally, other lentiviral systems of higher mammals (*e.g.* bovine leukaemia virus) may offer suitable packaging and expression systems, provided they are engineered to be immune to human serum. Much basic research is required in these areas.

Current limitations of retroviruses as packaging agents

One limitation of retroviruses as a delivery system is that of packaging capacity. As the maximum packageable mRNA is about 8–10 kb, genes whose cDNA is larger than this, such as dystrophin, cannot be packaged effectively in this vehicle.

Another major limitation concerns the effect of the chromosomal integration site on subsequent gene expression following infection of host cells. Much work in transgenic mice with the human globin cluster (74) and the CD2 gene (75) has indicated that sites far upstream or downstream of the coding sequences are required for integration-independent, tissue-specific gene expression. Such regions, termed dominant control regions (DCRs) or locus control regions (LCR) have been incorporated into retroviruses, but initial constructs were unstable, with multiple rearrangements during proviral transmission (76). A search for cryptic splice sites, polyadenylation sites, and direct repeat sequences led to rational mutagenesis studies, which have generated stably transmissible vectors showing tissue specificity (77). It is as yet unclear whether such considerations will be of importance in destructive anti-cancer gene therapy.

Another problem found by many investigators concerns the incorporation of tissue-specific regulatory elements within the context of retroviral vectors. The presence of strong enhancer elements within the commonly used retroviral LTRs may reduce the specificity of certain promoter elements such as the tyrosinase or albumin promoters, which in a plasmid context show strict inducibility or tissue specificity. This may perhaps be countered in three ways:

(1) by expressing the therapeutic gene in a transcriptional unit anti-sense to LTR-initiated transcription (78,79);

(2) using vectors carrying deletions in the 3′ LTR, the so-called self-inactivating (SIN) vectors, which generate proviruses devoid of LTR promoter elements (80–82);

(3) using naturally occurring or genetically modified viral vectors whose LTRs do not exhibit constitutive enhancer functions in the target cell type.

Maintaining high virus titres without sacrificing tissue specificity or inducibility of gene expression has been difficult and represents a major future challenge. None the less, there are several reports of successful eradication of tumours in laboratory animals following direct intratumoral injection of either retroviral producer cells or retroviral particles carrying pro-drug activating enzymes, and equally many examples of successful transgene expression in gene replacement therapies, albeit sometimes at low levels, so progress in the field is definitely visible.

The biggest challenge in the retroviral vector field, however, is the increase of titres to levels similar to that of the adenoviruses, i.e. from 10^7–10^9 up to 10^{11}–10^{13} p.f.u./ml. It seems unlikely that this will be possible using conventional technology, even with optimization of every stage of the process.

Another question of great importance concerns the incorporation of retroviral vectors into the germ line: whether regulatory authorities will balance this risk against patient death due to lack of treatment is a key ethical consideration. Perhaps if targeted integration of viruses was to become possible, then use in patients, even with potential for germ-line changes, would become more easily justifiable. Recent studies with fusions of retroviral integrase protein to sequence-specific DNA-binding proteins indicate that such an approach may be possible in the medium term (83), as retroviral integration could be directed, at least *in vitro*, to sites adjacent to the recognized DNA sequence.

Finally, in a medical era increasingly dominated by management and cost accountants, the cost of validating the production process for clinical grade viral vectors may, in the presence of alternative, equally effective technologies, limit some possible applications of retroviral vectors on financial grounds.

Adenoviral vectors

Introduction

Human adenovirus is the aetiological agent of many common respiratory infections. At least 42 serotypes exist, but all vectors in common use at present are based on serotypes 2 and 5. The structure of a typical adenovirus is

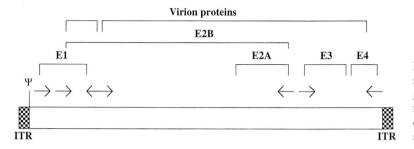

Figure 27.2. Schematic representation of the adenovirus genome. ITR, inverted terminal repeat; Ψ, packaging signal; arrows denote viral transcription initiation sites.

shown in Fig. 27.2. The genome is about 36 kb in length, a double-stranded linear DNA molecule which is bound at each end with an inverse terminal repeat (ITR) sequence, whose presence is required for DNA replication and the generation of infectious virus (84). At the extreme left-hand end of the viral genome map, as it is conventionally drawn, is the E1 region, which encodes the E1A and E1B groups of proteins. As the E1 regions transform cells and must therefore be deleted in any gene therapy vectors, as unique restriction sites exist within this region, and as a well characterized cell line which provides the E1 region functions in *trans* existed (293 cells) first generation vectors were produced using deletions in this region.

The chief advantages of these early adenoviral systems were:

(1) the ability to package genes within virus particles to high titre (up to 10^{12} p.f.u./ml) which will infect both dividing and non-dividing cells of a wide a variety of types;

(2) the efficient uptake and nuclear localization of the DNA vector, which allows highly efficient transient gene expression following infection;

(3) the extrachromosomal location of the adenoviral DNA, which therefore avoids potential dangers of integration events.

Balanced against these three advantages, however, were:

(1) the small coding capacity of such vectors (4–5 kb), thus placing a limit on the genes capable of being packaged in such constructs;

(2) the laborious nature of generating and identifying suitable recombinant adenoviral stocks;

(3) the generation, by recombination, of wild-type virus within such stocks.

For gene replacement therapies, another disadvantage is the immune response generated against the virus proteins resulting from expression of both early and late viral genes

following infection, which leads to a rapid loss of trans-gene expression, despite persistent transgene expression in athymic mice (85). However, in destructive gene therapy, this may be an advantage, as activating the host immune system represents one of the major strategies for anti-cancer gene therapy. As an example, E1-deficient adeno-viruses carrying the thymidine kinase gene have been shown, following direct intratumoral injection, to induce tumour regression of squamous cell carcinomas of the head and neck following ganciclovir treatment in nude mice (86); furthermore, delivery of the IL-2 gene via direct injection of adenovirus particles into mastocytomas in experimental mice led to significant tumour regression (87).

Improved adenoviral vectors

As to date, the development of cell lines expressing specific adenoviral genes has not occurred in a systematic way, increasing the size of genes packageable within adenoviral vectors has concentrated on finding other regions of the adenoviral genome, which are non-essential for viral replication *in vitro*.

One such region is the E3 region, which encodes proteins which interact with host proteins such as the MHC and diminishes the host response to infection. Deletion of this region allows for an extra capacity for inserts of just under 4 kb, thus raising the maximum size of inserts in a double E1–E3 mutant vector to 8.3 kb (88). This study also improved the frequency of formation of re-combinant viruses, by utilizing a packaging-defective viral mutant propagated within bacteria. However, mutation in the 19 kDa protein of the E3 region leads to greater lym-phocyte infiltration in the area of infection, as compared with viruses carrying a wild-type 19 kDa protein (89). Hence, deletion of the E3 region may be of use for cancer gene therapy, but of limited use in gene replacement strategies.

A recent report indicates efficient transfer and expression of marker genes to mesothelioma ascites following intraperitoneal injection of recombinant

E1+E3-deleted adenoviruses (90). Nevertheless, another recent report has indicated that generation of wild-type adenovirus following multiple passages of an E1–E3 mutant strain does occur (91), a significant point when considering such strains for clinical use.

A second modification in adenoviral vectors concerns the incorporation of a temperature-sensitive mutation into the E2a gene (92). When using the virus carrying a ts E2a gene, transgene expression persisted for a longer period (21 days versus <14 days) and infiltration of CD8+ T cells decreased, as compared with viruses carrying a wild-type E2a gene. However, levels of inflammation remained high, indicating the requirement for further alterations in virus structure in the future to enable gene replacement strategies to be successful.

In principle, adenoviral vectors could be used in which almost the entire sequences of adenovirus were deleted, if cell lines analogous to those used for retrovirus production could be developed. Vectors packaged in such systems might not induce immune responses and could thus be of great use in gene replacement strategies, although of less use in cancer gene therapies. This represents a long-term area of research. As a first step in this direction, Mitani et al. (93) have reported the development of a replication-deficient adenoviral plasmid carrying an ampicillin resistance gene and a bacterial origin of replication in the E1 region (which can hence be propagated as a plasmid in bacteria). This construct also lacks the coding sequences for L1, L2, VA I, VA II, and pTP (several of the virion proteins). When co-transfected into 293 cells with a helper virus, this plasmid DNA may be rescued as infectious virus. The next step in the development of improved methods of viral vector production is to complement the missing genes on plasmids, thus removing the requirement for a helper virus. Whether high titres of virus will be maintained in such systems is a key question for future work in this area.

As all adenoviral gene expression is normally induced by E1A and E1B proteins, and as E1-deficient adenoviruses are able to induce expression of adenoviral proteins, it appears that some host cells contain proteins which can complement the E1 mutations (94). Thus it is likely that expression of adenoviral genes following intro-

duction of viral vectors may vary between cell types. As a result of this, it may be difficult to generalize when trying to predict the efficacy of an adenoviral vector for a proposed specific gene therapy experiment.

It is as yet unclear what the optimal balance between expression of a toxic gene and the stimulation of the host immune response will be, if adenoviruses are to be used for cancer gene therapy.

The greatest potential barrier at present to successful human gene therapy using potentially toxic genes encoded within adenoviruses appears to be the lack of specificity of infection. However, in cases where specific tissues may be isolated, such as balloon catheterized arteries, or direct injection into accessible tumours such as melanomas, the efficient infectivity of the virus may be of use. While expression of the therapeutic gene may be placed under the control of a tissue-specific promoter (95), the expression of viral proteins and subsequent immune reaction may lead to difficulties when clinical applications for long-term gene replacement are being designed. However, in destructive gene therapy, such as the treatment of cancer, such immune reactions may be of value, as seen by the complete destruction of gliomas in experimental rats following direct injection of adenoviral particles expressing HSV tk (96).

Further modifications of vectors are needed to overcome such problems. These may include the modification of tissue tropism by incorporation of novel epitopes into the adenovirus fibre protein, which interreacts with the adenovirus receptor (97). In this regard a recent report has demonstrated the successful incorporation of an epitope of the gastrin-releasing peptide into the fibre protein (98), characterized by stable protein production and adoption of a correct quaternary trimeric structure. Whether the high titres of recombinant virus currently achievable will then be sacrificed remains to be seen.

Adeno-associated viral vectors

AAV virus type 2 is a 4.8 kb human parvovirus (reviewed recently in reference 99) whose structure is shown in Fig. 27.3. In order to replicate, it requires superinfection by either adenovirus or herpesvirus. In the absence of

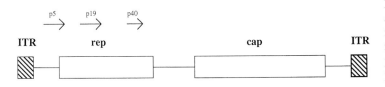

Figure 27.3. Structure of the adeno-associated virus genome. ITR, inverted terminal repeat; rep, AAV replication proteins; cap, AAV capsid proteins; arrows denote viral promoter initiation sites.

helper virus, no replication takes place and integration of the viral DNA occurs, often at a specific site on chromosome 19 (100). All human cells tested are capable of being infected with AAV and no human pathology has yet been associated with this virus.

The only sequences required in *cis* for viral replication and encapsidation are the inverted terminal repeats (ITRs) found at both ends of the genome. Hence, the maximum size of foreign DNA is of the order of 4.4 kb. Expression of the *rep* and *cap* proteins are also required for DNA replication and packaging of virions, although the precise nature of the adenoviral helper function is unclear.

Like adenovirus it will transduce both replicating and non-dividing cells (101), although it has been reported that transduction is more efficient in S-phase cells (102).

The chief differences between the AAV and the adenoviral vector system are:

(1) as integration of the AAV genome occurs following infection, a greater chance of long-term gene expression exists, as compared to the episomal adenoviral genome.

(2) all coding sequences for AAV proteins are eliminated from the vector containing the transgene, hence immunological responses to viral infection are likely to be less pronounced.

Until recently, a significant problem in AAV vector production has been the generation of wild-type virus, a factor which is likely to be a problem for obtaining approval for clinical uses. (The presence of wild-type adenovirus is not a problem, as adenovirus can be destroyed or removed by heat treatment and/or CsCl ultracentrifugation.) This was due to the co-transfection of AAV lacking packaging signals to provide the necessary AAV proteins in trans, much like the first-generation retroviral vectors.

The AAV-derived genes which must be provided in *trans* for AAV vector production are termed *rep* (which encodes proteins required for viral DNA replication) and *cap* (which encodes the virion capsid proteins). Hence an ideal packaging cell line would stably express such proteins. It has been claimed that long-term expression of the *rep* gene in cells has been impossible due to its toxic nature, thus preventing the development of packaging lines analogous to the retrovirus. Furthermore, expression of *rep* from its own promoter in transient transfection experiments is suboptimal due to inhibition of the AAV p5 promoter by the protein products of *rep*. However, Flotte *et al.* (103) have recently expressed the *rep* and *cap* proteins in *trans* under the control of the HIV LTR; this has led both to increased titres of recombinant virus (up to 2×10^{11} p.f.u./ml) as well as eliminating the presence of

wild-type AAV. Also, Clark *et al.* (104) have recently generated stable transfectants of HeLa cells expressing AAV rep, cap, and containing a recombinant AAV genome. When these cells are infected with recombinant adenovirus, rAAV particles are generated.

A tightly inducible expression system for *rep* and *cap* may be useful in the generation of a more efficient packaging system for AAV vectors, but it may be that the current transient transfection protocols will prove sufficient for regulatory authorities.

The chief limitations of the AAV system at present are:

(1) the small size of foreign DNA which can be inserted;

(2) the lack of any tissue specificity of infection.

The chief advantages of AAV appear to be:

(1) the stable incorporation of intron-containing expression systems, as no inadvertent splicing with other viral sequences will occur in such vectors;

(2) the apparent lack of any enhancer elements which may affect the design of inducible expression systems.

In this regard, a recent report (105) has described an AAV vector which demonstrates erythroid-specific expression of human β-globin at physiological levels in MEL cells. However, rearrangement of vector sequences was described in some clones and some integration–site- dependence of expression was noted. Further studies of such events may be necessary in the move towards clinical applications.

Detailed safety studies concerning germ-line transmission, the effect of an adenoviral infection following treatment with an AAV vector and the tissue distribution of virus following systemic delivery are at present most timely.

Viruses related to AAV may also be of use in the longer-term: in particular, the human parvovirus B19; the related mouse virus minute virus of mouse (MVM); and LuIII have promise as gene therapy vehicles (*e.g.* see references 106 and 107), although the association of B19 with spontaneous abortion, aplastic crisis, and occasional severe arthritis would need to be understood more fully before such vectors could reach clinical trials.

Route of administration and pharmacokinetic considerations

The efficacy of any gene therapy protocol will be affected by the time period of gene expression at the site of interest. For systemic delivery, there are a number of possible routes of delivery, including intravenous, intraperitoneal, or subcutaneously. The half-life of the medicine is also a key parameter, and this may be affected by the route of delivery. Finally, the age of the recipient (new-born, growing or adult), may also have a major effect on the efficacy of delivery.

Zhu et al. (25) demonstrated expression of the CAT gene in six different organs following injection of lipid encapsidated DNA into the tail vein. A study by Stratford-Perricaudet et al. (108) has demonstrated long-term expression of genes in muscle and heart following intra-venous injection of recombinant adenoviruses. A more detailed study by Lew et al. (109) monitored the rate of blood clearance of lipid-encapsidated DNA, persistence of that DNA in tissues for a period of up to 6 months, and expression of the gene HLA-B7 encoded by that DNA, fol-lowing a single dose via the tail vein. These studies indi-cated that although DNA was detectable by polymerase chain reaction (PCR) up to months post-injection in muscle, no protein was detectable immunohistochemically at any site within 7 days of injection. A recent study has compared routes of administration for the delivery of adenoviral-encoded lacZ (110). This was concerned with short-term expression (5 days post-delivery) via eight routes, including intramuscular, intravenous, intra-peritoneal, and via various sites of the alimentary canal. It was noteworthy that following tail vein delivery, a marked preference for delivery to the liver (in addition to the site of injection) was evident. However, no PCR-based methods for evaluating delivery were reported, a necessary step in the approval of such virus vectors as clinical materials.

Finally, a more specialized analysis of delivery to ocular tissues has compared delivery of adenovirus particles with the vitreous body, the anterior chamber or the peribulbar space. Delivery to different cell types within the eye was possible depending on the delivery route, which may lead to gene therapy applications for genes such as retinitis pigmentosa.

There is currently a great need for detailed pharmaco-kinetic studies of gene therapy delivery vehicles, not least to allow use of such reagents in human clinical trials.

Like conventional medicines, it is likely that gene thera-pies will have a window of useful dosage, where the beneficial effects outweigh possible risks. However, given the hereditable nature of DNA, strict controls of such materials may be necessary to prevent such recombinant material being transmitted vertically via meiotic processes.

Gene delivery to tumour endothelium

Several reports have described gene transfer to the endothelium. These range from in vitro studies showing that adenovirus can transfer genes and elicit expression in quiescent endothelium (112) to studies where either lipo-some-encapsulated DNA (25) or adenovirus (113) was administered in vivo and endothelial expression reported.

Despite these studies, specific gene delivery to the tumour vasculature via the general circulation remains a largely uncharted territory. None the less, it is clear that any specificity of gene delivery must result from specificity at one of the following levels:

(1) specificity of DNA uptake/transduction;

(2) specificity of gene expression within transduced cells.

The first option is particularly attractive, as it may allow lower doses of therapy to be administered, as there will not be a non-specific uptake of the gene in non-target tissues.

Modification of viral tropism

Although both retroviruses and adenoviruses are internal-ized via specific receptors (114–117), none of the as yet characterized viruses used as vectors, with the possible exception of HIV (which is internalized via the CD4 receptor), demonstrate tissue-specificity of infection.

While to date, no reports of modified adenoviral par-ticles have been published, several recent studies have addressed the modification of retroviral envelope proteins. The aim is to target retroviral binding to a cell-type specific surface receptor which will still allow endocytosis of the virus followed by successful uncoating, reverse transcription, and integration of the provirus. There is thus a limitation on the generality of such a method.

The earliest report of such a strategy involved the incorporation of the extracellular domain of the CD4 antigen into avian leukosis virus (ALV) virions. This was not designed to infect cells, but rather to neutralize HIV infection (118). Whilst incorporation of CD4 into virions was demonstrated, a significant amount of wild-type virus may well have also been present, as successful packaging required the presence of wild-type envelope proteins.

A more general strategy was reported by Russell et al. (119), who formed fusions of the env polypeptide of MoMuLV to functional single-chain antibody fragment raised against the hapten 4-hydroxy-5-iodo-3-nitro-phenacetyl caproate (NIP). They demonstrated that such fusion proteins could be packaged into functional viruses but no titres of such viruses were reported. A more ambitious approach was adopted to target retroviruses to cells expressing the erythropoietin (EPO) receptor (120) by fusing the coding sequences for EPO to the N-terminus of the MoMuLV amphotropic enveloped gene. Packaging of such a fusion protein into retroviral particles was achieved and infection of cells carrying EPO receptors (including HeLa transfectants) was demonstrated. However, no detailed titres were reported and again, it is unclear whether wild-type virus is also present, an important corollary for the targeting of toxic gene products. A similar approach was used by Chu and Dornburg (70) using the SNV retrovirus envelope for targeting a virus to tumour cells. They raised antibodies to a membrane fraction of a liver metastasis of a breast tumour and prepared a single-chain antibody cDNA (scFv). This was fused to the envelope sequences and packaged. Titres were reported to be $\approx=10^2$ c.f.u./ml, a drop of 10 000 compared with wild-type virus. Much basic work is therefore required before such an approach will be usable in a clinical setting.

A second approach has involved the chemical linking of ecotropic retroviruses (which are unable to infect non-murine cells) to molecules which bind specifically to particular cell types. Although such work is still in its early stages, Neda *et al.* (121) demonstrated transient expression of a lacZ marker gene in human hepatoma cells following chemical linkage of ecotropic, lacZ-encoding MoMuLV to lactose (which recognizes the liver-specific asialoglycoprotein receptors). In a more detailed study, Etienne-Julan *et al.* (122) analysed the infectivity of MoMuLV (as detected by selection for G418 resistance) cross-linked to a variety of compounds including EGF, antibodies to the EGF receptor, antibodies to the transferrin receptor and antibodies to the MHC class I, using a biotin–streptavidin adaptor. They were able to demonstrate a 1% infectivity rate of such modified viruses in human cells. Given production of high titre virus, such efficiencies may be sufficient to allow effective targeting in *in vivo* models, although no data are yet available in this regard.

Such an approach may be used in principle to target virions to the tumour vasculature, provided that appropriate target receptors may be identified. Currently, the most obvious candidates are those of the VEGF receptors kinase insert domain-containing receptor (KDR) and Fms-like-tyrosine kinase (flt)-1. These are receptors for the only currently known endothelial-cell-specific mitogen; and *KDR* is expressed highly on vessels in tumours (123,124), although it has also been reported to be expressed on normal sinusoidal endothelium in rat liver (125). *KDR* is also induced by hypoxia in endothelial cell cultures (J. Waltenberger (Ulm), European Vascular Biology Association meeting, Oxford, UK, 1995), which is found in many tumours. However, integrins, such as $\alpha_v\beta_3$ integrin, which has recently been shown to be upregulated on tumour endothelium (126) *or* adhesion molecules (such as E-selection or P-selectin), which have been shown to be up-regulated on tumour endothelium of breast tumours or melanomas (127,128) may also be useful. Whether such molecules will internalise following binding remains to be

determined. However, integrins have recently been shown to be involved in the uptake of adenovirus particles via an endocytic method (117), which gives hope for a successful internalization of viruses targeted to such molecules.

The greatest hurdles to overcome in the generation of material suitable for clinical use are:

(1) the ability to characterize the composition of such hybrid viruses;

(2) the development of methods which allow virus production using envelope fusion proteins in the absence of wild-type envelope proteins, or the ability to purify such modified viruses from wild-type counterparts without loss of infectivity;

(3) the generation of such viruses without loss of viral titre; and

(4) the generation of viruses which are internalized, replicated, and integrated into the host genome following cell-surface binding.

Antibody-based targeting

The ability to target DNA linked to antibodies to the tumour vasculature might avoid the safety concerns of viral particles. Advances in this area have been hindered by failure to identify cell-surface antigens whose tissue distribution is sufficiently specific to allow effective tumour targeting. Recently, however, the production of an antibody to oncofetal fibronectin, also known as BC-1, as a cell-surface marker which apparently has significant specificity for tumour endothelium (129,130; H. Turley and R. Bicknell, unpublished results) may be a way around the problem. It is unclear, however, whether such a molecule would allow internalization of the antibody/DNA complex. The best targets would be growth factor receptors known to internalize following ligand binding. In this regard the KDR, *flt-1, flt-4, tie* and *tek* gene products are worthy of further study (131–135). It has been hypothesized that the KDR, molecules may localize to the abluminal side of the cell, making them accessible to blood-borne therapies; this is consistent with the localization of VEGF, the ligand for KDR, to this area in immunohistochemical experiments (136). It is particularly important to understand both the tissue distribution of such receptors and their method of signalling following ligand binding, as internalization will be a prerequisite for an antibody-based delivery system.

The greatest challenges in this approach may ultimately concern effective uptake and nuclear localization of the DNA. Using liposomes and/or inactivated adenoviral particles may be necessary for a successful delivery.

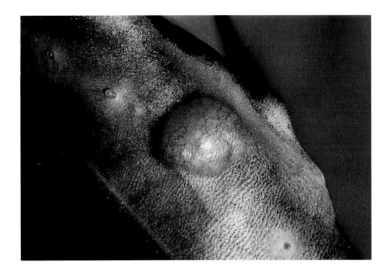

Figure 3.3. Photograph of a tumour formed from VEGF121 expressing MCF-7 cells. Note the large vessels present in the skin. These were never seen in tumours formed from wild type cells.

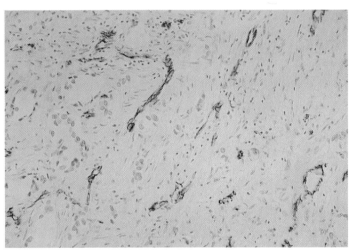

Figure 4.1. (a) Photograph showing a node-positive infiltrating ductal breast carcinoma with high IMD (>100 microvessels at the 'hotspot'). The patient with this tumour is in the subgroup of cases with the highest risk of recurrence and death. (b) A node-negative inflitrating ductal breast carcinoma with low IMD (<50 microvessels at the 'hotspot'). The patient with this tumour is in the subgroup of cases with the lowest risk of recurrence and death. Staining by the anti-CD31 antibody (clone JC/70A Dako) at the dilution 1:200 overnight and the streptavidin–biotin peroxidase complex. Microvessel counts performed using the method suggested by Weidner in a 200× field (0.74 mm² area).

(a)

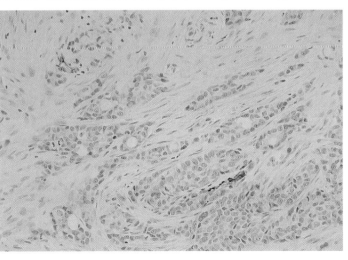

(b)

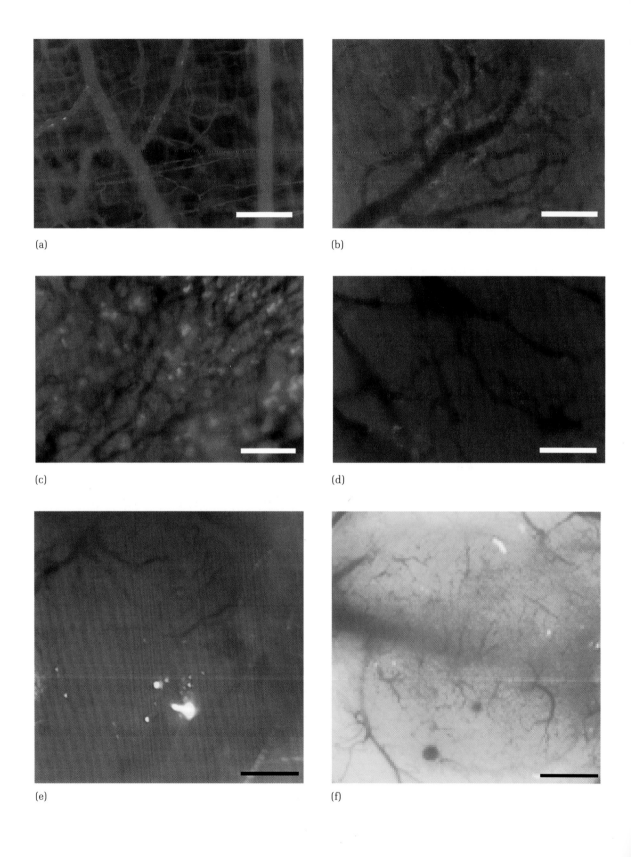

(a)

(b)

(c)

(d)

(e)

(f)

Figure 5.7. Transvascular transport in dorsal skin and tumours. (a) There is hardly any extravasation of 90 nm diameter liposomes from normal vessels. (b) Heterogeneous extravasation of 90 nm diameter liposomes from LS174T tumour vessels, 48 hours after injection. Note that some vessels are leaky as indicated by the yellow fluorescence for rhodamine, while others are not. Extravasated liposomes do not diffuse far from blood vessels. (Adapted from reference 14.) (c) Liposomes of 400 nm diameter (yellow fluorescent spots) extravasate adequately from LS174T tumour. (d) Liposomes of 600 nm diameter do not extravasate, suggesting that LS174T vessels have pore-size cut-off of about 500 nm. (Adapted from reference 62.) (e) The human glioma (HGL21) xenograft is permeable to Lissamin green (i.e. tumour tissue becomes green) when grown subcutaneously (Yuan and Jain, unpublished results). (f) The same glioma develops blood–brain barrier properties (i.e. impermeable to Lissamin green) when grown in the cranial window (Adapted from reference 14.)

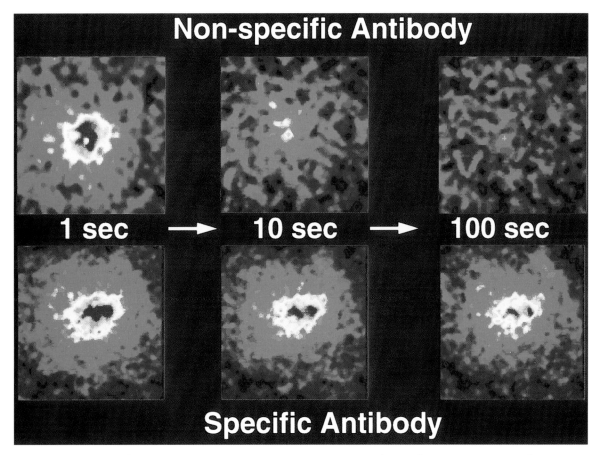

Figure 5.8. Role of binding in the interstitial transport in tumours, measured using fluorescence recovery after photobleaching. (a) Recovery of a photobleached spot is complete in about 100 s for a non-specific monoclonal antibody. (b) Recovery is incomplete for an antibody against carcino-embryonic antigen, present on the surface of many carcinoma cells. (Adapted from reference 84.)

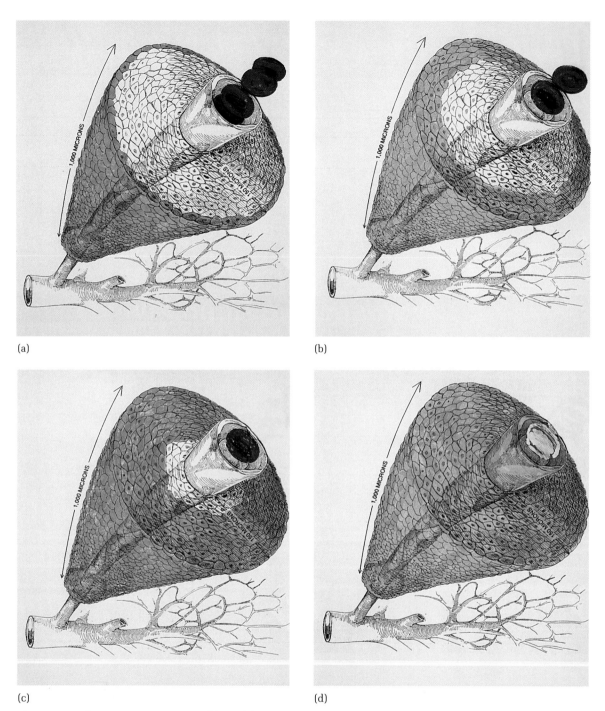

(a)

(b)

(c)

(d)

Figure 6.4. Schematic representations of four of the many possible scenarios relating erythrocyte flux and hypoxia in one cross-sectional area of a tumour vessel at a given instant in time. For illustrative purposes, the cells with a nominal level of oxygenation ($P_{O_2}<2.5$ mmHg) are shaded blue, oxygenated erythrocytes red and deoxygenated ones blue. (a) and (b) show the effect of varying erythrocyte flux (c) shows a scenario of a vessel which the erythrocytes are deoxygenated. It is also possible to have a status similar to (c) with no erythrocyte flux, just plasma perfusion (d). Moreover, it is possible that (a) and (c) represent scenarios at the arterial and venous end of the same capillary.

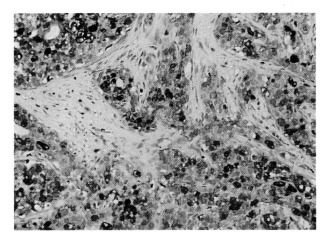

(a)

Figure 19.4. Immunohistochemical staining of thymidine phosphorylase in malignant human breast tissue. (a) An invasive ductal carcinoma which shows positive staining of the tumour cells with negative stroma. (b) An invasive ductal carcinoma which shows positive staining of the inflammatory and stromal cells, with negative neoplastic cells.

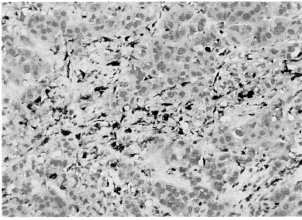

(b)

Figure 20.2. The vessels within the disc are usually recognized in ordinary planar sections. However, better definition can be obtained by the injection of Luconyl Blue 15 min prior to disc harvesting. The branching capillaries, in a disc stimulated by 1 ng of tumour necrosis factor α contrast with the pink trabeculae of the polyvinyl sponge. Some leukocytes and erythrocytes are also seen. Haematoxylin and eosin: ×300.

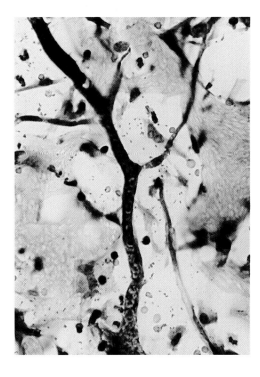

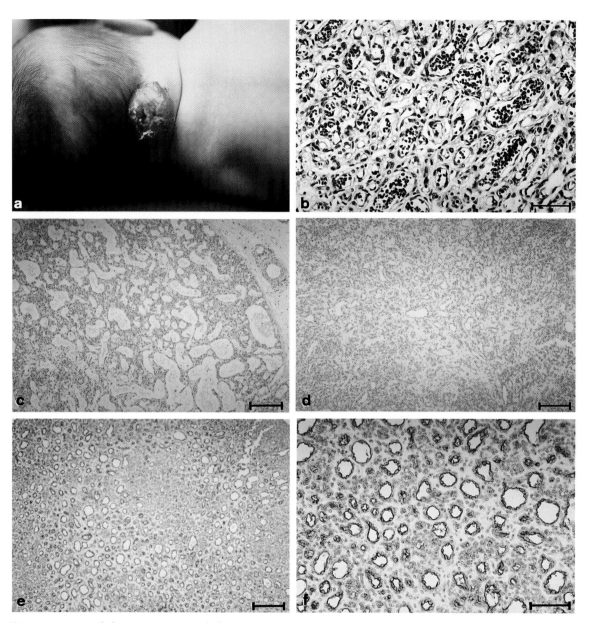

Figure 24.1. Juvenile haemangioma morphology. (a) Macroscopic view of a juvenile haemangioma in the nape of the neck of a neonate. It is several centimetres in size, is elevated above the surface, and bright red in colour. This haemangioma was surgically removed because of superficial ulceration and infection resulting from repeated mechanical abrasion due to its anatomical localization. (b) Histology of the haemangioma shown in (a). This is a typical capillary haemangioma composed of thin walled vessels which are heterogeneous in size, varying from capillaries to post-capillary and larger venules. The vessels are separated by scant connective tissue. (c) and (d) Low-power views of another juvenile haemangioma. This material was obtained by excision biopsy of a lesion for which definitive histological diagnosis was required. These images, which are from the same tumour, demonstrate the characteristic heterogeneity in vessel size in different regions of a single tumour. (e) and (f) Endothelial cells were identified in this lesion using the lectin *Ulex europaeus* as a histological marker. (f) Is a higher magnification of the upper left-hand region of (e). (b) and (f) Are at the same magnification; bars = 75 μm. (c)–(e) are at the same magnification; bars = 150 μm. [Parts (a) and (b) were kindly provided by Dr L. Schweigerer, Zentrum für Kinderheilkunde, University of Marburg, and parts (c–f) were prepared in collaboration with the Dermatology Clinic, Geneva Cantonal Hospital.]

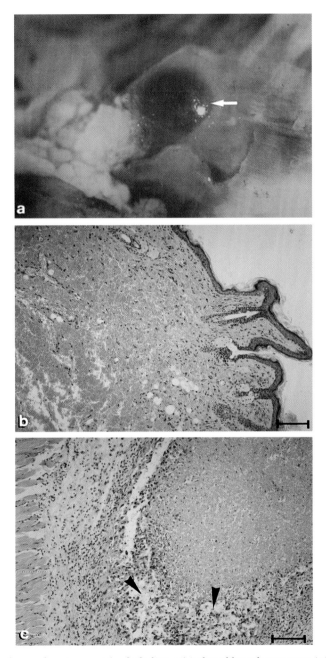

Figure 24.3. Morphology of secondary tumours (endotheliomas) induced by subcutaneous injection of PymT-transformed endothelial (End) cells. (a) Macroscopically, these tumours consist of large blood-filled cavernous or cystic structures. (b) A prominent histological feature in the early phase of tumour growth is massive haemorrhage, which may completely disrupt normal tissue architecture at the site of injection. (c) A more localized subcutaneous lesion in which a region of central necrosis containing red cell ghosts (seen at higher magnification) is surrounded by an intense inflammatory reaction with a well-developed neovascular response. Lumina of neovessels are indicated by arrowheads. Magnification in (b) and (c) is the same as in Fig. 24.1 c–e; bars = 150 μm. [Part (a) is from Williams *et al.*, 1989. With copyright permission from Cell Press.]

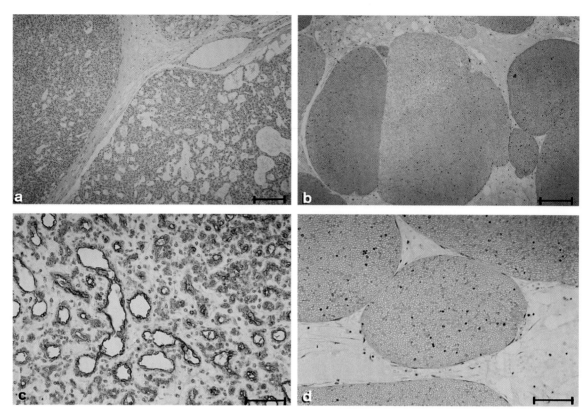

Figure 24.4. Morphological comparison between juvenile haemangioma and intraperitoneal endothelioma. (a) Juvenile capillary haemangioma composed of aggregates of vessels which are heterogeneous in size. Haemangiomas may be lobulated and surrounded by a pseudo-capsule. (b) Endothelioma induced following intraperitoneal injection of End cells into an adult mouse. Note the presence of large blood-filled cavernous or cystic lesions and the absence of an intense inflammatory reaction in the surrounding stroma as seen in Fig. 24.2(c) (a) and (b) are at the same magnification. (c) Endothelial cells in the haemangioma have been identified by *Ulex europaeus* lectin immunohistochemistry; note the presence of relatively uniform stromal cells with plump nuclei in the connective tissue separating the vessels. (d) Intraperitoneal End cell-induced endothelioma showing a large cavernous cystic-like structure lined by a single layer of flattened cells. (c) and (d) are at the same magnification. Magnification in (a) and (b) is the same as in Fig. 24.1(c–e) and 24.2(b,c); bars = 150 μm. Magnification of (c) and (d) is the same as in Fig. 24.1(b,f); bars = 75 μm.]Parts (a) and (c) were prepared in collaboration with the Dermatology Clinic, Geneva Cantonal Hospital.]

Vascular targeting of gene therapy using transcriptional control

The most commonly used route for the development of tissue-specific gene expression vectors involves the use of transcriptional control elements. For many cell types, the use of tissue culture systems and transgenic mice have delineated sequences necessary for either transient or stable gene expression. In particular, the transgenic mice have shown that sequences sufficient to generate physiological levels of tissue specific gene expression *in vitro*, are often very poor in inducing efficient expression *in vivo*. The identification of DNase I hypersensitive sites has correlated with the presence of sequences which mediate integration-independent high-level gene expression, in the presence of proximal promoter elements.

The analysis of endothelial-specific gene expression has largely been confined to transient reporter gene expression assays. This has been due to

(1) the short *in vitro* life span of the commonly used human umbilical vein endothelial cells, which precludes the generation of stable transfectants;

(2) the lack of efficient transfection systems for the longer life-span bovine endothelial cells of large vessel (bovine aortic endothelial cells) or microvessel (bovine adrenal capillary endothelium) origin;

(3) the fact that promoters for endothelial-specific genes have been isolated only relatively recently.

Several candidate promoters for tumour endothelial-specific expression may be of use. These include that of E-selectin/ELAM-1, which has been shown to be induced on cytokine-treated endothelial cells (137). The gene is also up-regulated on the endothelium of breast, melanoma, and bladder tumours (128). The minimal ELAM-1 promoter constructs (700–800 bp) which show cytokine-inducibility in endothelial cells *in vitro*, have also been shown to be active in the cervical cancer line HeLa (138). There is therefore a need to identify elements which mediate non-endothelial cell repression to allow truly endothelial-specific gene therapy constructs to be delivered.

Another potential promoter is that of the *KDR* gene; although this gene appears to be up-regulated in tumour endothelium, as this gene is expressed constitutively, albeit at a low level in most normal endothelial cells, it may be necessary to use this in conjunction with a prodrug-activating system, to introduce a means of controlling potentially toxic side-effects due to non-specific delivery of therapies to normal endothelium. It may also require the use of retroviruses to deliver the therapy more specifically to the dividing endothelial cells of the tumour.

The identification of promoters specific to proliferating endothelium may now, at least theoretically, be identified by using the PCR differential display technique (139).

One critical question which needs to be addressed is whether the selectivity of retroviral integration into proliferating cells means that promoters specific for microvascular endothelium, as opposed to tumour endothelium, will be sufficiently selective for safe therapies. If this is the case, then promoters such as that for von Willebrand factor, preproendothelin or angiotensin-converting enzyme may be suitable in such approaches.

The key developments in the success of a transcriptionally regulated gene therapy approach are efficient transfection systems for the analysis of promoters in endothelial cells of a variety of origins, and the analysis of such promoters in transgenic mice systems. For retrovirally based systems, development of systems which mask the dominant effects of LTR enhancer functions will be necessary, as will be the increase in titres currently achievable using tissue-specific promoter constructs — (10^4–10^5 p.f.u./ml). Development of adenoviruses with tumour endothelial-specific promoters would appear to be a fine anti-cancer strategy, but no reports in this field are yet available.

Conclusions and future prospects

Although a great deal of progress has been made towards the development of effective gene therapies, many important hurdles still need to be overcome, before such reagents become commonplace tools for clinicians. The next 10 years will give indications whether vascular-targeted anti-cancer gene therapy will be a viable future therapy, but it may well be well into the next millenium before such issues are fully resolved.

Acknowledgements

The authors gratefully acknowledge many helpful discussions with Professor Ted Friedmann, Center for Molecular Genetics, Department of Paediatrics, UCSD, La Jolla, CA during his tenure of the Newton Abraham Visiting Professorship, Oxford University. R. T .J. and R. B. are supported by the Imperial Cancer Research Fund.

References

1. Denekamp, J. (1993). Angiogenesis, neovascular proliferation and vascular pathophysiology as targets for cancer therapy. *Br. J. Radiol.*, **66**, 181–96.

2. Fan, T-P. D., Jaggar, R. T., and Bicknell, R. (1995). Controlling the vasculature: angiogenesis, anti-angiogenesis and vascular targeting of gene therapy. *TIPS*, **16**, 57–66.

3. Burrows, F. J. and Thorpe, P. E. (1993). Eradication of large solid tumors in mice with an immunotoxin directed against tumor vasculature. *PNAS*, **90**, 8996–9000.

4. Watanabe, N. Niitsu, Y., Umeno, H., Sone, H, Neda, H, Yamauchi, N., *et al.* (1988). Synergistic Cytotoxic and anti-tumor effects of recombinant human tumor necrosis factor and hyperthermia. *Cancer Res.*, **48**, 650–3.

5. Schweigerer, L., Malerstein, B., and Gospodarowicz, D. (1987). Tumour necrosis factor inhibits the proliferation of cultured capillary endothelial cells. *Biochem. Biophys. Res. Commun.*, **143**, 997–1004.

6. Sato, N., Goto, T., Haranaka, K., Satomi, N., Nariuchi, H., Mano-Hirano, Y., and Sawasaki, Y. (1986). Actions of tumor necrosis factor on cultured vascular endothelial cells: morphologic modulation, growth inhibition and cytotoxicity. *J. Nat Cancer Inst.*, **76**, 1113–21.

7. Robaye, B., Mosselmans, R., Fiers, W., Dumont, J. E., and Galand, P. (1991). Tumor necrosis factor induces apoptosis (programmed cell death) in normal endothelial cells *in vitro*. *Am. J. Pathol.*, **138**, 447–6.

8. Frater-Schroder, M., Risau, W., Hallman, P., Gautschi, R., and Bohlen, P. (1987). Tumor necrosis factor type alpha, a potent inhibitor of endothelial cell growth *in vitro*, is angiogenic *in vivo*. *PNAS*, **84**, 5277–81.

9. Leibovich, S. J., Polverini, P. J., Shepard, H. M., Wiseman, D. M., Shively, V., and Nuseir, N. (1987). Macrophage-induced angiogenesis is mediated by tumour necrosis factor-alpha. *Nature* **329**, 630–2.

10. Lienard, D., Ewalenko, P., Delmotte, J. J., Renard, N., and Lejeune, F. J. (1992). High dose recombinant tumour necrosis factor α in combination with interferon γ and melphalan in isolation perfusion of the limbs for melanoma and sarcoma. *J. Clin. Oncol.*, **10**, 52–60.

11. Hellerqvist, C. G., Thurman, G. B., Page, D. L., Wang, Y-F., Russell, B. A., Montgomerie, C. A., and Sundell, H. W. (1993). Antitumor effects of GBS toxin: a polysaccharide exotoxin from group B β-hemolytic streptococcus. *J. Cancer Res. Clin. Oncol.*, **120**, 63–70.

12. Borelli, E., Heyman, R., Hsi, M., and Evans, R. M. (1988). Targeting of an inducible toxic phenotype in animal cells. *J. Natl Acad. Sci. USA*, **85**, 7572–6.

13. Mullen, C. A., Kilstrup, M., and Blaese, R. M. (1992). Transfer of the bacterial gene for cytosine deaminase to mammalian cells confers lethal sensitivity to 5-fluorocytosine — a negative selection system. *Proc. Natl Acad. Sci. USA*, **89**, 33–7.

14. Moolten, F. L. and Wells, J. M. (1990). Curability of tumors bearing herpes thymidine kinase genes transferred by retroviral vectors. *J. Natl Cancer Inst*, **82**, 297–300.

15. Culver, K. W., Ram, Z., Walbridge, S., Ishii, H., Oldfield, E. H., and Blaese, R. M. (1992). *In vivo* gene transfer with retroviral vector producer cells for treatment of experimental brain tumors. *Science*, **256**, 1550–2.

16. Bi, W. L., Parysek, L. M., Warnick, R., and Stambrook, P. J. (1993). *In vitro* evidence that metabolic cooperation is responsible for the bystander effect observed with HSV tk retroviral gene therapy. *Hum. Gene Ther.*, **4**, 725–31.

17. Pitts, J. D. (1994). Cancer gene therapy: a bystander effect using the gap junctional pathway. *Mol.* Carcinogenesis, **11**, 127–30.

18. Horn, N. A., Meek, J. A., Budahazi, G., and Marquet, M. (1995). Cancer gene therapy using plasmid DNA: purification of DNA for human clinical trials. *Hum. Gene Ther.*, **6**, 565–73.

19. Plautz, G. E., Yang, Z-Y., Wu, B., Gao, X., Huang, L., and Nabel, G. J. (1993). Immunotherapy of malignancy by *in vivo* gene transfer into tumors. *Proc. Natl Acad. Sci. USA*, **90**, 4645–9.

20. Vile, R. G. and Hart, I. R. (1993). Use of tissue-specific expression of the herpes simplex virus thymidine kinase gene to inhibit growth of established murine melanomas following direct intratumoral injection of DNA. *Cancer Res.*, **53**, 3860–3864.

21. Nabel, G. J., Nabel, E. G., Yang, Z-Y., Fox, B. A., Plautz, G. E., Gao, X., *et al.* (1993). Direct gene transfer with DNA-liposome complexes in melanoma: expression, biologic activity, and lack of toxicity in humans. *Proc. Natl Acad. Sci. USA*, **90**, 11307–11.

22. Gao, X. and Huang, L. (1991). A novel cationic liposome reagent for efficient transfection of mammalian cells. *Biochem. Biophys. Res. Commun.*, **179**, 280–285.

23. Caplen, N. J., Alton, E. W. F. W., Middleton, P. G., Dorin, J. R., Stevenson, B. J., Gao, X., *et al.* (1995). *Nature Med.*, **1**, 39–46.

24. San, H., Yang, Z-Y., Pompili, V. J., Jaffe, M. L., Plautz, G. E., Xu, L., *et al.* (1993). Safety and short-term toxicity of a novel cationic lipid formulation for human gene therapy. *Hum. Gene Ther.*, **4**, 781–8.

25. Zhu, N., Liggitt, D., Liu, Y., and Debs, R. (1993). Systemic gene expression after intravenous DNA delivery into adult mice. *Science*, **261**, 209–11.

26. Lasic, D. D., Martin, F. J., Gabizon, A., Huang, S. K., and Papahadjopoulos, D. (1991). Sterically stabilized liposomes: a hypothesis on the molecular origin of the extended circulation times. *Biochem. Biophys. Acta*, **1070**, 187–92.

27. Vaage, J., Mayhew, E., Lasic, D., and Martin, F. (1992). Therapy of primary and metastatic mouse mammary carcinomas with doxorubicin encapsulated in long circulating liposomes. *Int. J. Cancer*, **51**, 942–8.

28. Gorman, C. (1995). *Cambridge Healthtech Institute meeting: Gene therapy: new technologies and applications.* Arlington, VA, USA.

29. Holmberg, E., Maruyama, K., Litzinger, D. C., Wright, S., Davis, M., Kabalka, G. W., *et al.* (1989). Highly efficient immunoliposomes prepared with a method which is compatible with various lipid compositions. *Biochem. Biophys. Res. Commun.*, **165**, 1272–8.

30. Son, K. and Huang, L. (1994). Exposure of human ovarian carcinoma to cisplatin transiently sensitizes the tumor cells for liposome-mediated gene transfer. *Proc. Natl Acad. Sci. USA*, **91**, 12669–72.

31. Nabel, G. J., (1994). Comment *Ann. N. Y. Acad. Sci.*, **716**, 34.

32. Wagner, E., Zenke, M., Cotten, M., Beug, H., and Birnstiel, M. L. (1990). Transferrin-polycation conjugates as carriers for DNA uptake into cells. *Proc. Natl Acad. Sci. USA*, **87**, 3410–14.

33. Wagner, E., Cotten, M., Foisner, R., and Birnstiel, M. L. (1991). Transferrin-polycation–DNA complexes: the effect of polycations on the structure of the complex and DNA delivery to cells. *Proc. Natl Acad. Sci. USA*, **88**, 4255–9.

34. Curiel, D. T., Agarwal, S., Wagner, E., and Cotten, M. (1991). Adenovirus enhancement of transferrin-polylysine-

mediated gene delivery. *Proc. Natl Acad. Sci. USA*, **88**, 8850–4.

35. Curiel, D. T. (1994). High–efficiency gene transfer mediated by adenovirus–polysine–DNA complexes. *Ann N. Y. Acad. Sci.*, **716**, 36–58.

36. Cotten, M., Wagner, E., Zatloukal, K., Phillips, S., Curiel, D. T., and Birnstiel, M. L. (1992). High-efficiency receptor-mediated delivery of small and large (48 kb) gene constructs using the endosome-disruption activity of defective or chemically inactivated adenovirus particles. *Proc. Natl Acad. Sci. USA*, **89**, 6094–8.

37. von Rüden, T., Stingl, L., Cotten, M., Wagner, E., and Zatloukal, K. (1995). Generation of high titer retroviral vectors following receptor-mediated, adenovirus-augmented transfection. *Biotechniques*, **18**, 484–9.

38. Zatloukal, K., Cotten, M., Berger, M., Schmidt, W., Wagner, E., and Birnstiel, M. L. (1994). *In vivo* production of human factor VIII in mice after intrasplenic implantation of primary fibroblasts transfected by receptor-mediated, adenovirus-augmented gene delivery. *Proc. Natl Acad. Sci. USA*, **91**, 5148–52.

39. Wu, G. Y. and Wu, C. H. (1987). Receptor-mediated *in vitro* gene transformation by a soluble DNA carrier system. *J. Biol. Chem.*, **262**, 4429–32.

40. Wu, C. H., Wilson, J. M., and Wu, G. Y. (1989). Targeting genes: delivery and persistent expression of a foreign gene driven by mammalian regulatory eements *in vivo*. *J. Biol. Chem.*, **264**, 16985–7.

41. Wu, G. Y., Wilson, J. M., Shalaby, F., Grossman, M., Shafritz, D. A., and Wu, C. H. (1991). Receptor-mediated gene delivery *in vivo*. *J. Biol. Chem.*, **266**, 14338–42.

42. Wilson, J. M., Grossman, M., Wu, C. H., Chowdury, N. R., Wu, G. Y., and Chowdury, J. R. (1992). Hepatocyte-directed gene transfer *in vivo* leads to transient improvement of hypercholesterolemia in low density lipoprotein receptor-deficient rabbits. *J. Biol. Chem.*, **267**, 963–7.

43. Wilson, J. M., Grossman, M., Cabrera, J. A., Wu, C. H., and Wu, G. Y. (1992). A novel mechanism for achieving transgene persistence *in vivo* after somatic gene transfer into hepatocytes. *J. Biol. Chem.*, **267**, 11483–9.

44. Perales, J. C., Ferkol, T., Beegen, H., Ratnoff, O. D., and Hanson, R. W. (1994). Gene transfer *in vivo*: sustained expression and regulation of genes introduced into the liver by receptor-targeted uptake. *Proc. Natl Acad. Sci. USA*, **91**, 4086–90.

45. Buschle, M., Cotten, M., Kirlappos, H., Mechtler, K., Schaffner, G., Zauner, W., *et al.* (1995). Receptor-mediated gene transfer into human T-lymphocytes via binding of DNA/CD3 antibody particles to the CD3-T-cell recptor complex. *Hum. Gene Ther.*, **6**, 753–61.

46. Peters, G., Brookes, S., Smith, R., and Dickson, C. (1983). Tumorigenesis by mouse mammary tumor virus: evidence for a common region for provirus integration in mammary tumors. *Cell*, **33**, 369–77.

47. Varmus, H. E. (1983). Using retroviruses as insertional mutagens to identify cellular oncogenes. *Prog. Clin. Biol. Res.*, **119**, 23–35.

48. Onions, D. (1987). Epidemiology of feline leukaemia virus infections. *Baillières Clin. Haematol.*, **1**, 45–58.

49. Danos, O. and Mulligan, R. C. (1988). Safe and efficient generation of recombinant retroviruses with amphotropic and ecotropic host ranges. *Proc. Natl Acad. Sci. USA*, **85**, 6460–4.

50. Markowitz, D., Goff, S., and Bank, A. (1988). A safe packaging line for gene transfer: separating viral genes on two different plasmids. *J. Virol.*, **62**, 1120–4.

51. Markowitz, D., Goff, S., and Bank, A. (1988). Construction and use of a safe and efficient amphotropic packaging cell line. *Virology* **167**, 400–6.

52. Miller, A. D. and Buttimore, C. (1986). Redesign of retrovirus packaging cell lines to avoid recombination leading to helper virus production. *Mol. Cell. Biol.*, **6**, 2895–902.

53. Pear, W. S., Nolan, G. P., Scott, M. L., and Baltimore, D. (1993). Production of high-titer helper-free retroviruses by transient transfection. *Proc. Natl Acad. Sci. USA*, **90**, 8392–6.

54. Yee, J. K., Miyanohara, A., LaPorte, P., Bouic, K., Burns, J. C., and Friedmann, T. (1994). A general method for the generation of high-titer, pantropic retroviral vectors: highly efficient infection of primary hepatocytes. *Proc. Natl Acad. Sci. USA*, **91**, 9564–8.

55. Yang, Y., Vanin, E. F., Whitt, M. A., Fornerod, M., Zwart, R., Schneiderman, R. D., *et al.* (1995). Inducible, high-level production of infectious murine leukemia retroviral vector particles pseudotyped with vesicular stomatitis virus G envelope protein. *Hum. Gene Ther.*, **6**, 1203–13.

56. Kotani, H., Newton III, P. B., Zhang, S., Chiang, Y. L., Otto, E., Weaver, L., *et al.* (1994). Improved methods of retroviral vector transduction and production for gene therapy. *Hum. Gene Ther.*, **5**, 19–28.

57. Dorner, A. J., Semler, B. L., Jackson, R. J., Hanecak, R., Duprey, E., and Wimmer, E. (1984). *In vitro* translation of poliovirus RNA: utilization of internal initiation sites in reticulocyte lysate. *J. Virol.*, **50**, 507–14.

58. Jang, S. K., Kräusslich, H-G., Nicklin, M. J. H., Duke, G. M., Palmenberg, A. C., and Wimmer, E. (1988). A segment of the 5′ non-translated region of encephalomy-ocarditis virus RNA directs internal entry of ribosome during *in vitro* translation. *J. Virol.*, **62**, 2636–43.

59. Levine, F., Yee, J-K., and Friedmann T. (1991). Efficient gene expression in mammalian cells from a dicistronic transcriptional unit in an improved retroviral vector. *Gene*, **108**, 167–74.

60. Adam, M. A., Ramesh, N., Miller, A. D., and Osbourne, W. R. A. (1991). Internal initiation of translation in retroviral vectors carrying picornavirus 5′ nontranslated regions. *J. Virol.*, **65**, 4895–990.

61. Zitvogel, L., Tahar, H., Cai, Q., Storkus, W. J., Muller, G., Wolf, S. F., *et al.* (1994). Construction and characterisation of retroviral vectors expressing biologically active human interleukin-12. *Hum. Gene Ther.*, **5**, 1493–506.

62. Welsh, R. M., Jensen, F. C., Cooper, N. R., and Oldstone, M. B. A. (1975). Inactivation of lysis of oncornaviruses by human serum. *Virology*, **74**, 432–40.

63. Russell, D. W., Berger, M. S., and Miller A. D. (1995). The effects of human serum and cerebrospinal fluid on retroviral vectors and packaging cell lines. *Hum. Gene Ther.*, **6**, 635–41.

64. Martinez, I. and Dornburg, R. (1995). Improved retroviral packaging lines derived from spleen necrosis virus. *Virology*, **208**, 234–41.

65. Watanabe, S. and Temin, H. (1983). Construction of a helper cell line for avian reticuloendotheliosis virus cloning vectors. *Mol. Cell. Biol.*, **3**, 2241–9.

66. Dornburg, R. (1995). Reticuloendotheliosis viruses and derived vectors. *Gene Ther.*, **2**, 301–10.

67. Miller, A. D., Garcia, J. V., von Suhr, N., Lynch, C. M., Wilson, C., and Eiden, M. V. (1991). Construction and properties of retrovirus packaging cells based on gibbon ape leukemia virus. *J. Virol.*, **65**, 2220–4.

68. Koo, H. M., Brown, A. C., Ron, Y., and Dougherty, J. P. (1991). Spleen necrosis virus, an avian retrovirus, can infect primate cells. *J. Virol.*, **65**, 4769–75.

69. Chu, T-H. T., Martinez, I., Sheay, W., and Dornburg, R. (1994). Cell targeting with retroviral vector particles containing antibody-envelope fusion proteins. *Gene Ther.*, **1**, 292–9.

70. Chu, T-H. T., and Dornburg, R. (1995). Retroviral vector particles displaying the antigen-binding site of an antibody enable cell-type-specific gene transfer. *J. Virol.*, **69**, 2659–63.

71. Ban, J., First, N. L., and Temin, H. M. (1989). Bovine leukemia virus packaging cell line for retrovirus-mediated gene transfer. *J. Gen. Virol.*, **70**, 1987–93.

72. Carroll, R., Lin, J. T., Dacquel, E. J., Mosca, J. D., Burke, D. S., and St Louis, D. C. (1994). A human immunodeficiency virus type 1 (HIV-1) based retroviral vector system utilizing stable HIV-1 packaging cell-lines. *J. Virol.*, **68**, 6047–51.

73. Aguzzi, A. (1993). The foamy virus family: molecular biology, epidemiology and neuropathology. *Biochem. Biophys. Acta.*, **1155**, 1–24.

74. Grosveld, F., van Assendelft, G. B., Greaves, D. R., and Kollias, G. (1987). Position-independent, high-level expression of the human beta-globin gene in transgenic mice. *Cell*, **51**, 975–85.

75. Lang, G., Wotton, D., Owen, M. J., Sewell, W. A., Brown, M. H., Mason, D., *et al.* (1988). The structure of the CD2 gene and its expression in transgenic mice. *EMBO J.*, **7**, 1675–82.

76. Novak, U., Harris, E. A. S., Forrester, W., Groudine, M., and Gelinas, R. (1990). High-level beta-globin expression after retroviral transfer of locus activation region-containing human beta-globin gene derivatives into murine erythroleukemia cells. *PNAS*, **87**, 3386–90.

77. Lebouch, P., Huang, G. M. S., Humphries, R. K., Oh, Y. H., Eaves, C. J., Tuan, D. Y. H., and London, I. M. (1994). Mutagenesis of retroviral vectors transducing human β-globin gene and β-globin locus control retion derivatives results in stable transmission of an active transcriptional structure. *EMBO J.*, **13**, 3065–76.

78. Huber, B. E., Richards, C. A., and Krenitsky, T. A. (1991). Retroviral-mediated gene therapy for the treatment of hepatocellular carcinoma: an innovative approach for cancer therapy. *Proc. Natl Acad. Sci. USA*, **88**, 8039–43.

79. Vile, R. A. and Hart, I. R. (1993). *In vitro* and *in vivo* targeting of gene expression to melanoma cells. *Cancer Res.*, **53**, 962–7.

80. Fu, S. F., von Rüden, T., Kantoff, P. W., Garber, C., Seiberg, M., Rüther, U., *et al.* (1986). Self-inactivating retroviral vectors designed for transfer of whole genes into mammalian cells. *Proc. Natl Acad. Sci. USA*, **83**, 3194–8.

81. Yee, J. K., Moores, J. C., Joly, D. J., Wolff, J. A., Respess, J. G., and Friedmann, T. (1987). Gene expression from transcriptionally disabled retroviral vectors. *Proc. Natl. Acad. Sci. USA*, **84**, 5197–201.

82. Olson, P., Nelson, S., and Dornburg, R. (1994). Improved self-inactivating retroviral vectors derived from spleen necrosis virus. *J. Virol.*, **68**, 7060–6.

83. Bushman, F. D. (1994). Tethering human immunodeficiency virus 1 integrase to a DNA site directs integration to nearby sequences. *Proc. Natl. Acad. Sci. USA*, **91**, 9233–7.

84. Stow, N. (1982). The infectivity of adenovirus genomes lacking DNA sequences from their left-hand termini. *Nucleic Acids Res.*, **10**, 5105–19.

85. Engelhardt, J. F., Yang, Y., Stratford-Perricaudet, L. D., Allen, E. D., Kozarsky, K., Perricaudet, M., *et al.* (1993). Direct gene transfer of human CFTR into human bronchial epithelia of xenografts with E1-deleted adenoviruses. *Nature Genet.*, **4**, 240–8.

86. O'Malley, B. W., Jr., Chen, S-H., Schwartz, M. R., and Woo, S. L. C. (1995). Adenovirus-mediated gene therapy for human head and neck squamous cell cancer in a nude mouse model. *Cancer Res.*, **55**, 1080–5.

87. Cordier, L., Duffour, M-T., Sabourin, J-C., Lee, M. G., Cabannes, J., Ragot, T., *et al.* (1995). Complete recovery of mice from a pre-established tumor by direct intratumoral delivery of an adenovirus vector harboring the murine IL-2 gene. *Gene Ther.*, **2**, 16–21.

88. Bett, A. J., Haddara, W., Prevec, L., and Graham, F. L. (1994). An efficient and flexible system for construction of adenovirus vectors with insertions or deletions in early regions 1 and 3. *Proc. Natl Acad. Sci. USA*, **91**, 8802–6.

89. Ginsberg, H. S., Lundhulm-Beauchamp, U., Horswood, R. L., Pernis, B., Wold, W. S. M., Chanock R. M., and Prince, G. A. (1989). Role of early region 3 (E3) in pathogenesis of adenovirus disease. *Proc. Natl Acad. Sci. USA*, **86**, 3823–7.

90. Brody, S. L., Jaffe, H. A., Han, S. K., Wersto, R. P., and Crystal R. G. (1994). Direct *in-vivo* gene-transfer and expression in malignant-cells using adenovirus vectors. *Hum. Gene Ther.*, **5**, 437–47.

91. Lochmüller, H., Jani, A., Huard, J., Prescott, S., Simoneau, M., Massie, B., *et al.* (1994). Emergence of early region 1-containing replication-competent adenovirus in stocks of replication-defective adenovirus recombinants (E1 –+ E3 –) during multiple passages in 293 cells. *Hum. Gene Ther.*, **5**, 1485–91.

92. Engelhardt, J. F., Litzky, L., and Wilson, J. M. (1994). Prolonged transgene expression in cotton rat lung with recombinant adenoviruses defective in E2a. *Hum. Gene Ther.*, **5**, 1217–29.

93. Mitani, K., Graham, F. L., Caskey, C. T., and Kochanek, S. (1995). Rescue, propagation and partial purification of a helper virus-dependent adenovirus vector. *Proc. Natl Acad. Sci. USA*, **92**, 3854–8.

94. Imperiale, M. J., Kao, H-T., Feldman, L. T., Nevins, J. R., and Strickland, S. (1984). Common control of the heat shock gene and early adenovirus genes: evidence for a cellular E1A-like activity. *Mol. Cell Biol.*, **4**, 867–74.

95. Karlsson, S., van Doren, K., Schweiger, S. G., Nienhuis, A. W., and Gluzman, Y. (1986). Stable gene transfer and tissue-specific expression of a human globin gene using adenoviral vectors. *EMBO J.*, **5**, 2377–86.

96. Chen, S-H., Shine, H. D., Goodman, J. C., Grossman, R. G., and Woo, S. L. C. (1994). Gene therapy for brain tumors: regression of experimental gliomas by adenovirus-mediated gene transfer *in vivo*, *Proc. Natl Acad. Sci. USA*, **91**, 3054–7.

97. Stevenson, S. C., Rollena, M., White, B., Weaver, L., and McClelland, A. (1995). Human adenovirus seroptype-3 and serotype-5′ and bind to 2 different cellular receptors via the fiber head domain. *J. Virol.*, **69**, 2850–57.

98. Michael, S. I., Hong, J. S., Curiel, D. T., and Engler, J. A. (1995). Addition of a short peptide ligand to the adenovirus fiber protein. *Gene Ther.*, **2**, 660–8.

99. Flotte, T. R. and Carter, B. J. (1995). Adeno-associated virus vectors for gene therapy. *Gene Ther.*, **2**, 357–62.

100. Kotin, R. M., Linden, R. M., and Berns, K. I. (1992). Characterisation of a preferred site on human chromosome 19q for integration of adeno-associated virus DNA by non-homologus recombination. *EMBO J.*, **11**, 5071–8.

101. Podsakoff, G., Wong, K. K. Jnr, and Chatterjee, S. (1994). Efficient gene transfer into non-dividing cells by adeno-associated virus-based vectors. *J. Virol.*, **68**, 5656–66.

102. Russell, D. W., Miller, A. D., and Alexander, I. E. (1994). Adeno-associated virus vectors preferentially transduce cells in S phase. *Proc. Natl Acad. Sci. USA*, **91**, 8915–19.

103. Flotte, T. R., Barraza-Ortiz, X., Solow, R., Afione, S. A., Carter, B. J., and Guggino, W. B. (1995). An improved system for packaging recombinant adeno-associated virus vectors capable of *in vivo* transduction. *Gene Ther.*, **2**, 29–37.

104. Clark, K. R., Voulgaropoulou, F., Fraley, D. M., and Johnson, P. R. (1995). Cell lines for the production of recombinant adeno-associated virus. *Hum. Gen. Ther.*, **6**, 1329–41.

105. Einerhand, M. P. W., Antoniou, M., Zolotukhin, S., Muzyczka, N., Berns, K. I., Grosveld, F., and Valerio, D. (1995). Regulated high-level human β-globin gene expression in erythroid cells following recombinant adeno-associated virus-mediated gene transfer. *Gene Ther.*, **2**, 336–43.

106. Maxwell, I. H., Maxwell, F., Rode, S. L.III, Corsini, J., and Carlson, J. O. (1993). Recombinant LuIII autonomous parvovirus as a transient transducing vector for human cells. *Hum. Gene. Ther.*, **4**, 441–50.

107. Corsini, J., Carlson, J. O., Maxwell, F., and Maxwell, I. H. (1995). Symmetrical-strand packaging of recombinant parvovirus LuIII genomes that retain only the terminal regions. *J. Virol.*, **69**, 2692–6.

108. Stratford-Perricaudet, L. D., Makeh, I., Perricaudet, M., and Briand, P. (1992). Widespread, long-term gene transfer to mouse skeletal muscles and heart. *J. Clin. Invest.*, **90**, 626–30.

109. Lew, D., Parker, S. E., Latimer, T., Abai, A. M., Kuwahara-Rundell, A., Doh, S. G., *et al.* (1995). *Hum. Gen. Ther.*, **6**, 553–64.

110. Huard, J., Lochmüller, H., Acsadi, G., Jani, A., Massie, B., and Karpati, G. (1995). The route of administration is a major determinant of the transduction efficiency of rat tissues by adenoviral recombinants. *Gene Ther.*, **2**, 107–15.

111. Mashkour, B., Couton, D., Perricaudet, M., and Briand, P. (1994). *In vivo* adenovirus-mediated gene transfer into ocular tissues. *Gene Ther.*, **1**, 122–6.

112. Lemarchand, P., Ari Jaffe, H., Danel, C., Cid, M. C., Kleinman, H. K., Stratford-Perricaudet, L. D., *et al.* (1992). Adenovirus-mediated transfer of a recombinant human alpha 1-antitrypsin cDNA to human endothelial cells. *Proc. Natl Acad. Sci. USA*, **89**, 6482–6.

113. Lemarchand, P., Jones, M., Yamada, I., and Crystal, R. G. (1993). *In vivo* gene transfer and expression in normal unin-jured blood vessels using replication-deficient recombinant adenovirus vectors. *Circ. Res.*, **72**, 1132–8.

114. Bates, P., Young, J. A. T., and Varmus, H. E. (1993). A receptor for subgroup A Rous Sarcoma Virus is related to the low-density-lipoprotein receptor. *Cell*, **74**, 1053–64.

115. Albritton, L. M., Tseng, L., Scadden, D., and Cunningham, J. M. (1989). A putative murine ecotropic retrovirus receptor gene encodes a multiple membrane-spanning protein and confers susceptibility to virus infection. *Cell*, **57**, 659–66.

116. Belin, M-T. and Boulanger, P. (1993). Involvement of cellular adhesion sequences in the attachment of adenovirus to the HeLa cell surface. *J. Gen. Virol.*, **74**, 1485–97.

117. Wickham, T. J., Mathias, P., Cheresh, D. A., and Nemerow, G. R. (1993). Integrin $\alpha_v\beta_3$ and integrin $\alpha_v\beta_5$ promote adenovirus internalization but not virus attachment. *Cell*, **73**, 309–19.

118. Young, J. A. T., Bates, P., Willert, K., and Varmus, H. E. (1990). Efficient incorporation of human CD4 protein into avian leukosis virus particles. *Science*, **250**, 1421–3.

119. Russell, S. J., Hawkins, R. E., and Winter, G. (1993). Retroviral vectors displaying functional antibody frag-ments. *Nucleic Acids Res.*, **21**, 1081–5.

120. Kasahara, N., Dozy, A. M., and Kan, Y. W. (1994). Tissue-specific targeting of retroviral vectors through ligand–receptor interactions. *Science*, **266**, 1373–6.

121. Neda, H., Wu, C. H., and Wu, G. Y. (1991). Chemical modification of an ecotropic murine leukemia virus results in redirection of its target cell specificity. *J. Biol. Chem.*, **266**, 14143–6.

122. Etienne-Julan, M., Roux, P., Carillo, S., Jeanteur, P., and Piechaczyk, M. (1992). The efficiency of cell targeting by recombinant retroviruses depends on the nature of the receptor and the composition of the artificial cell–virus linker. *J. Gen. Virol.*, **73**, 3251–5.

123. Brown, L. F., Berse, B., Jackman, R. W., Tognazzi, K., Manseau, E. J., Dvorak, H. F., and Senger, D. R. (1993). Increased expression of vascular permeability factor (vascular endothelial growth factor) and its receptors in kidney and bladder carcinomas. *Am. J. Pathol.*, **143**, 1255–62.

124. Plate, G. H., Breier, G., Weich, H. A., Mennel, H. D., and Risau, W. (1994). Vascular endothelial growth factor and glioma angiogenesis — coordinate induction of VEGF receptors, distribution of VEGF protein and possible *in vivo* regulatory mechanisms. *Int. J. Cancer*, **59**, 520–9.

125. Yamane, A., Seetherm, L., Yamaguchi, S., Gotoh, N., Takahashi, T., Neufeld, G., and Shibuya, M. (1994). A new communication system between hepatocytes and sinusoidal endothelial cells in liver through vascular endothelial growth factor and flt tyrosine kinase receptor family (flt-1 and kdr/flk-1). *Oncogene*, **9**, 2683–90.

126. Brooks, P. C., Montgomery, A. M. P., Rosenfeld, M., Reisfeld, R. A., Hu, T., Klier, G., and Cheresh, D. A. (1994). Integrin $\alpha_v\beta_3$ antagonists promote tumor regression by inducing apoptosis of angiogenic blood vessels. *Cell*, **79**, 1157–64.

127. Fox, S. B., Turner, G. D. H., Gatter, K. C., and Harris, A. L. (1996). The increased expression of adhesion molecules ICAM-3 and E- and P-selectins on breast cancer endo-thelium. *J. Pathol.*, **177**, 369–76.

128. Schadendorf, D., Heidel, J., Gawlik, C., Suter, L., and Czarnetzki, B. M. (1995). Association with clinical outcome of expression of VLA-4 in primary cutaneous malignant melanoma as well as P-selectin and E-selectin on intratumoral vessels. *J. Natl Cancer Inst.*, **87**, 366–71.

129. Nicolo, G., Salvi, S., Oliveri, G., Borsi, L., Castellani, P., and Zardi, L. (1990). Expression of tenascin and of the

ED-B containing oncofetal fibronectin isoform in human cancer. *Cell Differ. Dev.*, **32**, 401–8.

130. Kaczmarek, J., Castellani, P., Nicolo, G., Spina, B., Allemanni, G., and Zardi, L. (1994). Distribution of oncofetal fibronectin isoforms in normal, hyperplastic and neoplastic human breast tissues. *Int. J. Cancer*, **59**, 11–16.

131. Terman, B. I., Carrion, M. E., Kovacs, E., Rasmussen, B. A., Eddy R. L., and Shows, T. B. (1991). Identification of a new endothelial cell growth factor receptor tyrosine kinase. *Oncogene*, **6**, 1677–83.

132. Shibuya, M., Yamaguchi, S., Yamane, A., Ikeda, T., Tojo, A., Matsushime, H., and Sato, M. (1990). Nucleotide sequence and expression of a novel human receptor-type tyrosine kinase gene (flt) closely related to the fms family. *Oncogene*, **5**, 519–24.

133. Pajusola, K., Aprelikova, O., Korhonen, J., Kaipainen, A., Pertovaara L., Alitalo, R., and Alitalo, K. (1992). Flt4 receptor tyroisne kinase contains seven immunoglobulin-like loops and is expressed in multiple human tissues and cell lines. *Cancer Res.*, **52**, 5738–43.

134. Partanen, J., Armstrong, E., Mäkelä, T. P., Korhonen, J., Sandberg, M., Renkonen, R., *et al.* (1992). A novel endothelial cell surface receptor tyrosine kinase with extracellular epidermal growth factor homology domains. *Mol. Cell. Biol.*, **12**, 1698–707.

135. Dumont, D. J., Yamaguchi, T. P., Conlon, R. A., Rossant, J., and Breitman, M. L. (1992). Tek, a novel tyrosine kinase gene located on mouse chromosome 4, is expressed in endothelial cells and their presumptive precursors. *Oncogene*, **7**, 1471–80.

136. Dvorak, H. F., Sioussat, T. M., Brown, L. F., Berse, B., Nagy J. A., Sotrel, A., *et al.* (1991). Distribution of vascular permeability factor (vascular endothelial growth factor) in tumors: concentration in tumor blood vessels. *J. Exp. Med.*, **174**, 1275–78.

137. Bevilacqua, M. P., Stengelin, S., Gimbrone, J. M. A., and Seed, B. (1989). Endothelial leukocyte adhesion molecule 1: an inducible receptor for neutrophils related to complement regulatory proteins and lectins. *Science*, **243**, 1160–5.

138. Whelan, J., Ghersa, P., van Huijsduijnen, R. H., Gray, J., Chandra, G., Talabot, F., and DeLamarter, J. F. (1991). An NF-κB-like factor is essential but not sufficient for cytokine induction of endothelial leukocyte adhesion molecule 1 (ELAM-1) gene transcription. *Nucleic Acids Res.*, **19**, 2645–53.

139. Liang, P., and Pardee, A. (1992). Differential display of eukaryotic messenger RNA by means of the polymerase chain reaction. *Science*, **257**, 967–71.

140. Dzierzak, E. A., Papayannopoulou, T., and Mulligan, R. C. (1988). Lineage-specific expression of a human β-globin gene in murine bone marrow transplant recipients reconstituted with retrovirus-transducted stem cells. *Nature*, **331**, 35–41.

Index